EMERGENCY MEDICAL RESPONDER

First Responder in Action

Barbara Aehlert, RN

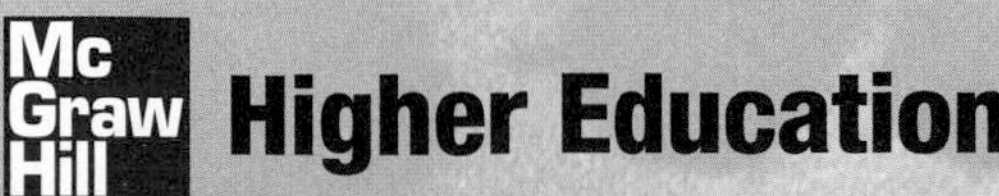

Boston Burr Ridge, IL Dubuque, IA Madison, WI New York San Francisco St. Louis
Bangkok Bogotá Caracas Kuala Lumpur Lisbon London Madrid Mexico City
Milan Montreal New Delhi Santiago Seoul Singapore Sydney Taipei Toronto

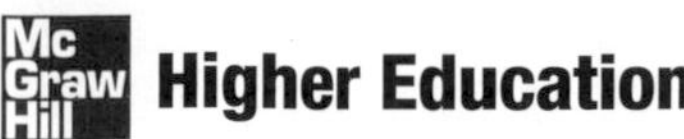

Higher Education

EMERGENCY MEDICAL RESPONDER: FIRST RESPONDER IN ACTION

Some ancillaries, including electronic and print components, may not be available to customers outside the United States.

This book is printed on recycled, acid-free paper containing 10% postconsumer waste.

1 2 3 4 5 6 7 8 9 0 QPD/QPD 0 9 8 7 6

ISBN-13 978-0-07-298644-0
ISBN-10 0-07-298644-1

Publisher, Career Education: *David T. Culverwell*
Senior Sponsoring Editor: *Claire Merrick*
Editorial Coordinator: *Michelle L. Zeal*
Outside Developmental Services: *Julie Scardiglia*
Senior Marketing Manager: *Lisa Nicks*
Senior Project Manager: *Mary E. Powers*
Senior Production Supervisor: *Laura Fuller*
Lead Media Project Manager: *Audrey A. Reiter*
Senior Media Producer: *Renee Russian*
Designer: *Laurie B. Janssen*
Cover Designer: *Ron Bissell*
(USE) Cover Image: © *The McGraw-Hill Companies, Inc./Rick Brady, photographer.*
Senior Photo Research Coordinator: *Lori Hancock*
Supplement Producer: *Tracy L. Konrardy*
Compositor: *TechBooks/GTS, Los Angeles, CA*
Typeface: *10/12 New Baskerville*
Printer: *Quebecor World Dubuque, IA*

Unless otherwise credited all photos © The McGraw-Hill Companies, Inc./Rick Brady, photographer.

We would like to thank the following organizations for their help in producing the photographs for this publication.
Maryland Fire and Rescue Institute; Prince George's County Fire and EMS Dept.; Whitetail Mountain Ski Patrol; Branchville Volunteer Fire Dept.; Greenbelt Volunteer Fire Dept.; College Park Volunteer Fire Dept.; Greenbelt Police Dept.; University of Maryland Police Department; Maryland Dept. of Natural Resources Police; Sandy Point State Park Beach Rescue; Anne Arundel County Community College; Montgomery County Fire and Rescue; Berwyn Heights Volunteer Fire Dept.

Medicine is an ever-changing science. As new research and clinical experience broaden our knowledge, changes in treatment are required. The authors and the publisher of this work have checked with sources believed to be reliable in their efforts to provide information that is complete and generally in accord with the standards accepted at the time of publication. However, in view of the possibility of human error or changes in medical sciences, neither the authors, the publisher, nor any other party who has been involved in the preparation or publication of this work warrants that the information contained herein is in every respect accurate or complete, and they are not responsible for any errors or omissions or for the results obtained from use of such information. Readers are encouraged to confirm the information contained herein with other resources.

Library of Congress Cataloging-in-Publication Data

Aehlert, Barbara.
Emergency medical responder : first responder in action / Barbara Aehlert. — 1st ed.
p. cm.
Includes index.
ISBN 978-0-07-298644-0 — 0-07-298644-1 (alk. paper)
1. Emergency medical technicians. 2. Emergency medical technicians—Study and teaching.
3. Medical emergencies. I. Title.

RC86.7.A352 2007
616.02'5—dc22

2005057657
CIP

www.mhhe.com

Dedication

For more than 45 years, I lived in urban communities with state-of-the-art Emergency Medical Services (EMS) provided by full-time, paid EMS professionals. In 2004, I moved to an area of rural Texas where EMS is provided by volunteer Emergency Medical Responders. This book is dedicated to Emergency Medical Responders who, paid or volunteer, choose to make the world a better place by providing EMS care to the members of their community.

Barbara Aehlert

About the Author

Barbara Aehlert is the president of Southwest EMS Education, Inc., in Phoenix, Arizona, and Pursley, Texas. She has been a registered nurse for more than 30 years, with clinical experience in medical/surgical and critical care nursing and, for the past 18 years, in prehospital education. Barbara is an active CPR, First Aid, ACLS, and PALS instructor and takes a special interest in teaching basic dysrhythmia recognition to nurses and paramedics. She is a consultant with the Southwest Ambulance paramedic program in Mesa, Arizona, and an active member of the Pursley, Texas, Volunteer Fire Department.

Brief Contents

Contents

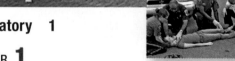

Foreword

Emergency Medical Responders (EMRs) respond to emergencies—and emergencies happen every minute of every day. These emergencies include medical problems, such as heart attacks. They also include traumatic injuries from motor vehicle crashes, industrial accidents, and violent crimes. In the past few years, we have also faced larger emergencies: cataclysmic hurricanes, terrorist attacks, and the fear of infectious disease outbreaks. In many of these situations, the EMR is the first medically trained person to care for critically ill or injured patients.

When my colleagues and I arrive at an emergency scene on a fire apparatus or an ambulance, there is often an EMR already on the scene—beginning care, gathering information, and helping us prepare our patient for transport. When not responding to an emergency, these everyday heroes can be found cruising in police cars, working on river barges, sailing ocean liners, toiling in industry, staffing fire apparatus, and studying on college campuses. They are ready to respond immediately to emergencies anywhere people live, work, or play.

One of the greatest challenges for any community is the ability to have enough appropriately trained EMS providers available to respond rapidly when an emergency arises. The need to train a larger number of competent EMRs has never been greater. These emergency healthcare professionals provide a bridge between the layperson and the rest of the emergency medical community. They are stationed within each community and are trained to provide rapid, timely care to sick or injured patients until other emergency care providers can arrive.

Emergency Medical Responders are often the first members of the EMS team to arrive on the scene of an emergency, size up the situation, and provide emergency care. They practice in a wider diversity of settings than almost anyone else in EMS—EMRs are everywhere in our communities, performing their EMR role as well as their regular jobs. These providers demonstrate pride and dedication in their role on the frontline of emergency care in this country.

Barbara Aehlert wrote this text with great depth and clarity. Students who use this book can feel confident that they have learned accurate, up-to-date, and complete information so that they can face emergencies and provide essential emergency care in their practice setting, whatever the emergency is and wherever it occurs.

Kim McKenna, RN, EMT-P
Chief Medical Officer
Florissant Valley Fire Protection District
Florissant, Missouri

Preface

This book and the materials that accompany it are designed to teach you how to safely and efficiently provide immediate care to an ill or injured person in accordance with the guidelines established by the Department of Transportation (DOT) First Responder National Standard Curriculum. Although they may be used alone to increase your awareness of what to do in an emergency situation, these materials are best used in an Emergency Medical Responder training program.

This book has been divided into seven modules (sections), which contain chapters with information relevant to each module. Each chapter begins with a list of knowledge, attitude, and skill objectives, which describe what you should be able to do after completing the chapter and related exercises.

Before studying a chapter, first read the knowledge objectives. These objectives will give you an idea of the information you should obtain from reading the material in this book. Next, read the attitude objectives to learn about the behaviors that you are expected to develop as a healthcare professional. Then, read the skill objectives to discover the procedures you should be able to perform after reading about, observing, and then practicing each skill.

After reviewing the objectives, begin reading the chapter. Each chapter contains illustrations, tables, and other features to help you understand the information presented. For example, the skills discussed in this book are also demonstrated on the DVD that accompanies this text. When you have finished reading the chapter, go through the objectives again to be sure that you have met them.

At the end of each module of the Emergency Medical Responder course, time is allowed for skill practice, review, and evaluation. Watch the skills on the DVD to help you learn and master each skill. Use the practice questions in this book to help you assess your mastery of the knowledge objectives presented in the course. Flashcards are provided on the DVD to help you prepare for the final examination.

Information that is related to your role as an Emergency Medical Responder, but is not part of the DOT First Responder Curriculum, is located in the appendices at the end of this book.

I hope you find this text helpful. If you have comments or suggestions about how I could improve this text, please visit my web site, http://www.swemsed.com, and drop me a line. I would like to hear from you.

Barbara Aehlert, RN

Southwest EMS Education, Inc.

Phoenix, Arizona/Pursley, Texas

Guided Tour

Features to Help You Study and Learn

Modules

The text is organized according to the First Responder National Standard Curriculum published by the U.S. Department of Transportation (DOT) and the National Highway Traffic Safety Administration (NHTSA).

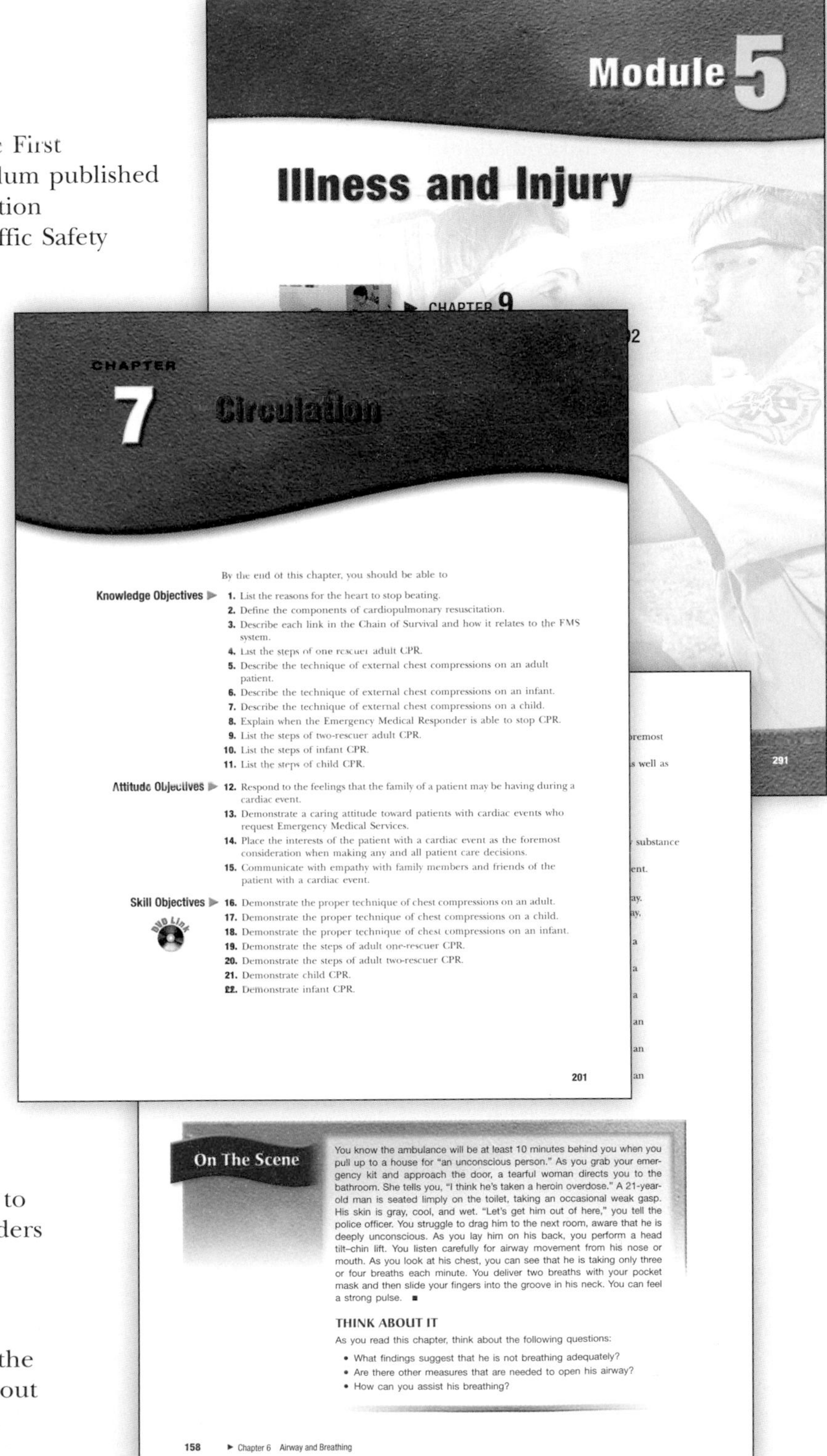

Module 5
Illness and Injury
CHAPTER 7
Circulation
By the end of this chapter, you should be able to
Knowledge Objectives
1. List the reasons for the heart to stop beating.
2. Define the components of cardiopulmonary resuscitation.
3. Describe each link in the Chain of Survival and how it relates to the EMS system.
4. List the steps of one-rescuer adult CPR.
5. Describe the technique of external chest compressions on an adult patient.
6. Describe the technique of external chest compressions on an infant.
7. Describe the technique of external chest compressions on a child.
8. Explain when the Emergency Medical Responder is able to stop CPR.
9. List the steps of two-rescuer adult CPR.
10. List the steps of infant CPR.
11. List the steps of child CPR.
Attitude Objectives
12. Respond to the feelings that the family of a patient may be having during a cardiac event.
13. Demonstrate a caring attitude toward patients with cardiac events who request Emergency Medical Services.
14. Place the interests of the patient with a cardiac event as the foremost consideration when making any and all patient care decisions.
15. Communicate with empathy with family members and friends of the patient with a cardiac event.
Skill Objectives
16. Demonstrate the proper technique of chest compressions on an adult.
17. Demonstrate the proper technique of chest compressions on a child.
18. Demonstrate the proper technique of chest compressions on an infant.
19. Demonstrate the steps of adult one-rescuer CPR.
20. Demonstrate the steps of adult two-rescuer CPR.
21. Demonstrate child CPR.
22. Demonstrate infant CPR.
DVD Link
201
On The Scene
You know the ambulance will be at least 10 minutes behind you when you pull up to a house for "an unconscious person." As you grab your emergency kit and approach the door, a tearful woman directs you to the bathroom. She tells you, "I think he's taken a heroin overdose." A 21-year-old man is seated limply on the toilet, taking an occasional weak gasp. His skin is gray, cool, and wet. "Let's get him out of here," you tell the police officer. You struggle to drag him to the next room, aware that he is deeply unconscious. As you lay him on his back, you perform a head tilt–chin lift. You listen carefully for airway movement from his nose or mouth. As you look at his chest, you can see that he is taking only three or four breaths each minute. You deliver two breaths with your pocket mask and then slide your fingers into the groove in his neck. You can feel a strong pulse. ■
THINK ABOUT IT
As you read this chapter, think about the following questions:
• What findings suggest that he is not breathing adequately?
• Are there other measures that are needed to open his airway?
• How can you assist his breathing?
158 ► Chapter 6 Airway and Breathing

Objectives Each chapter includes the knowledge, attitude, and skill objectives established by the DOT curriculum for the subject matter.

DVD Link This icon indicates the chapter skills presented on the student DVD located in the back of the text.

On The Scene These case studies represent emergency situations similar to those that Emergency Medical Responders may encounter in the field.

Think About It Questions related to the case study that readers should think about as they read each chapter or appendix.

Key Terms Key terms are bolded within the text so that readers can review their meaning within the Glossary.

Margin Notes Useful and additional information about the topic being discussed.

Objective References Each knowledge and attitude objective is referenced in the margin where it is covered in the chapter.

Stop and Think! Safety tips and practical advice for the EMR.

Remember This! Information and tips related to the EMR's role relative to other emergency care providers. This feature also provides information related to patient care.

You Should Know Interesting and useful statistics and information. This feature also presents additional information related to the EMR's providing patient care.

Making a Difference Information and tips to help the EMR provide excellent and/or specialized patient care.

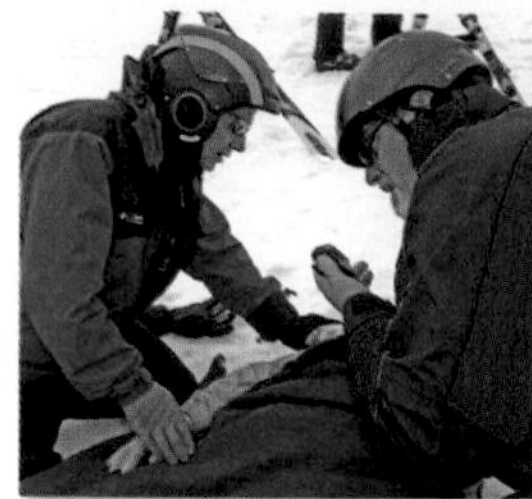

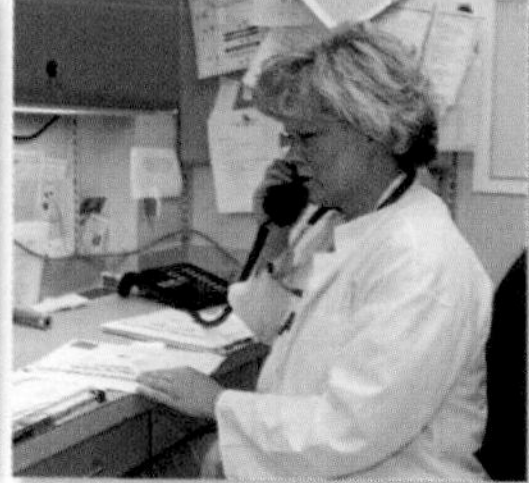

FIGURE 1-3 ▲ On-line medical direction is direct communication with a physician by radio or telephone or face-to-face communication at the scene.

Medical oversight is also referred to as medical control or medical direction.

Objective 4 ▸

The medical director is responsible for ensuring that the emergency care provided to ill or injured patients is medically appropriate.

The development of treatment protocols and standing orders are examples of prospective medical direction.

However, this authority varies by state law. In situations that require emergency medical care, it is very important that you request EMS personnel to the scene as soon as possible.

Medical oversight is the process by which a physician directs the emergency care provided by EMS personnel to an ill or injured patient. Every EMS system *must* have medical oversight. The physician who provides medical oversight is called the medical director. The two types of medical oversight are on-line and off-line medical direction.

On-Line Medical Direction

On-line medical direction, also called *direct* or *concurrent medical direction*, is direct communication with a physician by radio or telephone—or face-to-face communication at the scene—before performing a skill or providing care (Figure 1-3).

Off-Line Medical Direction

Off-line medical direction, also referred to as *indirect, prospective*, or *retrospective medical direction*, is the medical supervision of EMS personnel using policies, treatment protocols, standing orders, education, and quality management reviews.

Prospective Medical Direction **Prospective medical direction** includes activities performed by a physician medical director before an emergency call. It is impossible for the medical director to be physically present at every emergency. Therefore, the medical director develops treatment protocols and standing orders, usually with the assistance of a local EMS advisory group.

Treatment Protocols A **treatment protocol** is a list of steps to be followed when providing emergency care to an ill or injured patient. For example, a patient experiencing a heat-related illness may be treated using the steps outlined in the sample treatment protocol for heat-related emergencies.

10 ▸ Chapter 1 Introduction to the EMS System

(Figure 6-2). Because the tongue is attached to the lower jaw, moving the jaw forward will lift the tongue away from the back of the throat.

Stop and Think!

Because the risk of exposure to blood, vomitus, or potentially infectious material is high, you must remember to take appropriate body substance isolation precautions when managing a patient's airway.

Head Tilt–Chin Lift

The head tilt–chin lift maneuver is the most effective method for opening the airway in a patient with no known or suspected trauma to the head or neck. It requires no equipment and is simple to perform. When the procedure is done correctly, the base of the tongue will be displaced from blocking the back of the throat (Figure 6-3). Patients who are likely to need the head tilt–chin lift maneuver include

- An unresponsive patient with no known or suspected trauma to the head or neck
- A patient who is not breathing with no known or suspected trauma to the head or neck
- A patient who is not breathing and has no pulse (cardiac arrest) with no known or suspected trauma to the head or neck

Remember This!

Never use the head tilt–chin lift maneuver to open the airway if trauma to the head or neck is suspected. Damage to the patient's spinal cord can result.

162 ▸ Chapter 6 Airway and Breathing

center (Figure 1-5). In these centers, specially trained personnel and equipment are available 24 hours a day to care for patients with serious injuries.

Other types of specialty centers include burn, heart/cardiovascular, hyperbaric, pediatric, perinatal, poison, spinal cord injury, and stroke centers (Table 1-3).

You Should Know

In both urban and rural areas, a patient may be stabilized at a closer hospital and then transferred to a specialty center if the patient requires care beyond that available at the initial receiving facility.

Rehabilitation Services

Soon after their condition has been stabilized and they have been moved from the hospital emergency department, some patients will require the services of healthcare professionals who specialize in rehabilitation. These healthcare professionals include rehabilitation nurses, physicians, physical therapists, occupational therapists, and social workers. They work with the patient and the patient's family to return the ill or injured patient to his or her previous state of health.

Making a Difference

To ensure that your patient receives the best possible care for his or her illness or injury, you must be familiar with the capabilities of the medical facilities in your area.

FIGURE 1-5 ▸ A trauma center is a specialty facility with trained personnel and equipment available 24 hours a day to care for seriously injured patients.

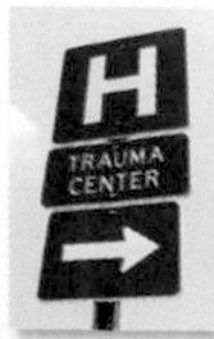

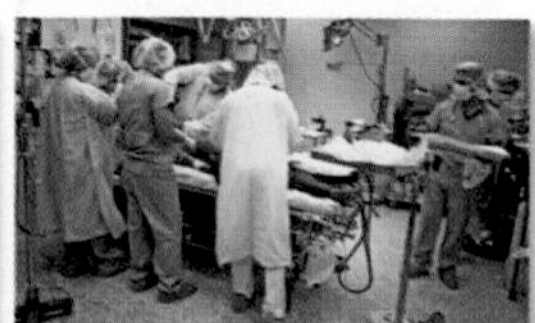

12 ▸ Chapter 1 Introduction to the EMS System

Skill Drills Procedures and skills essential to the EMR's role.

Skill Drill 2-1

Removing Gloves

STEP 1 Using your index finger and thumb on one hand, pull the bottom (cuff) of the glove away from your other hand.
Peel the glove off your hand, being careful not to touch the skin of your wrist or hand with the outside surface of the glove. As you begin to remove the glove, it will turn inside out. This action helps prevent exposure to blood or other possibly infectious fluids on the gloves.

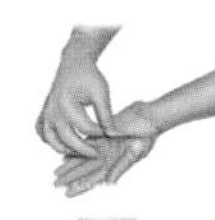

STEP 2 Place your fingers inside the bottom (cuff) of the other glove. Pull the glove off by turning it inside out.

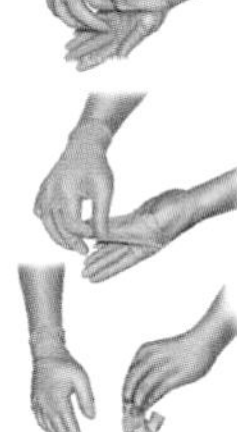

ontainer. Wash

al. If you have a latex allergy, wear gloves made of a nonlatex
e. If you have a cut on your hand or wrist, apply a bandage
g on gloves. Check the condition of the gloves before putting
hem if they have small holes or tears in them.
es between contacts with different patients. If a glove tears
t care, remove it as soon as you can and replace it with a
y contaminated gloves and other PPE in clearly labeled
tainers.
gloves, keep in mind that the outer surface of the gloves
inated. Do not let the outside surface of the gloves come
in. Be careful not to let the gloves snap when taking them
germs may become airborne and contact your eyes, mouth,
echnique for removing gloves is shown in Skill Drill 2-1.

Skill Drill 11-3

Applying a Bipolar Traction Splint

STEP 1
- Adjust the traction splint to the proper length. Position the splint next to the patient's uninjured leg using the bony prominence of the buttock as a landmark. Extend the splint 6–12 inches beyond the patient's uninjured heel. Lock the splint in position.
- Position the support straps at the midthigh, above the knee, below the knee, and above the ankle. Open the straps and fasten them under the splint.

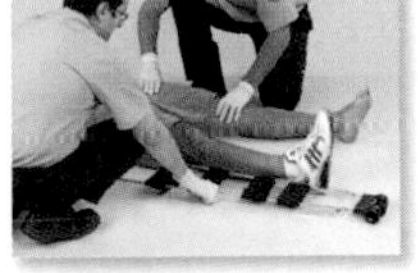

STEP 2 Stabilize the injured leg so that it does not move while an assistant fastens the ankle hitch around the patient's foot and ankle.

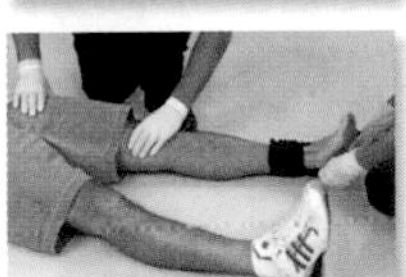

STEP 3
- While your assistant continues to apply gentle manual traction, position the splint under the injured leg. The ischial pad should rest against the bony prominence of the buttocks.
- Raise the heel stand after the splint is in position.

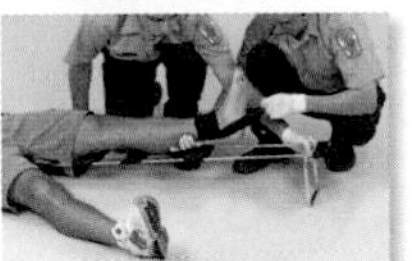

STEP 4
- Pad the groin area.
- Attach the ischial strap. Secure the strap over the groin and thigh.

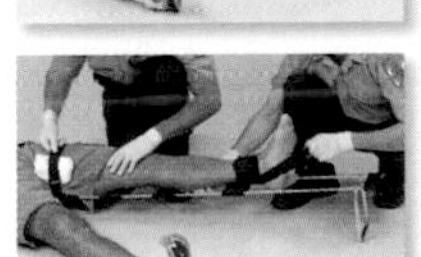

Continued on next page

s

e legislatures. Every state has
describe how its EMS person-
ing of a written authorization
to perform medical acts and
n. **Certification** is a designa-
d requirements to perform a

s and functions that can be
rofessional, called the **scope**
to state, ask your instructor
as an Emergency Medical

ertification

number of agencies, including
cians (NREMT) (Figure 1-19),
Safety and Health Institute
ire the successful completion
follows the DOT curriculum.
edical Responder requires you
to successfully complete a written and practical skills examination.

Certification as an Emergency Medical Responder is good for a limited time—usually two years. Participating in CE courses or an Emergency Medical Responder refresher course is required for recertification.

FIGURE 1-19 ▲ Emergency Medical Responders can be certified by a number of agencies, including the National Registry of Emergency Medical Technicians (NREMT).

You Should Know

National Registry of Emergency Medical Technicians

The NREMT helps develop professional standards. It also verifies the skills and knowledge of EMS professionals by preparing and conducting examinations.

On The Scene

Wrap-Up

In responding to the scenario, you recall the standard procedures for your team and have someone activate the EMS system by dialing 9-1-1. You turn off the engine and free your patient's hand. You then lay him down in a safe area and control the bleeding.

The ambulance crew, staffed with an EMT and a Paramedic, arrive quickly. You give them a brief report and assist them in assessing and caring for the patient. After they start an intravenous line to give the patient pain medicine, his face relaxes. He is then transported to the trauma center, where two of his fingers are successfully reattached. He stops in to thank you two weeks later on his way home from a rehabilitation session. ■

On The Scene: Wrap-Up Using the information presented in the chapter, this feature presents a wrap-up of the case study from the beginning of the chapter.

Sum It Up A bulleted list of the key information covered in the chapter.

Tracking Your Progress Readers can check off the objectives they have mastered after learning the chapter content.

Chapter and Appendix Quizzes
This workbook-type feature includes a full range of question types: multiple choice, true or false, matching, short answer, and sentence completion. Each quiz allows readers to ensure that they have mastered the information before moving on to the next chapter.

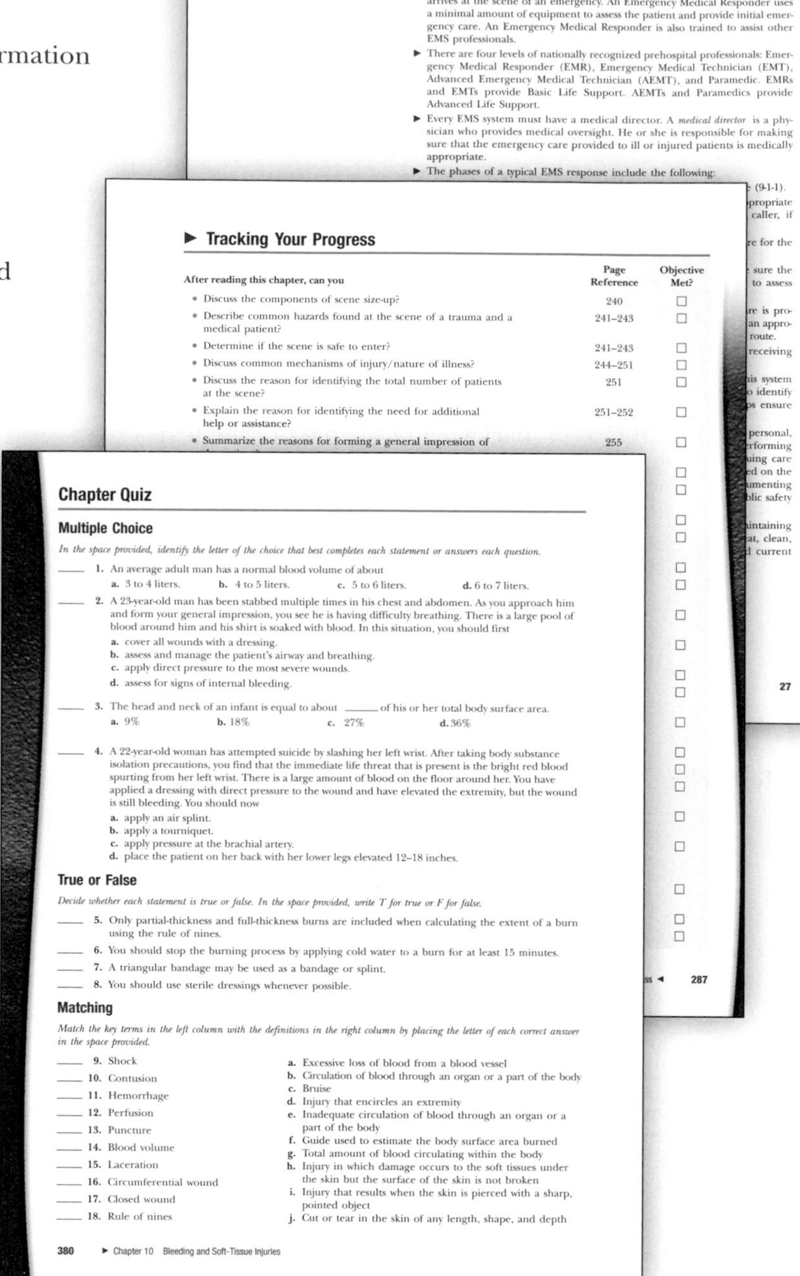

Sum It Up

► The *Emergency Medical Services (EMS) system* is part of the healthcare system. It consists of a coordinated network of resources that provides emergency care and transportation to victims of sudden illness and injury.
► An *Emergency Medical Responder* is the first person with medical training who arrives at the scene of an emergency. An Emergency Medical Responder uses a minimal amount of equipment to assess the patient and provide initial emergency care. An Emergency Medical Responder is also trained to assist other EMS professionals.
► There are four levels of nationally recognized prehospital professionals: Emergency Medical Responder (EMR), Emergency Medical Technician (EMT), Advanced Emergency Medical Technician (AEMT), and Paramedic. EMRs and EMTs provide Basic Life Support. AEMTs and Paramedics provide Advanced Life Support.
► Every EMS system must have a medical director. A *medical director* is a physician who provides medical oversight. He or she is responsible for making sure that the emergency care provided to ill or injured patients is medically appropriate.
► The phases of a typical EMS response include the following:

27

► Tracking Your Progress

After reading this chapter, can you	Page Reference	Objective Met?
• Discuss the components of scene size-up?	240	☐
• Describe common hazards found at the scene of a trauma and a medical patient?	241–243	☐
• Determine if the scene is safe to enter?	241–243	☐
• Discuss common mechanisms of injury/nature of illness?	244–251	☐
• Discuss the reason for identifying the total number of patients at the scene?	251	☐
• Explain the reason for identifying the need for additional help or assistance?	251–252	☐
• Summarize the reasons for forming a general impression of	255	☐

287

Chapter Quiz

Multiple Choice

In the space provided, identify the letter of the choice that best completes each statement or answers each question.

____ 1. An average adult man has a normal blood volume of about
a. 3 to 4 liters. b. 4 to 5 liters. c. 5 to 6 liters. d. 6 to 7 liters.

____ 2. A 23-year-old man has been stabbed multiple times in his chest and abdomen. As you approach him and form your general impression, you see he is having difficulty breathing. There is a large pool of blood around him and his shirt is soaked with blood. In this situation, you should first
a. cover all wounds with a dressing.
b. assess and manage the patient's airway and breathing.
c. apply direct pressure to the most severe wounds.
d. assess for signs of internal bleeding.

____ 3. The head and neck of an infant is equal to about ____ of his or her total body surface area.
a. 9% b. 18% c. 27% d. 36%

____ 4. A 22-year-old woman has attempted suicide by slashing her left wrist. After taking body substance isolation precautions, you find that the immediate life threat that is present is the bright red blood spurting from her left wrist. There is a large amount of blood on the floor around her. You have applied a dressing with direct pressure to the wound and have elevated the extremity, but the wound is still bleeding. You should now
a. apply an air splint.
b. apply a tourniquet.
c. apply pressure at the brachial artery.
d. place the patient on her back with her lower legs elevated 12–18 inches.

True or False

Decide whether each statement is true or false. In the space provided, write T for true or F for false.

____ 5. Only partial-thickness and full-thickness burns are included when calculating the extent of a burn using the rule of nines.
____ 6. You should stop the burning process by applying cold water to a burn for at least 15 minutes.
____ 7. A triangular bandage may be used as a bandage or splint.
____ 8. You should use sterile dressings whenever possible.

Matching

Match the key terms in the left column with the definitions in the right column by placing the letter of each correct answer in the space provided.

____ 9. Shock	a. Excessive loss of blood from a blood vessel
____ 10. Contusion	b. Circulation of blood through an organ or a part of the body
____ 11. Hemorrhage	c. Bruise
____ 12. Perfusion	d. Injury that encircles an extremity
____ 13. Puncture	e. Inadequate circulation of blood through an organ or a part of the body
____ 14. Blood volume	f. Guide used to estimate the body surface area burned
____ 15. Laceration	g. Total amount of blood circulating within the body
____ 16. Circumferential wound	h. Injury in which damage occurs to the soft tissues under the skin but the surface of the skin is not broken
____ 17. Closed wound	i. Injury that results when the skin is pierced with a sharp, pointed object
____ 18. Rule of nines	j. Cut or tear in the skin of any length, shape, and depth

380 ► Chapter 10 Bleeding and Soft-Tissue Injuries

Appendices

Address important and timely topics related to the EMR's role.

Glossary

Provides a full definition of the key terms bolded within each chapter and appendix.

Supplements

For the Student

Student DVD

- A DVD of DOT skills packaged in the back of the text
- Includes Digital Flashcards

Student CD

Includes

- 200-Question Exam with Answer Key
- 100-Question Sample Final Exam with Answer Key
- McGraw-Hill's *Spanish Guide to Patient Assessment for the Emergency Medical Responder*
- Test-Taking Preparation for the Emergency Medical Responder Certification Exam

Pocket Guide

Portable, essential information Emergency Medical Responders need to provide initial emergency medical care in the field

For the Instructor

Instructor CD

Includes

- Instructor's Manual/Lesson Plans
- PowerPoint Slides
- Computerized Test Banks provided in EZ Test format
  - Instructor Questions—questions created exclusively for the instructor
  - Student Questions—student text quiz questions provided in a computerized test bank

Acknowledgments

No book is published without the assistance of many people. This book is certainly no exception. From its inception so many months ago, I have been delighted to be able to work once again with David Culverwell, Claire Merrick, and Julie Scardiglia. Dave and Claire have always been the "global" thinkers. Their energy and vision were and are astounding. Julie and I are two halves that join as one when working on a project. At any hour of the day or night, I know that, if I have a question, Julie is there on the other end of the computer or telephone to provide an answer. My sincerest thanks for handling the details, sending gentle reminders, and making sure I was given space from time to time to step away from the computer. In addition, sincere thanks to Michelle Zeal, Connie Kuhl, Shannon Cox, and Lisa Nicks for all their invaluable assistance. Many thanks to Mary Powers, Laurie Janssen, Lori Hancock, and Laura Fuller of McGraw-Hill for their excellent work in the production and design of this book; thanks also to Renee Russian, Audrey Reiter, and Tracy Konrardy of McGraw-Hill for their assistance with the student CD, student DVD, instructor CD, and Pocket Guide. Their excellent work and meticulous attention to many details are very much appreciated.

The contributors for this book and the materials that accompany it were personally selected because of their experience in EMS. Whether a physician, nurse, or paramedic, they treat their patients with compassion and respect and display professionalism every day they are on the job. Their commitment to excellence and professionalism in EMS is evident throughout this book. Thank you to Gary Smith, MD; Lynn Browne-Wagner, RN; Andrea Legamaro, RN; Terence Mason, RN; Suzy Coronel, CEP; Paul Honeywell, CEP; Captain Randy Budd, CEP; Captain Holly Button, CEP; Captain Sean Newton, CEP; Captain Jeff Pennington, CEP; and Major Raymond Burton. Special thanks to Janet Fitts, RN, and Edith Valladares for their invaluable contributions to the *Spanish Guide to Patient Assessment for the Emergency Medical Responder,* featured on the student CD.

Kim McKenna, RN, read every word in this book and provided scenarios, questions, and activities for the text and instructor's materials. After reviewing it once, she painstakingly reviewed the material again for accuracy. Thanks for your attention to detail, suggestions, and time for this project in the midst of your busy schedule. Steve Kidd and the staff of Delve Productions worked very hard to ensure that the DVD that accompanies this book is easy to use and useful for Emergency Medical Responders. Rick Brady did an outstanding job taking the photos that appear in this book. Thanks to Carin Marter, CEP; the City of Mesa Fire Department; the City of Tempe Fire Department; and AirEvac Services (Phoenix, Arizona) for providing additional photos.

Thanks to the many EMS professionals who reviewed this text and the materials that accompany it. Each reviewer provided valuable comments and suggestions, which were carefully read and discussed. Modifications have been made where needed based on their comments.

Barbara Aehlert, RN

Southwest EMS Education, Inc.
Phoenix, Arizona/Pursley, Texas

Contributors

Lynn Browne-Wagner, RN
Phoenix, AZ

Randy Budd, RRT, CEP
EMS Captain, Mesa Fire Dept.
Mesa, AZ

Major Raymond W. Burton (Retired)
Plymouth Academy/Plymouth County Sheriff's Academy
Plymouth, MA

Holly Button, CEP
Wellness Program Captain, Mesa Fire Dept.
Mesa, AZ

Suzy Coronel, MICP, NREMT-P
Operations Manager, Sportsmedicine Fairbanks
Fairbanks, AK

Janet Fitts, RN, EMT-P, Educational Consultant
Prehospital and Emergency Medical Services
Pacific, MO

Paul Honeywell
Director of Field Training, Southwest Ambulance
Mesa, AZ

Terence Mason, RN
EMS Coordinator, Mesa Fire Dept.
Mesa, AZ

Kim McKenna, RN, EMT-P
Chief Medical Officer, Florissant Valley Fire Protection District
Florissant, MO

Sean Newton, CEP
EMS/Fire Captain, City of Scottsdale Fire Dept.
Scottsdale, AZ

Jeff Pennington, CEP
Gilbert Fire Dept.
Gilbert, AZ

Gary Smith, MD
Medical Director: Apache Junction, Gilbert, and Mesa Fire Departments
Apache Junction, Gilbert, and Mesa, AZ

Edith Valladares
Director, Foreign Languages and Academic ESL
Central Piedmont Community College
Charlotte, NC

Reviewers

Paul A. Bishop
Monroe Community College
Rochester, NY

Anthony N. Brown
National Ski Patrol System Emergency Care Advisor/Trainer
Idaho Falls, ID

Major Raymond W. Burton (Retired)
Plymouth Academy/Plymouth County Sheriff's Academy
Plymouth, MA

David S. Farrow
S.W. EMS
Phoenix, AZ

Janet Fitts, RN, EMT-P, Educational Consultant
Prehospital and Emergency Medical Services
Pacific, MO

Franklin R. Hubbell, DO
SOLO
Conway, NH

Edward Kalinowski, MED, PhD
University of Hawaii, Department of Emergency Medical Services
Honolulu, HI

Barbara Klingensmith, PhD, NREMT-P
Florida State Fire College
San Antonio, FL

Kim McKenna, RN, EMT-P
Florissant Valley Fire Protection District
Florissant, MO

Keith Monosky, MPM, EMT-P
The George Washington University
Washington, DC

Keith A. Ozenberger
UTMB–Galveston
Galveston, TX

Douglas A. Pratt
Weber State University
Ogden, UT

William Seifarth
MIEMSS
Baltimore, MD

Jeanne Shepard
Mesa Fire Department
Mesa, AZ

Tom Vines
Carbon County Sheriff's SAR
Red Lodge, MT

Maryalice Witzel
Banner Good Samaritan Medical Center
Phoenix, AZ

Module 1

Preparatory

CHAPTER

1 Introduction to the EMS System

By the end of this chapter, you should be able to

Knowledge Objectives ▶

1. Define the components of Emergency Medical Services (EMS) systems.
2. Differentiate the roles and responsibilities of the Emergency Medical Responder from other prehospital care providers.
3. Define medical oversight and discuss the Emergency Medical Responder's role in the process.
4. Discuss the types of medical oversight that may affect the medical care of an Emergency Medical Responder.
5. State the specific statutes and regulations in your state regarding the EMS system.

Attitude Objectives ▶

6. Accept and uphold the responsibilities of an Emergency Medical Responder in accordance with the standards of an EMS professional.
7. Explain the rationale for maintaining a professional appearance when on duty or when responding to calls.
8. Describe why it is inappropriate to judge a patient based on a cultural, gender, age, or socioeconomic model, and to vary the standard of care rendered as a result of that judgment.

Skill Objectives ▶ No skill objectives are identified for this lesson.

On The Scene

Minutes from quitting time, you are startled by an overhead page for a "blue team" response to the maintenance building. Grabbing the emergency kit you carefully checked this morning, you walk quickly to the scene. Fellow employees recognize your emergency team shirt and wave you to the back of the building. A worker has been injured while repairing a gear in a lawn tractor. His hand is stuck in the engine, which still roars loudly. He is in severe pain and is soaked in sweat. Several of his fingers have been cut off. Blood is pooling on his forearm and dripping to the floor. Your coworkers gather around, waiting for you to take action. ■

THINK ABOUT IT

As you read this chapter, think about the following questions:

- What is your most important concern as you approach this and all emergencies?
- How will you call for additional emergency care?
- Which Emergency Medical Responder skills might you need in this situation? What other skills may need to be provided by an Emergency Medical Technician or a Paramedic?
- How can your medical protocols assist in this situation?
- What components of the emergency care system is this patient likely to need?

Introduction

The Emergency Medical Responder

You, the Emergency Medical Responder, are an important and essential part of the Emergency Medical Services (EMS) system. An **Emergency Medical Responder** is an individual with medical training who is the first to arrive at the scene of an emergency, such as a motor vehicle crash, a life-threatening medical situation, or a disaster. Emergency Medical Responders may be paid or volunteer and may work in the following positions:

- Fire department personnel
- Law enforcement officers
- Military personnel
- Members of the ski patrol
- Teachers
- Lifeguards
- Designated industrial or commercial medical response teams
- Truck drivers
- Park rangers
- Coaches
- Athletic trainers

As an Emergency Medical Responder, you will be tasked with providing medical assistance and enlisting the aid of other emergency caregivers as needed. You will often have a limited amount of equipment with which to assess a patient, provide emergency care, and assist other healthcare professionals. The Department of Transportation (DOT) developed the Emergency Medical Responder National Standard Curriculum to help you gain the knowledge, attitude, and skills necessary to be a competent, productive, and valuable member of the healthcare team. This curriculum was developed by representatives of federal and state agencies, professional medical organizations, and education experts. Emergency Medical Responder training programs follow guidelines established by this curriculum.

Making a Difference

The Goals of Emergency Medical Responder Training

When you successfully complete an Emergency Medical Responder training program, you will have gained the knowledge, attitudes, and skills to do the following:

- Recognize and assess the seriousness of a patient's condition or the extent of injuries to determine the emergency medical care a patient requires
- Safely and efficiently provide initial emergency medical care for a victim of a sudden illness or injury

The Emergency Medical Services System

The Origins of EMS

The Emergency Medical Services system is part of the healthcare system.

A **healthcare system** is a network of people, facilities, and equipment designed to provide for the general medical needs of the population. The **Emergency Medical Services (EMS) system** is a coordinated network of resources that provides emergency care and transportation to victims of sudden illness or injury. As an Emergency Medical Responder, you are a part of the EMS system.

EMS has developed from the days when volunteers were untrained in emergency care and provided minimal stabilization at the scene of an emergency. At that time, patients were taken to the nearest hospital by funeral homes, taxis, and automobile towing companies as an optional service.

This document is commonly called the "White Paper."

In 1966, the National Academy of Sciences—National Research Council (NAS/NRC) published a paper called "Accidental Death and Disability, The Neglected Disease of Modern Society." This paper exposed problems within the EMS system, including

- A lack of standardized training of emergency responders (e.g., ambulance attendants, police, and fire personnel)
- Inadequate medical direction
- Outdated and/or inadequate transport vehicles
- A lack of local government support of EMS
- A lack of citizen first aid knowledge

The paper called for more government support of prehospital services. It also suggested improvements, such as guidelines for EMS system development, training for prehospital personnel, and the upgrading of transport vehicles and their equipment. Some of the suggested changes included

- Improving citizen knowledge of basic first aid
- Changing the emergency vehicles used
- Improving the training of emergency responders (e.g., ambulance attendants, police, and fire personnel)
- Providing physician oversight (medical direction)
- Improving the care provided by hospital emergency departments
- Improving communications and record keeping
- Increasing local government support to provide the best possible EMS

The Highway Safety Act of 1966 charged the DOT National Highway Traffic Safety Administration (NHTSA) with the responsibility of improving EMS. This act provided funding for the development of highway safety programs to reduce the number of deaths related to highway accidents. This act also established national standards for training Emergency Medical Technicians and the minimum equipment required on an ambulance.

EMS System Components

Objective 1 ►

In 1988, NHTSA established the Technical Assessment Program. This program identified 10 essential parts of an EMS system and the methods used to assess these areas (Table 1-1). States use the standards set by NHTSA to determine how effective their EMS systems are.

TABLE 1-1 Ten Components of an EMS System

• Regulation and policy	• Medical oversight
• Resource management	• Trauma systems
• Human resources and training	• Facilities
• Communications	• Public information and education
• Transportation	• Evaluation

Regulation and Policy

To ensure the delivery of quality emergency medical care for adults and children, each state must have laws in place that govern its EMS system. As an Emergency Medical Responder, you must be familiar with your state and local EMS regulations and policies.

Resource Management

Each state must make sure that all victims of medical or traumatic emergencies have equal access to appropriate emergency care. This includes making sure enough vehicles, equipment, supplies, and trained personnel are available to meet the needs of local EMS systems.

Human Resources and Training

Individuals working in an EMS system should be trained to a minimum standard. Training programs should be monitored regularly. In addition, instructors should meet certain requirements and the curriculum should be made standard throughout the state.

Levels of Prehospital Training

Objective 2 ►

There are four levels of nationally recognized prehospital professionals: Emergency Medical Responder (EMR), Emergency Medical Technician (EMT), Advanced Emergency Medical Technician (AEMT), and Paramedic (Table 1-2).

Emergency Medical Responder (EMR) An Emergency Medical Responder (EMR) is a person who has the basic knowledge and skills necessary to provide lifesaving emergency care while waiting for the arrival of additional EMS help. An Emergency Medical Responder is also trained to assist other EMS professionals.

Emergency Medical Technician (EMT) An Emergency Medical Technician (EMT) is a member of the EMS team who provides prehospital emergency care. An EMT has taken a minimum of a 110-hour course and is more skilled than an Emergency Medical Responder. At the scene of an emergency, EMTs continue the care begun by Emergency Medical Responders. This care includes stabilizing the patient and preparing the patient for transport.

Advanced Emergency Medical Technician (AEMT) An Advanced Emergency Medical Technician (AEMT) has additional training in skills such as patient assessment, giving intravenous (IV) fluids and medications, performing advanced airway procedures, and assessing abnormal heart rhythms through electrocardiogram (ECG) monitoring.

Paramedic A Paramedic can perform the skills of an AEMT and has had additional instruction in pathophysiology (changes in the body caused by disease), physical examination techniques, and invasive procedures.

You Should Know

EMRs and EMTs provide basic emergency care and are referred to as Basic Life Support (BLS) personnel. Because AEMTs and Paramedics provide more advanced care than EMRs and EMTs, they are often referred to as Advanced Life Support (ALS) personnel.

TABLE 1-2 Levels of EMS Training

Basic Life Support (BLS)	**Emergency Medical Responder (EMR)**	• Is the first person with medical training at the scene of an emergency
		• Provides initial emergency care
		• Skills include
		  • Patient assessment
		  • Opening and maintaining an airway
		  • Ventilating patients
		  • Performing CPR
		  • Controlling bleeding
		  • Bandaging wounds
		  • Stabilizing the spine and injured arms and legs
		  • Assisting with childbirth
		  • Assisting other EMS professionals

	Emergency Medical Technician (EMT)	• Is more skilled than an Emergency Medical Responder
		• Continues the care begun by Emergency Medical Responders
		• Can perform all Emergency Medical Responder skills
		• Additional skills include
		  • Assisting patients with specific prescribed medications
		  • Giving oral glucose and activated charcoal when needed

Advanced Life Support (ALS)	**Advanced Emergency Medical Technician (AEMT)**	• Is more skilled than an EMT
		• Can perform all EMT skills
		• Additional skills include
		  • More training in patient assessment
		  • Ability to give intravenous (IV) fluid and medications
		  • Advanced airway procedures
		  • Electrocardiogram (ECG) monitoring

	Paramedic	• Is more skilled than an AEMT • Has more education about diseases, physical examination techniques, and invasive procedures

Communications

An EMS communications network must reliably allow citizens to access the EMS system (usually by dialing 9-1-1). To ensure adequate EMS system response and coordination, the following are essential:

- A means for dispatch to emergency vehicle communication
- Communication between emergency vehicles
- Communication from the emergency vehicle to the hospital
- Hospital-to-hospital communication
- Communication between agencies, such as between EMS and law enforcement personnel

You Should Know

National Incident Management System (NIMS)

In situations involving a large number of patients, rescuers, and equipment, an **Incident Management System** is often used to control, direct, and coordinate the activities of multiple agencies. In 2003, President Bush directed the Secretary of Homeland Security to develop and administer a National Incident Management System (NIMS). NIMS provides a consistent, nationwide plan to allow all government, private-sector, and nongovernment organizations to work together during domestic incidents.

Activating the EMS System

Under a federal law enacted in 1999, 9-1-1 is replacing all other emergency telephone numbers.

The 9-1-1 network is an important part of our nation's emergency response and disaster preparedness system. Because there is no "11" on a telephone pad, 9-1-1 should always be referred to as "nine-one-one," not "nine-eleven." 9-1-1 is easily remembered, even by young children.

When an emergency occurs, your response to the scene will often depend on the environment in which you work. For example, law enforcement and fire department personnel are typically dispatched to the scene of an emergency after the patient or a bystander calls 9-1-1. However, if you are a lifeguard, teacher, hotel employee, truck driver, or coach, you may see the event occur and be on the scene, providing patient care, before additional help arrives. If you are the first medical person on the scene, you must know how to activate the EMS system and request assistance.

9-1-1 is the official national emergency number in the United States and Canada. When the numbers 9-1-1 are dialed, the caller is quickly connected to a single location, called a Public Safety Answering Point (PSAP). The PSAP dispatcher is trained to route the call to local emergency medical, fire, and law enforcement agencies. Although EMS is usually activated by dialing 9-1-1, other tools for activating an emergency response include emergency alarm boxes, citizen band radios, and wireless telephones.

Enhanced 9-1-1, or E9-1-1, is a system that routes an emergency call to the 9-1-1 center closest to the caller. This system automatically displays the caller's phone number and address. Most 9-1-1 systems that exist today are E9-1-1 systems. The Federal Communications Commission (FCC) has created a program that requires wireless telephone carriers to provide E9-1-1 services. When this program is fully put into practice, wireless E9-1-1 will provide the precise location of a 9-1-1 call from a wireless phone—within 50-100 meters, in most cases. Wireless E9-1-1 should be completed in late 2005.

You Should Know

9-1-1

According to the National Emergency Number Association (NENA), 99% of the population of the United States is covered by some type of 9-1-1 service. Ninety-three percent of that coverage is E9-1-1. Approximately 96% of the geographic United States is covered by some type of 9-1-1 system.

If a 9-1-1 caller does not speak English, the 9-1-1 call taker can add an interpreter from an outside service to the line. Communications centers that answer 9-1-1 calls also have special telephones for responding to 9-1-1 calls from callers who are deaf, hearing-impaired, or speech-impaired.

You Should Know

Voice over Internet Protocol (VoIP)

Voice over Internet Protocol (VoIP), also known as Internet Voice, is technology that allows users to make telephone calls by means of a broadband Internet connection instead of a regular telephone line.

Companies offering this service have different features. Some services allow you to call only other people using the same service. Others allow you to call anyone who has a telephone number. Some services do not work during power outages and may not offer backup power. Some offer E9-1-1 support as an optional service. Subscribers register and pay a fee for E9-1-1. With a subscription, an emergency call is automatically routed to the PSAP that handles 9-1-1 emergencies. If the subscriber is unable to speak, the PSAP operator will know the subscriber's location and be able to dispatch the emergency. If the user declines E9-1-1 service, he or she does not have direct access to emergency personnel via Internet Voice.

Transportation

Emergency transportation is the process of moving a patient from the scene of an emergency to an appropriate receiving facility. All patients who need transport must be moved safely in an appropriately staffed and equipped vehicle. Most patients can be moved effectively in a ground ambulance staffed by qualified emergency medical personnel (Figure 1-1). Patients with more serious injuries or illnesses may require rapid transportation by air medical services (Figure 1-2).

Medical Oversight

Objective 3 ▶

A physician oversees all aspects of patient care in an EMS system. In the United States, the medical care provided to patients is closely governed by laws called **medical practice acts.** These laws vary greatly from state to state. EMTs, AEMTs, and Paramedics act as chosen agents of a physician **medical director.** The care these EMS professionals give is generally considered an extension of the physician's license to practice medicine. As an Emergency Medical Responder, you *may* be a designated agent of the physician. Therefore, the emergency care you provide *may* be considered an extension of the medical director's authority.

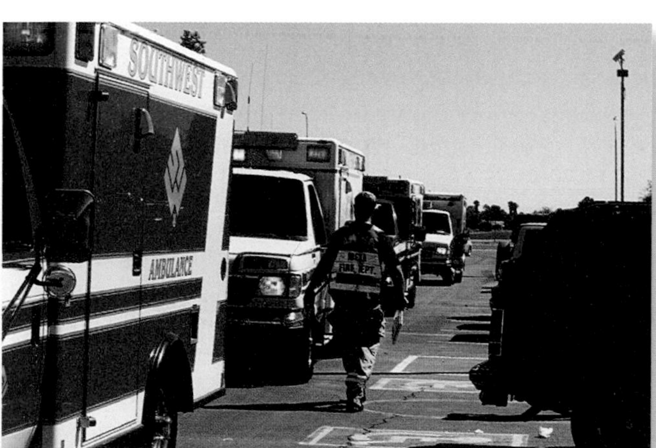

FIGURE 1-1 ▲ Most patients can be moved effectively in a ground ambulance staffed by qualified EMS personnel. © The McGraw-Hill Companies, Inc./Carin Marter, photographer

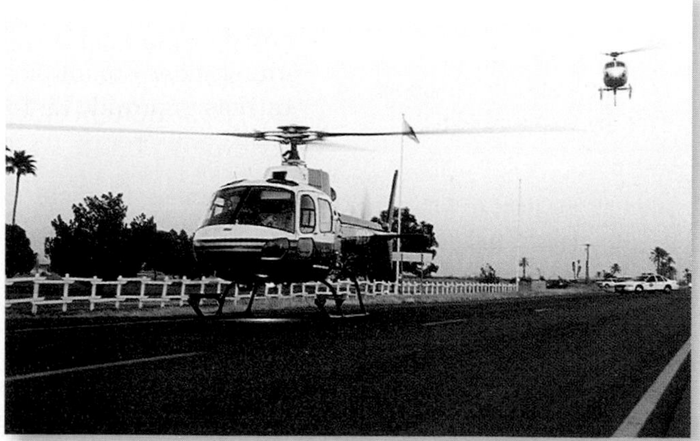

FIGURE 1-2 ▲ Patients with more serious injuries or illnesses may need to be moved rapidly by air medical services. © Courtesy of Air Evac Services, Phoenix, Arizona

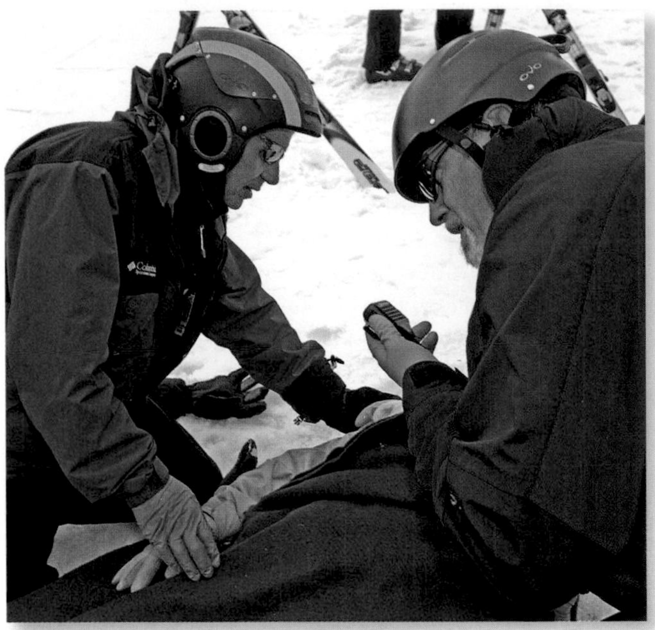

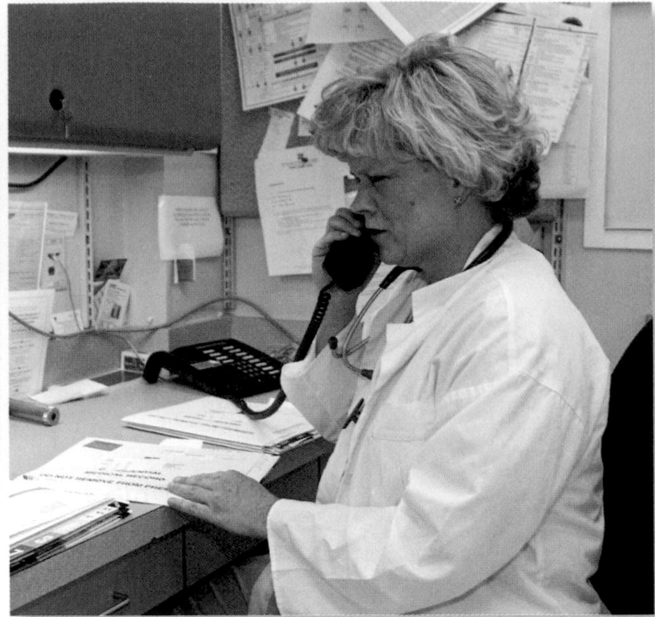

FIGURE 1-3 ▲ On-line medical direction is direct communication with a physician by radio or telephone or face-to-face communication at the scene.

Medical oversight is also referred to as medical control or medical direction.

However, this authority varies by state law. In situations that require emergency medical care, it is very important that you request EMS personnel to the scene as soon as possible.

Objective 4 ▶

Medical oversight is the process by which a physician directs the emergency care provided by EMS personnel to an ill or injured patient. Every EMS system *must* have medical oversight. The physician who provides medical oversight is called the medical director. The two types of medical oversight are on-line and off-line medical direction.

The medical director is responsible for ensuring that the emergency care provided to ill or injured patients is medically appropriate.

On-Line Medical Direction

On-line medical direction, also called *direct* or *concurrent medical direction,* is direct communication with a physician by radio or telephone—or face-to-face communication at the scene—before performing a skill or providing care (Figure 1-3).

Off-Line Medical Direction

Off-line medical direction, also referred to as *indirect, prospective,* or *retrospective medical direction,* is the medical supervision of EMS personnel using policies, treatment protocols, standing orders, education, and quality management reviews.

The development of treatment protocols and standing orders are examples of prospective medical direction.

Prospective Medical Direction **Prospective medical direction** includes activities performed by a physician medical director before an emergency call. It is impossible for the medical director to be physically present at every emergency. Therefore, the medical director develops treatment protocols and standing orders, usually with the assistance of a local EMS advisory group.

Treatment Protocols A **treatment protocol** is a list of steps to be followed when providing emergency care to an ill or injured patient. For example, a patient experiencing a heat-related illness may be treated using the steps outlined in the sample treatment protocol for heat-related emergencies.

Sample Treatment Protocol: Heat-Related Illness

If the patient has moist, pale, skin that is normal to cool in temperature, follow these steps:

1. Remove the patient from the hot environment.
2. Administer oxygen.
3. Remove as much of the patient's clothing as possible. Loosen clothing that cannot be easily removed.
4. Cool the patient by fanning him or her. Do not cool the patient to the point of shivering.
5. Elevate the patient's legs 8–12 inches (shock position).
6. Consult medical direction for further instructions.

Standing Orders **Standing orders** are written orders that authorize EMS personnel to perform certain medical procedures before establishing direct communication with a physician. Most protocols and standing orders are consistent with state and national standards, as well as regional guidelines.

Standing orders are used in critical situations in which delaying treatment would most likely harm the patient. They may also be used when technical or logistical problems delay establishing on-line communication. Direct communication with a physician should be established as soon as the patient's condition allows, as soon as is possible.

Retrospective Medical Direction **Retrospective medical direction** refers to actions performed by a physician after an emergency call. The physician may review the documentation related to the call. This review is done as part of an ongoing quality management program to make sure that appropriate medical care was given to the patient.

Trauma Systems

States must develop a system of specialized care for the triage (sorting) and transfer of trauma patients, including designated trauma centers.

Facilities

The medical facility closest to the scene of an emergency is not always the most appropriate facility.

Seriously ill or injured patients must be moved in a timely manner to the closest *appropriate* medical facility. Hospital care includes many specialties and patient care resources. When the patient arrives at the hospital by ambulance, healthcare professionals from the hospital's emergency department continue the care begun by Emergency Medical Responders (Figure 1-4). The patient is usually first seen by a nurse, who quickly assesses the severity of the patient's illness or

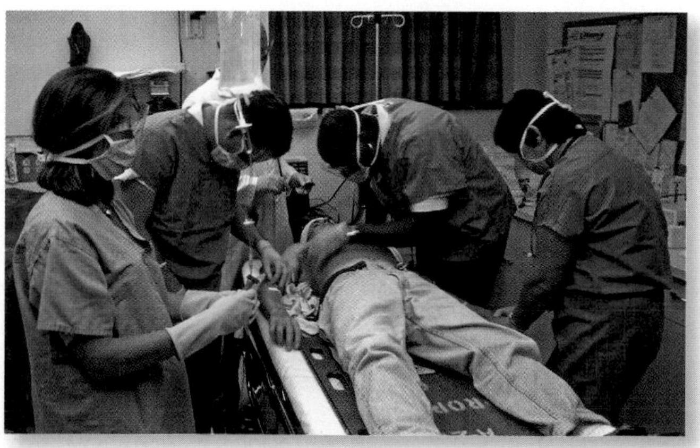

FIGURE 1-4 ▶ When the patient arrives at the hospital by ambulance, healthcare professionals from the hospital's emergency department continue the care begun by Emergency Medical Responders.

injury, and then by a physician. Depending on the patient's illness or injury, the patient may be seen by other members of the healthcare team.

An ill or injured patient receives definitive care in the hospital.

Members of the healthcare team that are available at most hospitals include

- Physicians
- Physician assistants
- Nurses and nurse practitioners
- Respiratory therapists
- Laboratory and radiology technicians
- Physical therapists

Additional resources available within the hospital include surgery and intensive care, among many others.

Specialty Centers

Some hospitals provide routine and emergency care but may specialize in the care of certain conditions or emergencies. Specialty centers have resources available, such as trained personnel and equipment, to help provide the best possible care for the patient's illness or injury. A trauma center is one type of specialty center (Figure 1-5). In these centers, specially trained personnel and equipment are available 24 hours a day to care for patients with serious injuries.

Other types of specialty centers include burn, heart/cardiovascular, hyperbaric, pediatric, perinatal, poison, spinal cord injury, and stroke centers (Table 1-3).

You Should Know

In both urban and rural areas, a patient may be stabilized at a closer hospital and then transferred to a specialty center if the patient requires care beyond that available at the initial receiving facility.

Rehabilitation Services

Soon after their condition has been stabilized and they have been moved from the hospital emergency department, some patients will require the services of healthcare professionals who specialize in rehabilitation. These healthcare professionals include rehabilitation nurses, physicians, physical therapists, occupational therapists, and social workers. They work with the patient and the patient's family to return the ill or injured patient to his or her previous state of health.

Making a Difference

To ensure that your patient receives the best possible care for his or her illness or injury, you must be familiar with the capabilities of the medical facilities in your area.

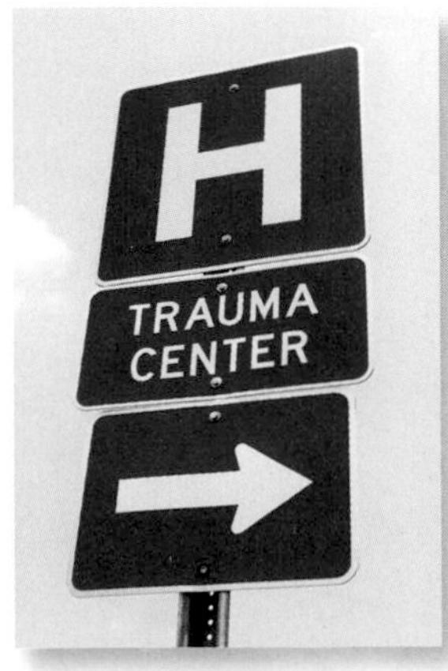

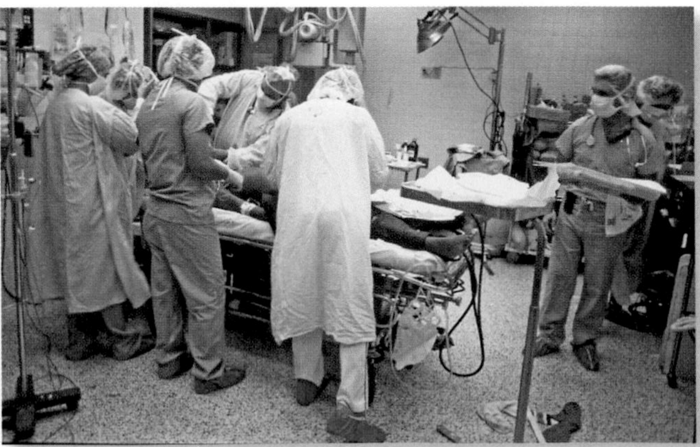

FIGURE 1-5 ▶ A trauma center is a specialty facility with trained personnel and equipment available 24 hours a day to care for seriously injured patients.

TABLE 1-3 Types of Specialty Centers

Burn Centers	Burn centers specialize in the care of burns, ranging from relatively mild to life-threatening burn injuries. Services include helping the patient and family with the emotional stress that often comes with a burn injury. They also provide daily assistance with exercise, scar control, wound care, splinting, and the activities of daily living.
Heart/Cardiovascular Centers	Heart/cardiovascular centers specialize in treating disorders of the heart and blood vessels.
Hyperbaric Centers	Hyperbaric centers specialize in hyperbaric oxygen (HBO) therapy, which uses 100% oxygen given at a controlled pressure (greater than sea level) for a set amount of time. Carbon monoxide poisoning and smoke inhalation are two conditions that may be treated with HBO therapy.
Pediatric Centers	Pediatric centers specialize in the treatment of children. Children are not just small adults. Their bodies are different, and the illnesses and injuries they experience often produce signs and symptoms that differ from those of an adult. Pediatric centers have professionals trained to recognize the medical, developmental, and emotional needs of children.
Perinatal Centers	Perinatal centers specialize in the care of high-risk pregnancies.
Poison Centers	Poison centers specialize in providing information in the treatment of poisonings and drug interactions. Some poison centers also provide education programs for medical professionals and the public about responding to biological and chemical terrorist incidents. They also provide education about nonterrorist incidents, such as epidemics and hazardous material incidents.
Spinal Cord Injury Centers	Spinal cord injury centers specialize in the medical, surgical, rehabilitative, and long-term follow-up care of patients with spinal cord injuries.
Stroke Centers	Stroke centers specialize in diagnosing and treating disease of the blood vessels of the brain. The staff at a stroke center works very quickly to determine the cause and location of the stroke and to give appropriate care.

Public Information and Education

As an Emergency Medical Responder, you should be actively involved in educating the public on how to access the EMS system and how to prevent injuries (Figure 1-6). Injury prevention programs, such as those on bicycle safety, the use of child safety seats, poisoning prevention, and drowning prevention, often lead to better use of EMS resources. Cardiopulmonary resuscitation (CPR) and first aid programs can improve a citizen's ability to recognize an emergency and provide appropriate care until more advanced care arrives.

You Should Know

- Accidental injuries are the leading cause of death in children from 1–21 years of age.
- Each year, between 20% and 25% of all children sustain an injury that is severe enough to require medical attention or bed rest or that results in missed school.
- Motor vehicle injuries are the leading cause of death among children at every age after their first birthday.
- Of children aged 0–12 years who were killed in motor vehicle crashes during 1999–2000, 52% were unrestrained, 18% were incorrectly restrained, and 35% were riding in the front seat.

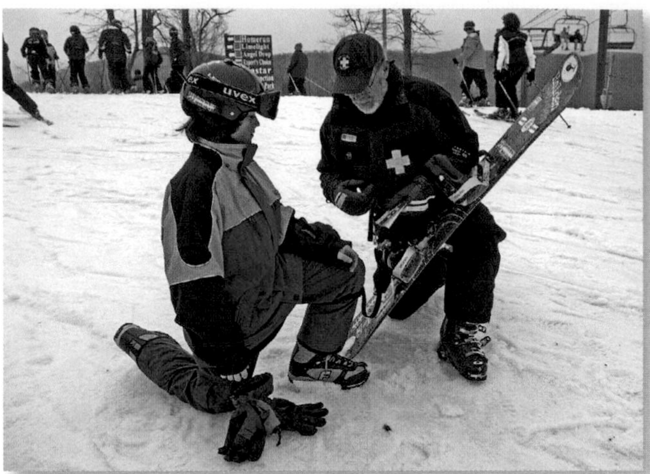

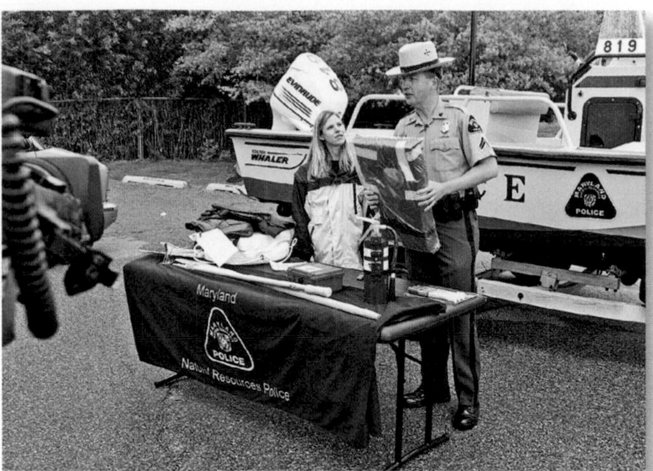

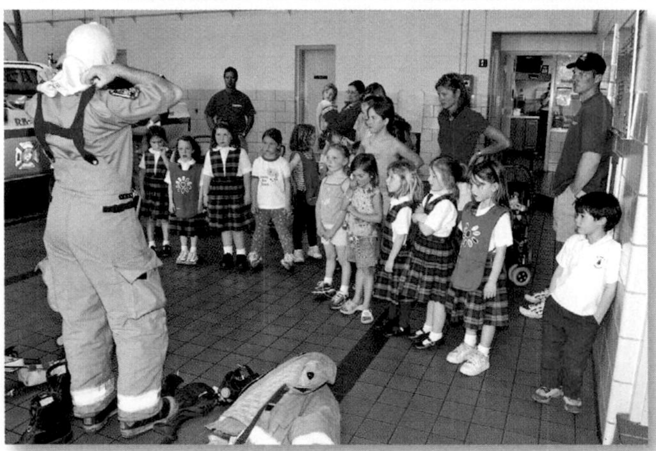

FIGURE 1-6 ▲ Emergency Medical Responders should educate the public about accessing the EMS system and preventing injuries.

Evaluation

Each state must have a program to review and improve the effectiveness of its EMS services provided to adult and pediatric patients. **Quality management** is a system of internal and external reviews and audits of all aspects of an EMS system. It is used to identify the areas of the EMS system needing improvement. Quality management also ensures that patients receive the highest quality medical care.

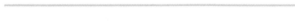

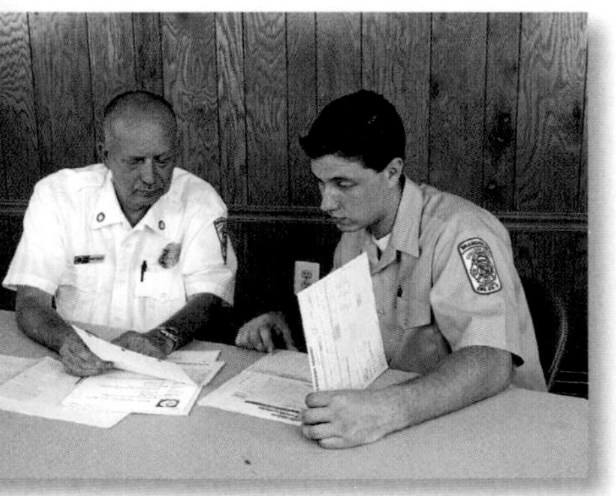

FIGURE 1-7 ▲ Quality management is an important part of EMS. It involves the constant monitoring of performance, including reviewing call documentation.

> **You Should Know**
>
> **EMS Quality Management**
>
> The goal of an EMS quality management program is to consistently provide timely medical care that is appropriate, compassionate, cost effective, and beneficial for the patient.

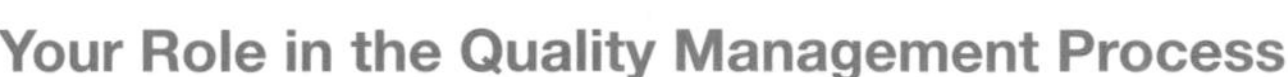

Your Role in the Quality Management Process

Quality management is an important part of EMS; it involves the constant monitoring of performance. Quality management includes

- Obtaining information from the patient, other EMS professionals, and facility personnel about the quality and appropriateness of the medical care you provided
- Reviewing and evaluating your documentation of an emergency call (Figure 1-7)
- Evaluating your ability to perform skills properly

- Evaluating your professionalism during interactions with the patient, EMS professionals, and other healthcare personnel
- Evaluating your ability to follow policies and protocols
- Evaluating your participation in continuing education opportunities

Making a Difference

Participating in the Quality Management Process

Your commitment to and participation in the quality management process is important in improving the EMS system. Your medical director or another healthcare professional will provide you with feedback about an area monitored by the process. When you receive the feedback, make sure to maintain a positive and professional attitude. Use the information shared as an opportunity for personal and professional growth.

The Phases of a Typical EMS Response

When an emergency occurs, a bystander frequently recognizes the event and activates the EMS system by calling 9-1-1 or another emergency number (Figure 1-8). The EMS dispatcher gathers information and activates an appropriate EMS response based on the information received. The bystander is often provided with instructions about how to provide basic first aid, including cardiopulmonary resuscitation (CPR) if necessary (Figure 1-9).

On the way to the scene, the Emergency Medical Responders prepare for the patient and situation based on the information given by the dispatcher. They consider a number of factors, including

- The number of patients
- Possible problems in gaining access to the patient
- Scene safety
- Potential complications based on the patient's reported illness or injury
- The equipment and supplies that will need to be taken to the patient to begin emergency care

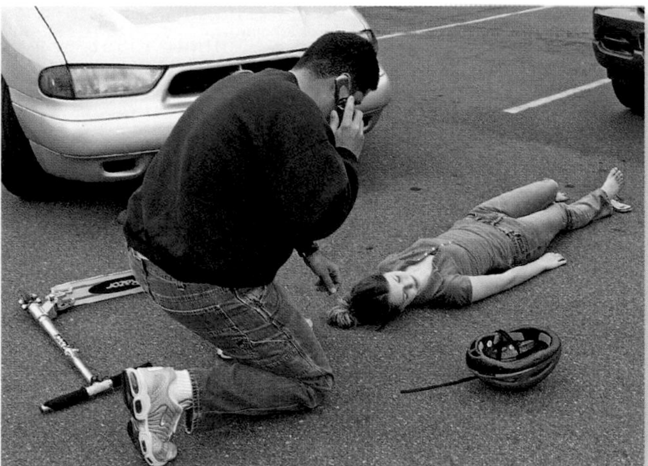

FIGURE 1-8 ▲ When an emergency occurs, a bystander frequently recognizes the event and activates the EMS system.

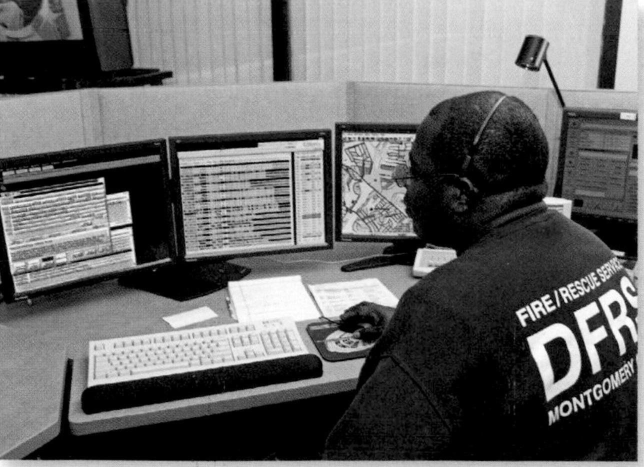

FIGURE 1-9 ▲ While in contact with the EMS dispatcher, the bystander is often provided with instructions regarding how to administer basic first aid.

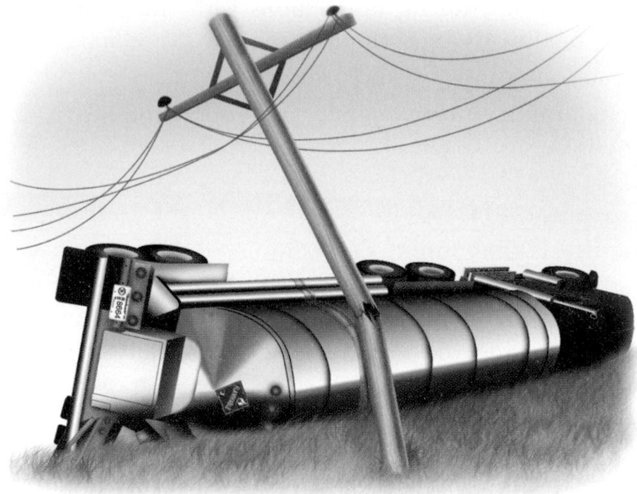

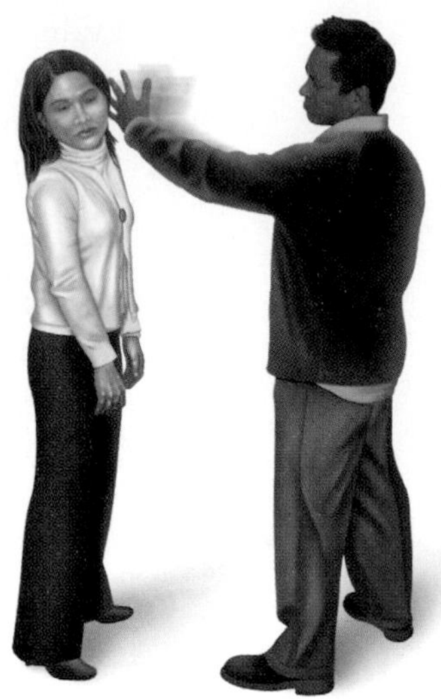

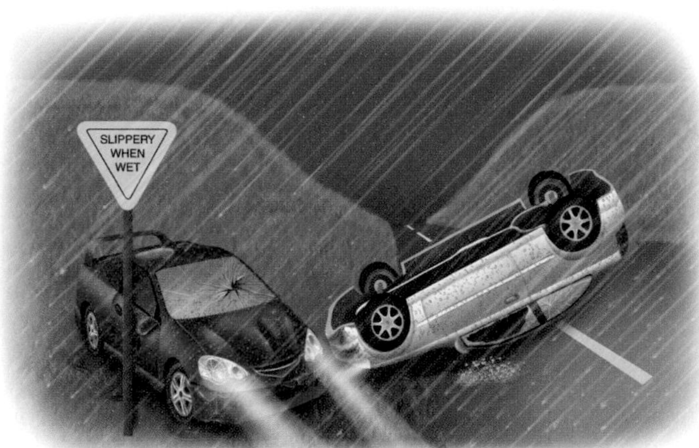

FIGURE 1-10 ▲ Arriving Emergency Medical Responders will quickly evaluate the safety of the scene, looking for hazards or potential hazards.

On arrival, Emergency Medical Responders will quickly evaluate the safety of the scene. The Emergency Medical Responders will be looking for hazards or potential hazards, such as downed electrical lines, possible hazardous materials, traffic hazards, unstable vehicles, signs of violence or potential violence, and weather hazards (Figure 1-10).

The phases of a typical EMS response are listed in Table 1-4 and shown in Figure 1-11.

TABLE 1-4 Phases of a Typical EMS Response

1. Detection of the emergency
2. Reporting the emergency (the call made for assistance, dispatch)
3. Response (medical resources sent to the scene)
4. On-scene care
5. Care during transport
6. Transfer to definitive care

FIGURE 1-11 ▶ The phases of a typical EMS response.

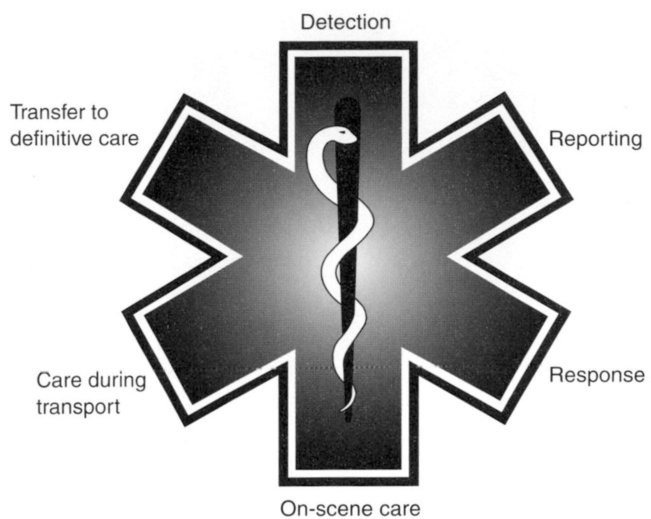

Stop and Think!

If the scene is not safe and you cannot make it safe, *do not enter*. If a safe scene becomes unsafe, leave. Lives have been lost when a well-meaning rescuer has attempted to assist in an emergency without enough training, assistance, or equipment. Wait for the arrival of additional resources.

This assessment is important to determine the emergency medical care the patient requires.

After making sure that the scene is safe, Emergency Medical Responders quickly perform a **patient assessment** to determine the seriousness of the patient's condition or the extent of injuries (Figure 1-12). Emergency Medical Responders will safely and efficiently provide emergency medical care for life-threatening emergencies at the scene until additional EMS resources arrive.

When more highly trained medical professionals arrive, Emergency Medical Responders provide the arriving personnel with a brief description of the emergency and a summary of the care provided before transferring patient care (Figure 1-13). If the patient's condition requires further emergency care, the

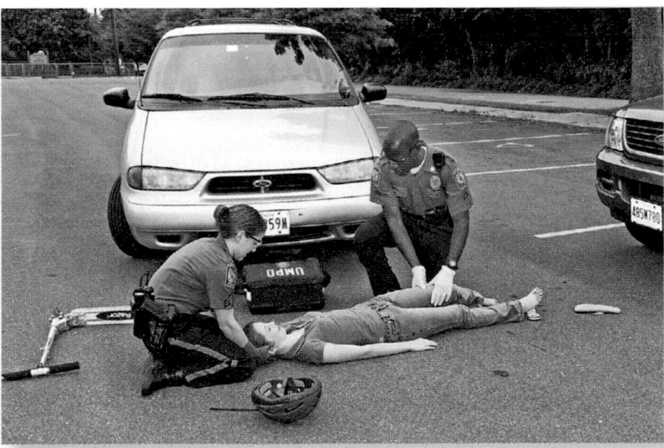

FIGURE 1-12 ▲ After ensuring the scene is safe, Emergency Medical Responders quickly assess the patient to determine the seriousness of the patient's condition or the extent of injuries.

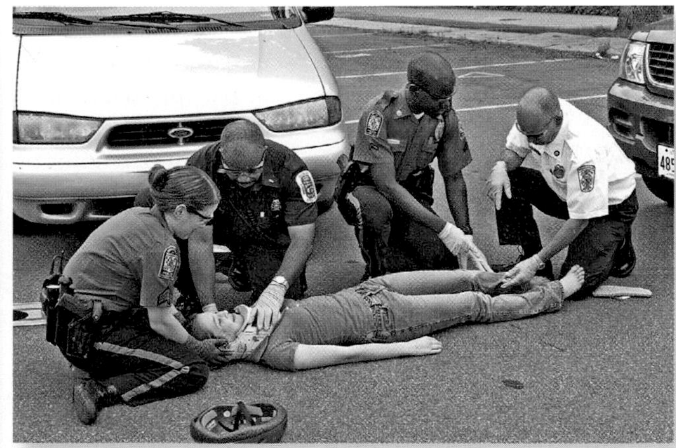

FIGURE 1-13 ▲ Before transferring care, Emergency Medical Responders provide more highly trained personnel with a brief description of the emergency and a summary of the care provided.

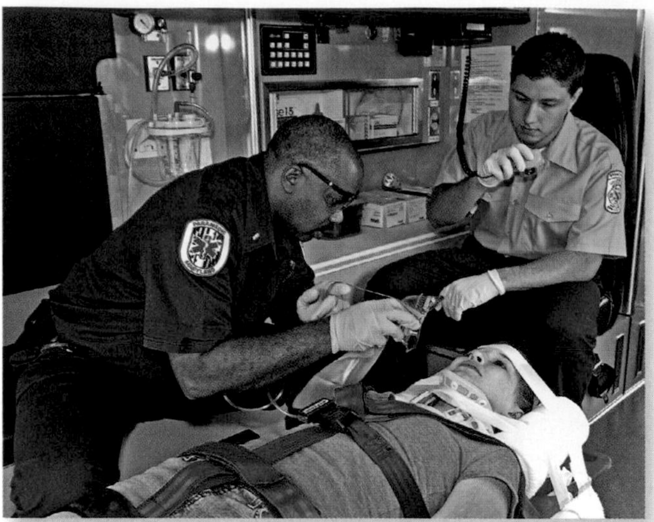

FIGURE 1-14 ▲ The patient is loaded into an ambulance and transported to an appropriate receiving facility, such as a hospital.

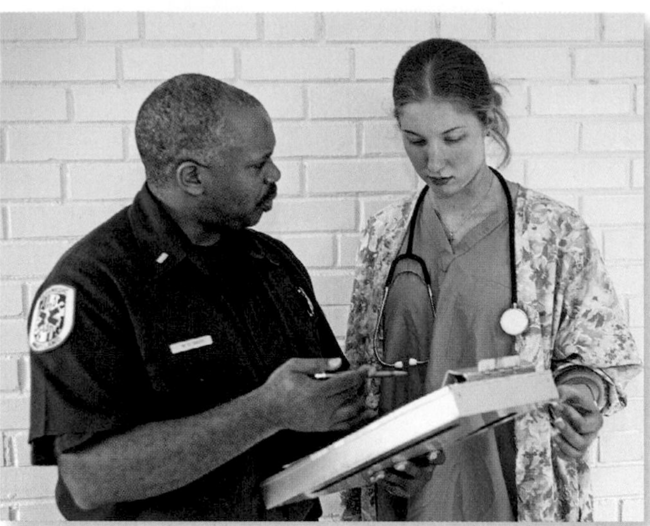

FIGURE 1-15 ▲ A brief description of the emergency and a summary of the care provided are given to emergency department personnel.

patient is placed into an ambulance and taken to an appropriate receiving facility, such as a hospital, for definitive care (Figure 1-14). On arrival at the receiving facility, a brief description of the emergency and a summary of the care provided are given to a healthcare professional with the same or greater level of medical training (Figure 1-15). Patient care is then transferred. Documentation of the call is finished, supplies are restocked, and the emergency vehicle is prepared for the next call. After the call is completed, a review may be held to discuss what went well. The review also identifies opportunities for improving patient care at the scene and during transport.

Your Roles and Responsibilities as an Emergency Medical Responder

You have many roles and responsibilities as an Emergency Medical Responder. Some Emergency Medical Responders, such as firefighters and law enforcement personnel, work for public safety agencies and are required to respond to the scene of an emergency. Other Emergency Medical Responders, such as lifeguards, members of the ski patrol, and teachers, may be called on to provide emergency care when a sudden illness or injury occurs.

Regardless of his or her primary profession, an Emergency Medical Responder is expected to provide a standard of care in an emergency. **Standard of care** refers to the minimum level of care expected of similarly trained healthcare professionals.

Your Roles as an Emergency Medical Responder

Safety

Although the patient's well-being is an important concern at the scene of an emergency, your personal safety *must* be your primary concern, followed by the safety of your crew, patients, and bystanders. Before approaching the patient, make sure the scene is safe for you to provide care. Then put on appropriate personal protective equipment (PPE) to minimize your risk of exposure to potentially infectious body fluids or other infectious agents (see Chapter 2).

When you are notified of an emergency, prepare for the patient and the situation based on the information given to you. Respond safely and in a timely manner to the address or location given.

When you arrive at the scene and before you initiate patient care, size up the scene. First determine if the scene is safe. Then identify the mechanism of the injury or the nature of the illness, identify the total number of patients, and request additional help if necessary. If law enforcement personnel are not present on the scene, create a safe traffic environment.

Gaining Access to the Patient

You must gain access to the patient in order to perform a **patient assessment** and provide emergency care. In some situations, you may need additional resources at the scene, such as law enforcement personnel, the fire department, the utility company, or a special rescue team. In these situations, be sure to notify the dispatcher as soon as possible of the need for these resources.

Patient care comes before extrication, unless a delay in movement would endanger the life of the patient or rescuer.

If the patient has been involved in a motor vehicle crash, you must make sure the scene is safe and provide necessary care to the patient before **extrication**. You must also make sure that the patient is removed in a way that minimizes further injury. To accomplish these tasks, you will need to work closely with the rescuers responsible for extrication.

Remember This!

Basic Equipment for an Emergency Kit

As an Emergency Medical Responder, you should have appropriate equipment and supplies available in case of an emergency (Figure 1-16). Be sure to check the contents of your emergency kit regularly and replace items as they become outdated.

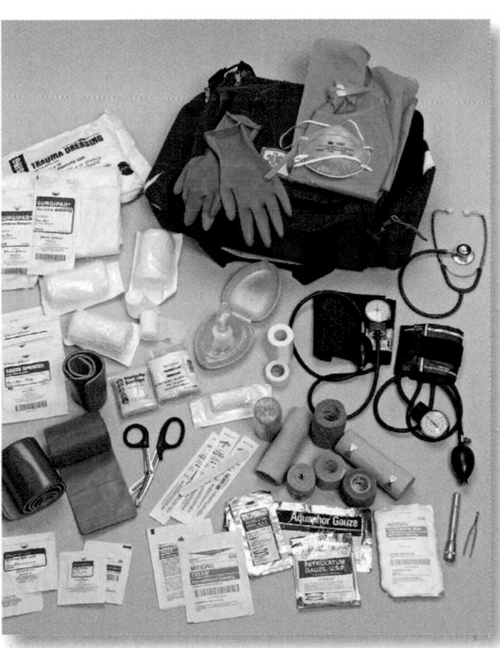

FIGURE 1-16 ▲ Basic equipment and supplies for an emergency kit.

Personal protective equipment (PPE)	Two pairs of latex gloves (or other gloves, if you are allergic to latex) Masks and barrier devices for ventilating patients, including high-efficiency particulate air (HEPA) masks Goggles or face shields Gowns
Wound management	Trauma shears, adhesive tape, and bandages and dressings, including triangular bandages, roller-type bandages, universal dressings or gauze pads, and occlusive dressings (such as petroleum gauze) for making an airtight seal Upper- and lower-extremity splints Stick (for a tourniquet) Eye protector (such as a paper cup or cone) Tweezers Antiseptic wipes

Vital signs	Wristwatch with a second hand or a digital watch that shows seconds Stethoscope Blood pressure cuff (adult and pediatric) if you are expected to take a blood pressure
Extrication tools and devices	Jack and jack handle, pliers, a hammer, screwdrivers, and a rope Blanket and pillow Disposable chemical cold pack Bag or case for equipment

Additional Emergency Equipment

You may want to include these additional items in your emergency kit (or in a separate kit) if you have been trained in their use and are permitted to use them according to your local protocol:

- Oral airways (adult and pediatric)
- Bag-valve masks (adult and pediatric)
- Biohazard bag
- Flashlight (aluminum or heavy-duty)
- Seatbelt cutter
- Two-way hand-held radio and/or cellular telephone
- Notebook or clipboard with black ink pen, emergency phone numbers, radio frequencies, and copies of your protocols
- Hand-operated suction device
- Obstetrics (OB) kit (for emergency childbirth)
- Raincoat or poncho (for wet weather)
- Safety vest (for visibility)
- Bag or case for equipment
- Window punch
- Flares and/or chemical light sticks
- Local maps and/or Global Positioning System (GPS) unit

Patient Assessment

Gather information about the emergency by observing the scene, speaking with the patient and bystanders, and assessing the patient.

After reaching the patient, you must perform a systematic assessment to determine what is wrong and quickly identify life-threatening conditions. As an Emergency Medical Responder, you will give emergency medical care to adults, children, and infants based on your findings. Depending on the patient's illness or injury, you may need to perform certain skills, including

- Opening and maintaining an airway
- Ventilating the patient
- Providing CPR
- Operating an automated external defibrillator (AED; an AED delivers an electrical shock to the heart)
- Providing emergency medical care for victims of trauma, such as controlling bleeding, bandaging wounds, and manually stabilizing injured limbs
- Providing emergency medical care to assist in childbirth
- Managing general medical complaints, altered mental status, seizures, environmental emergencies, behavioral emergencies, and psychological crises

While waiting for EMS professionals to arrive, reassess the patient frequently and provide additional emergency care as needed.

Making a Difference

Once you begin emergency care, you must continue that care until

- An individual with medical training equal to or greater than your own assumes responsibility for the patient *or*
- You are physically unable to continue providing care due to exhaustion *or*
- There is a change in the scene that weakens or endangers your physical well-being

Continuation of Care Through Additional EMS Resources

Remember the four *C*s when giving a verbal report: *c*ourteous, *c*lear, *c*omplete, and *c*oncise.

When personnel with more advanced medical training arrive on the scene, first identify yourself as an Emergency Medical Responder. Then give them a brief explanation about what happened, the position in which the patient was found, your assessment findings, the emergency care you gave, and the patient's response to the treatment given (Figure 1-17).

When they arrive on the scene, the medical personnel with more advanced training will assume responsibility for the patient. Your assistance may be needed in the following situations:

- Protecting an entrapped patient from injury during extrication procedures
- Performing emergency moves
- Lifting the stretcher and placing it in the ambulance
- Making sure that the patient and stretcher are secured

Making a Difference

Providing a Verbal Report

When transferring patient care to a healthcare professional with medical training equal to or greater than your own, be sure to include the following elements in your verbal report:

- Identify yourself as an Emergency Medical Responder.
- Describe what happened and the position in which the patient was found.
- Describe your assessment findings.
- Report any medical history you obtained from the patient.
- Describe the emergency medical care you gave.
- Describe the patient's response to the treatment given.

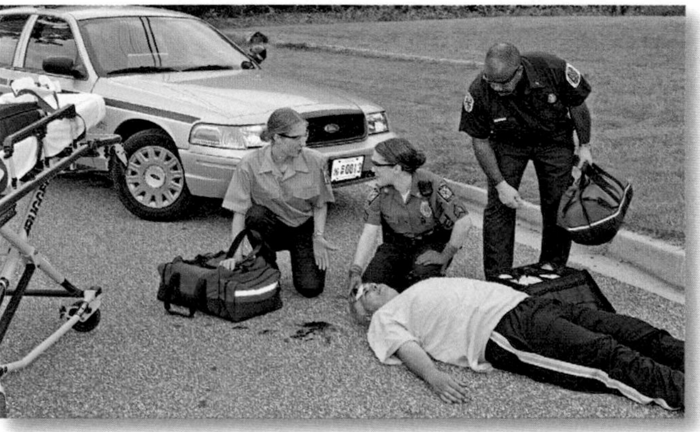

FIGURE 1-17 ► When personnel with more advanced medical training arrive on the scene, identify yourself as an Emergency Medical Responder and give a brief verbal report.

Documentation

You may be required by state law or your agency to document what you saw and heard at the scene. You may also have to document the emergency care you provided and the patient's response to that care.

Public Safety Liaison

As an Emergency Medical Responder, you will be working with public safety personnel, including law enforcement officers, firefighters, and other EMS professionals. The information you give them about the first few minutes after the emergency may be important to the healthcare professionals who will provide further patient care.

Making a Difference

Roles of the Emergency Medical Responder

- Personal, crew, patient, and bystander safety
- Gaining access to the patient
- Patient assessment to identify life-threatening conditions
- Continuation of care through additional EMS resources
- Initial patient care based on assessment findings
- Assisting with additional emergency care
- Documentation of the emergency per local and state requirements
- Public safety liaison

Your Responsibilities as an Emergency Medical Responder

Objective 6 ▶ You will be expected to accept and uphold the responsibilities of an Emergency Medical Responder according to the standards of an EMS professional. These standards include preserving life, relieving suffering, promoting health, and doing no harm. You must respect and keep private all information of a confidential nature that is obtained in the course of your work as an Emergency Medical Responder, unless required by law to report the information.

Objective 8 ▶ Every patient has the right to expect competent, considerate, respectful care from every member of the healthcare team at all times and under all circumstances (Figure 1-18). It is not appropriate to judge a patient or vary the care you provide based on a patient's race, ethnicity, national origin, religion, gender, age, mental or physical disability, sexual orientation, or ability to pay for the care provided.

Making a Difference

The emergency medical care you provide as an Emergency Medical Responder must be based on need and without regard to the patient's race, ethnicity, national origin, religion, gender, age, mental or physical disability, sexual orientation, or ability to pay for the care provided.

Many patient complaints about medical care result from the patient's belief that he or she was not treated with respect. As an EMS professional, you have an obligation to do the following:

FIGURE 1-18 ▶ Healthcare personnel, including Emergency Medical Responders, must give all patients competent, considerate, and respectful care at all times and under all circumstances.

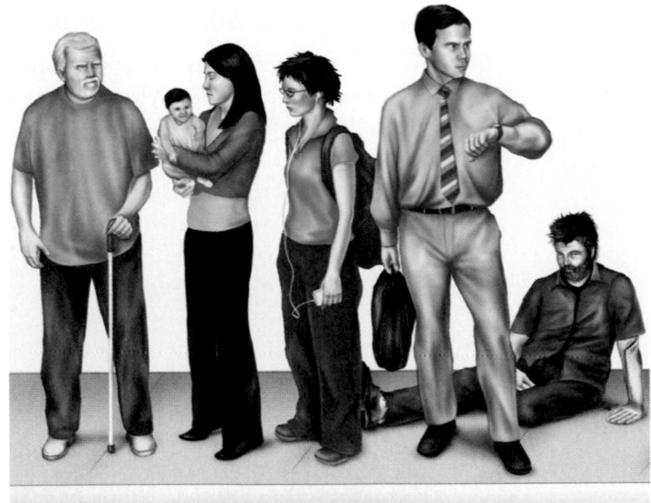

- Respect each patient as an individual.
- Provide emergency medical care to every patient to the best of your ability.
- Listen attentively to your patients and take their concerns and complaints seriously.
- Provide clear explanations.
- Provide patients with emotional support to help ease fear and anxiety.
- Preserve each patient's dignity during examinations.

Personal Health and Safety

Your job as an Emergency Medical Responder has physical demands that require stamina and endurance. You will have to walk, stand, and assist in lifting and carrying ill or injured patients who weigh more than 125 pounds. Climbing and balancing may be required to gain access to the patient, such as on stairs or a hillside. You may also have to help transport the patient safely. In some situations, the patient may be found in a location where patient assessment is possible only if you stoop, kneel, crouch, or crawl.

To make sure that your well-being, as well as that of the patient and your coworkers, is not at risk in these situations, you must first take care of yourself. Maintain your health by exercising regularly. Exercise prepares you to handle the physical demands of the job by improving muscle tone and circulation. Exercise also provides a physical release for stress. Getting enough sleep, rest, and good nutrition are important to staying healthy and doing your job well. Also keep your immunizations up to date.

Making a Difference

Personal Traits of an EMS Professional

- Professional appearance, attitude, and conduct
- Professional oral and written communications
- Mastery of EMS knowledge and skills
- Confidence and leadership abilities
- Compassionate patient advocate
- Good moral character
- Ability to adapt to situations using sound judgment

An older adult should be addressed using his or her last name with Mr., Mrs., or Ms.

Attitude and Communication

As an Emergency Medical Responder, it is important that you possess and maintain a caring attitude. When you arrive at the patient's side, begin by introducing yourself: "Hello. My name is _______, and I am an Emergency Medical Responder. I am here to help you. What is your name?" Be considerate of your patient's personal space, physical condition, and feelings.

Personal space is the invisible area immediately around you that you interpret as your own. The size of your personal space can change, depending on whom you are with, and you may feel threatened when others invade your personal space without your consent. When talking with a patient, it is important to consider the distance between you and the patient and recognize that a "comfortable distance" differs among cultures. For example, the Japanese typically have a larger personal space than North Americans do, while Italians have a much smaller one. Examples of the personal space common in the United States are listed in Table 1-5.

Many of the tasks you will perform as an Emergency Medical Responder will occur within the boundaries of another's personal space. It is helpful to take the time to explain procedures that intrude on another's personal space before beginning them. If you do not, the patient may become agitated, nervous, or even aggressive because of your actions.

Composure

Many emergency calls involve minor injuries and the medical care that is required is straightforward. However, you will come across situations involving life-threatening injuries as well as patients and family members who are upset. As an Emergency Medical Responder, others will look to you as the person in control of the situation. Even though you may feel anxious, you must be able to adapt to these situations, remain calm, and display confidence.

Making a Difference

Your contact with the patient, family, bystanders, and other members of the healthcare team must be respectful and professional, even in stressful or chaotic situations.

TABLE 1-5 Common Zones of Personal Space in the United States

Zone	Distance	Notes
Public space	12 feet or more	Impersonal contact with others occurs in this space.
Social space	4–12 feet	Much of a patient interview occurs at this distance.
Personal space	1½–4 feet	Much of a physical assessment occurs at this distance.
Intimate space	Touching to 1½ feet	This space is best for assessing breath and other body odors.

Tamparo CT, Lindh WQ. Therapeutic Communications for Health Professionals, 2nd ed. Thomson Learning, 2000, pages 31–32. (printed in Canada).

Appearance

Objective 7 ▶

It has been said that you never get a second chance to make a good first impression. As an Emergency Medical Responder, you will meet individuals who are experiencing a medical emergency. In 30 seconds or less, they will form an opinion about you based on what they see, hear, and sense. When you approach a patient and prepare to provide needed emergency care, you are expecting the patient to place his or her trust in you. Presenting a neat, clean, and professional appearance invites trust. It also instills confidence, enhances cooperation, and brings a sense of order to an emergency.

Making a Difference

The patient, the patient's family, and bystanders often view the attention you pay to your appearance as a reflection of your care. If you are courteous, are respectful, and present a professional appearance, they are reassured that you will provide quality patient care. If you are ill mannered or your appearance is untidy, they may assume that the care you provide will be of poor quality.

Good personal hygiene is essential to presenting a professional appearance. It includes the following:

- Bathing daily and keeping your teeth clean
- Using a deodorant or an antiperspirant
- Making sure your hair is clean and, if long, restrained, so that is will not fall into open wounds
- Making sure that your fingernails are clean and neatly trimmed

Good grooming includes making sure that your uniform is clean, mended, and fits well. Shoes should be clean and comfortable, provide support, and fit properly. You should wear a watch with a second hand for timing things such as a patient's heart rate, breathing rate, and labor pains. Because they may be offensive and nauseating to patients, fragrances should not be worn.

Maintaining Knowledge and Skills

Your Emergency Medical Responder education does not end with completing the Emergency Medical Responder course. As a healthcare professional, you must keep your knowledge and skills current through continuing education (CE) and refresher courses. CE and refresher courses are helpful because they help you keep the skills and knowledge you learned during your initial training. CE and refresher courses also provide information about advances in medicine, skills, and equipment. In addition, they educate you about changes in local protocols and national guidelines that affect EMS.

CE occurs in different forms, including skill labs, lectures and workshops, conferences and seminars, case reviews and/or quality management reviews, reading professional journals, and reviewing videotapes and/or audiotapes.

Making a Difference

Responsibilities of the Emergency Medical Responder

- Personal health and safety
- Composure and a caring attitude
- Neat, clean, and professional appearance
- Up-to-date knowledge and skills
- Current knowledge of local, state, and national issues affecting EMS

Specific Statutes and Regulations

Objective 5 ►

Statutes are laws established by Congress and state legislatures. Every state has statutes that establish an EMS regulatory body and describe how its EMS personnel are licensed or certified. **Licensure** is the granting of a written authorization by an official or a legal authority. It allows a person to perform medical acts and procedures not permitted without the authorization. **Certification** is a designation that ensures a person has met predetermined requirements to perform a particular activity.

State laws also detail the medical procedures and functions that can be performed by a licensed or certified healthcare professional, called the **scope of practice.** Because EMS statutes vary from state to state, ask your instructor about the laws in your area that affect you as an Emergency Medical Responder.

Emergency Medical Responder Certification

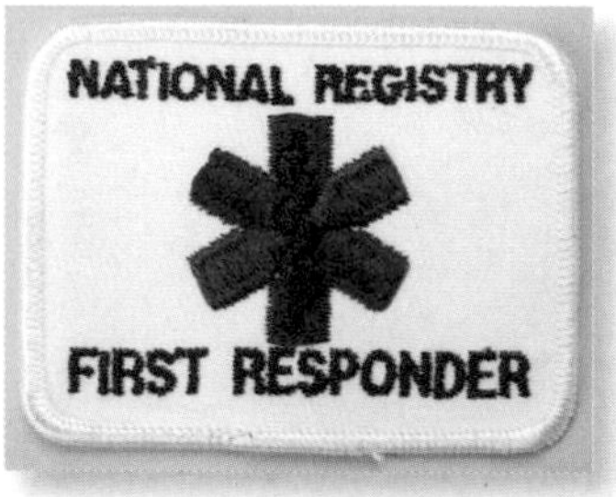

FIGURE 1-19 ▲ Emergency Medical Responders can be certified by a number of agencies, including the National Registry of Emergency Medical Technicians (NREMT).

Emergency Medical Responders can be certified by a number of agencies, including the National Registry of Emergency Medical Technicians (NREMT) (Figure 1-19), the National Safety Council (NSC), the American Safety and Health Institute (ASHI), and state agencies. Most state agencies require the successful completion of an Emergency Medical Responder course that follows the DOT curriculum. Recognition as a nationally registered Emergency Medical Responder requires you to successfully complete a written and practical skills examination.

Certification as an Emergency Medical Responder is good for a limited time—usually two years. Participating in CE courses or an Emergency Medical Responder refresher course is required for recertification.

You Should Know

National Registry of Emergency Medical Technicians

The NREMT helps develop professional standards. It also verifies the skills and knowledge of EMS professionals by preparing and conducting examinations.

On The Scene

Wrap-Up

In responding to the scenario, you recall the standard procedures for your team and have someone activate the EMS system by dialing 9-1-1. You turn off the engine and free your patient's hand. You then lay him down in a safe area and control the bleeding.

The ambulance crew, staffed with an EMT and a Paramedic, arrive quickly. You give them a brief report and assist them in assessing and caring for the patient. After they start an intravenous line to give the patient pain medicine, his face relaxes. He is then transported to the trauma center, where two of his fingers are successfully reattached. He stops in to thank you two weeks later on his way home from a rehabilitation session. ■

Sum It Up

- The *Emergency Medical Services (EMS) system* is part of the healthcare system. It consists of a coordinated network of resources that provides emergency care and transportation to victims of sudden illness and injury.
- An *Emergency Medical Responder* is the first person with medical training who arrives at the scene of an emergency. An Emergency Medical Responder uses a minimal amount of equipment to assess the patient and provide initial emergency care. An Emergency Medical Responder is also trained to assist other EMS professionals.
- There are four levels of nationally recognized prehospital professionals: Emergency Medical Responder (EMR), Emergency Medical Technician (EMT), Advanced Emergency Medical Technician (AEMT), and Paramedic. EMRs and EMTs provide Basic Life Support. AEMTs and Paramedics provide Advanced Life Support.
- Every EMS system must have a medical director. A *medical director* is a physician who provides medical oversight. He or she is responsible for making sure that the emergency care provided to ill or injured patients is medically appropriate.
- The phases of a typical EMS response include the following:
  1. When an emergency occurs, a call is made for emergency assistance (9-1-1).
  2. The EMS dispatcher gathers information and activates the appropriate EMS response. The dispatcher provides instructions to the caller, if needed, before the EMS providers arrive.
  3. On the way to the scene, Emergency Medical Responders prepare for the patient and the situation.
  4. On arriving at the scene, Emergency Medical Responders make sure the scene is safe. The Emergency Medical Responders then begin to assess the patient, providing initial emergency care.
  5. When additional EMS resources arrive, additional emergency care is provided at the scene. If transport is required, the patient is moved to an appropriate receiving facility. Continued emergency care is provided en route.
  6. On arriving at the hospital, patient care is transferred to the receiving facility's personnel.
- *Quality management* is a system of internal and external reviews. This system reviews all aspects of an EMS system. Quality management is used to identify areas of the EMS system that need improvement. This system helps ensure that the patient receives the highest-quality medical care.
- The roles of an Emergency Medical Responder include ensuring personal, crew, patient, and bystander safety; gaining access to the patient; performing a patient assessment to identify life-threatening conditions; continuing care through additional EMS resources; providing initial patient care based on the assessment findings; assisting with additional emergency care; documenting the emergency per local and state requirements; and acting as a public safety liaison.
- The responsibilities of an Emergency Medical Responder include maintaining personal health and safety; a caring attitude and composure; a neat, clean, and professional appearance; up-to-date knowledge and skills; and current knowledge of local, state, and national issues affecting EMS.

► Tracking Your Progress

After reading this chapter, can you	Page Reference	Objective Met?
• Define the components of Emergency Medical Services (EMS) systems?	5–15	☐
• Differentiate your roles and responsibilities as an Emergency Medical Responder from those of other prehospital care providers?	6–7	☐
• Define medical oversight and discuss your role in the process?	9–10	☐
• Discuss the types of medical oversight that may affect the medical care you provide?	9–11	☐
• State the specific statutes and regulations in your state regarding the EMS system?	9	☐
• Accept and uphold your responsibilities as an Emergency Medical Responder in accordance with the standards of an EMS professional?	22–25	☐
• Explain the rationale for maintaining a professional appearance when on duty or when responding to calls?	25	☐
• Describe why it is inappropriate to judge a patient based on a cultural, gender, age, or socioeconomic model and to vary the standard of care rendered as a result of that judgment?	22–23	☐

Chapter Quiz

Multiple Choice

In the space provided, identify the letter of the choice that best completes each statement or answers each question.

_____ **1.** The Emergency Medical Responder National Standard Curriculum was developed by the
- **a.** National Research Council.
- **b.** Department of Transportation.
- **c.** National Association of EMTs.
- **d.** National Registry of EMTs.

_____ **2.** Which of the following organizations contributes to the development of professional standards and verifies the skills and knowledge of EMS professionals by preparing and conducting examinations?
- **a.** National Association of State EMS Directors
- **b.** National Council of State EMS Training Coordinators
- **c.** National Association of Emergency Physicians
- **d.** National Registry of Emergency Medical Technicians

_____ **3.** You arrive on the scene of a motor vehicle crash involving a minivan. You observe heavy damage to the vehicle. Your *primary* concern at the scene should be
- **a.** the well-being of the patient.
- **b.** personal safety.
- **c.** bystander safety.
- **d.** determining the total number of patients.

_____ **4.** Before approaching the patient in the crash described in question 3, you should
- **a.** await the arrival of personnel with more advanced medical training.
- **b.** contact a physician for instructions about how to proceed.
- **c.** put on personal protective equipment and size up the scene.
- **d.** determine the location of the nearest hospital.

_____ **5.** The EMS system is usually activated by using

a. pagers.
b. telephones.
c. citizen band radios.
d. emergency alarm boxes.

_____ **6.** Which of the following tasks correctly reflects skills that may be performed by an Emergency Medical Responder?

a. Giving an injection
b. Performing advanced airway procedures
c. Controlling bleeding
d. Giving oral medications

_____ **7.** The process by which a physician directs the emergency care provided by EMS personnel to an ill or injured patient is called

a. certification.
b. system regulation.
c. medical oversight.
d. resource management.

_____ **8.** When medical personnel with more advanced training arrive, you should

a. ask them to obtain information from bystanders.
b. instruct them to stand back and wait until you have completed your assessment of the patient.
c. immediately leave the scene.
d. identify yourself and give a courteous, clear, complete, and concise verbal report.

_____ **9.** The four nationally recognized levels of prehospital professionals, *from least to most advanced*, are

a. Paramedic, Advanced Emergency Medical Technician, Emergency Medical Technician, and Emergency Medical Responder.
b. Emergency Medical Technician, Emergency Medical Responder, Advanced Emergency Medical Technician, and Paramedic.
c. Emergency Medical Responder, Advanced Emergency Medical Technician, Emergency Medical Technician, and Paramedic.
d. Emergency Medical Responder, Emergency Medical Technician, Advanced Emergency Medical Technician, and Paramedic.

_____ **10.** Removing patients from entrapment is called

a. stabilization.
b. extrication.
c. triage.
d. immobilization.

_____ **11.** Two patients have been found trapped inside a vehicle. The patients are assessed and medical control is then contacted by telephone. This communication is an example of

a. prospective medical control.
b. off-line medical control.
c. on-line medical control.
d. retrospective medical control.

_____ **12.** One of the patients in question 11, a 30-year-old man, has experienced severe injuries. To which of the following specialty centers should he be transported for definitive care?

a. stroke center
b. trauma center
c. rehabilitation center
d. poison center

_____ **13.** States use the standards set by which of the following organizations to evaluate the effectiveness of their EMS system?

- **a.** National Highway Traffic Safety Administration
- **b.** American College of Surgeons
- **c.** American College of Emergency Physicians
- **d.** Federal Communications Commission

_____ **14.** Enhanced 9-1-1

- **a.** sends medical personnel to an emergency scene without the assistance of a dispatcher.
- **b.** locates and dispatches the closest appropriate public safety vehicle.
- **c.** prioritizes emergency calls.
- **d.** routes an emergency call to the 9-1-1 center closest to the caller and displays the caller's phone number and address.

True or False

Decide whether the statement is true or false. In the space provided, write T for true or F for false.

_____ **15.** A scene size-up is performed to sort patients by the seriousness of their injuries.

Matching

Match the key terms in the left column with the definitions in the right column by placing the letter of each correct answer in the space provided.

_____ **16.** Medical director

_____ **17.** On-line medical direction

_____ **18.** Scope of practice

_____ **19.** Personal space

_____ **20.** Healthcare system

_____ **21.** Quality management

_____ **22.** Emergency Medical Responder

_____ **23.** Treatment protocol

_____ **24.** Standing orders

_____ **25.** Prospective medical direction

_____ **26.** Medical practice act

_____ **27.** Emergency Medical Services (EMS) system

- **a.** Written instructions that authorize EMS personnel to perform certain medical interventions before establishing direct communication with a physician
- **b.** Activities performed by a physician before an emergency call
- **c.** State law that grants authority to provide medical care to patients and determines the scope of practice for healthcare professionals
- **d.** Individual with medical training who is the first to arrive at the scene of an emergency
- **e.** List of steps to be followed when providing emergency care to an ill or injured patient
- **f.** Coordinated network of resources that provides emergency care to and transportation of victims of sudden illness and injury
- **g.** Specific medical procedures and functions that can be performed by a licensed or certified healthcare professional
- **h.** Invisible area immediately around each of us that we interpret as our own
- **i.** Physician who provides medical oversight and is responsible for ensuring that actions taken on behalf of ill or injured people are medically appropriate
- **j.** System of internal and external reviews of all aspects of an EMS system; this system is used to identify the aspects that need improvement to ensure that the public receives the highest quality of prehospital care
- **k.** Network of people, facilities, and equipment designed to provide for the general medical needs of the population
- **l.** Direct communication with a physician (or his or her designee) by radio or telephone, or face-to-face communication at the scene, before performing a skill or administering care

Short Answer

Answer each question in the space provided.

28. List the 10 essential components of an Emergency Medical Services (EMS) system.

1. ______________________ 6. ______________________

2. ______________________ 7. ______________________

3. ______________________ 8. ______________________

4. ______________________ 9. ______________________

5. ______________________ 10. ______________________

29. List six responsibilities of an Emergency Medical Responder.

1. ______________________

2. ______________________

3. ______________________

4. ______________________

5. ______________________

6. ______________________

30. Explain how the role of a Paramedic differs from your role as an Emergency Medical Responder.

____

____

____

31. List the six phases of a typical EMS response.

1. ______________________

2. ______________________

3. ______________________

4. ______________________

5. ______________________

6. ______________________

32. Why is it important to maintain a professional appearance when on duty or when responding to calls?

____

____

____

CHAPTER

2 The Well-Being of the Emergency Medical Responder

By the end of this chapter, you should be able to

Knowledge Objectives ▶

1. List possible emotional reactions that the Emergency Medical Responder may experience when faced with trauma, illness, death, and dying.
2. Discuss the possible reactions that a family member may exhibit when confronted with death and dying.
3. State the steps in the Emergency Medical Responder's approach to the family confronted with death and dying.
4. State the possible reactions that the family of the Emergency Medical Responder may exhibit.
5. Recognize the signs and symptoms of critical incident stress.
6. State possible steps that the Emergency Medical Responder may take to help reduce/alleviate stress.
7. Explain the need to determine scene safety.
8. Discuss the importance of body substance isolation (BSI) precautions.
9. Describe the steps the Emergency Medical Responder should take for personal protection from airborne and bloodborne pathogens.
10. List the personal protective equipment necessary for each of the following situations: hazardous materials, rescue operations, violent scenes, crime scenes, electricity, water and ice, exposure to bloodborne pathogens, exposure to airborne pathogens.

Attitude Objectives ▶

11. Explain the importance of serving as an advocate for the use of appropriate protective equipment.
12. Explain the importance of understanding the response to death and dying and communicating effectively with the patient's family.
13. Demonstrate a caring attitude toward any patient with illness or injury who requests emergency medical services.
14. Show compassion when caring for the physical and mental needs of patients.
15. Participate willingly in the care of all patients.
16. Communicate with empathy to patients being cared for, as well as with family members, and friends of the patient.

Skill Objectives ▶

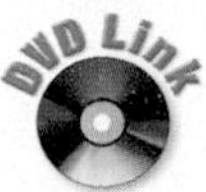

17. Given a scenario with potential infectious exposure, the Emergency Medical Responder will use appropriate personal protective equipment. At the completion of the scenario, the Emergency Medical Responder will properly remove and discard the protective garments.

18. Given the above scenario, the Emergency Medical Responder will complete disinfection/cleaning and all reporting documentation.

On The Scene

Your spouse looks frustrated as the familiar beep of your volunteer fire department pager gets progressively louder. "Not again," she groans as you grab your gear and move quickly to your truck. I have to go, you think, noting the address of a close friend and the message on your pager. You radio your response status and the dispatcher advises you that police have secured the scene. As you walk into the living room past his wife, you see him. Your best friend is slumped forward at the kitchen table, lying in a pool of blood. A large, gaping hole is visible on the back of his head. His hunting rifle lies on the floor beside him. You can feel your heart racing. Your hand trembles violently as you reach for the carotid pulse that you know will not be there. ■

THINK ABOUT IT

As you read this chapter, think about the following questions:

- In this situation, what emotional reactions would you expect from the patient's family?
- How might you respond emotionally to this call?
- How will you approach the patient's wife?
- What methods will you use to tell if you should begin resuscitation?
- What personal protective equipment will you need in this situation?

Introduction

Your Well-Being as an Emergency Medical Responder

You will encounter many stressful situations when providing emergency medical care to patients. Some of these situations include child abuse, trauma, and death. The patients you interact with may be seriously ill or injured. They may be angry, frightened, violent, or withdrawn.

In this chapter, you will learn how to help the patient, the patient's family, your own family, and other Emergency Medical Responders deal with stress. You will learn to recognize the signs of stress. This chapter will offer you information about how to manage stress through changes in your lifestyle and work environment. You will also learn about the professional resources that you can use to help you deal with stress. Finally, you will learn how to determine that a scene is safe, which will help you lessen your chance of being exposed to infectious disease.

Emotional Aspects of Emergency Medical Care

Stress is a chemical, physical, or emotional factor that causes bodily or mental tension. When dealing with an ill or injured person, the patient, the patient's family and friends, and bystanders will expect you to provide excellent medical care. They will also depend on you for emotional support. Each of us responds

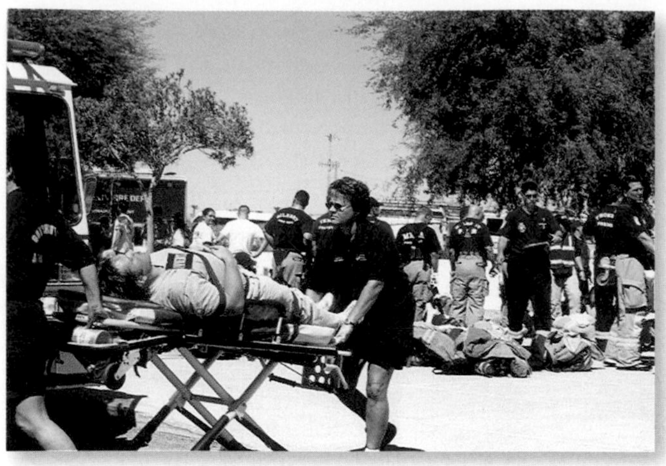

FIGURE 2-1 ▶ Emergency Medical Responders respond to many different types of stressful situations. © Courtesy of City of Tempe Fire Department, Tempe, Arizona

differently to an emergency. It is important that you learn how to anticipate and recognize the signs and symptoms of stress in yourself and others. You should also know how to manage stress when it occurs.

Stressful Situations

Objective 1 ▶

Although stress is part of everyone's life, the discussion of stress in this chapter focuses on stress in EMS.

As an Emergency Medical Responder, you will encounter stressful situations when providing emergency medical care (Figure 2-1). Examples of stressful situations are listed in Table 2-1.

The delivery of emergency medical care has an emotional impact on the patient, the patient's family, bystanders, and you. You will rarely witness the actual mishap or violent act that occurred. However, you will be repeatedly exposed to the human suffering and tragedies that result from them.

You may feel emotions such as joy, pride, and contentment when you are able to make a positive difference in a patient's life (Figure 2-2). You may experience emotions such as anger, anxiety, frustration, fear, grief, and helplessness when you are unable to relieve a patient's suffering or when a patient dies despite your best efforts to resuscitate him or her. You may feel sick at the sight of a severe injury. You may feel sad or anxious when dealing with a dying patient. These emotions are common and expected. You should not feel embarrassed or ashamed when these situations affect you. As you gain experience, you will learn to recognize

TABLE 2-1 Stressful Situations and Additional Factors That May Cause Stress

Examples of Stressful Situations	Additional Factors That May Cause Stress
• Mass casualty incidents • Infant and child trauma • Death, **terminal illness** • Amputations • Violence • Death of a child • Infant, child, elder, or spousal abuse • Death or injury of a coworker or other public safety personnel • Emergency response to illness or injury of a friend or family member	• Facing dangerous situations • Working in challenging locations and terrain • Dealing with weather conditions • Operating under severe time pressures • Handling media attention

FIGURE 2-2 ▶ The delivery of emergency medical care has an emotional impact on the patient, the patient's family, bystanders, and you.

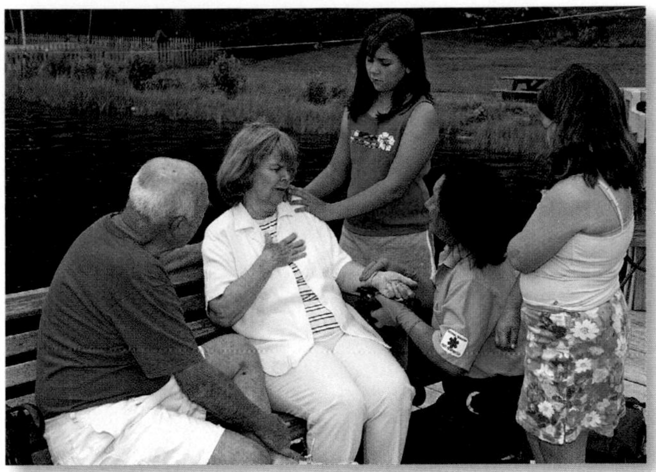

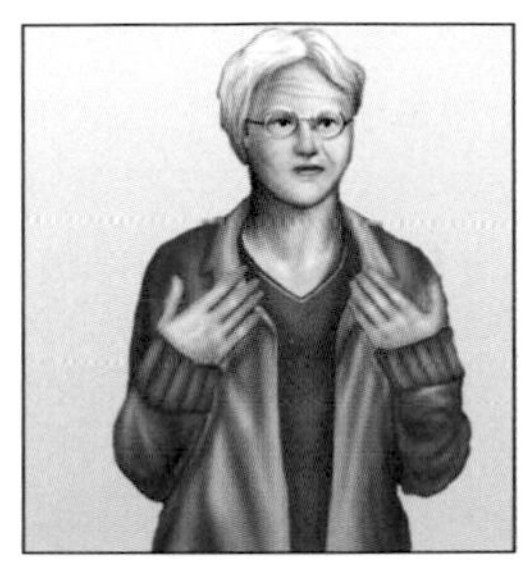

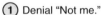

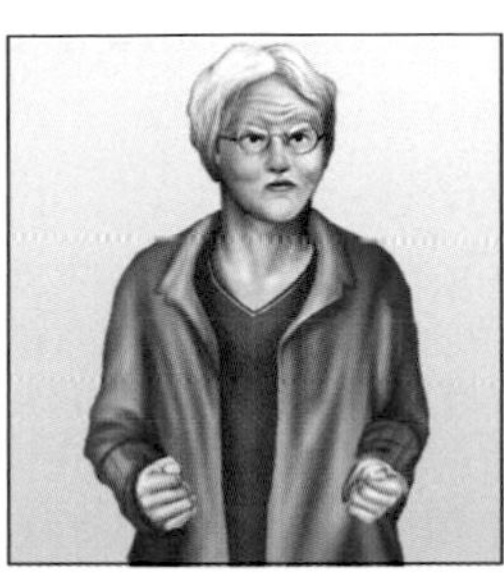

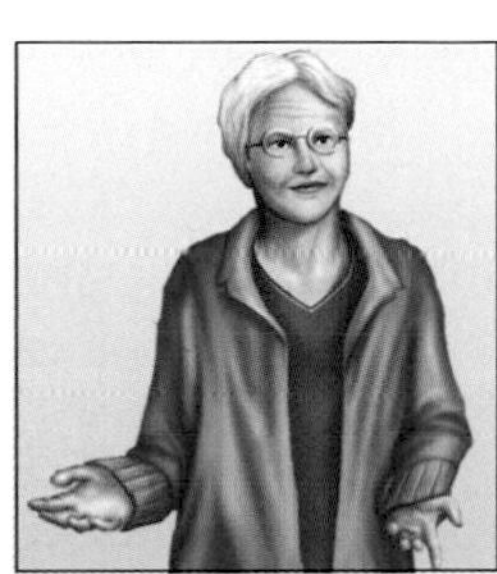

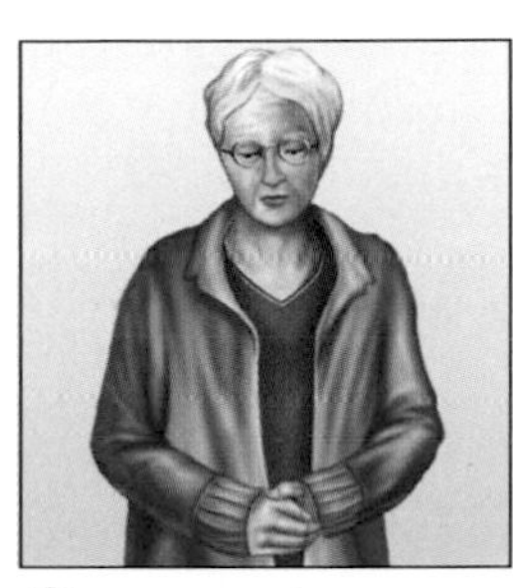

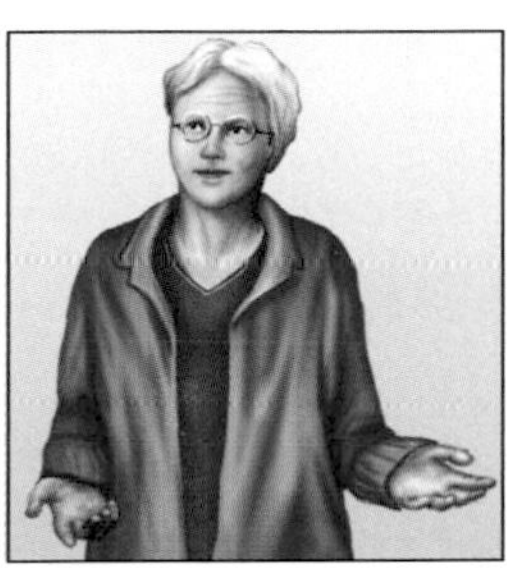

(1) Denial "Not me." (2) Anger "Why me?" (3) Bargaining "OK, but first let me..." (4) Depression "I don't care anymore." (5) Acceptance "OK, I am not afraid."

FIGURE 2-3 ▲ *Any* change of circumstance can initiate the process of grief.

and control these feelings while caring for patients. Despite the situation, you must act professionally. You must also be able to work quickly and confidently, think clearly, and make appropriate decisions about your patient's care.

The Stages of Grief

Critically ill or injured patients may experience grief. They may not recognize that they are reacting to the loss of something that was important to them.

Grief is a normal response that helps people cope with the loss of someone or something that had great meaning to them. While grief is most often associated with death, *any* change of circumstance can cause us to go through this process (Figure 2-3). How deeply a person feels grief and for how long depends on how important the person believes the loss is. Knowing about the stages of grief will help you provide appropriate care.

You Should Know

Changes in Circumstances That Contribute to Grief

- Loss of or change in status or environment (for example, retirement or relocation)
- Loss of personal possessions (such as a home destroyed by fire)
- Change in a relationship (such as separation, divorce, or death)
- Loss of a significant other (for example, a partner, child, parent, close friend, or pet)
- Loss of or change in health (including a body part or function, physical or mental capacity)
- Loss of or change in security (financial, social, occupational, or cultural)

Grief is a natural, inevitable part of our journey through life.

Grief is a very personal, individual process. However, Elizabeth Kübler-Ross, a world-famous authority on death and dying, developed a model of the stages of grief that a person typically experiences. Although five stages of grief are presented here, a person may move back and forth between stages (see the *You Should Know* box). An individual may also skip a stage, go through two or three stages at the same time, go through each stage more than once, or stay in one stage of the process for minutes, hours, days, or longer. Cultural differences will also affect how a person experiences grief.

You Should Know

The Five Stages of Grief

1. Denial
2. Anger
3. Bargaining
4. Depression
5. Acceptance

Denial

"Not me."

Denial is the first phase of the grieving process. Denial is a defense mechanism. It is used to create a buffer against the shock of dying or dealing with an illness or injury. During this stage of the grief process, the person is unable or refuses to believe the reality of what has happened. The patient may try to ignore or deny the seriousness of the illness or injury. The patient may dismiss the symptoms with words such as *only* or *a little.* During the denial stage, common reactions from the patient or family include "Not me" and "This can't be happening." During this stage, the patient or family member often does not grasp the information you provide about the illness or injury.

When dealing with a patient in this stage of the grief process, try to find a family member or close friend who can give you more information about the patient's illness or injury. The information you receive can help you make appropriate decisions regarding the patient's care.

Anger

Anger is the second stage of the grief process. The ill or injured person's anger comes from several sources. It can be related to her discomfort, a limitation of activity, or an inability to control the situation. Family, friends, and medical professionals are common targets for blame. The person often experiences guilt and blames herself for either taking or failing to take specific actions ("If only I had . . .").

"Why me?"

In the anger stage, common reactions from the person (or the family) include "Why is this happening to me?" The person's anger may be marked by the following:

- Abusive language
- Criticism of anyone who offers help
- Resentment (particularly of those who are healthy)
- Irritability
- Becoming demanding or impatient

Stop and Think!

When dealing with an angry person, remember that your safety is your priority. If the scene is not safe and you cannot make it safe, *do not enter.*

When dealing with an angry person, do not take anger or insults personally. Also, do not become defensive. Be tolerant, be empathetic, and use good listening and communication skills. Speak to the person in a calm, controlled tone. It is not necessary to agree with the person, but do not challenge how he is feeling. Briefly and honestly explain what he can expect from you, as well as what you expect from him.

Bargaining

"Okay, but first let me . . ."

Bargaining is the third stage of the grief process. During this stage, the person is willing to do anything to change what is happening to her. The person may bargain with herself, her family, God, or medical professionals. Bargaining reflects the person's need for time to accept the situation. Bargaining is marked by statements such as the following:

- "I promise I'll be a better person if . . ."
- "If I could live to . . ."
- "Okay, but first let me . . ."

Depression

"I don't care anymore."

Depression is the fourth stage of the grief process. Depression is a normal response to the loss of a significant other or the loss of a bodily function. Depression may also result from feeling a loss of control over one's destiny.

A depressed person

- Is sad and usually silent
- Appears withdrawn and indifferent
- May take a long time to perform routine activities
- May have difficulty concentrating and following instructions
- May reject your attempts to help
- May accept your help and then fail to react to your interventions
- Shows a lack of interest

You may feel confused, annoyed, defensive, frustrated, or even angry because of the patient's behavior. It is important to recognize these feelings. However, do not communicate them while caring for your patient. Be supportive and nonjudgmental. Provide whatever care is needed.

Acceptance

"Okay, I am not afraid."

The fifth and final stage of the grief process is acceptance. The person has come to terms with his loss or change in circumstances and is learning to live with it. In the case of a dying patient, he realizes his fate and understands that death is certain. Acceptance does not mean that the patient is happy about dying. Instead, the patient believes that he has done all that is possible in preparing to die. For example, the patient has said what needed to be said and has completed any unfinished business. Acceptance is marked by statements such as "I am ready for whatever comes" and "Okay, I am not afraid." Friends and family members may need more support than the patient during this stage.

Making a Difference

As an EMS professional, you must accept every call for assistance without prejudice. Provide the best emergency care you can for every patient—without questioning the validity of the complaint.

The Patient's Response to Illness and Injury

Objective 13 ▶

Objective 15 ▶

What a patient considers an emergency may not appear to be an emergency to a person with medical training. Some medical personnel become irritated or annoyed when they feel they have been summoned to assist a person who does appear particularly ill or who has a minor complaint. Keep in mind that pain is what the *patient* says it is and an emergency is what the *patient* perceives it to be. As an EMS professional, you must accept every call for assistance without prejudice. Provide the best emergency care you can for every patient—without questioning the validity of the complaint.

Making a Difference

An emergency is what the *patient* perceives it to be.

Because patients react differently to an illness or injury, you must be prepared for a variety of emotions and behaviors (Figure 2-4). Depending on the nature of the illness or the severity of the injury, your patient may experience a number of emotions. Your patient's response to these emotions may be seen as distrust, resentment, despair, anger, or regression. **Regression** is a return to an earlier or former developmental state. For example, an adult patient's behavior may appear childlike. This reaction is common and natural because an ill or injured patient, like a child, depends on others for his or her survival.

You Should Know

Common Patient Responses to Illness and Injury

Fear	Anxiety
Embarrassment	Anger
Frustration	Sorrow
Pain	Depression
Regression	Guilt, shame, or blame
Feeling of being powerless or helpless	

It is important to understand these emotions in order to be tolerant of them. For example, a busy executive experiences a heart attack. He may feel helpless because he finds himself dependent on medical professionals, whose

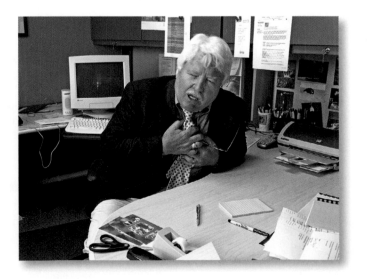

FIGURE 2-4 ▶ As an Emergency Medical Responder, you must be prepared for a variety of emotions and behaviors from your patients.

experience and skills he cannot easily evaluate. He may be angry because his life has been disrupted. He may experience fear and anxiety because his independence is threatened. He may also wonder what the next few minutes, hours, days, and months will bring. His concerns might include the following:

- "Why is this happening to me?"
- "Am I going to be disabled?"
- "How will I provide for my family if I can't work?"
- "Am I going to die?"

Objective 14 ▶

Dealing with Ill and Injured Patients

Introduce Yourself

Identify yourself and establish your role by saying, "My name is _____. I am an Emergency Medical Responder trained to provide emergency care. I am here to help you."

Treat the Patient with Respect

Recognize the patient's need for privacy, preserve her dignity, and treat her with respect. Most patients are uncomfortable about being examined. In our culture, clothing is ordinarily removed in front of another in situations of trust or intimacy. Be aware that your patient will be anxious about having her clothing removed and having an examination performed by a stranger. Some patients will view these actions as an invasion of their privacy. Help ease your patient's fears by explaining what you are about to do and why it must be done (Figure 2-5). When performing a physical examination, be sure to properly drape or shield an unclothed patient from the stares of others. Conduct the examination professionally and efficiently. Talk with the patient throughout the procedure. These actions will build trust and help reduce the patient's anxiety. If your patient is a child, ask for help from a parent or family member to lessen the child's anxiety.

Making a Difference

Do not assume that an unresponsive patient cannot hear what is being said. If your patient is unresponsive, speak in a normal tone of voice. Talk to him as if he were awake. Provide reassurance, offer words of comfort, and explain what you are doing. Many healthcare professionals have been embarrassed when a patient is successfully resuscitated and is able to relay accurately what was said by those caring for him.

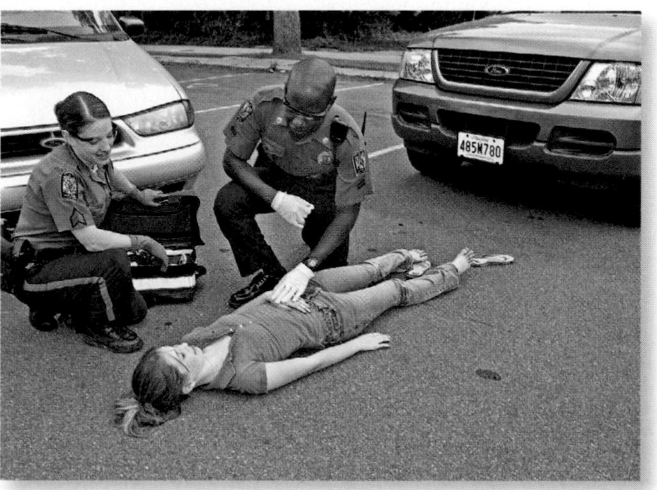

FIGURE 2-5 ▶ Explaining what you are about to do and why it must be done will help ease your patient's fears.

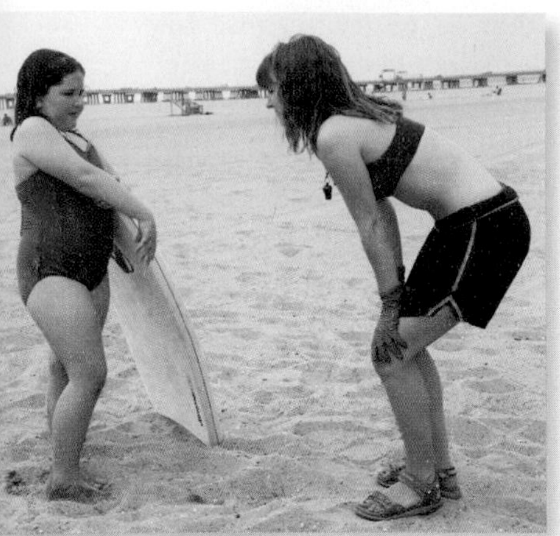

FIGURE 2-6 ▲ Effective listening requires concentration.

Recognize the Patient's Need for Control

Although many patients will feel a sense of relief when you arrive, the lights, sirens, and flurry of activity involved in providing emergency care can be frightening. Even though your patient may be ill or injured, she will usually feel the need to show her independence. When possible, allow the patient to make choices, such as the hospital to which she prefers to be transported.

Listen with Empathy

Remain calm, be sympathetic, and listen with empathy. To listen with **empathy** means to understand, be aware of, and be sensitive to the feelings, thoughts, and experience of another. Effective listening requires concentration (Figure 2-6). Do not interrupt your patient before he has finished telling you what his problem is. Do not anticipate what he is going to say and finish his sentences for him. Allow him time to explain what is wrong in his own words.

Do Not Give False Hope or Reassurance

Do not give false hope or reassurance. You should not say, "Everything is going to be okay," when it is obvious that it will not. Similarly, you should not say you understand when you have not had the same experience as your patient. Instead, reassure the patient by saying, "We will do everything we can to help."

Use a Reassuring Touch

If appropriate, use a reassuring touch. Touch is a sensitive means of communication. It can be used to express feelings that cannot be expressed well with words. It is important to assess your level of comfort and that of your patient regarding the use of touch. Some healthcare professionals are uncomfortable touching patients to display concern, caring, and reassurance. Most patients will accept a reassuring touch and will respond positively to it. Others are uncomfortable when touched in this way and may misunderstand your intentions. Be sensitive to the patient's acceptance of touch. Learn to recognize when the use of compassionate touch is appropriate.

Making a Difference

Cultural Considerations

Effective communication with persons of different cultures requires sensitivity and awareness. It is important to refrain from using offensive language and avoid speaking in ways that are disrespectful to your patient's cultural beliefs. For example, you should be aware of the amount of personal space, eye contact, and touching that is considered acceptable.

- When speaking with most patients, 18 inches between people is usually considered a comfortable distance. Hispanics, Asians, and people from the Middle East generally stand closer together when talking.
- Many Native Americans and patients of Mexican descent avoid direct eye contact to show respect. Sustained direct eye contact is considered rude or disrespectful. Mexican Americans have a high respect for authority and the elderly. They should be addressed formally (by title). The Vietnamese avoid eye contact when speaking with someone they consider an authority figure or someone who is older. European Americans use firm eye contact and look for the impact of what is being said.

- Hispanics typically find a touch on the arm, shoulder, or back comforting. Asian and Arab patients generally find touch acceptable only between members of the same gender, except within the family. Because Asians consider the area of the body below the waist private, it is almost never exposed. In addition, Asian Americans prefer to be addressed by position and role, such as "mother" or "teacher." An individual's name is considered private and is used only by family and close friends.
- Mexican American women may be reluctant to undress, even in the presence of a healthcare professional of the same gender.
- Pacific Islanders (native Hawaiians and Samoans) and Asian Americans are often reluctant to ask questions or express emotion to others. They may be overly agreeable in their communications. Arab Americans may be reluctant to reveal information about themselves to strangers. Many Hispanic Americans are vocal about illness and pain.

The Responses of Family, Friends, and Bystanders to Injury or Illness

Objective 16 ▶

Family members, friends, or bystanders at the scene of an ill or injured patient may have many of the same responses as the patient. Depending on the nature of the illness or the severity of the patient's injury, family members, friends, and bystanders may be anxious, angry, sad, demanding, or impatient. A bystander's anger often results from feelings of guilt. At the scene, the family, friends, or bystanders may pressure you to move the patient to the hospital before you have completed your assessment and provided initial emergency care.

Dealing with family members, friends, and bystanders requires many of the same approaches you use in dealing with patients:

- Identify yourself and take control of the situation. Use a gentle but firm tone of voice and explain what you are doing to help the patient.
- Allow them to have and express their emotions, but do not let them distract you from treating the patient's illness or injury. Accept their concerns and recognize that their behavior stems from grief.
- Comfort them by being sympathetic, listening empathetically, and reassuring them that everything that can be done to help will be done.
- Do not give false hope or reassurance.
- Keep emotionally distraught individuals away from the patient. If possible, assign another Emergency Medical Responder to care for them and their grief. You can reduce interference by well-meaning family, friends, and bystanders by assigning them a simple task to keep them occupied. Feeling useful frequently helps lessen a person's anxiety.

Death and Dying

Dealing with death and with dying patients is part of the work of an EMS professional. A person's attitude about death is influenced by his or her culture, experiences, religion, and age. Your reaction to a situation involving the death of a patient will also depend on the circumstances surrounding the event. It is important to look at your own fears, attitudes, and beliefs about death and dying. Doing so can help you understand the needs of the dying patient and his or her family.

Dying is a process. Death is an event.

You will encounter situations in which you must determine if a patient is dead or requires emergency medical care. Dying is a process that may take minutes, hours, days, weeks, or months. As a patient dies, changes occur in the patient's level of responsiveness, breathing, and circulation.

Death occurs when the patient's organs stop functioning. When the patient's heart stops (cardiac arrest), brain death will occur within four to six minutes unless circulation is rapidly restored. For this reason, cardiopulmonary resuscitation (CPR) is most effective when started immediately after a cardiac arrest occurs. When you arrive at the scene of a cardiac arrest, CPR should be started immediately if the person is unresponsive, breathless, and without a pulse (heartbeat). CPR should not be started if a valid Do Not Resuscitate (DNR) order is present or in cases of obvious death.

You Should Know

In some Latin American and Asian-Pacific cultures, a patient may not be told he or she has a terminal illness. It is believed to upset the patient's inner harmony and that it may hasten the progression of disease or death.

Advance Directives and Do Not Resuscitate Orders

Some patients, such as those who have been diagnosed with a terminal illness, may not want aggressive efforts aimed at reviving them when they are dying. These patients may have an advance directive or a Do Not Resuscitate (DNR) order. An **advance directive** is a legal document that details a person's health-care wishes when she becomes unable to make decisions for herself. A **Do Not Resuscitate order** is an order written by a physician. It instructs medical professionals not to provide medical care to a patient who has experienced a cardiac arrest.

Call for additional EMS personnel as soon as possible.

If you arrive on the scene of a cardiac arrest, begin CPR if

- A DNR order is not present
- There are no signs of obvious death
- A DNR order is present but the DNR documentation is unclear
- A DNR order is present but you are not sure the order is valid

If you arrive on the scene of a cardiac arrest and a DNR order is present,

- Make sure the form clearly identifies the person to whom the DNR applies.
- Make sure the patient is the person referred to in the DNR document.
- Make sure the document is of the correct type approved by your state and local authorities.

If you determine the DNR order is valid, follow the instructions outlined in the document. This may include stopping resuscitation if it has already been started. Call Advanced Life Support personnel to the scene to confirm that the patient is dead.

Signs of Obvious Death

Be sure to let the police know about your observations.

In some situations, it will be clear that a person has been dead for some time. One obvious sign of death is decapitation (beheading). Other signs include putrefaction, dependent lividity, and rigor mortis.

If a person shows signs of obvious death, do not disturb the body or scene. The police or medical examiner will need to authorize removal of the body. It will be important for you to observe and document the following:

- The position of the patient/victim
- The patient's vital signs and injuries
- The conditions at the scene
- Statements of persons at the scene
- Statements of the patient/victim before death

Putrefaction

Putrefaction is the decomposition of organic matter, such as body tissues.

Dependent Lividity

Dependent lividity is the settling of blood in dependent areas. Dependent areas are those areas on which the body has been resting. Dependent lividity is considered an obvious sign of death only when there are widespread areas of discolored skin (reddish-purple skin) in dependent areas of an unresponsive, breathless, and pulseless person. In some EMS systems, both lividity and rigor mortis must be present to be considered signs of obvious death. Lividity is harder to detect on a person with dark skin pigmentation. In addition, lividity may be absent if there was major blood loss before death.

Rigor Mortis

The onset of rigor mortis is usually delayed in a cold environment and sped up in a hot one.

Rigor mortis is the stiffening of body muscles that occurs after death. This stiffening occurs because of chemical changes in muscle tissue. After death, the muscles of the body normally are relaxed for about 3 hours. They stiffen between 3 hours and 36 hours, then become relaxed again. The condition of the body, the environmental temperature, and the amount of work the muscles performed just before death affect how quickly rigor mortis occurs. A high level of muscle activity increases acid production. The presence of acid speeds up the onset of rigor mortis.

Rigor mortis begins in the muscles of the face. It then spreads downward to other parts of the body. Rigor may be more difficult to detect with obese individuals. The state of rigor usually lasts about 24–36 hours or until muscle decay occurs.

You Should Know

Signs of Obvious Death

- Decapitation or other obvious mortal injury
- Putrefaction (decomposition)
- Extreme dependent lividity
- Rigor mortis

Helping the Dying Patient

Most people fear dying alone.

As an Emergency Medical Responder, you may arrive to find a patient has died or is dying. A dying patient may ask to talk with his family. If the family is not at the scene, it is appropriate to offer to pass on important messages. Write down the information. Be sure to follow through with the patient's request. A dying patient may want to express his feelings and concerns to you (Figure 2-7). Just being there and listening is often all that the patient wants from you. Remember to preserve the patient's dignity and treat him with respect.

FIGURE 2-7 ▶ The dying patient may want to express his or her feelings and concerns to you.

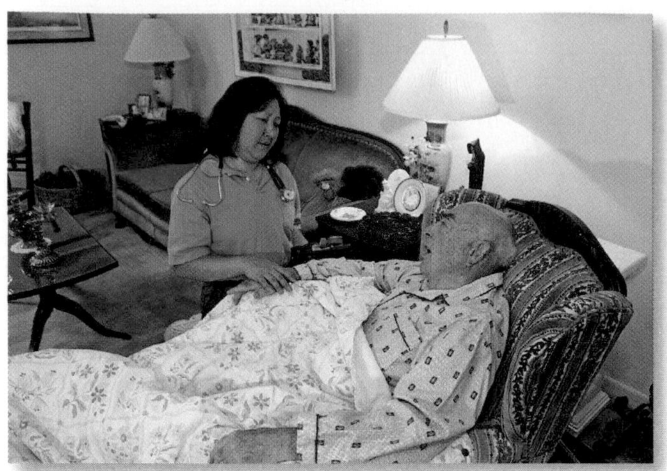

Making a Difference

Dealing with a Dying Patient and Family Members

- Patient needs include dignity, respect, sharing, communication, privacy, and control.
- Allow family members to express their feelings.
- Listen empathetically.
- Do not falsely reassure.
- Use a gentle tone of voice.
- Let the patient know that everything that can be done to help will be done.
- Use a reassuring touch, if appropriate.
- Comfort the family.

Helping the Dying Patient's Family

Objective 12 ▶

When conveying news about a patient's death, speak slowly and in a quiet, calm voice. You might begin by saying, "This is hard to tell you, but . . ." Tactfully explain that the patient is dead. Use the word *death, dying,* or *dead* instead of phrases such as "passed on," "no longer with us," or "has gone to a better place." An empathetic response such as "You have my sincere sympathy" may be used to express your feelings.

Objective 2 ▶

The patient's family will go through the grief process. If the patient had a prolonged illness, family members may have had an opportunity to share important messages. They may also have been able to resolve conflict before the patient died. When a person dies suddenly, family members and friends may experience intense grief and guilt. This may be particularly true if messages were left unsaid or harsh words were spoken before death.

Objective 3 ▶

Family members' reactions to a loved one's death may include anger, rage, withdrawal, disbelief, extreme agitation, guilt, or sorrow. In some cases, there may be no visible response or the response may seem inappropriate. Be sensitive to the needs of those who have suffered a loss by acknowledging their grief. They have a right to these feelings.

After a death, family members and close friends will often try to make sense of what has happened to their loved one. Many will want to learn the details surrounding the death. They will want to talk to those who were present at the time of death. They will also want to view the body. At a possible crime scene, do not disturb the body or the scene.

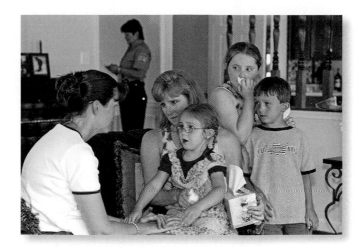

FIGURE 2-8 ▶ Many EMS agencies have arrangements with counselors who can provide grief support for family on the scene.

Some EMS agencies have arrangements with counselors who can be called to the scene to provide grief support for the family (Figure 2-8). Remain with the family until law enforcement personnel or the medical examiner assumes responsibility for the body. In addition, if available in your area, stay with the family until grief support personnel are on the scene to assist them. If counselors or grief support personnel are not available, give the family information packets so that they can seek help from mental health professionals.

Taking care of ill or injured people is emotionally demanding. Make sure to assess your own physical and emotional response to the situation when the call is over. It may be helpful for you to talk with other EMS professionals afterwards. You may find it helpful to discuss your feelings if the call involved death or dying.

Stress and Stress Management

As an EMS professional, you will experience personal stress and will encounter patients and bystanders in severe stress. A **stressor** is any event or condition that has the potential to cause bodily or mental tension. Common stressors associated with working in EMS are shown in Table 2-2.

TABLE 2-2 Common Stressors Associated with Working in EMS

Environmental Stressors	Psychosocial Stressors	Personal Stressors
• Lights, siren, alarm noise • Long hours and shifts • Absence of challenge between calls • Weather conditions and temperature extremes • Confined work spaces • Emergency driving and rapid scene response • Demanding physical labor • Multiple role responsibilities • Dangerous situations	• Family relationships • Conflicts with supervisors or coworkers • Agitated, combative, or abusive patients • Dealing with critically ill and injured or dying patients • Patients under the influence of drugs or alcohol • Incompatibility with partner	• Life-and-death decision making • Personal expectations • Feelings of guilt and anxiety • Dealing with death and dying

FIGURE 2-9 ▶ The fight-or-flight response prepares the body to protect itself.

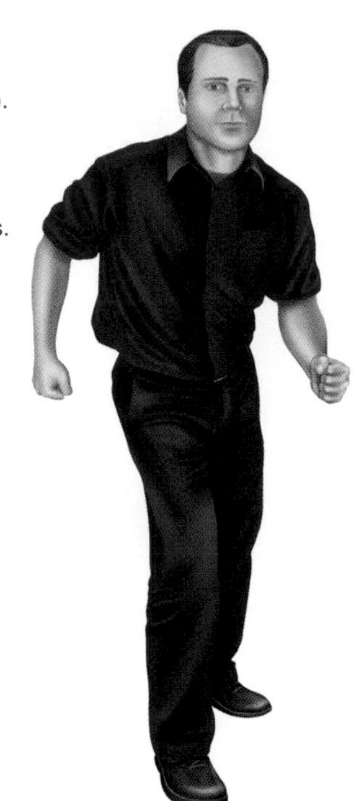
Pupils widen (dilate).
Heart rate increases.
Skeletal muscle strength increases.
Mental alertness increases.
Breathing passages dilate.
The force with which the heart contracts increases.

When you encounter a stressor, your brain tells the rest of your body how to adjust to it. The part of your body that is first aware of the stressor, such as your eyes or nose, sends a message along your nerves to your brain. Your brain receives the message and tells specific body organs to release chemicals. These chemicals activate the body's fight-or-flight response (Figure 2-9).

When the stressor is removed, the body should return to its normal state. If the stress does not stop, the brain keeps the body in a state of high alert and the body becomes exhausted. Over time, this state takes its toll on the body. Stress-induced illnesses result.

You Should Know

Examples of Stress-Induced Illnesses

- Headache
- Upset stomach
- Rash
- Insomnia
- Ulcers
- High blood pressure
- Heart disease
- Stroke

Recognizing the Warning Signs of Stress

Become aware of your stressors and your responses to them.

Stress can affect your emotional well-being and the way in which you interact with your patients and family. The signs of stress may be physical, behavioral, mental, or emotional (Table 2-3). Recognizing the warning signs and sources of stress will help you develop a plan about what to do to avoid or decrease its occurrence.

You Should Know

Common Signs and Symptoms of Stress

- Irritability toward coworkers, family, or friends
- Inability to concentrate
- Difficulty sleeping or nightmares
- Anxiety
- Indecisiveness
- Guilt
- Loss of appetite
- Loss of interest in sexual activities
- Isolation
- Loss of interest in work

Managing Stress

Lifestyle Changes

In EMS, cumulative stress is often referred to as *burnout.*

Cumulative stress is common in EMS. It results from repeated exposure to smaller stressors that build up over time. Cumulative stress may result from lack of sleep for several days in a row, job-related problems, or family and relationship issues.

TABLE 2-3 Signs of Stress

Physical Signs	Behavioral Signs	Mental Signs	Emotional Signs
• Increased heart rate • Pounding/racing heart • Elevated blood pressure • Sweaty palms • Tightness of the chest, neck, jaw, and back muscles • Headache • Diarrhea, constipation • Trembling, twitching • Stuttering, other speech difficulties • Nausea, vomiting • Sleep disturbances • Fatigue • Dryness of the mouth or throat • Susceptibility to minor illness	• Crying spells • Hyperactivity or underactivity • Changes in eating habits • Increased substance use or abuse, including smoking, alcohol consumption, use of medications and illegal substances • Excessive humor or silence • Violence, aggressive behavior (such as driving aggressively) • Withdrawal • Hostility • Proneness to accidents • Impatience	• Inability to make decisions • Forgetfulness • Reduced creativity • Lack of concentration • Diminished productivity • Lack of attention to detail • Attention deficit • Disorganized thoughts • Lack of control or a need for too much control	• Irritability • Angry outbursts • Hostility • Depression • Jealousy • Restlessness • Withdrawal • Anxiousness • Diminished initiative • Feelings of unreality or overalertness • Reduction of personal involvement with others • Tendency to cry • Tendency to be critical of others • Nightmares • Impatience • Reduced self-esteem

You Should Know

Signs of Cumulative Stress

- Physical and emotional exhaustion
- Negative attitude toward others
- Disrespectful attitude toward patients
- Increased absences
- Emotional outbursts
- Decreased work performance

Objective 6 ▶

There are several things you can do to manage stress in a healthy way. These steps include developing good dietary habits, exercising, and practicing relaxation techniques.

Developing Good Dietary Habits

An excess of certain substances, such as caffeine, sugar, fatty foods, and alcohol, can exaggerate your body's response to stress. These substances can also influence your behavior. Good dietary habits include reducing or avoiding the intake of sugar, caffeine, alcohol, and foods that are high in fat.

Exercising

Regular exercise is important to keeping physically fit. It helps you meet the physical requirements of your responsibilities. Sustained aerobic activity causes the body to release endorphins. These natural chemicals can relieve stress and bring about a sense of well-being. Exercise also allows you to "burn off" pent-up emotions.

Practicing Relaxation Techniques

Meditation, deep-breathing exercises, yoga, reading, music, and visual imagery can be used to help reduce stress.

Creating Balance

To manage the stress associated with caring for ill or injured people, you must learn to balance work, family and friends, fitness, and recreation (Figure 2-10). Consider the following suggestions to help you maintain balance in your life:

- Develop a recreational outlet or hobby.
- Get away when you can to recharge your emotional reserves.

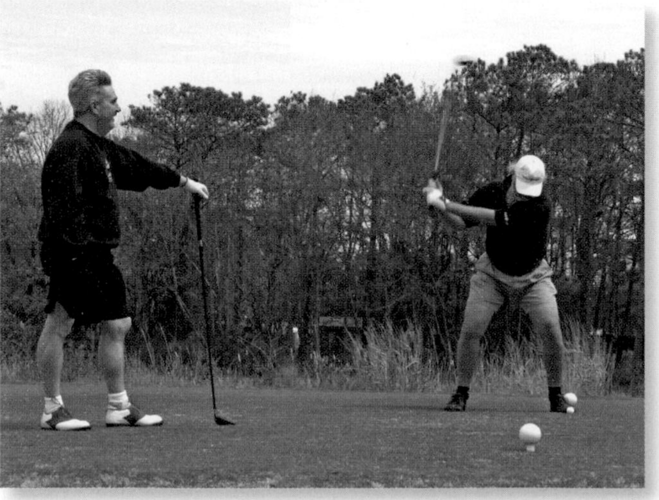

FIGURE 2-10 ▶ Learning to create balance in your life will allow you to manage the stress associated with EMS work.

- Learn to say no when you need time for yourself.
- Make sure to get adequate sleep. Be as consistent with your sleep schedule as possible.
- Develop mutually supportive friendships and relationships.

Family and Friends

Objective 4 ▶

Your role as an EMS professional can take a toll on those close to you. Family and friends may not understand the stressors that are a part of EMS work. After a particularly difficult call, you may arrive home too emotionally drained to take part in family activities. Family and friends may not understand the closeness and trust that develop among EMS professionals. Those who are close to you may become frustrated when you do the following:

- Eat, breathe, and sleep EMS
- Work long hours
- Sleep away from home
- Are on call when you are at home
- Agree to work yet another shift
- Miss important family events because of your shift schedule

The spouses of many EMS professionals frequently feel that they are of secondary importance, that the job comes first.

EMS professionals may find it hard to discuss their feelings about their work with others, especially loved ones. Some Emergency Medical Responders want to protect their loved ones from the horrors of the job. They may also need to protect confidential information. In addition, EMS professionals may be unwilling to expose themselves as being vulnerable. Family and friends become frustrated because they sense something is wrong and want to share your pain, but you refuse to do so. They may feel ignored and fear separation when you withdraw from them. These feelings often worsen if you prefer to talk with your coworkers about your feelings or spend your free time with your coworkers instead of with your family.

You Should Know

Responses to Stress by the Family and Friends of EMS Workers

- Lack of understanding of prehospital care
- Fear of separation or of being ignored
- Frustration caused by the on-call nature of the job and the inability to plan activities
- Frustration caused by wanting to share

Although you should do your best to leave your work at work, doing so is not always realistic. Your family and friends are a base of support for you. They can help you cope with the stressors associated with EMS work (Figure 2-11). *Do not assume they will not understand.* They can appreciate your feelings about a good or difficult call without knowing the details. Consider the following examples:

- "I had a tough call today. A two-year-old drowned in a backyard pool."
- "You won't believe what happened today! I performed abdominal thrusts on a person who was choking. The patient coughed up a piece of chicken and is going to be fine."

Make it a point to talk about your day with your loved ones. Actively listen to what they have to say when they tell you about theirs. Plan time for your family and friends. Say no when another request would require you to alter those plans.

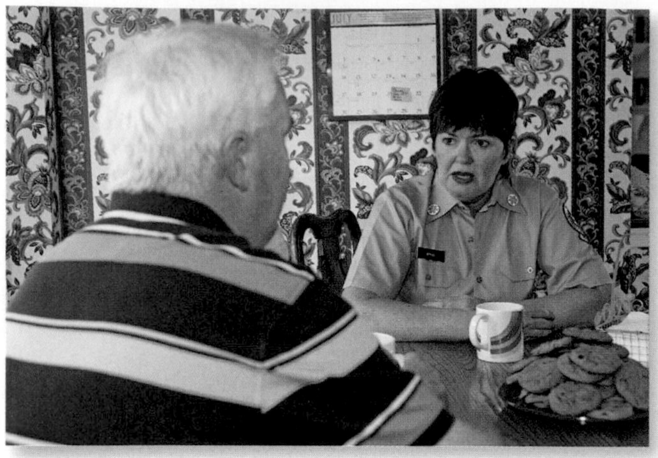

FIGURE 2-11 ▶ Your family and friends are a base of support and can help you cope with the stressors associated with caring for ill or injured people.

Work Environment Changes

To help you balance work and family, request work shifts that allow you more time for relaxation with family and friends. If you recognize the warning signs of stress, consider asking for a temporary rotation to a less stressful assignment.

Professional Help

When you need help coping with stress, seek assistance from a mental health professional, social worker, or member of the clergy. Many organizations have employee assistance programs. These programs offer confidential counseling to prehospital professionals. These resources can help you understand and effectively deal with stress.

Critical Incident Stress Management (CISM)

A **critical incident** is a situation that causes a healthcare provider to experience unusually strong emotions. This type of incident may interfere with the provider's mental ability to cope and function either immediately or later. Critical incident stress is a normal stress response to abnormal circumstances. Critical incident stress can affect all levels of EMS personnel. It can also affect law enforcement officers, dispatchers, nurses, physicians, and other healthcare workers.

Objective 5 ▶

One of the signs and symptoms of critical incident stress is exhaustion. This exhaustion often results from disturbing elements, such as the sounds, smells, or sights that occur at the incident. When awake, a person may have flashbacks of the disturbing elements. Nightmares may occur during sleep. Other signs and symptoms include anxiety, depression, irritability, an inability to concentrate, indecisiveness, and either hyperactivity or underactivity.

Learn how to access your local CISM response team.

Critical Incident Stress Management (CISM) is a program developed to assist emergency workers in coping with stressful situations. Its goal is to speed up the normal recovery process after a critical incident has been experienced. CISM uses the expertise of specially trained teams of peer counselors and mental health professionals. A comprehensive CISM program includes the following:

- Pre-incident stress education
- On-scene peer support
- One-on-one support
- Disaster support services

- Defusings
- Critical Incident Stress Debriefing (CISD)
- Follow-up services
- Spouse and family support
- Community outreach programs
- Wellness programs

CISM should be accessed when any of the following occur:

- Line-of-duty death or serious injury
- Mass casualty incident
- Suicide of a coworker
- Serious injury or the death of a child
- Events with excessive media interest or criticism
- Victims are known to you
- Any event that has an unusual impact on personnel
- Any disaster

Techniques used by the CISM team include debriefings and defusings.

Critical Incident Stress Debriefing (CISD)

CISM can successfully reduce stress, because feelings are expressed quickly after the event and the debriefing or defusing environment is nonthreatening.

A **Critical Incident Stress Debriefing (CISD)** is a formal group meeting led by a mental health professional and peer counselors. The three goals of CISD are

1. To reduce the impact of a critical incident
2. To speed up the normal recovery process after experiencing a critical incident
3. To prevent the development of post-traumatic stress disorder.

The benefits of CISD include

- Allowing emergency workers to share thoughts, feelings, and emotions
- Providing emotional reassurance
- Educating emergency workers about stress reduction and coping techniques

A CISD should be held within 24–72 hours of a critical incident. Usually, all emergency workers involved in the incident participate in a CISD. Sessions are nonthreatening and confidential.

Defusing

The defusing process concentrates on the most seriously affected workers.

A **defusing** is a shorter, less formal version of a debriefing. It is held for rescuers immediately or within a few hours after a critical incident. The goal of a defusing is to stabilize emergency workers so that they can return to service. If workers are at the end of their shift, the defusing helps them return home without unusual stress. The benefits of defusing include

- Allowing emergency workers to share thoughts, feelings, and emotions
- Providing emotional reassurance
- Educating emergency workers about stress reduction and immediate management techniques

Defusings are usually led by peer counselors, but they may be led by a mental health professional. A defusing may eliminate the need for a formal debriefing. It may also enhance the effectiveness of a debriefing, if one becomes necessary.

You Should Know

Critical Incident Stress Management

Critical Incident Stress Management was introduced to EMS in 1983. Since then, it has become widely used in EMS, fire departments, police departments, and other agencies. The effectiveness of CISM has been questioned in recent journal articles, however. The results of some studies raise doubts about the effectiveness of CISM. Check with your instructor about local practices following exposure to a critical incident.

Scene Safety

Objective 7 ▶

An Emergency Medical Responder is responsible for ensuring his or her own safety as well as the safety of the crew, patient, and bystanders. Part of this responsibility includes being aware of the risks associated with emergency medical care.

Disease Transmission

Signs of illness or disease may or may not be obvious.

As an Emergency Medical Responder, you will provide emergency care to persons who are ill or injured. When providing care, one of the most serious risks to which you will be exposed is infection. An **infection** results when the body is invaded by **pathogens** (germs capable of producing disease), such as bacteria and viruses. A **communicable** (contagious) **disease** is an infection that can be spread from one person to another. The germs multiply and cause tissue damage, which may result in illness and disease.

You Should Know

Factors That Increase Susceptibility to Infection

- Age (the very young and the elderly)
- Poor nutrition
- Excessive stress or fatigue
- Chronic illness
- Poor hygiene
- Alcoholism
- Body damage due to trauma
- Crowded or unsanitary living conditions
- Use of drugs that decrease the body's ability to fight infection

Methods of Disease Transmission

Communicable diseases can be spread in various ways. Contact with drainage from an open sore is an example of *direct* contact. Germs can also be spread through *indirect* contact with contaminated materials or objects, such as needles, toys, drinking glasses, eating utensils, and bandages. Using gloves can help prevent the spread of disease from direct and indirect contact. Germs can also be transmitted in droplets suspended in the air through coughing, talking, and sneezing. Using a mask can help prevent the spread of infection from droplets. Using a mask that shields the eyes offers even better protection.

Classification of Communicable Diseases

Communicable diseases may be classified as airborne, bloodborne, foodborne, or sexually transmitted (Figure 2-12):

FIGURE 2-12 ► Communicable diseases may be classified as airborne, bloodborne, foodborne, or sexually transmitted.

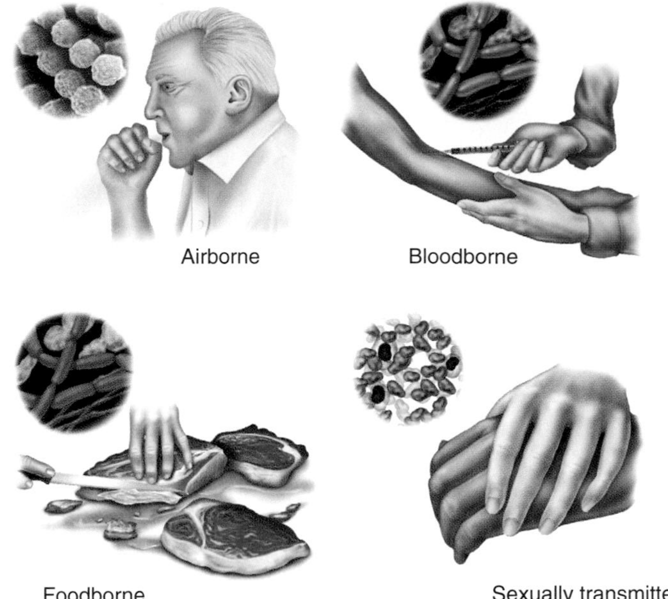

- **Airborne diseases** are spread by droplets produced by coughing or sneezing. Examples include tuberculosis, measles, meningitis, rubella, smallpox, and chicken pox (varicella).
- **Bloodborne diseases** are spread by contact with the blood or body fluids of an infected person. Examples include hepatitis B virus (HBV), hepatitis C, human immunodeficiency virus (HIV), and syphilis.
- **Foodborne diseases** are spread by the improper handling of food or by poor personal hygiene. Examples include salmonella (food poisoning) and hepatitis A.
- **Sexually transmitted diseases** are spread by either blood or sexual contact. Examples include chlamydia, gonorrhea, and HIV.

You Should Know

The hepatitis B virus can survive up to one week outside the human body. HIV can survive only a short time (hours) outside the body.

Learn More About It

To find out more information about communicable diseases, visit the web site for the Centers for Disease Control and prevention (CDC): http://www.cdc.gov/ncidod/diseases/hepatitis.

Infection Control

Objective 8 ►

An **exposure** is direct or indirect contact with infected blood, body fluids, tissues, or airborne droplets. An accidental exposure to infectious material can occur when your skin is pricked or cut, allowing the entry of germs. Germs can also enter your body through nicks or scrapes on your skin or through mucous membranes (such as your eyes, nose, and mouth). An exposure to a communicable disease does not automatically result in infection.

BSI precautions protect you and the patient.

Body substance isolation precautions have been developed by the **Centers for Disease Control and Prevention (CDC)** to reduce the risk of exposure to infection. These standards have been adopted by the **Occupational Safety and**

Health Administration (OSHA), which is the branch of the federal government responsible for safety in the workplace. The term **body substance isolation (BSI) precautions** refers to self-protection against all body fluids and substances. These fluids and substances include blood, urine, semen, feces, vaginal secretions, tears, and saliva. Precautions include handwashing and the use of personal protective equipment. They also include the proper cleaning, disinfecting, and disposing of soiled materials and equipment.

Stop and Think!

When caring for patients, assume that all human blood and body fluids are infectious. For your safety, use appropriate BSI precautions during *every* patient contact.

Remember This!

BSI Precautions

- Handwashing
- Use of personal protective equipment
- Cleaning, disinfecting, and disposing of soiled materials and equipment

Handwashing

Handwashing is the single most important method you can use to prevent the spread of communicable disease (Figure 2-13). Frequent handwashing removes germs picked up from other people or from contaminated surfaces. Wash your hands before and after contact with a patient (even if gloves were worn), after removing your gloves, and between patients.

It is the soap combined with the scrubbing action that helps dislodge and remove germs.

Proper handwashing begins with removing all jewelry from your hands and arms. Using soap and warm water, briskly rub your hands together to work up a lather. Continue washing for 10–15 seconds, washing the palm and back surface of each hand, your wrists, and exposed forearms. Scrub under and around your fingernails with a brush. With your fingers pointing downward, rinse your wrists, hands, and fingers with running water. Use a paper towel to dry them. Also use a paper towel to turn off the faucet. Avoid touching any part of the sink.

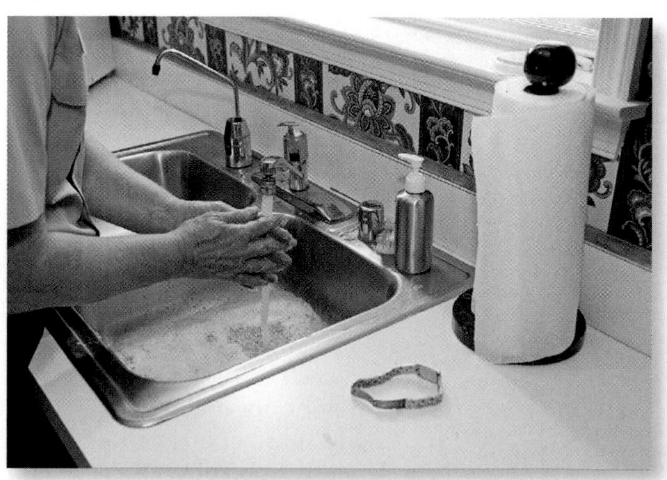

FIGURE 2-13 ▶ Hand-washing is the single most important method you can use to prevent the spread of disease.

Stop and Think!

Handwashing

- Wearing gloves does *not* eliminate the need for handwashing after each patient contact.
- Wash your hands immediately after exposure to blood and/or body fluids and after removing disposable gloves.
- Spend more time washing your hands after providing care to a patient at high risk for infection. Wash your hands for 30 seconds if you wore gloves and had contact with body fluids or other contaminants. If you were not wearing gloves and had contact with blood or body fluids, wash your hands for at least 2 minutes.

A waterless hand-cleansing solution can be used initially on the scene if you do not have access to soap and running water. Follow with a complete handwashing using soap and water as soon as possible after completing patient care.

Personal Protective Equipment (PPE)

Objective 9 ▶

Objective 11 ▶

Personal protective equipment (PPE) and BSI precautions are a part of scene safety. PPE includes eye protection, protective gloves, gowns, and masks. These items provide a barrier between you and infectious material. The infectious condition of a patient is usually unknown. Therefore, you *must* wear PPE when an exposure to blood or other potentially infectious material is likely, especially since this type of exposure can occur when it is not expected. Make it a habit to put on appropriate PPE before providing any patient care.

Eye Protection Eye protection should be worn when body fluids may be splashed into your face or eyes. This splashing can occur during childbirth, when suctioning an airway, or with a coughing or spitting patient. Available eyewear includes goggles and face shields (Figure 2-14). If you wear prescription eyeglasses, removable side shields should be applied to them or form-fitting goggles placed over them. To prevent the transfer of germs, remove protective eyewear without touching your face.

Gloves You should put on disposable gloves before physical contact with *every* patient. When providing patient care, use gloves made of vinyl, latex, or another

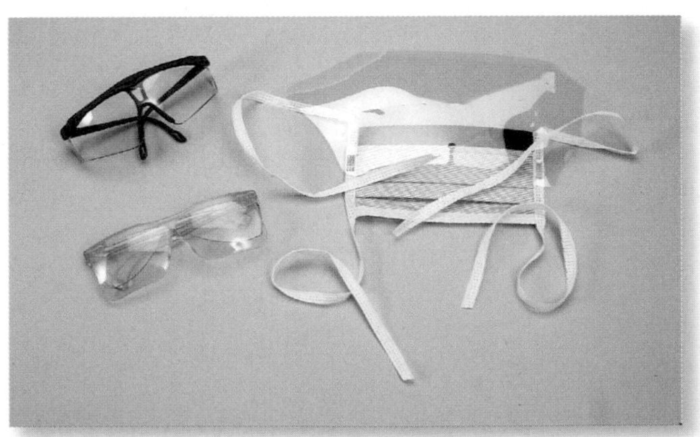

FIGURE 2-14 ▶ Goggles and face shields are types of protective eyewear.

Skill Drill 2-1

Removing Gloves

STEP 1 ▶ Using your index finger and thumb on one hand, pull the bottom (cuff) of the glove away from your other hand.

Peel the glove off your hand, being careful not to touch the skin of your wrist or hand with the outside surface of the glove. As you begin to remove the glove, it will turn inside out. This action helps prevent exposure to blood or other possibly infectious fluids on the gloves.

STEP 2 ▶ Place your fingers inside the bottom (cuff) of the other glove. Pull the glove off by turning it inside out.

STEP 3 ▶ Dispose of the gloves in an appropriate container. Wash your hands thoroughly.

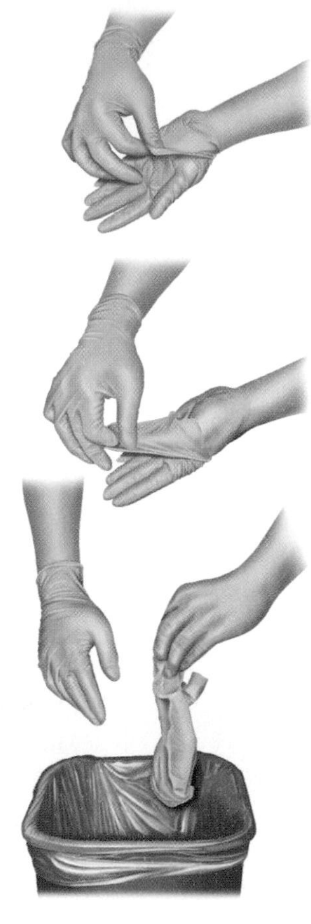

type of synthetic material. If you have a latex allergy, wear gloves made of a nonlatex material, such as nitrile. If you have a cut on your hand or wrist, apply a bandage to the cut before putting on gloves. Check the condition of the gloves before putting them on. Do not use them if they have small holes or tears in them.

Never reuse disposable gloves.

Change your gloves between contacts with different patients. If a glove tears while providing patient care, remove it as soon as you can and replace it with a new one. Throw away contaminated gloves and other PPE in clearly labeled biohazard bags or containers.

When removing gloves, keep in mind that the outer surface of the gloves are considered contaminated. Do not let the outside surface of the gloves come in contact with your skin. Be careful not to let the gloves snap when taking them off. If the gloves snap, germs may become airborne and contact your eyes, mouth, or skin. The proper technique for removing gloves is shown in Skill Drill 2-1.

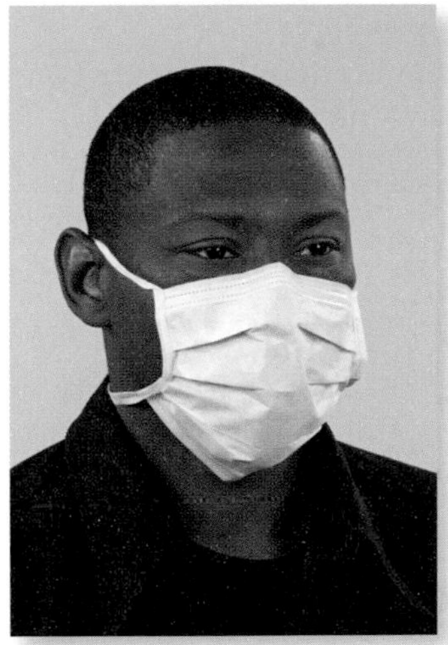

FIGURE 2-15 ▲ A surgical-type mask should cover your mouth, nose, and chin. To keep the mask from slipping, pinch the metal band at the top of the mask. This causes the mask to conform to the shape of your nose.

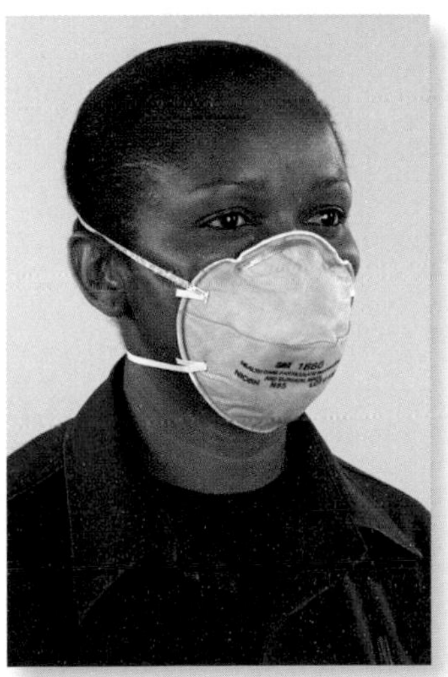

FIGURE 2-16 ▲ Wear a high-efficiency particulate air (HEPA) mask if you know or suspect that your patient has tuberculosis.

Stop and Think!

Using Gloves in Patient Care

- *Always* put on disposable gloves before physical contact with every patient.
- *Always* change gloves before caring for another patient.
- *Always* dispose of gloves properly.
- *Always* wash your hands after removing your gloves.

Gowns Disposable, fluid-resistant gowns should be used in situations in which large splashes of blood or body fluids might occur. Examples of such situations include childbirth, vomiting, and massive bleeding. After patient care activities are complete, properly dispose of the gown. If a gown is not available and you were exposed to the patient's body fluids when providing care, change your clothes and take a hot shower as soon as possible after contact with the patient. Wash your clothes in hot, soapy water for at least 25 minutes. Launder your clothes at work, if possible. If you have to take them home, wash them in a separate load.

Masks Wear a surgical-type facemask to protect against the possible splatter of blood or other body fluids. Also wear a facemask in situations in which an airborne disease is suspected (Figure 2-15). The mask should be changed if it becomes moist. If you know or suspect that your patient has tuberculosis, wear an N-95 or a high-efficiency particulate air (HEPA) mask (Figure 2-16). During ambulance transport of a patient with known or suspected tuberculosis, follow these safety measures:

- Wear a HEPA mask.
- Keep the windows of the vehicle open, if possible.
- Set the vehicle's ventilation system to a nonrecycling mode.

Refer to Table 2-4 for guidelines on using personal protective equipment.

Remember This!

Personal Protective Equipment (PPE)

- Eye protection
- Gloves
- Gowns
- Masks

TABLE 2-4 Guidelines for Using Personal Protective Equipment

Personal Protective Equipment	Guidelines for Use
Gloves	Any situation in which the potential for contacting blood or other body fluids exists
Gloves and chin-length plastic face shield (or mask and protective eyewear)	Any situation in which the splashing or spattering of blood or other body fluids is likely (such as in suctioning or with a coughing or spitting patient)
Gloves, chin-length plastic face shield (or mask and protective eyewear), and gown	Any situation in which the splashing or spattering of blood or other body fluids is likely and clothing is likely to be soiled (such as childbirth and arterial bleeding)

Immunizations

An infection can cause serious medical problems. Immunizations help your body fight infection. It is important to keep your immunizations current:

- Tetanus prevention (booster every 10 years)
- Hepatitis B vaccine
- Influenza vaccine (yearly)
- Measles, mumps, and rubella (MMR) vaccine (if needed)

Tetanus Tetanus (lockjaw) is a serious disease caused by a germ that enters the body through a cut or wound. Tetanus causes serious, painful spasms of all muscles. It can lead to "locking" of the jaw, so that the patient cannot open his or her mouth or swallow. The tetanus vaccine can prevent tetanus. This vaccine is usually given beginning at the age of 2 months. After receiving three doses of the vaccine (usually during childhood), a booster shot is needed every 10 years.

Hepatitis B Hepatitis B is a serious disease caused by the hepatitis B virus (HBV). This virus is spread through contact with the blood and body fluids of an infected person. A person can be infected in several ways:

- Having unprotected sex with an infected person
- Sharing needles
- Being stuck with a used needle while treating an infected patient
- Having blood splashed into your eyes or mouth or onto a skin wound
- Giving birth, when the virus passes from an infected mother to her baby

HBV can cause a loss of appetite, diarrhea and vomiting, tiredness, jaundice (yellow skin or eyes), stomach pain, and pain in muscles and joints. HBV can also cause long-term illness that leads to liver damage (cirrhosis), liver cancer, and death.

The hepatitis B vaccine can prevent hepatitis B. Everyone 18 years of age and younger and adults over 18 who are at risk should receive the HBV vaccine. Adults at risk for HBV infection include

- Healthcare workers and public safety workers who might be exposed to infected blood or body fluids
- People who have more than one sex partner in six months
- Men who have sex with other men
- People who have sexual contact with infected individuals
- People who inject illegal drugs
- People who have household contact with individuals who have chronic hepatitis B virus infection
- Hemodialysis patients

You Should Know

Hepatitis B

According to the Centers for Disease Control and Prevention,

- About 1.25 million people in the United States have chronic hepatitis B infection.
- About one third of people who are infected with hepatitis B in the United States do not know how they got it.

Each year, it is estimated that

- Eighty thousand people, mostly young adults, are infected with HBV
- More than 11,000 people have to stay in the hospital because of hepatitis B
- Between 4,000 and 5,000 people die from chronic hepatitis B

Influenza Influenza ("flu") is caused by a virus that spreads from infected persons to the nose or throat of others. Influenza can cause fever, sore throat, chills, cough, headache, and muscle aches. Most people are ill for only a few days. However, some people get much sicker and may need to be hospitalized. According to the Centers for Disease Control and Prevention, influenza causes an average of 36,000 deaths each year in the United States, mostly among the elderly. All healthcare workers who breathe the same air as a person at high risk for complications of influenza and do not have a contraindication to the flu vaccine should receive an influenza vaccination every year. The flu season usually peaks from January through March. Therefore, the best time to get the flu vaccine is in October or November.

Measles, Mumps, and Rubella Measles, mumps, and rubella are serious diseases that are spread from person to person through the air. The measles virus causes rash, cough, runny nose, eye irritation, and fever. The mumps virus causes fever, headache, and swollen glands. Rubella (German measles) is caused by the rubella virus. It causes a rash and mild fever. If a woman gets rubella while she is pregnant, she could have a miscarriage or her baby could be born with serious birth defects (Table 2-5).

The measles, mumps, and rubella (MMR) vaccine can prevent these diseases. Generally, anyone 18 years of age or older who was born after 1956 should get at least one dose of the MMR vaccine unless he or she can show that he or she has had either the vaccine or the diseases. Persons born before 1957 are generally considered immune to measles.

In the United States, about 100 people die each year from chicken pox.

Chicken Pox (Varicella) Chicken pox (varicella) is a common childhood disease that is usually mild. However, this disease can be serious, especially in young infants and adults. Chicken pox is caused by a virus, which is spread from person

TABLE 2-5 Signs, Symptoms, and Complications of Some Airborne Diseases

Disease	Signs and Symptoms	Complications
Measles	Rash Cough Runny nose Eye irritation Fever	Ear infection Pneumonia Seizures Brain damage Death
Mumps	Fever Headache Swollen glands	Deafness Meningitis (infection of the brain and spinal cord covering) Painful swelling of the testicles or ovaries Death (rare)
Rubella (German measles)	Rash Mild fever	Possible serious birth defects
Chicken pox (varicella)	Rash Itching Fever Tiredness	Severe skin infection Scars Pneumonia Brain damage Death

to person through the air or by contact with fluid from chicken pox blisters. The virus causes a rash, itching, fever, and tiredness.

Most people who get the varicella vaccine will not get chicken pox. However, if someone who has been vaccinated does get chicken pox, it is usually very mild. All healthcare workers should be immune to varicella, either due to having had chicken pox or from receiving two doses of the varicella vaccine.

Tuberculosis (TB) Tuberculosis (TB) is a disease caused by bacteria that usually attack the lungs. It is spread through the air when a person with TB coughs or sneezes. You may become infected with TB if you breathe in these bacteria. To determine if you have been exposed to tuberculosis, you should have a tuberculin skin test at least yearly.

Documenting and Managing an Exposure

If you are exposed to blood or body fluids, immediately wash the affected area with soap and water. Notify your designated infection control officer, medical director, or other designated individual as soon as possible. Get a medical evaluation and proper immunizations if necessary. Make sure to document the following:

- The date and time of the exposure
- The circumstances surrounding the exposure
- The type, source, and amount of body fluid to which you were exposed
- The actions you took to reduce the chances of infection

Know your local protocols about when and how soon to have a medical follow-up after an exposure incident. As a rule, exposure follow-up should be done immediately after the exposure. If the patient has HIV or hepatitis B, preventive care is most effective when given quickly.

Cleaning, Disinfecting, and Sterilizing Equipment

Do not reuse disposable equipment.

Germs can be killed or inactivated by cleaning, disinfecting, or sterilizing. Different chemicals or combinations of chemicals kill or inactivate different germs. When providing patient care, use disposable equipment whenever possible. Reusable equipment used in the care of a patient with intact skin usually requires only cleaning or disinfecting.

When dealing with contaminated materials, place them in appropriately labeled, leak-proof containers or bags. Double-bag disposable items if the patient is known to have a communicable disease.

Cleaning **Cleaning** is the process of washing a contaminated object with soap and water. An item must be cleaned before it is disinfected or sterilized. To clean equipment, begin by rinsing the item with cold water to remove obvious body fluid or tissue. Then wash the item with hot, soapy water. If the item has grooves or narrow spaces, use a stiff-bristled brush to clean it. Rinse it well with moderately hot water and then dry it. The item is now considered clean.

Physically removing germs by scrubbing is as important as the effect of the agent you use for cleaning or disinfecting.

Disinfecting **Disinfecting** is cleaning with chemical solutions, such as alcohol or chlorine. These agents destroy some types of germs that may be left after washing. Depending on the type and degree of contamination, items such as stethoscopes, blood pressure cuffs, backboards, and splints usually need only cleaning followed by disinfection. Isopropyl (rubbing) alcohol is often used to disinfect surfaces. However, rubbing alcohol may discolor, swell, harden, and crack rubber and certain plastics after prolonged and repeated use. When chlorine bleach is used as a disinfectant, it must be diluted. A solution of 1 part bleach and 10 parts water or 1 part bleach and 100 parts water may be used. The solution used will depend on the amount of material (such as blood, mucus, or urine) present on the surface to be cleaned and disinfected. Many commercially available disinfectants are available. Follow the manufacturer's instructions to disinfect equipment.

FIGURE 2-17 ► A placard is a diamond-shaped sign that is displayed on trucks, railroad cars, and large containers carrying hazardous materials.

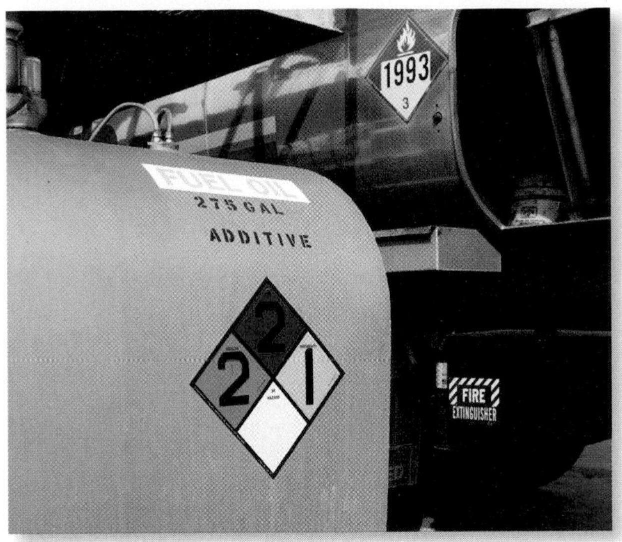

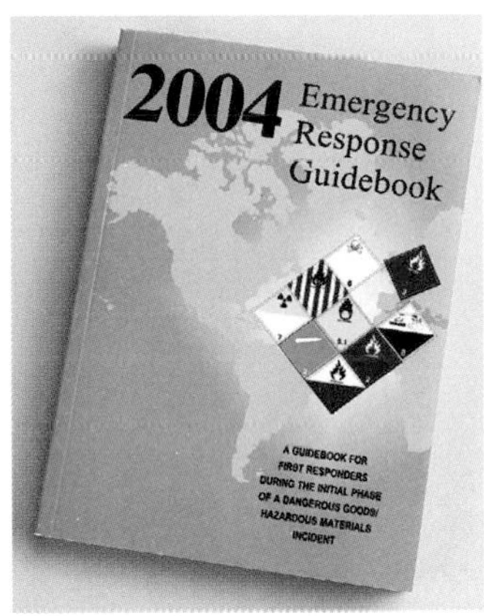

FIGURE 2-18 ▲ The four-digit identification number on a hazardous materials placard can be used to find information about the material in the *Emergency Response Guidebook*.

Sterilizing **Sterilizing** is a process that uses boiling water, radiation, gas, chemicals, or superheated steam to destroy all of the germs on an object. Reusable equipment that is inserted into a patient's body should always be sterilized.

Stop and Think!

Chemical solutions can be harmful. Always protect yourself by wearing gloves and goggles.

Hazardous Materials Scenes

You may be required to respond to situations involving hazardous materials. The National Fire Protection Association (NFPA) defines a **hazardous material** as a substance (solid, liquid, or gas) that, when released, is capable of creating harm to people, the environment, and property. (*Reprinted with permission from NFPA 1991–2005, Vapor Protective Ensembles for Hazardous Materials Emergencies, Copyright © 2005 National Fire Protection Association*). A hazardous materials scene may involve liquids, solids, or gases that are toxic. To prevent further injury, you must be able to recognize that a hazardous materials situation exists.

Use binoculars to identify possible hazards before approaching the scene. Look for signs or placards that provide information about the contents. A placard is a four-sided, diamond-shaped sign. It is displayed on trucks, railroad cars, and large containers that carry hazardous materials (Figure 2-17). The placard will contain a four-digit identification number to guide you to reference information found in the *Emergency Response Guidebook*, which is published by the United States Department of Transportation (Figure 2-18). The guidebook provides information to help you identify the type of hazardous material involved. In addition, it outlines basic initial actions to take at the scene. The placard will also contain a class or division number, which indicates whether the material is flammable, radioactive, explosive, or poisonous.

Learn how to contact your local hazardous materials team.

If you are the first person on the scene of an incident involving a hazardous material, *do not enter the scene.* Contact law enforcement and your local hazardous materials response team immediately. Stay upwind and on higher ground than the incident site. Keep unnecessary people away from the area.

Hazardous materials incidents require specialized protective equipment that is not commonly available to Emergency Medical Responders. In general, protective

Objective 10 ▶

clothing for a hazardous materials scene includes a hazardous materials suit and a Self-Contained Breathing Apparatus (SCBA) (Figure 2-19). Do not enter the scene unless you are trained to handle hazardous materials, are fully protected with the proper equipment, and know how to use that equipment. Provide emergency care only after the scene is safe and the patient is decontaminated.

Motor Vehicle Crashes and Rescue Scenes

Remember: Your personal safety is your number one priority. *Think* before entering a scene.

The scene of a motor vehicle crash may involve potential threats to your safety. It may also threaten the safety of your crew, the patient, and bystanders. Study the scene before entering and determine if it is safe to approach the patient. Determine the number and type of vehicles and the extent of damage. Also note the approximate number of persons injured and look for hazards. Assess the need for additional resources, such as a hazardous materials team or extrication equipment.

You Should Know

Potential Hazards at a Motor Vehicle Crash Scene

- Traffic
- Blood
- Gasoline spills
- Hazardous materials
- Undeployed air bags (especially with side curtains)
- Sharp edges and fragments
- Exposed or downed electrical wires
- Fire or potential for fire
- Explosive materials
- Unstable vehicle or structure
- Environmental conditions (such as heavy rain, heavy snowfall, and flash floods)

Traffic

Traffic is a common danger at a crash scene. If you arrive at a crash scene in a vehicle, be very careful when preparing to exit, especially if your door will open into traffic. Put on appropriate reflective gear, if available. Make sure that the vehicle is in park or that the brake is set. Check your rearview mirror for traffic and open the door slowly. Request the help of law enforcement personnel to investigate and assist with traffic control. If the fire department responds to the scene, its large trucks are often positioned in a specific way. This positioning is done to shield the collision site and to provide protection while you care for the patient.

Power Lines

Objective 10 ▶

Look for downed or exposed power lines, which are a potential source of electrocution. You *must* assume that any downed wire is dangerous. Contact the power company and fire department immediately. Do not attempt to move the downed wire and make sure not to touch any metal object or water in contact with it. Wait for the power company to shut off the power to the downed line before approaching the patient. If a downed wire is in contact with the vehicle, tell those inside the vehicle to remain inside until additional help arrives.

Fire Hazards

Look for fire or potential fire hazards, such as leaking fuel. Do not approach a burning vehicle unless you are trained to handle such situations and are fully protected with proper equipment.

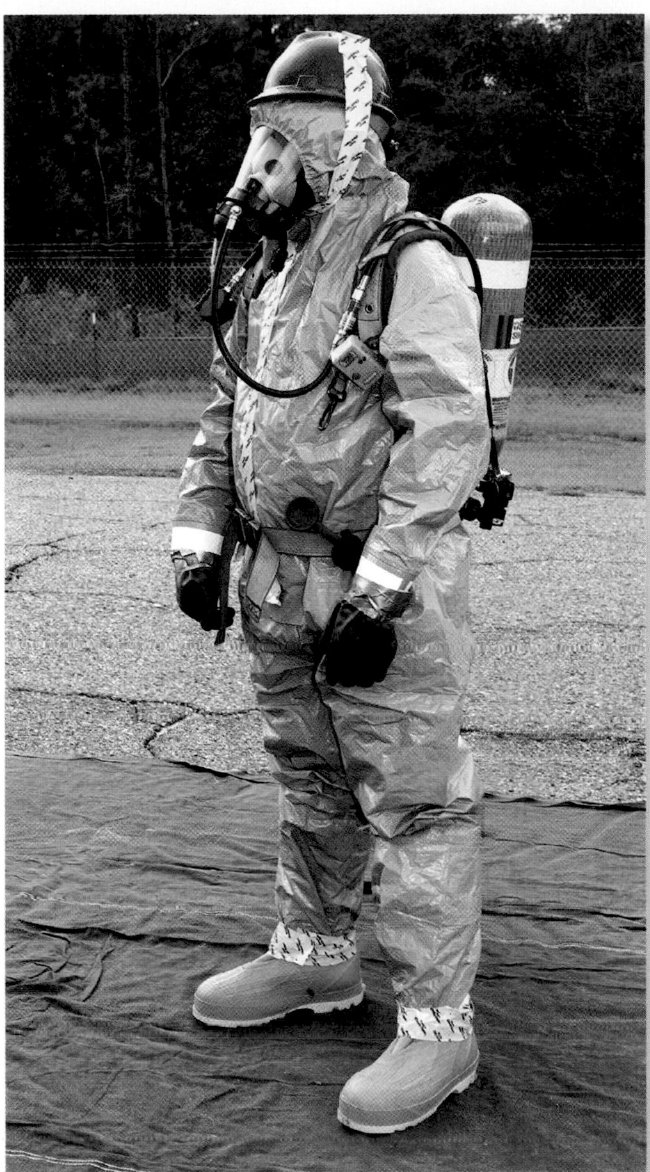

FIGURE 2-19 ▲ Protective clothing for a hazardous materials scene generally includes a hazardous materials suit and a Self-Contained Breathing Apparatus (SCBA).

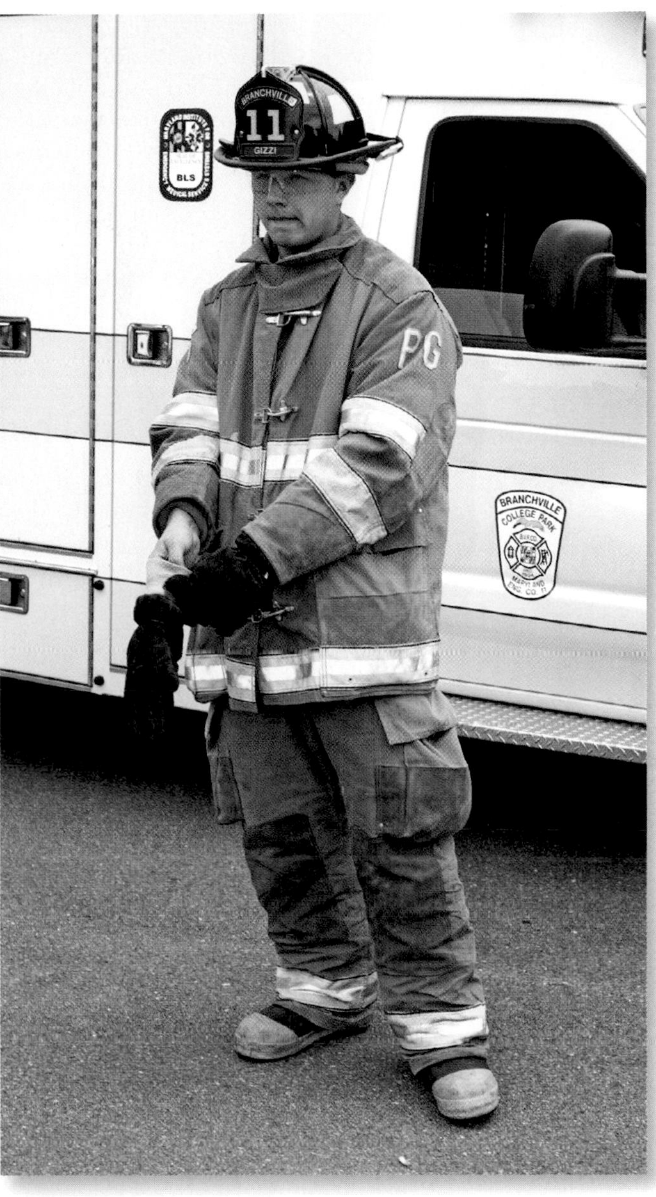

FIGURE 2-20 ▲ Protective clothing for a rescue scene typically includes turnout gear, puncture-proof gloves, a helmet, eye protection (such as safety glasses or goggles), and boots with steel toes.

Entrapped Victims

Look for entrapped victims. Request special rescue teams when an extensive or a complex rescue is needed. Protective clothing for a rescue scene typically includes turnout gear, puncture-proof gloves, a helmet, eye protection (safety glasses or goggles), and boots with steel toes (Figure 2-20). In cold weather, consider wearing long underwear, a warm head covering, and gloves. In wet weather, you may want to wear waterproof boots and slip-resistant gloves.

Violent Scenes

Violence may occur even when police are present on the scene.

Scenes involving armed or potentially hostile persons are among the most dangerous for emergency care providers and law enforcement personnel. EMS personnel may be mistaken for law enforcement officials because of their uniform or badge. The scene should *always* be secured by law enforcement before you provide patient care. However, a scene that has been declared safe does not mean that it will *continue* to be safe. Reassess scene safety often. Notify law enforcement personnel on the scene if a condition concerning scene safety comes to your attention. Table 2-6 lists some of the warning signs of danger.

Objective 10 ▶ Some EMS professionals wear body armor (bulletproof vests). Body armor does not cover the entire body. The areas of the body that are not covered are still vulnerable to injury. Body armor protects covered areas from most handgun bullets and most knives. It does not offer protection from high-velocity (rifle) bullets, from thin or dual-edged weapons (such as an ice pick), or when it is not worn. Body armor provides reduced protection when wet.

Stop and Think!

NEVER enter a potential crime scene or a scene involving a family dispute, a fight, an attempted suicide, alcohol, drugs, or weapons until law enforcement personnel have secured the scene and declared it safe for you to enter and provide patient care.

At a crime scene, law enforcement personnel are responsible for gathering the evidence that is needed for investigation and prosecution. EMS personnel are responsible for patient care. Do not disturb the scene unless absolutely necessary for medical care. Evidence includes fingerprints, footprints, blood and body fluid, hair, and carpet and clothing fibers. Avoid disturbing evidence by

- Being observant
- Touching only what is required for patient care
  - If it is necessary to touch something, remember what you touched and tell the police.
- Wearing gloves
  - Wearing gloves helps provde infection control and prevents you from leaving your fingerprints at the scene. However, it will not prevent you from smudging other fingerprints.

TABLE 2-6 Warning Signs of Danger

Residences	Street Scenes	Highway Encounters
• Unusual silence or a darkened residence • History of problems or violence • Known drug or gang area • Loud noises or items breaking • Acts of violence • Alcohol or other drug use • Evidence of dangerous pets	• Crowds (large groups of people may quickly become large and unpredictable) • Voices becoming louder • Pushing, shoving • Hostility toward others at the scene (perpetrator, police, victim) • Rapid increase in crowd size • Inability of law enforcement to control crowds	• Disabled vehicles; calls for "man slumped over wheel"; motor vehicle crashes • Suspicious movements within a vehicle • Grabbing or hiding of items • Arguing or fighting between passengers • Lack of activity where activity is likely • Signs of alcohol or drug use • Open or unlatched trunks (may hide people)

- Taking the same path in and out of the scene
- Avoiding stepping on bloodstains or splatter
- Disturbing the victim and the victim's clothing as little as possible
- Avoiding cuts to the victim's clothing that may have been caused by a knife, a bullet, or another penetrating weapon
- Saving the victim's clothing and personal items in a paper bag

Stop and Think!

Scene Safety in Violent Scenes

- Communicate with dispatch and law enforcement.
- Know an alternate way out of the scene.
- Have a prearranged panic code with dispatch and your partner(s).

On The Scene

Wrap-Up

Your friend has no pulse. His jaw and limbs are rigid and cold, and you decide not to resuscitate him. Paramedics arrive moments later and confirm that he is dead. You sit down next to his wife, put your arm around her shoulders, and tell her that her husband is dead. She screams and pushes you away angrily, asking why you didn't do anything to save him. Moments later, she moans and says she shouldn't have gone to work; she knew he'd been depressed.

You go back to the station after the call and tearfully explain to the crew about your lifelong friendship with the patient. Later that week, a debriefing is held. Because of your ongoing dreams about the event, you visit a counselor to help you cope with the strong emotions you are feeling. ■

Sum It Up

- As an Emergency Medical Responder, you will encounter many stressful situations. Whatever the situation, you must act professionally. It is important that you learn how to recognize the signs and symptoms of stress in yourself and others.
- Critically ill or injured patients may experience *grief,* which is a normal response to a loss of any kind. The five stages of grief are denial, anger, bargaining, depression, and acceptance. Remember that a person going through grief may skip a stage, go through more than one stage at the same time, or go through each stage more than once. Cultural factors influence how a person experiences grief.
- Patients may experience any number of emotions in response to their illness or injury. As an Emergency Medical Responder, you must be respectful of each patient. Listen with empathy to the patient's concerns, but do not give the patient false hope. In dealing with the patient's family or friends or with bystanders, you may need to use many of the same approaches you use in dealing with patients.
- Some patients may not want aggressive efforts aimed at reviving them when they are dying. These patients may have an *advance directive* or a *Do Not Resuscitate (DNR) order.* An advance directive is a legal document that details a

person's healthcare wishes when he or she becomes unable to make decisions for him- or herself. A Do Not Resuscitate order is written by a physician. It instructs medical professionals not to provide medical care to a patient who has experienced a cardiac arrest.

- The signs of obvious death include decapitation (beheading), putrefaction (decomposition), dependent lividity, and rigor mortis. If a person shows signs of obvious death, do not disturb the body or scene. The police or medical examiner will need to authorize removal of the body. You should document the victim's position and his or her injuries. You should also document the conditions at the scene, as well as statements of persons at the scene.
- As an EMS professional, you will experience personal stress and will encounter patients and bystanders in severe stress. A *stressor* is any event or condition that has the potential to cause bodily or mental tension. In order to be an effective Emergency Medical Responder, you must learn to recognize the physical, behavioral, mental, and emotional signs of stress.
- You should manage stress through lifestyle changes. These changes include developing good dietary habits, exercising, and practicing relaxation techniques. You should also seek to create balance in your life, including time with family and friends.
- Professional help may be needed to help you cope with stress. Many organizations have employee assistance programs that offer confidential counseling to prehospital professionals.
- *Critical Incident Stress Management (CISM)* is a program that assists emergency workers in coping with stressful situations. A *Critical Incident Stress Debriefing (CISD)* is a formal group meeting led by a mental health professional and peer counselors. A *defusing* is a shorter, less formal version of a debriefing. The goal of these forms of stress management is to speed up the normal recovery process after a critical incident. The results of some studies raise doubts about the effectiveness of CISM.
- An Emergency Medical Responder is responsible for ensuring the safety of the crew, the patient, and bystanders. However, an Emergency Medical Responder's first priority is ensuring his or her own safety at all scenes. This responsibility includes protecting oneself against disease transmission, which includes using personal protective equipment (PPE) and getting the proper vaccinations. It also involves safety at hazardous materials scenes, motor vehicle crashes and rescue scenes, and violent scenes.

▶ Tracking Your Progress

After reading this chapter, can you	Page Reference	Objective Met?
• List possible emotional reactions that you may experience when faced with trauma, illness, death, and dying?	34–35	☐
• Discuss the possible reactions that a family member may exhibit when confronted with death and dying?	41	☐
• State the steps in your approach to the family confronted with death and dying?	41	☐
• State the possible reactions that your family may exhibit?	49	☐
• Recognize the signs and symptoms of critical incident stress?	51	☐
• State possible steps that you may take to help reduce/alleviate stress?	47–50	☐
• Explain the need to determine scene safety?	52	☐

• Discuss the importance of body substance isolation (BSI) precautions?	53–54	☐
• Describe the steps you should take for personal protection from airborne and bloodborne pathogens?	54–57	☐
• List the personal protective equipment necessary for each of the following situations: hazardous materials, rescue operations, violent scenes, crime scenes, electricity, water and ice, exposure to bloodborne pathogens, exposure to airborne pathogens?	55–57	☐
• Explain the importance of serving as an advocate for the use of appropriate protective equipment?	55	☐
• Explain the importance of understanding the response to death and dying and communicating effectively with the patient's family?	44	☐
• Demonstrate a caring attitude toward any patient with illness or injury who requests emergency medical services?	38–40	☐
• Show compassion when caring for the physical and mental needs of patients?	39–40	☐
• Participate willingly in the care of all patients?	38	☐
• Communicate with empathy to patients being cared for, as well as with family members, and friends of the patient?	41	☐

Chapter Quiz

Multiple Choice

In the space provided, identify the letter of the choice that best completes each statement or answers each question.

_____ **1.** You respond to a residence for a possible drowning. You arrive to find law enforcement personnel performing CPR on a 3-year-old male. The child was found floating facedown in the pool. He was last seen 10 or 15 minutes ago. Before approaching the patient, you should

a. locate the child's parents and ask about the child's medical history.
b. contact the closest hospital to let them know they will be receiving a patient.
c. quickly survey the scene for possible hazards and put on appropriate personal protective equipment.
d. take a moment to wash your hands before beginning patient care.

_____ **2.** How should you approach the child's mother?

a. Let her know that everything that can be done to help will be done.
b. Using a gentle tone of voice, tell her that everything is going to be okay.
c. Calmly but firmly tell her that it appears her son will not survive.
d. Ask her how she could have let something like this happen.

_____ **3.** Body substance isolation (BSI) precautions consist of

a. self-protection against all body fluids and substances.
b. procedures used by EMS personnel when dealing with a violent patient.
c. the rescue equipment that should be worn at the scene of a motor vehicle crash.
d. procedures used by EMS personnel when relaying the news about a patient's death.

_____ **4.** The single most important method you can use to prevent the spread of communicable disease is

a. handwashing.
b. wearing vinyl or latex gloves.
c. keeping your immunizations current.
d. following a balanced diet.

_____ 5. Hepatitis B virus (HBV) and human immunodeficiency virus (HIV) are examples of

a. airborne diseases.
b. bloodborne diseases.
c. foodborne diseases.
d. sexually transmitted diseases.

_____ 6. You should wear a high-efficiency particulate air (HEPA) mask when providing care to a patient known or suspected to be infected with

a. hepatitis B.
b. measles.
c. tuberculosis.
d. tetanus.

True or False

Decide whether the statement is true or false. In the space provided, write T for true or F for false.

_____ 7. Body substance isolation precautions include handwashing, the use of personal protective equipment, and the proper cleaning, disinfecting, and disposing of soiled materials and equipment.

Matching

Match the key terms in the left column with the definitions in the right column by placing the letter of each correct answer in the space provided.

_____ 8. Terminal illness
_____ 9. Critical Incident Stress Debriefing
_____ 10. Do Not Resuscitate order
_____ 11. Pathogens
_____ 12. Stress
_____ 13. Airborne disease
_____ 14. Empathy
_____ 15. Grief
_____ 16. Rigor mortis
_____ 17. Communicable disease
_____ 18. Regression
_____ 19. Dependent lividity
_____ 20. Cumulative stress
_____ 21. Advance directive
_____ 22. Exposure
_____ 23. Cleaning
_____ 24. Critical incident
_____ 25. Stressor
_____ 26. Occupational Safety and Health Administration

a. Cleaning with chemical solutions, such as alcohol or chlorine
b. Repeated exposure to smaller stressors that build up over time
c. To understand, be aware of, and be sensitive to the feelings, thoughts, and experience of another
d. Normal response that helps a person cope with the loss of someone or of something that had great meaning to the person
e. Legal document that specifies a person's healthcare wishes when he or she becomes unable to make decisions for him- or herself
f. A return to an earlier developmental state
g. Washing a contaminated object with soap and water
h. Settling of blood in areas on which the body has been resting
i. Event or condition that has the potential to cause bodily or mental tension
j. Illness or injury for which there is no reasonable expectation of recovery
k. Group meeting led by a mental health professional and peer support personnel to allow rescuers to share thoughts, emotions, and other reactions to a critical incident
l. Substance that causes or may cause adverse effects on the health or safety of employees, the general public, or the environment
m. Infection that can be spread from one person to another
n. Situation that causes a healthcare provider to experience unusually strong emotions and that may interfere with the provider's psychological ability to cope and function immediately or later
o. Germs capable of producing disease
p. Using boiling water, radiation, gas, chemicals, or superheated steam to destroy all of the germs on an object
q. Stiffening of body muscles that occurs after death
r. Branch of the federal government responsible for safety in the workplace
s. Self-protection against all body fluids and substances
t. Specialized clothing or equipment worn for protection against a hazard
u. Contact with infected blood, body fluids, tissues, or airborne droplets, either directly or indirectly

_____ **27.** Disinfecting

_____ **28.** Body substance isolation precautions

_____ **29.** Sterilizing

_____ **30.** Hazardous material

_____ **31.** Personal protective equipment

v. Chemical, physical, or emotional factor that causes bodily or mental tension

w. Written physician order that instructs medical professionals not to provide medical care to a patient who has experienced a cardiopulmonary arrest

x. Infection spread by droplets produced by coughing or sneezing

Short Answer

Answer each question in the space provided.

32. You respond to a residence for a possible drowning. You arrive to find law enforcement personnel performing CPR on a 3-year-old male. The child was found floating facedown in the pool. He was last seen 10 or 15 minutes ago. The child's mother has arrived on the scene. Describe the mother's possible reactions to this situation.

____

____

____

33. The child in question 32 is transported to the hospital. Despite continued efforts to resuscitate him, he is pronounced dead. List the emotional reactions that you may experience because of this situation.

____

____

____

34. List six stressful situations you may encounter as an Emergency Medical Responder.

1. ______________________ 4. ______________________

2. ______________________ 5. ______________________

3. ______________________ 6. ______________________

35. A mother has been told of her child's death. List the five stages of the grief process in the order that most people experience them.

1. ______________________

2. ______________________

3. ______________________

4. ______________________

5. ______________________

36. You are called to the scene of a motor vehicle crash. A patient requires removal from one of the vehicles involved in the crash. List four items of protective clothing that should be worn in this situation.

1. ______________________________

2. ______________________________

3. ______________________________

4. ______________________________

37. List three lifestyle changes you can make to help reduce stress.

1. ______________________________

2. ______________________________

3. ______________________________

CHAPTER

3 Legal and Ethical Issues

By the end of this chapter, you should be able to

Knowledge Objectives ▶

1. Define the Emergency Medical Responder scope of care.
2. Discuss the importance of Do Not Resuscitate [DNR] (advance directives) and local or state provisions regarding EMS application.
3. Define consent and discuss the methods of obtaining consent.
4. Differentiate between expressed and implied consent.
5. Explain the role of consent of minors in providing care.
6. Discuss the implications for the Emergency Medical Responder in patient refusal of transport.
7. Discuss the issues of abandonment, negligence, and battery and their implications to the Emergency Medical Responder.
8. State the conditions necessary for the Emergency Medical Responder to have a duty to act.
9. Explain the importance, necessity, and legality of patient confidentiality.
10. List the actions that an Emergency Medical Responder should take to assist in the preservation of a crime scene.
11. State the conditions that require an Emergency Medical Responder to notify local law enforcement officials.
12. Discuss issues concerning the fundamental components of documentation.

Attitude Objectives ▶

13. Explain the rationale for the needs, benefits, and usage of advance directives.
14. Explain the rationale for the concept of varying degrees of DNR.

Skill Objectives ▶ There are no skill objectives identified for this lesson.

On The Scene

"The scene is safe. Proceed in," the dispatcher calls over the radio. A hunter has evidently shot himself while cleaning his gun. Your patient, an adult male, is sitting in a chair in the living room. He is awake, alert, and oriented, but he looks very pale. He is holding his upper leg, where you can see a small hole in his jeans. You carefully avoid touching the small handgun that is sitting on the table near the patient. The upholstery on the chair under him is soaked with blood. You introduce yourself and prepare to care for the patient, but he says, "No—don't touch me. I'm okay." You recognize that he is a reporter for the local news station. You carefully explain the danger of refusing care and that he may develop shock and die if he does not receive care. He insists that no care be given, so you contact your medical director for advice while you wait for the ambulance to arrive. ■

THINK ABOUT IT

As you read this chapter, think about the following questions:

- Can the patient refuse to allow you to care for him?
- What can you be accused of if you try to care for him without his consent?
- Is it okay to talk about his case to other coworkers because he is a reporter?
- Could you be accused of negligence in this situation?

Introduction

The Importance of Legal and Ethical Care

As an EMS professional, you will face many situations involving medical, legal, and ethical questions. Consider the following examples.

- You have completed your Emergency Medical Responder training and are heading home after a busy day at work. While driving through town, you come upon an automobile crash that apparently happened moments ago. You can see a middle-aged man slumped over the steering wheel. Should you stop and provide emergency care—even though you are off duty?
- You are on shift as an Emergency Medical Responder and receive a call from an attorney. The attorney is representing a patient who was involved in a fall while at work. You provided emergency care for the patient about two months ago. Should you release patient information to the attorney on the telephone?
- You are on shift as an Emergency Medical Responder and are called to a local park, where a seven-year-old child has fallen off a piece of playground equipment. Her arm appears to be broken. The next-door neighbor, an adult, is present on the scene. The child's parents cannot be reached. Can you provide emergency care for this child?

You will face situations like these and other legal and ethical questions every day. You must know how to make correct decisions when these questions arise.

The first and most basic principle for any healthcare professional is to *do no harm.* As an Emergency Medical Responder, you have certain legal and ethical duties to your patients, your medical director, and the public. Your patients, your medical director, and the public also have certain expectations of you. If you act in good faith and to an appropriate standard of care, you should be able to satisfy these duties and obligations. In this chapter, we will explore common legal definitions and the expectations of your career and practice as an Emergency Medical Responder.

Scope of Care

Legal Duties

Objective 1 ▶

As an Emergency Medical Responder, you have a legal duty to your patients, your medical director, and the public. You must provide for the well-being of your patients by providing necessary medical care outlined in the **scope of care.**

Make sure to check your state rules and regulations to find out the specific skills you are allowed by law to perform.

The scope of care (also called the **scope of practice**) includes the emergency care and skills an Emergency Medical Responder is legally allowed and expected to perform when necessary. These duties are set by state laws and regulations. They are also based on generally accepted standards. States often use the United States Department of Transportation Emergency Medical Responder Curriculum to define the Emergency Medical Responder's scope of care. Some states modify an Emergency Medical Services (EMS) professional's scope of care to fit the states' needs or desires. As a result, what is accepted EMS practice in one state may not be so in another. A medical director and/or your local, regional, or state EMS community may broaden or limit an Emergency Medical Responder's scope of care by using **standing orders** and **protocols.**

Regardless of your primary occupation, as an Emergency Medical Responder, you are expected to provide the same **standard of care** in an emergency as another Emergency Medical Responder with similar training and experience in similar circumstances. As an Emergency Medical Responder, the laws of the state in which you practice define your scope of care. Common skills that are within the Emergency Medical Responder's scope of care include

- Patient assessment
- Insertion of oral and nasal airways
- Upper airway suctioning
- Bag-valve-mask ventilation
- Supplemental oxygen therapy
- Cardiopulmonary resuscitation (CPR)
- Automated external defibrillation
- External hemorrhage control
- Bandaging wounds
- Manual stabilization of painful, swollen, and deformed extremities
- Assisting in childbirth
- Assisting in lifting and moving patients

In many states, your legal right to function as an Emergency Medical Responder may depend on **medical oversight.** This means that for you to practice as an Emergency Medical Responder, a physician must oversee your training and practice. A physician acting as medical oversight may allow you to carry out certain medical treatments in specific situations. Alternately, the physician may not allow you to provide emergency care without first making telephone or radio contact with a person of higher medical authority than you (such as a paramedic, nurse, or physician). When you practice under medical oversight, you are, in effect, practicing under the physician's license.

Making a Difference

Legal Duties of an Emergency Medical Responder

- Provide for the well-being of the patient by giving emergency medical care as outlined in the scope of care
- Provide the same standard of care as another Emergency Medical Responder with similar training and experience in similar circumstances
- Before providing emergency care, make telephone or radio contact with the medical oversight authority (if required to do so)
- Follow standing orders and protocols approved by medical oversight or the local EMS system
- Follow orders received from medical oversight

Ethical Responsibilities

Ethics are principles of right and wrong, good and bad, and the consequences of human actions. In other words, ethics are what a person *ought* to do. As a healthcare professional, you have an ethical responsibility to make your patient's physical and emotional needs a priority. While in contact with a patient, your patient must be your primary concern. Your patient may be from a different ethnic or social background or be a criminal. None of these circumstances can be allowed to interfere with the care you give.

You must treat all patients with respect. Give each patient the best care you are capable of giving. To do this, you have an ethical responsibility to practice and master your skills. This includes taking advantage of continuing education and refresher programs. After a call, review how you did and look for areas in which you can improve. For example, look for ways to improve your response times, patient outcomes, and your communication skills.

Value judgments about a patient's character have no place at any level of medical care.

You must be honest and accurate in your written and verbal communications. You must also respect your patients' right to privacy. Much of the information you will get from your patients is considered **protected health information (PHI).** Federal laws forbid the sharing of patient information that you receive in the course of your work as an Emergency Medical Responder without the patient's consent. These laws are discussed in more detail later in this chapter.

As a healthcare professional, you also have a responsibility to work cooperatively with other emergency care professionals. This includes other EMS professionals, law enforcement personnel, fire department and ambulance personnel, and hospital staff members. Make sure that your communications and actions with others are professional and respectful.

Making a Difference

Ethical Responsibilities of an Emergency Medical Responder

- Responding with respect to the physical and emotional needs of every patient
- Maintaining mastery of skills
- Participating in continuing education and refresher programs
- Critically reviewing your performance and seeking improvement
- Reporting (written and verbal) honestly and accurately
- Respecting confidentiality
- Working cooperatively with and with respect for other emergency care professionals

Making a Difference

Treat any patient with the same care and respect you would want a member of your family to receive.

Competence

Before a patient can accept or refuse the care you wish to provide, you must determine if the patient is capable of making the decision (competent). **Competence** is the patient's ability to understand the questions you ask him. It also means the patient can understand the result of the decisions he makes about his care. A patient is considered **incompetent** if he does not have the ability to understand the questions you ask. He is also considered incompetent if he does not understand the possible outcome of the decisions he makes about his care.

Because state laws vary, check with your instructor to find out the requirements for legal competence in your state.

How do you determine if a patient is competent? Well-known EMS attorneys have suggested a three-part test for determining a patient's competence:

1. *Legal competence.* Determine if the patient is legally competent. In most states, this means that your patient is at least 18 years of age, is a minor who is married or pregnant, is economically independent, or is a member of the armed forces.
2. *Mental competence.* Determine if the patient is alert and oriented by asking specific questions. Evaluate the patient's orientation to the following:
   - Person—the patient can tell you her name
   - Place—the patient can tell you where she is
   - Time—the patient can tell you the day, date, or time
   - Event—the patient can tell you what happened

   Find out if the patient has a mental condition, such as Alzheimer's disease, mental retardation, or dementia, which could affect her ability to make an informed decision.
3. *Medical/situational competence.* Some illnesses and injuries can temporarily affect a patient's ability to make an informed decision about her care. For example, head trauma, low blood sugar (hypoglycemia), shock, or low blood oxygen (hypoxia) can affect a patient's ability to think clearly.

In some situations, it may be difficult or impossible to determine if your patient is competent. An adult is generally considered incompetent if she:

- Has an altered mental status
- Is under the influence of drugs or alcohol
- Has a serious illness or injury that affects her ability to make an informed decision about her care
- Has a known mental disorder

"Under the influence of drugs" includes legal and prescription drugs.

A patient who has an altered level of consciousness is often referred to as "altered."

Serious injuries, such as head injuries or injuries that can lead to shock, can cause a change in the patient's mental status or unresponsiveness. Medical conditions such as diabetes or epilepsy can also alter a patient's mental status.

It is generally believed that any amount of alcohol or drugs can affect a patient's judgment. A patient under the influence of drugs or alcohol is assumed to have an altered level of consciousness. In most cases, a patient who is under the influence of drugs or alcohol is considered incompetent. However, determining competence can be tricky. Is a person who has had one drink or two beers intoxicated or incompetent? The person may not meet the legal definition of intoxicated by blood alcohol content. Your own state laws and medical oversight authority can help you determine the definitions of *altered* and *intoxicated.*

Some patients may be judged by the courts to be mentally incompetent. Someone who is truly mentally incompetent or legally mentally incompetent is rarely alone. A guardian who is able to allow or refuse care for the patient is usually present.

Consent

Objective 3 ▶

When your patient allows you to provide emergency care, he is giving you permission, or consent. You must have **consent** before assessing or treating a patient. Any competent patient has the right to decide about his care. The patient's consent is based on the information you give him about his condition. It is also based on the treatment you will provide and the patient's understanding of that information.

Expressed Consent

Objective 4 ▶

Consent may be expressed or implied. You must obtain expressed consent from *every* mentally competent adult before you provide any medical care. Expressed consent is given by a patient who is of legal age and competent to give consent. **Expressed consent** is a type of consent in which a patient gives specific permission for care and transport to be provided. Expressed consent may be given verbally, in writing, or nonverbally. Examples of nonverbal expressed consent include allowing care to be given, or a gesture, such as a nod or walking to the ambulance.

Expressed consent must be **informed consent.** This means that you must give the patient enough information to make an informed decision; otherwise, the patient's expressed consent may be not considered valid. You must tell the patient what you are going to do, how you are going to do it, the possible risks, and the possible outcome of what will be done. To obtain expressed consent, do the following.

- Identify yourself and your level of medical training.
- Explain all treatments and procedures to the patient.
- Identify the benefits of each treatment or procedure.
- Identify the risks of each treatment or procedure.

You must give the patient explanations using words and phrases that the patient can understand. Do not use confusing medical terms. If the patient speaks a language different from your own, you must make every attempt to find someone who can translate for you. Remember, in order for expressed consent to be valid, the patient must understand what you are saying. You must also understand what the patient is saying to you.

Remember This!

A competent adult can withdraw consent at any time during care and transport.

A competent adult may agree to some medical treatments but not to others. For example, a patient with a cut on her leg may allow you to look at the injury and bandage it but refuse transport for further care. If this situation should occur, call advanced medical personnel to the scene to evaluate the patient and the situation.

Implied Consent

Implied consent is sometimes called the *emergency rule.*

Implied consent is consent assumed from a patient requiring emergency care who is mentally, physically, or emotionally unable to provide expressed consent. Implied consent is based on the assumption that the patient would consent to lifesaving treatment if able to do so. It is effective only until the patient no longer requires emergency care or regains competence to make decisions. For example, an unresponsive diabetic patient with low blood sugar may be treated under implied consent. It is assumed that a patient with low blood sugar would want someone to give him sugar if he were unable to do this for himself. Implied consent does not allow you to treat a competent adult for a condition that is not life-threatening.

Special Situations

Objective 5 ▶

Children and mentally incompetent adults must have a parent or guardian give consent for treatment. Each state has its own laws about when a minor child becomes of legal age to consent to his or her own treatment. State laws also

A minor is a child under the age of 18 years.

Even if there is written parental consent to treat a child, make every attempt to contact the child's parents as soon as possible.

address emancipated minors. An emancipated minor is a person who is less than the legal age of consent but who, due to special circumstances, is given the rights of adults. Mental incompetence is also determined by state laws and sometimes involves court hearings and judgments. You must be familiar with your own state laws.

In some situations, parents may grant permission to another person or an agency to allow medical care for their child in an emergency. For example, many parents sign a form allowing their child's school, coach, or daycare provider to authorize care in an emergency. A life-threatening emergency may exist for a child or a mentally incompetent adult when no parent or guardian is present. In these cases, you may treat the patient under implied consent.

Refusals

Objective 6 ▶

All competent adults have the right to refuse emergency care. If your patient is a child or mentally incompetent adult, only a parent or legal guardian can refuse care on behalf of the patient. If a patient refuses treatment or transport, you must inform him or her of the following:

- The nature of the illness or injury
- The treatment that needs to be performed
- The benefits of that treatment
- The risks of not providing that treatment
- Any alternatives to treatment
- The dangers of refusing treatment (including transport)

Remember to use words and phrases the patient can understand.

You must make sure that the patient fully understands your explanation and the consequences of refusing treatment or transport. Call advanced medical personnel to the scene as soon as possible to evaluate the patient. While waiting for the arrival of additional EMS personnel, make multiple attempts to try to convince the patient to accept care. The patient's refusal may stem from a lack of understanding because of the effects of the illness or injury, pain, or drugs or alcohol. If you have doubts about your patient's competence, contact the medical director unless the situation is life-threatening and you have begun treatment under implied consent.

Remember This!

As an Emergency Medical Responder, you cannot make a decision on your own not to treat or transport a patient. You must consult with medical direction or leave this decision to advanced medical personnel on the scene.

Know your EMS system's policy regarding a patient's refusal of care.

Some refusals of care carry a higher risk of legal liability than others. A patient may stumble, fall to the grass, and then refuse care because she is certain she is not injured. Considering the nature of the fall, the surface the patient fell on, and the lack of signs of trauma, you may agree that the patient is competent and uninjured. In situations like this, contact the medical director or call Advanced Life Support personnel to the scene to assess the patient.

A patient involved in a high-speed motor vehicle crash may also claim he has no injuries. As a trained Emergency Medical Responder, you know that, even though there are no visible injuries or signs of trauma, there may be hidden internal injuries that require transport and a physician's evaluation. If this patient chose to refuse emergency care, it would be considered a high-risk refusal because it is likely that the patient has experienced an injury.

You Should Know

Examples of High-Risk Refusals

- Abdominal pain
- Chest pain
- Severe electrical shock
- Foreign body ingestion
- Poisoning
- Pregnancy-related complaints
- Water-related incidents
- Falls > 20 feet
- Head injury
- Vehicle rollovers
- High-speed auto crashes
- Auto-pedestrian or auto-bicycle injury with major impact (> 5 mph)
- Pedestrian thrown or run over
- Motorcycle crash > 20 mph or with the separation of the rider from the bike
- Pediatric patient with a vague medical complaint

Most EMS systems require an Emergency Medical Responder to contact his or her medical oversight authority for high-risk refusals. Some systems require this contact for *any* situation in which a patient refuses treatment or transport. When contacting your medical direction authority, make sure that you clearly describe the events and your assessment. Your medical direction authority may allow the patient to refuse care. In some cases, such as those involving drugs or alcohol, medical direction may instruct you to treat and transport the patient against his or her wishes. In these situations, ask law enforcement personnel to help you. Remember to document carefully your findings and treatment.

If the patient refuses to allow his or her vital signs to be taken or will not answer your questions, make sure to document it in your report.

If you are unable to persuade the patient, parent, or guardian to receive care, you must carefully document the patient's refusal of care. Your documentation should include the patient's name, age, chief complaint, and medical history, as well as two complete sets of vital signs. You should also document details about the patient's mental status. These details include the patient's appropriate behavior, cooperation, and ability to follow instructions or commands. Document your physical examination findings and the patient's reason for refusing treatment and/or transport. The patient's signature should be obtained on a refusal form that notes the advice the patient was given, the patient's understanding of the risks of the refusal, and the patient's understanding of the possible outcome if the advice given is not followed.

The patient's signature should be witnessed by a law enforcement officer, family member, or friend. If the patient refuses to sign the form, document this and attempt to get a law enforcement officer, if possible, to sign as a witness.

You Should Know

Chief Complaint

In many cases, the patient's chief complaint will be the reason you were called to the scene. However, the patient's chief complaint may turn out to be different from the reason you were called. For example, a family member may call 9-1-1 and tell the dispatcher that the patient is complaining of difficulty breathing. When you arrive and speak directly to the patient, you may find that the patient is complaining of chest pain but has no complaint of difficulty breathing. Document the chief complaint using the patient's description of what is wrong.

Advance Directives and Do Not Resuscitate (DNR) Orders

Objective 2 ▶

Any competent patient can refuse resuscitation. What about a patient who is unresponsive? Should all unresponsive patients be treated under implied consent, regardless of the circumstances?

Objective 13 ▶

Some patients who have been diagnosed with a terminal illness may not want further medical care, even if it could prolong their life. The patient may argue that instead of prolonging her life, you are, in fact, prolonging her death. Continued pain and suffering, a loss of dignity, and artificial life support are some of the reasons a competent patient may not want treatment or resuscitation. Whatever the reason, if it is properly documented and the documentation is available to you, you must honor the patient's request. These legal documents are called **advance directives** and Do Not Resuscitate (DNR) orders. A DNR order is a type of advance directive that is used when patients wish to outline their care for when they are terminally ill. Patients often fill out advance directive forms or ask their physicians to write DNR orders. In some cases, the patient's next of kin or legal guardian will begin this process for an unresponsive or a mentally incompetent patient. When this occurs, it is generally based on what the patient would want if he were able to do this for himself.

Some patients who have a DNR do not have a terminal illness.

Objective 14 ▶

All 50 states have laws or protocols to address advance directives and DNR orders. A situation may occur in which you have doubts about the legality of the order or it does not fit within the protocols of your agency. In this case, it is best to err on the side of caution and begin resuscitation. If the patient or family members on the scene request resuscitation efforts in the presence of a questionable advance directive, immediately begin resuscitation.

If you arrive on the scene to find that a patient is not breathing, the patient has no pulse, and an advance directive is present,

Call Advanced Life Support personnel to the scene to confirm that the patient is dead.

- Make sure the form clearly identifies the person to whom the DNR applies
- Make sure the patient is the person referred to in the document
- Make sure the document you are viewing is the correct type approved by your state and local authorities

If you determine that the document is valid, follow the instructions outlined in the document.

Different types of DNR orders exist. In some states, a DNR order may specify that the patient does not want CPR or a shock to the heart if his or her heart stops beating. However, the patient may want (and expect) oxygen to be given. The patient may also want medications (given by Advanced Life Support personnel). Alternately, a DNR order may specifically state that the patient does not want any resuscitative measures, including CPR, heart shocks, and medications.

Some states recognize only a specific form of advance directive for EMS personnel, regardless of similar forms issued by private physicians or hospitals. Figure 3-1 is an example of the Prehospital Medical Care Directive form currently used in Arizona. This form is considered valid if it is printed on an orange background and includes specific wording on the form. Arizona EMS personnel are not required to accept or interpret medical care directives that do not meet these specific requirements. A person who has a valid Prehospital Medical Care Directive may wear an identifying bracelet on either the wrist or the ankle. In Arizona, the bracelet must be on an orange background and state three specific pieces of information: (1) Do Not Resuscitate, (2) the patient's name, and (3) the patient's physician. You must be familiar with the laws of your own state and the protocols of your agency and medical direction authority.

PREHOSPITAL MEDICAL CARE DIRECTIVE

IN THE EVENT OF CARDIAC OR RESPIRATORY ARREST, I REFUSE ANY RESUSCITATION MEASURES INCLUDING CARDIAC COMPRESSION, ENDOTRACHEAL INTUBATION AND OTHER ADVANCED AIRWAY MANAGEMENT, ARTIFICIAL VENTILATION, DEFIBRILLATION, ADMINISTRATION OF ADVANCED CARDIAC LIFE SUPPORT DRUGS AND RELATED EMERGENCY MEDICAL PROCEDURES.

Patient: ______________________ Date: ______________________

(Signature or mark)

Attach recent photograph here or provide all of the following information below:

(Attach photo here)

Date of Birth ______________________

Sex __________ Race ______________

Eye Color ______________________

Hair Color ______________________

Hospice Program (if any) ______________________

Name and telephone number of patient's physician ______________________

____

I have explained this form and its consequences to the signer and obtained assurance that the signer understands that death may result from any refused care listed above.

______________________ Date: ______________________

(Licensed health care provider)

I was present when this was signed (or marked). The patient then appeared to be of sound mind and free from duress.

______________________ Date: ______________________

(Witness)

FIGURE 3-1 ▲ Sample Prehospital Medical Care Directive form.

Remember This!

Although a patient may have an advance directive, you must obtain consent for medical treatment from the patient as long as she is able to make decisions about her healthcare.

Assault and Battery

Objective 7 ►

When you hear the words *assault* and *battery*, you may think of some form of physical aggression or attack by one person on another. In medicine, assault and battery are not necessarily defined as attacking or physically striking a patient. Touching a competent adult patient without his or her consent can be considered assault or battery.

There are no universal definitions of assault and battery. Each state has its own laws and definitions. In most states, **assault** is considered threatening, attempting, or causing a fear of offensive physical contact with a patient or another person. **Battery** is the unlawful touching of another person without consent. Check your local protocols and definitions concerning these terms. To protect yourself from possible legal action, clearly explain your intentions to your patient and obtain his or her consent before beginning patient care.

Abandonment

Objective 7 ►

Abandonment is terminating patient care without making sure that care will continue at the same level or higher. You can be charged with abandonment if you turn over the patient to another healthcare professional with less medical training than you have. You can also be charged with abandonment if you stop patient care when the patient still needs and desires additional care and has not expressly requested termination of care.

Stop and Think!

If a scene is unsafe, it is not abandonment if you leave the scene for your safety, with the intention of returning as soon as the scene is made safe. Responder safety comes first.

Once you have begun patient care, you must complete it to the best of your ability. Patient care may be transferred to another healthcare professional if that person accepts the patient and his or her medical qualifications are equal to or greater than yours.

Remember This!

Once you have begun patient care, you must continue to provide care until it is no longer needed or until patient care is transferred to another healthcare professional whose medical qualifications are equal to or greater than yours.

Negligence

Objective 7 ►

Negligence is a deviation from the accepted standard of care, resulting in further injury to the patient. When a healthcare professional is negligent, he or she fails to act as a reasonable, careful, similarly trained person would act under similar circumstances. Negligence is the cause of most lawsuits against EMS personnel. Four elements must be present to prove negligence: (1) there was a duty to act, (2) the healthcare professional breached that duty, (3) injury and/or damages (physical or psychological) were inflicted, and (4) the actions or inactions of the healthcare professional caused the injury and/or damage (proximate cause). A successful negligence lawsuit can result in loss of the healthcare professional's certification or licensure and financial penalties.

You Should Know

Components of Negligence

- You had a duty to act.
- You breached that duty.
- Injury and/or damages were inflicted.
- Your actions or lack of actions caused the injury and/or damage.

Duty to Act

Objective 8

The first element of negligence is a duty to act. The duty to act may be either a formal, contractual duty or an implied duty. A formal duty occurs when an EMS service has a written contract to provide services. For example, an EMS service may have a formal contract with a community that requires a response to 9-1-1 calls. An ambulance service may have a formal contract with a long-term care facility. Written contracts usually contain clauses that state when service to a patient must be provided or may be refused.

An implied duty occurs, for example, when a patient calls 9-1-1 and the dispatcher confirms that an Emergency Medical Responder will be sent. If you are the Emergency Medical Responder sent to the scene, you have an implied legal obligation (duty) to care for the patient. When you begin patient care, you have established an implied contract with the patient.

Check your EMS agency's policies and procedures regarding your obligation to provide care if you are off duty.

A legal duty to act may not exist. In some states, an off-duty Emergency Medical Responder has no legal duty to act if he or she observes or comes upon an emergency. In other states, an off-duty healthcare professional is required to stop and provide care. In some states, any citizen must stop. You must know your specific state regulations regarding the duty to act. Although a legal duty to act may not exist, a moral or an ethical duty to act may exist. You must decide if you are morally or ethically bound to provide care in emergency situations.

Making a Difference

Whether you provide care to a patient when you are on or off duty, the care you provide must be the same as another reasonable, prudent (sensible), similarly trained person would provide under similar circumstances.

Breach of Duty

Whatever the situation, you must act as a similarly trained Emergency Medical Responder would in a similar situation.

The second element that must be proved in a negligence lawsuit is that a breach of duty occurred. A healthcare professional can only perform skills and provide treatment within his or her scope of care. Performing skills or treatments outside your scope of care can lead to a breach of duty.

A breach of duty may be proved if you failed to act or you acted inappropriately. If you are dispatched to a scene to assist a patient and choose not to respond to the call, you are failing to act. If you respond to the call and act outside your scope of care or do not complete an assessment or perform all treatments indicated, you are failing to act appropriately.

Damages

The third element that must be proved in a negligence case is injury or damage done to the patient. Damages occur if the patient is injured, either physically or psychologically, by your breach of duty.

Proximate Cause

Proximate cause is established when

- Your action or inaction was either the cause of or contributed to the patient's injury
- You could reasonably foresee that your action or inaction would result in the damage

Attorneys usually use statements (testimony) from expert witnesses to prove that an Emergency Medical Responder either failed to act or acted inappropriately and that these actions or inactions were the cause of the patient's injury. Expert witnesses can include other Emergency Medical Responders, EMTs, Paramedics, nurses, and doctors.

You can protect yourself against negligence claims by

- Maintaining a professional attitude and conduct
- Providing care and treatment within your scope of care
- Maintaining mastery of your skills
- Participating in continuing education and refresher programs
- Following instructions provided by your medical oversight authority
- Following your standing orders or protocols
- Providing your patients with a consistently high standard of care
- Making sure your documentation is thorough and accurate

Confidentiality

Objective 9 ▶

The HIPAA privacy rules are very complex. Be sure to check with your EMS agency about its policies regarding patient confidentiality.

Health Insurance Portability and Accountability Act (HIPAA)

The **Health Insurance Portability and Accountability Act (HIPAA)** went into effect in 2003. This law was passed by Congress in 1996 to ensure the confidentiality of a patient's health information. HIPAA does the following:

- Provides patients with control over their health information
- Sets boundaries on the use and release of medical records
- Ensures the security of personal health information
- Establishes accountability for the use and release of medical records

Individuals who break HIPAA privacy rules face criminal and civil penalties. Some important points about HIPAA include the following:

- Patients have the right to review and copy their medical records. Patients can also request amendments and corrections to these records.
- Healthcare providers (and plans) must tell patients with whom they are sharing their information and how it is being used.

Stop and Think!

A breach of a person's health privacy can have a major impact beyond the physical health of that person. This breach can result in the loss of a job, the alienation of family and friends, the loss of health insurance, and public humiliation.

The effects of HIPAA are widespread in medicine. As an Emergency Medical Responder, you must protect and keep confidential any health-related information about your patients. You must keep confidential any medical history given to you in a patient interview. You must also keep private any findings you discover during your patient assessment and any care that you provide.

Protected Health Information (PHI)

Protected health information (PHI) is information that

- Relates to a person's physical or mental health, treatment, or payment
- Identifies the person or gives a reason to believe that the individual can be identified
- Is transmitted or maintained in *any* format, including oral statements, electronic information, written material, and photographic material

You may use and disclose the patient's protected health information for three purposes without any written consent, authorization, or other approvals from the patient. These purposes are treatment, payment, and healthcare operations. If the patient's PHI is used or disclosed for any reason other than treatment, payment, or healthcare operations, a signed authorization form must be obtained from the patient or the patient's authorized representative.

In some situations, you can disclose specific PHI without the patient's authorization. These situations require an opportunity for the patient to agree verbally or object to the disclosure of information. These situations include

- Disclosures to the patient's next-of-kin or to another person (designated by the patient) involved in the patient's healthcare
- Notification of a family member (or the patient's personal representative) of the patient's location, general condition, or death
- Disaster situations

Remember This!

Be sure to follow your agency's policies when disclosing any protected health information. If you are in doubt, contact your supervisor or ask the patient's permission before you release any information.

Persons involved in the patient's care and other contact persons include blood relatives, spouses, roommates, boyfriends and girlfriends, domestic partners, neighbors, and colleagues. In these situations, disclose only the minimum amount of information necessary. The information you share should be directly related to the person's involvement with the patient's healthcare.

If the patient is injured or in cases of an emergency, you may use your professional judgment to decide if sharing PHI is in the patient's best interest. For example, you may tell your patient's relatives or others involved in the patient's care that he or she may have experienced a heart attack. You may also provide updates on the patient's condition. In these situations, reveal only the PHI that is directly relevant to the person's involvement with the patient's healthcare.

The patient's consent, authorization, or opportunity to agree or object to the release of PHI is not required in some situations. Examples of these situations include the following:

- Situations in which you are required by law to provide this information
- Public health activities, such as injury/disease control and prevention
- Situations involving victims of abuse, neglect, or domestic violence
- Judicial and administrative proceedings
- Specific law enforcement situations
- Situations in which you wish to avoid a serious threat to health or safety

Accidentally revealing PHI may occur when caring for a patient. Accidental disclosures usually occur during a radio or face-to-face conversation between healthcare professionals. You may freely discuss all aspects of your patient's medical condition, the treatment you gave, and any of the patient's health information you have with others involved in the patient's medical care. However, when discussing patient information with another healthcare professional, take a moment to look around you. Be sensitive to your level of voice. Make sure that persons who do not need to know this information are not able to hear what is said.

An accidental disclosure may also occur when information about a patient is left out in the open for others to access or see. For example, a prehospital care report may be left on a desk or may be visible on a computer screen when you leave to respond to another call. You must maintain the confidence and security of all material you create or use that contains patient care information. Prehospital care reports should not be left in open bins or on desktops or other surfaces. Store them in safe and secure areas. When using a computer, be aware of those who may be able to view the monitor screen. Take simple steps to shield the screen from unauthorized persons.

Special Situations

Medical Identification Devices

You may respond to a call and find the patient wearing medical identification. This identification device may be in the form of a bracelet, a necklace, or an identification card. Medical identification is used to alert healthcare personnel to a patient's particular medical condition. For example, the patient may have diabetes, epilepsy, a heart condition, or a specific allergy. You must consider this information while performing your assessment and patient interview.

Remember This!

Even though the patient is wearing a medical identification device, you must always perform a thorough patient assessment. The reason you were called may be completely different from the condition described by the medical identification device the patient is wearing or carrying.

Crime Scenes

Objective 10 ▶

During your career as an Emergency Medical Responder, you may be dispatched to a crime scene. Your dispatcher should notify you of the potential crime scene at the time you are sent to the call. You may be required to stage (remain at a safe distance) and wait for an "all clear" from law enforcement personnel before entering the scene and providing patient care. Even after law enforcement

A crime scene is the responsibility of law enforcement personnel. As an Emergency Medical Responder, your responsibilities are to ensure your own safety and then provide care for the patient.

personnel have declared the scene safe to enter, you must always assess the scene yourself to ensure your safety. Once you are certain the scene is safe, your first priority is patient care.

Making a Difference

It is important to understand your obligations in providing patient care and balancing your other responsibilities on the scene. For example, a law enforcement officer may need to delay your treatment of patients until a crime scene has been secured.

Crime scenes demand certain actions and responsibilities from medical personnel. For example, you should protect potential evidence by leaving intact any holes in clothing from bullets or stab wounds. Do not disturb any item at the scene unless emergency care requires it. You should always be alert and observe and document anything unusual on a call. These actions are especially important at a crime scene. You may be called to testify in court about what you observed at the scene.

Consider talking with law enforcement personnel on the scene to discuss various crime scene issues:

- Possible victim and suspect statements
- Evidence you observe
- Shoe prints collected from Emergency Medical Responders for comparison
- The names of all personnel on the scene, including Emergency Medical Responders, fire personnel, and so on

Objective 11 ▶

Generally, you will report special situations to law enforcement or emergency department staff.

Special Reporting Requirements

State or local laws and regulations or agency protocols require you to report certain situations or conditions that you know or suspect have occurred. For example, you are required to report known or suspected abuse of a child, an elderly person, and, in some locations, a spouse. You must also report injuries that may have occurred while committing a crime, such as gunshot and knife wounds. EMS agencies require you to report exposure to an infectious disease. Because state and local reporting requirements vary, you must learn the requirements for your area and act accordingly.

Organ Donation

An organ donor is a person who has signed a legal document to donate his or her organs in the event of his or her death. This document may be an organ donor card that the patient carries. Alternately, the patient may have indicated an intent to be a donor on his or her driver's license. Family members may also tell you that the patient is an organ donor. A patient who is a potential organ donor should not be treated differently than any other patient who requires your care. Your responsibilities include

- Providing any necessary emergency care
- Notifying EMS or hospital personnel that the patient is a potential organ donor when you transfer patient care

Documentation

Objective 12 ▶

Pay attention to time intervals when documenting.

Every organization that employs healthcare professionals has documentation requirements. As an Emergency Medical Responder, you may or may not be required to complete a prehospital care report (PCR). Most EMS agencies have a documentation form, which you must complete for each patient you encounter. It is important to document information in an organized, systematic manner.

The Uses of a Prehospital Care Report

A prehospital care report has many uses. The medical uses of a PCR include helping ensure continued patient care. The PCR may be the only source of information that hospital personnel can refer to later. This report may include important information about the scene, the patient's condition on arrival at the scene, the emergency medical care provided or attempted, and any changes in the patient's condition.

The PCR is a legal document and is considered an official record of the care provided by EMS personnel. The PCR may be used in legal proceedings. In general, the person who completed the form must go to court with the form. In many cases, the PCR may be your only reference source about a patient encounter.

The PCR may be used for billing purposes and for collecting agency or service statistics. It may also be used for educational purposes to show proper documentation and how to handle unusual calls. Data obtained from the PCR may be collected and used for research purposes. For example, the PCR may be used to determine how often specific patient care procedures are performed. It may also be used to determine continuing education needs.

The PCR is often used in quality management programs. The PCR is reviewed to assess how well information is documented, compliance with local rules and regulations, and the appropriateness of the medical care provided.

You Should Know

The Uses of a Prehospital Care Report

- Medical use (to ensure continued patient care)
- Legal record
- Administrative use (billing as well as agency/service statistics)
- Education
- Research (data collection)
- Quality management

Documentation Guidelines

Providing false information on the PCR may lead to your being suspended, having your certification revoked, and experiencing other legal action.

When documenting a patient encounter, you must be careful to record information honestly and accurately. It is not appropriate to record your opinion or impression about a patient or situation. You must document the facts. For example, write down important things that you observe at the scene, such as empty pill bottles, the presence of a suicide note, or weapons. Document your assessment findings, the emergency care provided to the patient, and the patient's response to your care. If you contacted medical direction and were given instructions, be sure to write down the instructions you were given and the results of carrying out those instructions.

On The Scene

Wrap-Up

As the Paramedics arrive on the scene, the patient vomits and then says, "I don't feel so good; maybe I should go to the hospital." You quickly cut away his jeans, being careful to avoid the area the bullet has penetrated. As you are controlling the bleeding, he admits that his girlfriend shot him during an argument. The paramedic in charge asks you to set up an IV for him. You quickly explain that you are not trained to perform that skill.

A few hours later, a reporter from the local news station calls to check on the patient and find out what happened. You politely tell the reporter that you are not able to share any information about the patient care due to privacy laws. The reporter is not happy with your answer and says she will call the hospital to get the information she wants. ■

Sum It Up

- The *scope of care* (also called the scope of practice) includes the emergency care and skills an Emergency Medical Responder is allowed and expected to perform. These duties are set by state laws and regulations. As an Emergency Medical Responder, you have a legal duty to ensure the well-being of your patients by providing necessary medical care. Your ethical responsibilities include treating all patients with respect and giving each patient the best care you are capable of giving. You must also determine if the patient is competent (that is, if he or she can understand the questions you ask and the results of the decisions the patient makes about his or her care).
- A competent patient must give you his or her *consent* (permission) before you can provide emergency care. *Expressed consent* is one in which a patient gives specific permission for care and transport to be provided. Expressed consent may be given verbally, in writing, or nonverbally. *Implied consent* is consent assumed from a patient requiring emergency care who is mentally, physically, or emotionally unable to provide expressed consent. Implied consent is based on the assumption that the patient would consent to lifesaving treatment if he or she were able to do so.
- Patients have the right to refuse care and transport. As an Emergency Medical Responder, you must make sure that the patient fully understands your explanation and the consequences of refusing treatment or transport. Call advanced medical personnel to the scene as soon as possible to evaluate the patient. In high-risk situations in which the patient's injuries may not be obvious, you must contact the medical director or call Advanced Life Support personnel to the scene to assess the patient.
- An *advance directive* is a form filled out by the patient. It outlines patients' wishes for care if they are not able to express them. A *Do Not Resuscitate (DNR) order* is written by a physician and details patients' wishes for care when they are terminally ill.
- *Assault* is considered threatening, attempting, or causing a fear of offensive physical contact with a patient or another person. *Battery* is the unlawful touching of another person without consent. Because each state has its own definitions of assault and battery, you should check your local protocols concerning these terms. To protect yourself from possible legal action, clearly explain your intentions to your patient and obtain his or her consent before beginning patient care.

- *Abandonment* is terminating patient care without making sure that care will continue at the same level or higher. You can also be charged with abandonment if you stop patient care when the patient still needs and desires additional care.
- When a healthcare professional is negligent, he or she fails to act as a reasonable, careful, similarly trained person would act under similar circumstances. *Negligence* includes the following four elements: (1) the duty to act, (2) a breach of that duty, (3) injury or damages (physical or psychological) that result, and (4) proximate cause (the actions or inactions of the healthcare professional that caused the injury or damages).
- A medical identification device is used to alert healthcare personnel to a patient's particular medical condition. This identification device may be in the form of a bracelet, a necklace, or an identification card.
- If you are sent to a crime scene, you must wait for law enforcement personnel to declare that the scene is safe to enter. After you are certain the scene is safe and have ensured your safety, your first priority is patient care. You should be alert and document anything unusual on the call.
- An organ donor is a person who has signed a legal document to donate his or her organs in the event of his or her death. The patient may have an organ donor card or may have indicated his or her intent to be a donor on his or her driver's license.
- A *prehospital care report (PCR)* is a legal document that is used in a number of ways: (1) for medical uses (to ensure continued patient care), (2) as a legal record, (3) for administrative uses (billing as well as agency/service statistics), (4) for education, and (5) for research (data collection).

▶ Tracking Your Progress

After reading this chapter, can you	**Page Reference**	**Objective Met?**
• Define the Emergency Medical Responder scope of care?	72–73	☐
• Discuss the importance of Do Not Resuscitate [DNR] (advance directives) and local or state provisions regarding EMS application?	79	☐
• Define consent and discuss the methods of obtaining consent?	75–77	☐
• Differentiate between expressed and implied consent?	76–77	☐
• Explain the role of consent of minors in providing care?	76–77	☐
• Discuss the implications for the Emergency Medical Responder in patient refusal of transport?	77–78	☐
• Discuss the issues of abandonment, negligence, and battery and their implications in your role as an Emergency Medical Responder?	81–82	☐
• State the conditions necessary for you to have a duty to act?	82–83	☐
• Explain the importance, necessity, and legality of patient confidentiality?	83–85	☐
• List the actions that you should take to assist in the preservation of a crime scene?	85–86	☐
• State the conditions that require you to notify local law enforcement officials?	86	☐
• Discuss issues concerning the fundamental components of documentation?	87	☐
• Explain the rationale for the needs, benefits, and usage of advance directives?	79	☐
• Explain the rationale for the concept of varying degrees of DNR?	79	☐

Chapter Quiz

Multiple Choice

In the space provided, identify the letter of the choice that best completes each statement or answers each question.

_____ **1.** Terminating patient care without making sure that care will continue at the same level or higher is called

a. breach of duty.
b. abandonment.
c. damages.
d. failure to act.

_____ **2.** You are dispatched to a private residence for an "ill man." You arrive to find a 40-year-old man unresponsive on the living room floor. The patient's 14-year-old daughter states she arrived home a few minutes ago and found her father in this condition. She immediately called 9-1-1 and then called her mother, who is at work. Your general impression is that the patient appears to be unresponsive. You can see that he is breathing. There are no obvious signs of trauma. Select the *correct* statement about this situation.

a. You cannot provide care for this patient if he is unable to give you verbal consent to treat him.
b. You can provide care for this patient based on the child's request that you provide care to her father.
c. You may provide care for this patient using implied consent.
d. You may provide care for this patient only if the medical director authorizes you to do so.

_____ **3.** When assessing the patient in question 2 and attempting to learn the reason he is unresponsive, you should

a. immediately contact medical direction for any information about the patient in hospital records.
b. see if you can locate a neighbor who might have information that will help you.
c. attempt to locate the patient's wife to find out the patient's medical history.
d. look for a medical identification device; look in the immediate area for signs of a fall, drug overdose, or alcohol use; and ask the patient's daughter about the patient's medical history.

True or False

Decide whether each statement is true or false. In the space provided, write T for true or F for false.

_____ **4.** The emergency care and skills an Emergency Medical Responder is legally allowed and expected to perform are set by state laws and regulations.

_____ **5.** Individuals who violate rules regarding a patient's protected health information may face criminal and civil penalties.

_____ **6.** Implied consent requires that the patient be of legal age and able to understand the consequences of his or her decision.

_____ **7.** You must have written consent from the patient to discuss the patient's health information with other healthcare professionals involved in the medical care of the patient.

_____ **8.** A potential organ donor should not be treated differently than any other patient who requires your care.

Matching

Match the key terms in the left column with the definitions in the right column by placing the letter of each correct answer in the space provided.

_____ **9.** Assault

_____ **10.** Advance directive

_____ **11.** Negligence

_____ **12.** Abandonment

_____ **13.** Battery

_____ **14.** Implied consent

_____ **15.** Expressed consent

_____ **16.** Duty to act

a. Unlawful touching of another person without consent

b. Terminating care of a patient without ensuring that care will continue at the same level or higher

c. Consent in which a patient gives specific authorization for care and transport

d. Formal contract or implied legal obligation to provide care to a patient requesting services

e. Threatening, attempting, or causing fear of offensive physical contact with a patient or another individual

f. Deviation from the accepted standard of care, resulting in further injury to the patient

g. Consent based on the assumption that the patient would consent to lifesaving interventions if he or she were able to do so

h. Legal document that specifies a person's healthcare wishes when the person becomes unable to make decisions for him- or herself

Short Answer

Answer each question in the space provided.

17. When can patient care be transferred to another healthcare professional?

____

____

____

18. List the four elements that must be proved in a negligence case.

1. ______________________________

2. ______________________________

3. ______________________________

4. ______________________________

19. A 48-year-old man is involved in a high-speed motor vehicle crash. The patient was not restrained. He is alert and oriented to person, place, time, and event. Obvious injuries include minor bleeding from a cut on his forehead and a large bruise on his chest. The patient is refusing treatment and transport to the hospital. Advanced Life Support personnel are en route to the scene. What information must you give the patient regarding his refusing care?

____

____

____

20. Briefly explain how you should obtain expressed consent from a patient.

____

____

____

Sentence Completion

In the blanks provided, write the words that best complete each sentence.

21. ______________ ______________ ______________ consists of the emergency care and skills an Emergency Medical Responder is legally allowed and expected to perform when necessary.

22. A written document that specifies a person's healthcare wishes when he or she becomes unable to make decisions for him- or herself is known as a(n) ______________ ______________.

CHAPTER

4 The Human Body

By the end of this chapter, you should be able to

Knowledge Objectives ▶

1. Describe the anatomy and function of the respiratory system.
2. Describe the anatomy and function of the circulatory system.
3. Describe the anatomy and function of the musculoskeletal system.
4. Describe the components and function of the nervous system.

Attitude Objectives ▶ There are no attitude objectives identified for this lesson.

Skill Objectives ▶ There are no skill objectives identified for this lesson.

On The Scene

It has already been a tough assignment for your unit on this security detail. Then, just after lunch, while patrolling the perimeter of your area, you hear a blast and the sound of glass breaking. An initial team goes to investigate and then you are sent in to check out the one officer injured by the explosion. Your patient is lying on the ground, awake and moaning. He was struck by flying debris and thrown approximately 12 feet from an armored carrier during the blast.

His spine position is maintained while you quickly perform your initial assessment. He has strong radial and carotid pulses and you find no immediate life threats. As you wait for the EVAC unit, you continue your head-to-toe assessment. He has several open cuts superior to his right eyebrow. His face is tender over the mandible area and he is having trouble speaking because of the pain. There is tenderness to the cervical spine area. You note bruising on his chest lateral to his right nipple and his ribs are tender. He jumps with pain when you palpate over his sternum but says he is not having any difficulty breathing. When you palpate the left upper quadrant of his abdomen, the patient pushes your hand away. There is deformity in the area of his femur. Luckily, you can feel a strong dorsalis pedis pulse in both feet, and normal movement and sensation is present distal to the injury. ■

THINK ABOUT IT

As you read this chapter, think about the following questions:

- Based on your physical exam, what underlying structures may be injured?
- Which injuries could lead to trouble with breathing or circulation?
- Where are the mandible, the cervical spine, the sternum, and the femur located?
- Where are the carotid, radial, and dorsalis pedis pulses found?

Introduction

Understanding the Structure and Function of the Body

Anatomy is the study of the structure of an organism, such as the human body. **Physiology** is the study of the normal functions of an organism, such as the human body. As an Emergency Medical Responder, you must be familiar with the structure and function of the human body so that you can better assess an injured or ill patient. For example, if a patient were stabbed in the right upper area of the abdomen and you had an understanding of anatomy and physiology, you would then know the organs possibly affected. You would understand their function in the body and could anticipate possible complications. The knife blade could have injured the liver, gallbladder, intestines, blood vessels, diaphragm, lungs, and kidneys, depending on the length of the blade and the direction of the stab (for example, whether it was upward, straight, or downward). Your understanding of the human body is essential in order to give proper emergency care.

Body Systems

Cells are the basic units of all living tissue.

The human body is made up of billions of **cells,** the basic building blocks of the body. Cells that cluster together to perform a specialized function are called **tissues.** For example, nervous tissue is specialized to receive and conduct electrical signals over long distances in the body. Muscle tissue is a group of similar cells that can contract, usually in response to an electrical signal from a nerve. An **organ** is made up of at least two types of tissue that work together to perform a particular function. Examples of organs are the brain, stomach, and liver. **Vital organs** are organs, such as the brain, heart, and lungs, that are essential for life. An **organ system** (also called a body system) is made up of tissues and organs that work together to perform a common function. The human body consists of 10 major organ systems:

- Circulatory
- Digestive
- Endocrine
- Integumentary
- Muscular
- Nervous
- Reproductive
- Respiratory
- Skeletal
- Urinary

Homeostasis

Homeostasis is also called a "steady state." Illness and injury alter this sensitive internal balance.

Organ systems rely on each other to maintain a constant internal environment (**homeostasis**) and perform the required functions of the entire body. The human body has various "check and balance" systems to maintain homeostasis.

For example, the body's organ systems require a relatively constant temperature to function properly. If the body's temperature is too low, the muscles shiver to produce heat. If the body's temperature is too high, blood vessels near the skin's surface dilate (expand). This dilation brings more blood to the body surface and allows heat to be passed off into the environment. Sweating is another means of cooling the body through evaporation.

The balanced state that the body requires to function properly is very sensitive to changes caused by illness or injury.

When an organ system does not function properly due to illness or injury, other body functions are affected. For example, the circulatory and respiratory systems need the kidneys to perform their function in order for the body to maintain its balanced environment. If the kidneys fail to produce urine, the circulatory system will retain too much fluid within the bloodstream. This will cause a backup of fluid into the lungs and affect the patient's breathing, disrupting the body's internal balance.

Remember This!

Remember that, as an Emergency Medical Responder, you are a healthcare professional. Healthcare professionals use medical terms to communicate information to other healthcare professionals about a patient's illness or injury. To relay correctly what you are seeing and what the patient is saying in your written and verbal reports, you must know medical terms and their meanings.

Body Positions and Directional Terms

Medical terms are used to convey to other healthcare professionals the location of a patient's injury or symptoms, so that further care can be given. Directions are applied to the body when it is in the **anatomical position.** In the anatomical position, a person is standing, arms to the sides with the palms turned forward, feet close together and pointed forward, the head pointed forward, and the eyes open (Figure 4-1). The following are definitions and examples of common directional terms:

- *Superior/inferior.* **Superior** means above or in a higher position than another portion of the body. The head is the most superior part of the body. The neck is superior to the chest because it is closer to the head. **Inferior** means in a position lower than another. The soles of the feet are the most inferior part of the body. The knees are inferior to the pelvis because they are closer to the feet.
- *Anterior/posterior.* **Anterior,** or ventral, represents the front portion of the body or body part. The heart is anterior to the spine. **Posterior,** or dorsal, is the back side of the body or body part. The spine is posterior to the heart.

These terms are most often used when referring to an extremity (arm or leg).

- *Proximal/distal.* **Proximal** means closer to the midline, or center area, of the body. When this term is used to reference an extremity, it means nearer to the point of attachment to the body. The knees are proximal to the toes. **Distal** means farthest from the midline, or center area, of the body. With reference to an extremity, it means farthest from the point of attachment to the body. The elbow is distal to the shoulder.
- *Midline.* The **midline** is an imaginary line down the center of the body that divides the body into right and left sides. Using the midline as a reference point will assist in describing whether an injury is **lateral** (toward the side) or **medial** (toward the midline). The breastbone (sternum) is medial to the left nipple. The armpit (axilla) is lateral to the sternum.

FIGURE 4-1 ▶ The anatomical position and directional terms. (a) Front (anterior) view. (b) Back (posterior) view.

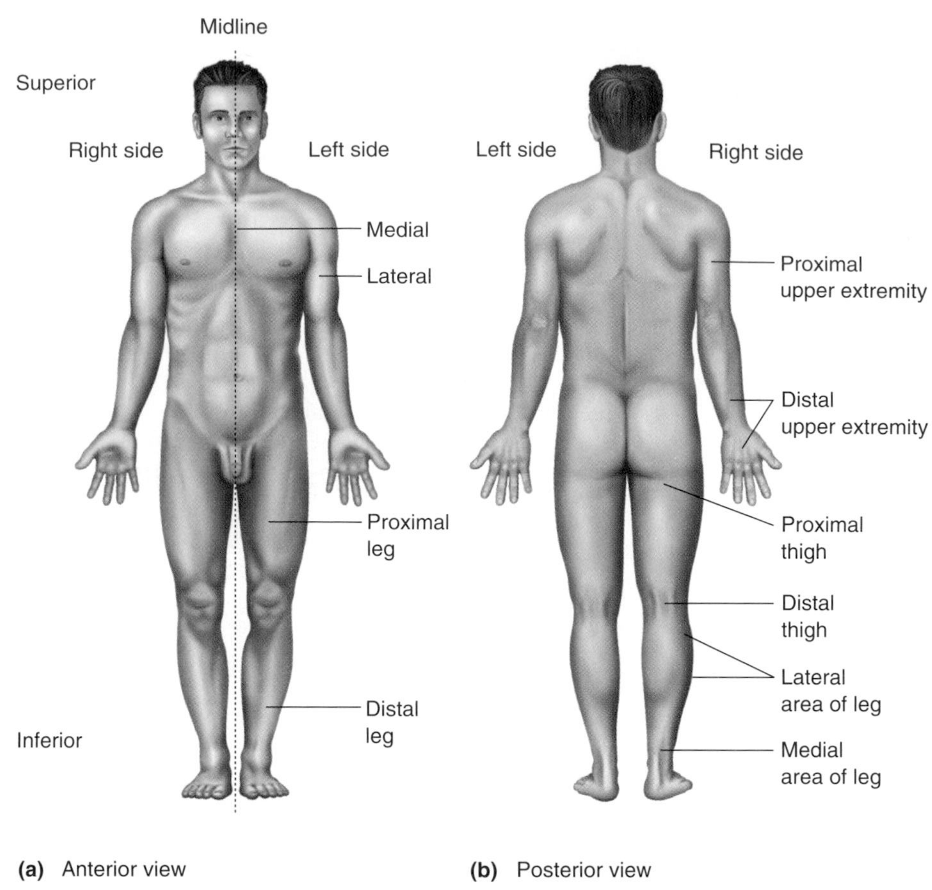

Remember This!

- When you look at a patient in the anatomical position, describe the patient's injuries from the patient's perspective. In other words, *right* and *left* always refer to the *patient's* right and left.
- If you forget the proper medical term for something, use a plain, understandable description instead. For example, if you forget that the back is posterior, then refer to the "back of the patient." Do not make up terms—it could be embarrassing.

It is important to use these terms properly, so that you can describe the position in which the patient is found and transported.

Ill and injured patients are found in many positions. When a person is standing upright, he is said to be **erect.** A person lying flat on his back (face up) is said to be in a **supine** position. A person lying face down and flat is in a **prone** position. If a person is found on his side, he is in a **lateral recumbent position.** If he is found on his left side, he is in a left lateral recumbent position. If he is on his right side, he is in a right lateral recumbent position.

As an Emergency Medical Responder, you may choose to place a patient in a specific position based on the patient's condition. For example, a patient with signs of shock may be placed in the shock position. The **shock position** is lying on the back with the feet elevated approximately 8–12 inches. In the **Trendelenburg position,** the patient is lying on her back with the head of the bed lowered and her feet raised in a straight incline. **Fowler's position** is lying on the back with the upper body elevated at a 45- to 60-degree angle. A patient who is short of breath is often placed in this position.

Body Cavities

A **body cavity** is a hollow space in the body that contains internal organs (Figure 4-2). The **cranial cavity** is located in the head. It contains the brain and is protected by the skull. The **spinal cavity** extends from the bottom of the skull to the lower back. It contains the spinal cord and is protected by the vertebral (spinal) column. The brain and spinal cord make up the central nervous system. This system allows the body to carry electrical signals from the body's organ systems to the brain and spinal cord, as well as to the various organ systems of the body.

The **thoracic (chest) cavity** is located below the neck and above the diaphragm and is protected by the rib cage. The thoracic cavity contains the heart, major blood vessels, and the lungs. The heart is surrounded by another cavity, the **pericardial cavity.** The lungs are surrounded by the **pleural cavities.** The right lung is located in the right pleural cavity; the left lung is located in the left pleural cavity.

The abdominal and pelvic cavities are often called the abdominopelvic cavity.

The **abdominal cavity** is located below the diaphragm and above the pelvis. The abdominal cavity contains the stomach, intestines, liver, gallbladder, pancreas, and spleen. Although not separated by any kind of wall, the area below the abdominal cavity is called the **pelvic cavity.** The pelvic cavity contains the urinary bladder, part of the large intestine, and reproductive organs.

Knowing the organs found within each of the four quadrants will help you describe the location of the injury or the symptoms of a sick or injured patient.

To make things easier when identifying the abdominal organs and the location of pain or injury, the abdominal cavity is divided into four quadrants (Figure 4-3). These quadrants are created by drawing an imaginary line that intersects with the midline through the navel (umbilicus). The right upper quadrant (RUQ) contains the liver, gallbladder, portions of the stomach, the right kidney, and major blood vessels. The left upper quadrant (LUQ) contains the stomach, spleen, pancreas, and left kidney. The right lower quadrant (RLQ) contains the appendix. The left lower quadrant (LLQ), along with the other three quadrants, contains the intestines. In females, the right and left lower quadrants contain the ovaries and fallopian tubes. The uterus is in the midline above (superior to) the pelvis and just behind (posterior to) the bladder.

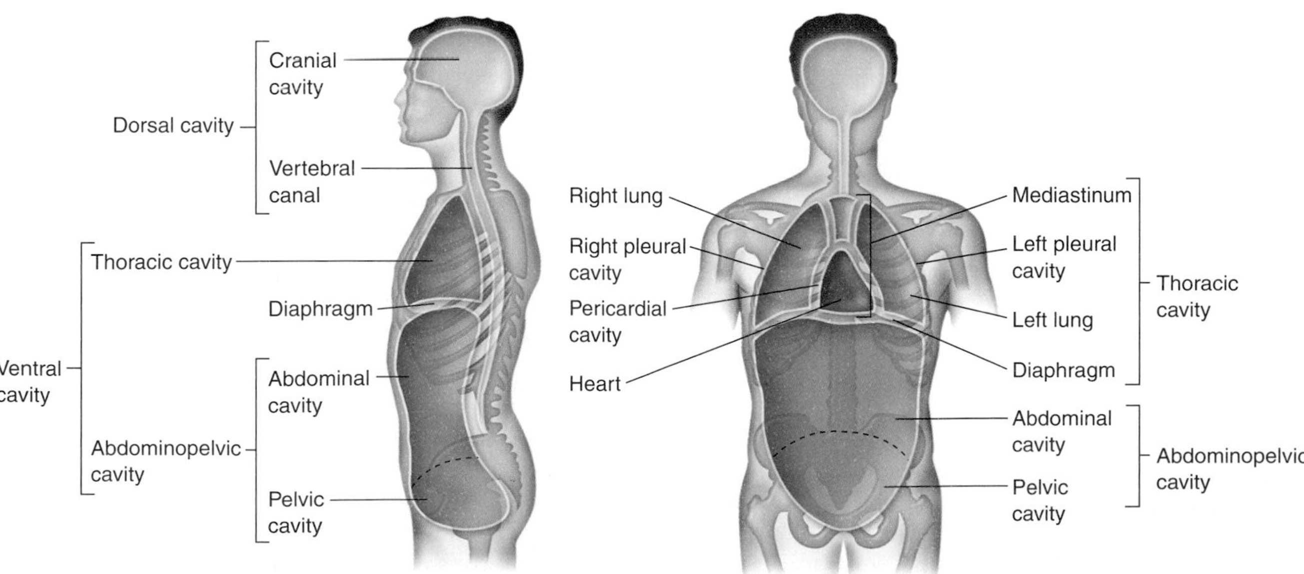

FIGURE 4-2 ▲ Body cavities.

FIGURE 4-3 ► The abdominal area is divided into four quadrants.

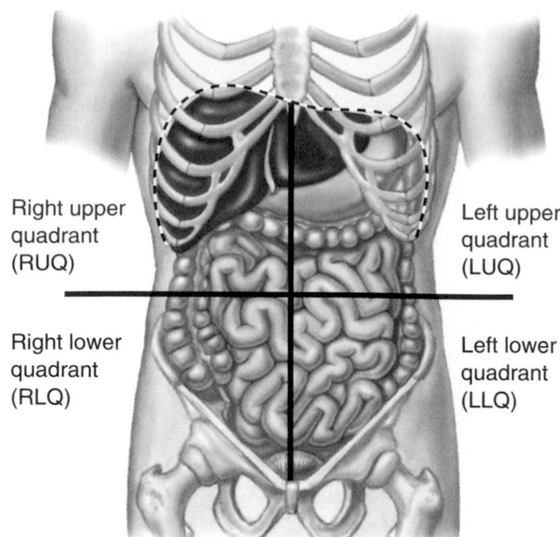

The Musculoskeletal System

Objective 3 ►

The musculoskeletal system gives the human body its shape and ability to move, and it protects the major organs of the body. It consists of the skeletal system (bones) and the muscular system (muscles).

The Skeletal System

The skeletal system consists of 206 bones of various types. Bones store minerals for the body, such as calcium and phosphorus. Many bones have a hollow cavity, which contains a substance called bone marrow. Bone marrow produces the body's blood cells—the red blood cells, white blood cells, and platelets.

The skeletal system is divided into two groups of bones. The **axial skeleton** is the part of the skeleton that includes the skull, spinal column, sternum, and ribs. The **appendicular skeleton** is made up of the upper and lower extremities (arms and legs), the shoulder girdle, and the pelvic girdle (Figures 4-4 and 4-5). The **shoulder girdle** is the bony arch formed by the collarbones (clavicles) and shoulder blades (scapulae). The **pelvic girdle** is made up of bones that enclose and protect the organs of the pelvic cavity. It provides a point of attachment for the lower extremities and the major muscles of the trunk. It also supports the weight of the upper body.

Bones are classified by their shape and size—long, short, flat, and irregular (Figure 4-6). Long bones are the relatively cylindrical bones of the upper and lower extremities, such as the humerus of the upper arm. Short bones can be found in the carpal bones of the hand and the tarsal bones of the feet. The shoulder blade (scapula) is an example of a flat bone. The vertebrae are examples of irregular bones.

The Skull

The mandible is the largest and strongest bone of the face and is the only movable bone of the face.

The skull is made up of 29 bones (Figure 4-7). The most important bones of the skull are the cranial bones, which house and protect the brain; the upper jaw (maxilla); the lower jaw (mandible); and the cheekbones (zygomatic bones). The skull is supported by the neck, which receives its strength from the vertebrae. Attached to the skull are many facial bones. Attached to these

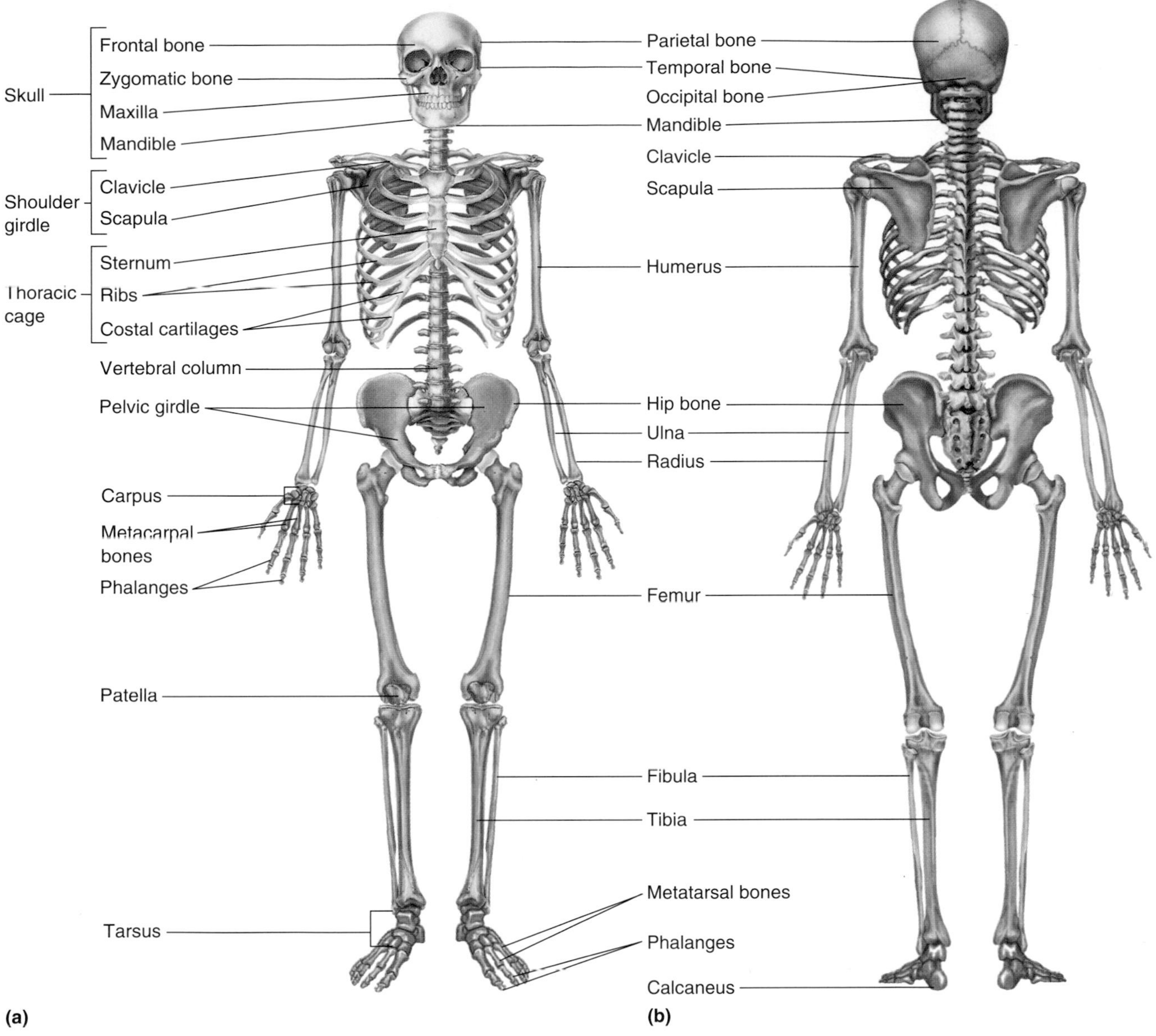

FIGURE 4-4 ▲ The adult skeleton. (a) Anterior view. (b) Posterior view. The appendicular skeleton is shaded in blue; the rest of the skeleton is the axial skeleton.

bones are muscles that allow eye movements and facia l expressions. These muscles also allow the tongue to be held in position so that the airway remains open. Without these important mouth muscles, a person would not be able to swallow food or fluids without gagging and choking.

The Spine

The spine (vertebral column) is made up of 32–33 vertebrae, which are arranged in regions (Figure 4-8 and Table 4-1). The vertebrae of each region have a distinctive shape. The vertebral column is made up of 7 cervical (neck) vertebrae, 12 thoracic vertebrae, 5 lumbar vertebrae, 5 fused vertebrae that form the sacrum, and 3–4 fused vertebrae that form the coccyx (tailbone). The vertebral column provides rigidity to the body while allowing movement. It also encloses and protects the spinal cord. It extends from the base of the skull to the coccyx.

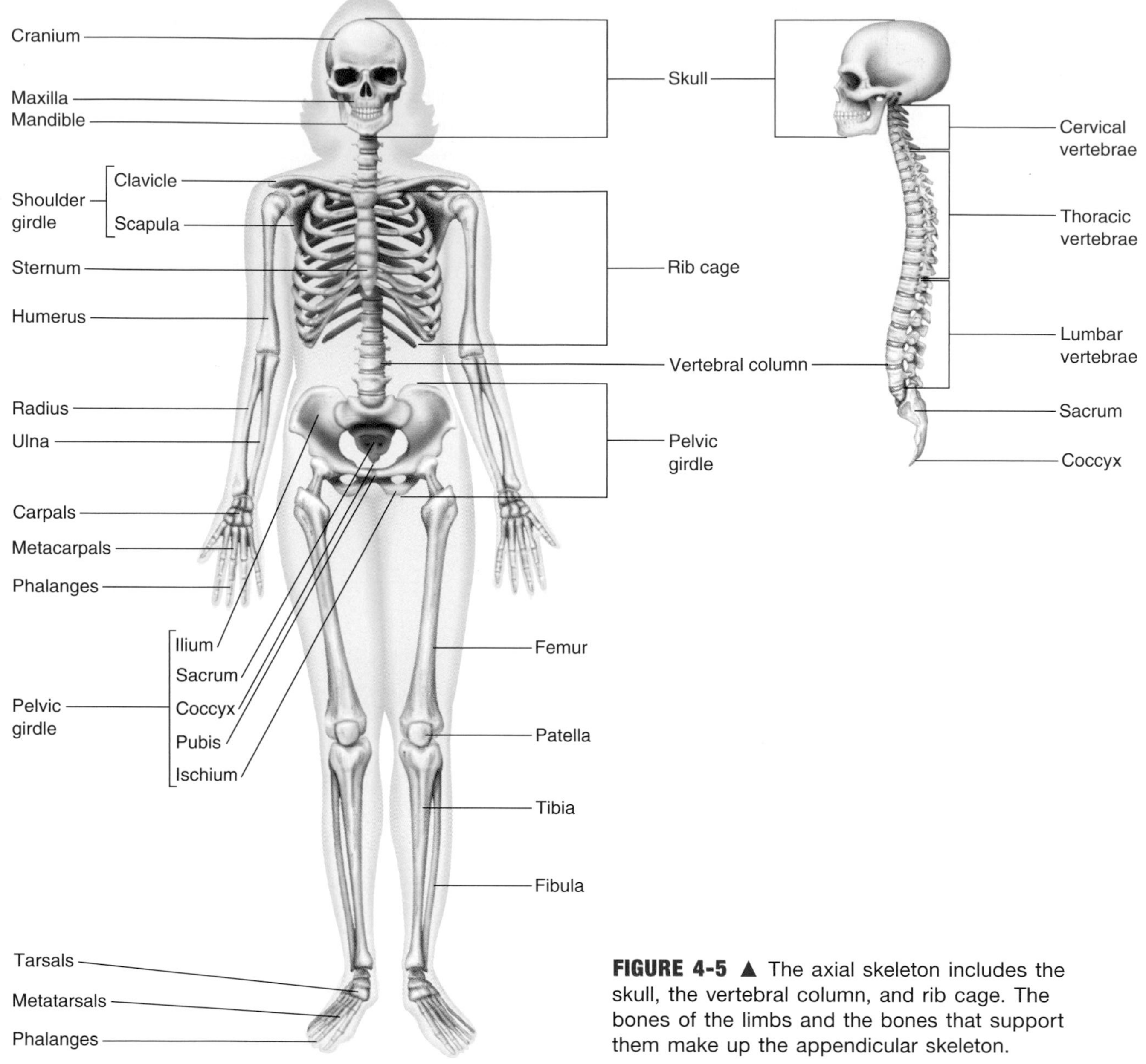

FIGURE 4-5 ▲ The axial skeleton includes the skull, the vertebral column, and rib cage. The bones of the limbs and the bones that support them make up the appendicular skeleton.

> On the scene of an emergency, rescuers often refer to the cervical spine as the *c-spine.*

The 7 cervical vertebrae of the neck hold up the head and allow it to rotate left and right as well as backward, forward, and side to side. The first cervical vertebra, the atlas, supports the skull. The second cervical vertebra is called the axis. The 12 thoracic vertebrae form the upper back and posterior portion of the thorax. Below the thoracic vertebrae are 5 lumbar vertebrae. The lumbar vertebrae are the largest and strongest of the vertebrae, because they carry the bulk of the body's weight. Below the lumbar vertebrae are 5 fused vertebrae, which form the sacrum (the back wall of the pelvis), and eventually attach to the 3 or 4 fused vertebrae that form the coccyx. The fused sacral vertebrae are connected to the pelvis, which attaches the lower appendicular skeleton to the axial skeleton.

FIGURE 4-6 ► Bones are classified by their shape and size.

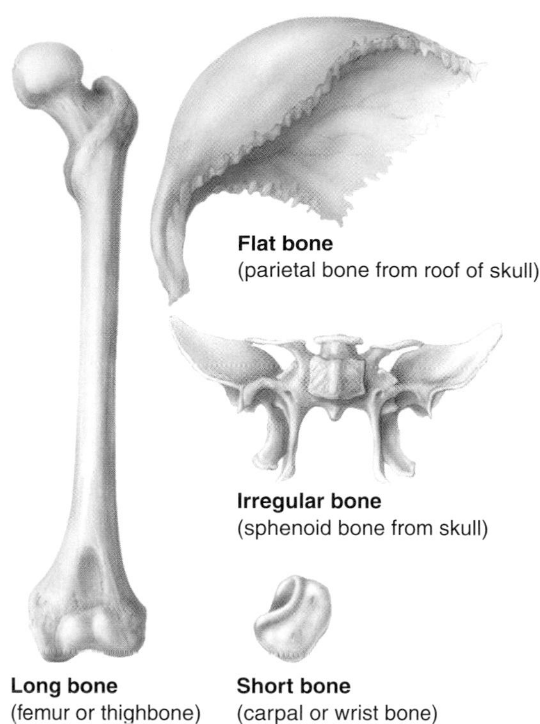

FIGURE 4-7 ► The anterior view of the skull.

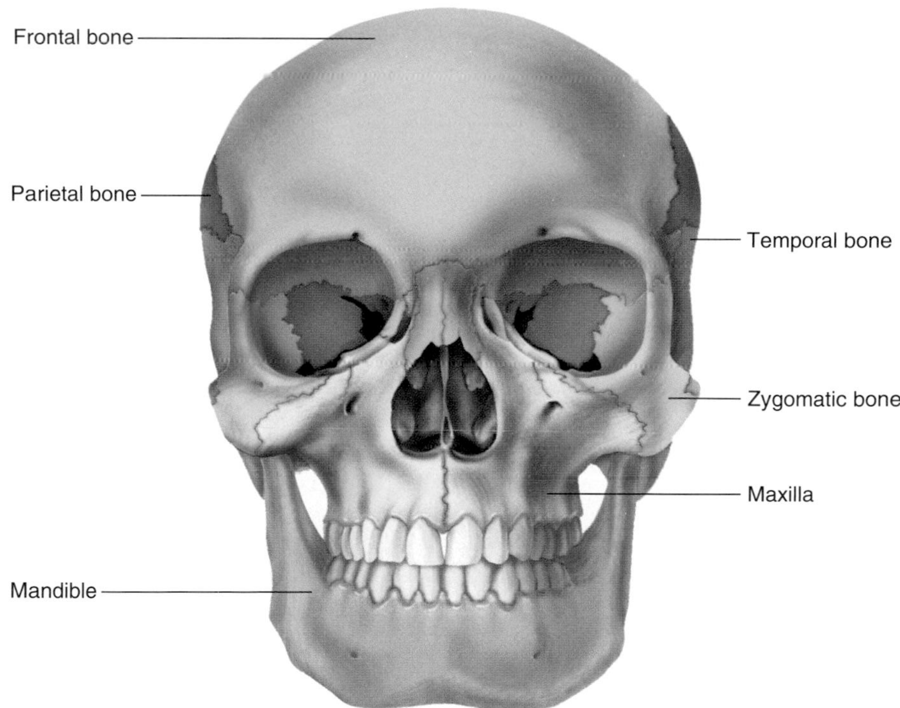

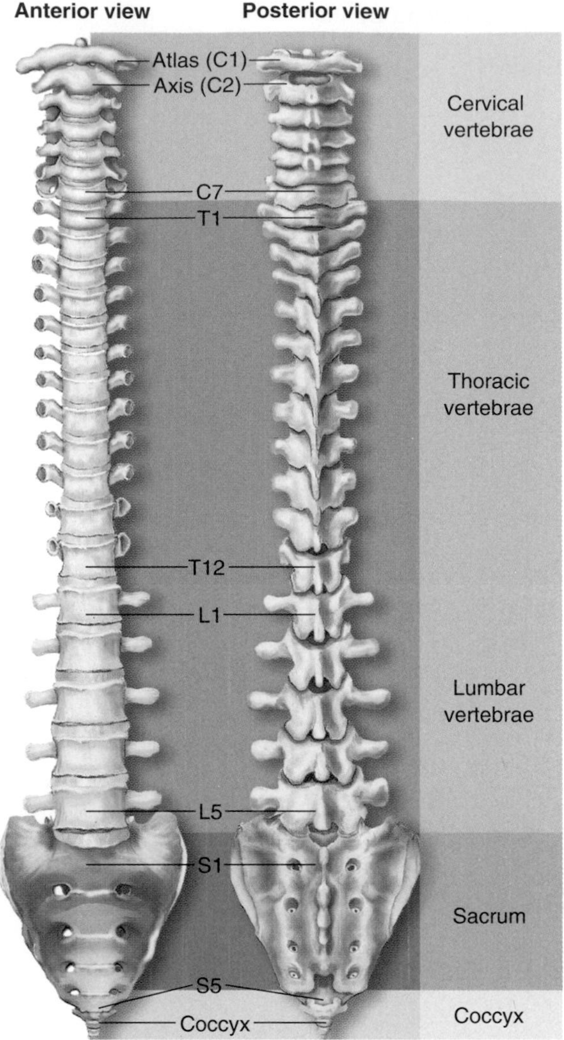

FIGURE 4-8 ▶ The vertebral column (spine), anterior and posterior views.

You Should Know

The adult spinal cord is approximately 16–18 inches long and approximately 3/4 inch in diameter in the midthorax. The spinal cord is shorter than the bony vertebral column. It extends down to only about the second lumbar vertebra. In the cervical and thoracic regions of the vertebral column, the spinal cord lies very close to the walls of the vertebrae. The spinal cord is at risk for injury in these areas.

TABLE 4-1 Regions of the Spinal Column

Region	Number of Vertebrae
Cervical spine (neck)	7
Thoracic spine (chest, upper back)	12
Lumbar spine (lower back)	5
Sacrum	5 (fused)
Coccyx	3–4 (fused)

FIGURE 4-9 ► The vertebral column (spine), with detail of the spinal cord and discs.

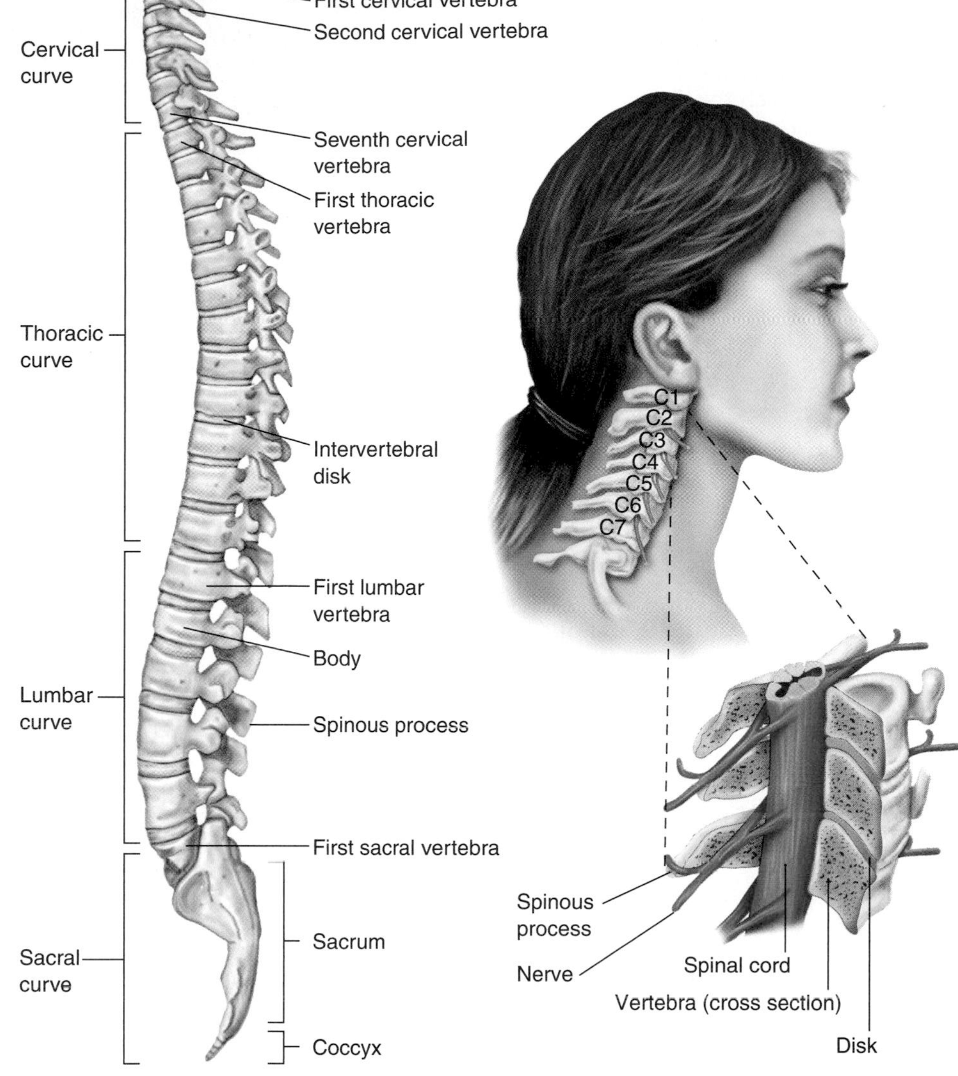

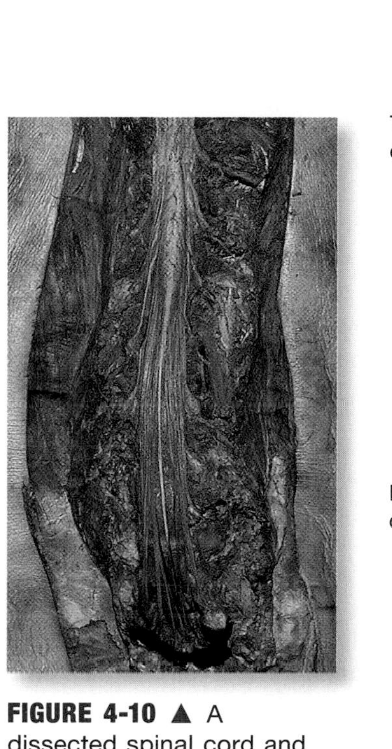

FIGURE 4-10 ▲ A dissected spinal cord and roots of the spinal nerves.
© The McGraw-Hill Companies, Inc./Karl Rubin, photographer

The discs between the vertebrae are soft and rubbery, acting as shock absorbers.

Between the vertebrae are discs. Each disc is a tiny pad, which is made up mainly of water (Figure 4-9). These discs cushion the vertebrae. They also help protect the spinal nerves. The spinal nerves exit the spinal cord at openings between the vertebrae. They send signals to the body's muscles and organs (Figure 4-10).

The Chest

The chest (thorax) is made up of the 12 thoracic vertebrae, 12 pairs of ribs, and the breastbone (sternum) (Figure 4-11). These structures form the thoracic cage, protecting the organs within the thoracic cavity, such as the heart, the lungs, and major blood vessels. All of the ribs are attached posteriorly to the thoracic vertebrae by ligaments. Pairs 1 through 10 are attached to the front of the sternum. Pairs 1 through 7 are attached to the front of the sternum by cartilage and are called **true ribs.** Rib pairs 8 through 10 are attached to the cartilage of the seventh ribs. These ribs are called **false ribs.** Pairs 11 and 12 are not attached to the front of the sternum; these ribs are called **floating ribs.**

The sternum is attached to the ribs and collarbones (clavicles).

The sternum (breastbone) consists of three sections. The **manubrium** is the uppermost (superior) portion; it connects with the clavicle and first rib. The body is the middle portion. The **xiphoid process** is a piece of cartilage that

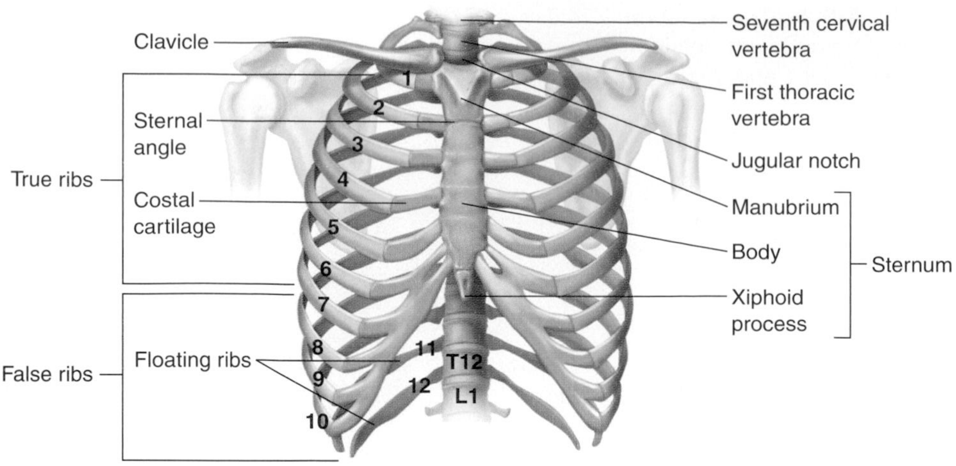

FIGURE 4-11 ▶ The thoracic cage (anterior view). The thoracic cage includes 12 pairs of ribs and the 12 thoracic vertebrae with which they join. The thoracic cage also includes the breastbone (stemum).

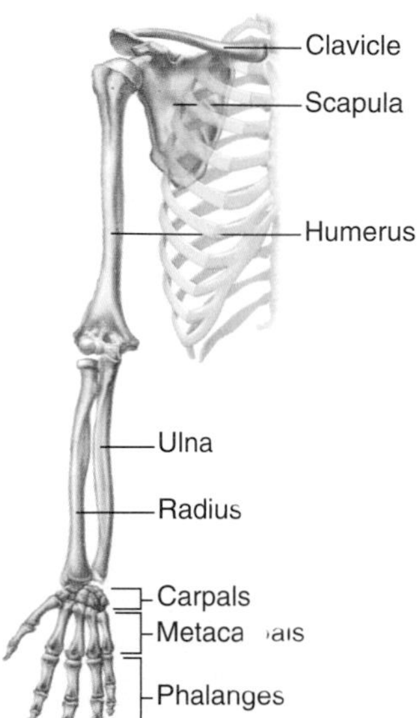

FIGURE 4-12 ▲ The shoulder girdle consı ts of two pairs of bones that attach the upper limb to the body: each pair is composed of a scapuıa (shoulder blade) and a clavicle (collarbone).

makes up the inferior portion. This landmark is important when determining the proper hand position for chest compressions in CPR. The superior portion of the sternum is attached to the clavicles, which joins the axial skeleton to the appendicular skeleton.

The Upper Extremities

The upper extremities are made up of the bones of the shoulder girdle, the arms, the forearms, and the hands. The **humerus** is the upper arm bone where the biceps and triceps muscles are attached, allowing the shoulder to rotate, flex, and extend (Figure 4-12). The clavicles (collarbones) and the scapulae (shoulder blades) form the capsule into which the proximal portion of the humerus inserts to form the shoulder joint. The forearm contains two bones, the **radius** (lateral, th:ımb side) and the **ulna** (medial side). The ulna is the longer of the two bones. The elbow is the joint where the humerus connects with the radius and the ulna. The forearm is connected to the wrist **(carpals)** and then to the hand **(metacarpals)** and the fingers **(phalanges).** There are multiple bones and joints within the wrist and hand, allowing humans to have a great deal of flexibility, movement, and use.

The humerus is the largest bone of the upper extremity and is the second longest bone in the body.

In general, the bones of the lower extremities are thicker, heavier, and longer than the upper-extremity bones.

The knee is the largest joint in the body.

The Lower Extremities

The lower extremities are made up of the bones of the pelvis, upper legs, lower legs, and feet (Figure 4-13). These bones support the body and are essential for standing, walking, and running. The **pelvis** is a bony ring formed by three separate bones that fuse to become one in an adult. The lower extremities are attached to the pelvis at the hip joint. The hip joint is formed by the socket of the hip bone and the head of the thigh bone **(femur).** The head of the femur is the upper end of the bone and is shaped like a ball. The femur is the longest, heaviest, and strongest bone of the body.

The knee is a hinge joint that allows the distal leg to move in flexion and extension. It is protected anteriorly by the kneecap **(patella)** and attaches the femur to the two lower leg bones, the **tibia** (shinbone) and the **fibula.** The tibia is the larger of the two bones of the lower leg. The lower leg attaches to the foot by the ankle, which is similar to the wrist of the upper extremities. Like the hand, the foot contains several smaller bones and joints, allowing free movement of the foot at the ankle. The **tarsal** bones make up the back part of the foot and heel. The **metatarsal** bones make up the main part of the foot. The toes (phalanges) are the foot's equivalent of the fingers, but without the same movements. The toes move in flexion and extension only.

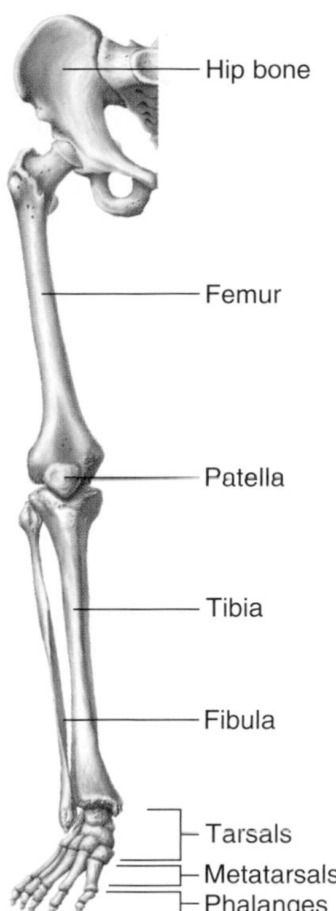

FIGURE 4-13 ▲ The lower extremity bones.

When a skeletal muscle contracts, it shortens, pulling on the structure next to it to cause movement.

The Muscular System

The muscular system performs several functions for the body:

- Gives the body shape
- Protects internal organs
- Provides for movement of the body
- Maintains posture
- Helps stabilize joints
- Produces body heat

Muscles allow you to smile, open your mouth, breathe, speak, blink, walk, talk, and move food through your digestive system. The heart is a muscle that pumps blood through the body.

Muscles are classified according to their structure and function: skeletal (voluntary) muscle, smooth (involuntary) muscle, and cardiac muscle.

Skeletal Muscles

Skeletal muscles move the skeleton, produce the heat that helps maintain a constant body temperature, and maintain posture. Skeletal muscles are *voluntary* because you can determine how they move. Most skeletal muscles are attached to bones by means of **tendons.** Tendons firmly attach the end of a muscle to a bone. The tendons of many muscles cross over joints, which helps stabilize the joint. Skeletal muscles produce rapid, forceful contractions but do not contract unless they are stimulated by a nerve. Although the contractions are forceful, skeletal muscle tires easily and must rest after short periods of activity. Regular exercise maintains or increases the size and strength of skeletal muscles. When contraction occurs, the bones work together with the muscles to produce body movement. For example, when the forearm bends or straightens at the elbow, the bones and muscles function as a lever (Figure 4-14).

Even when you are not moving, your muscles are in a state of partial contraction. This state is referred to as **muscle tone.** Because of electrical signals sent from nerve cells, some muscle fibers are continuously contracted at any given time. This state of constant tension keeps your head in an upright position, your back straight, and the muscles of your body prepared for action.

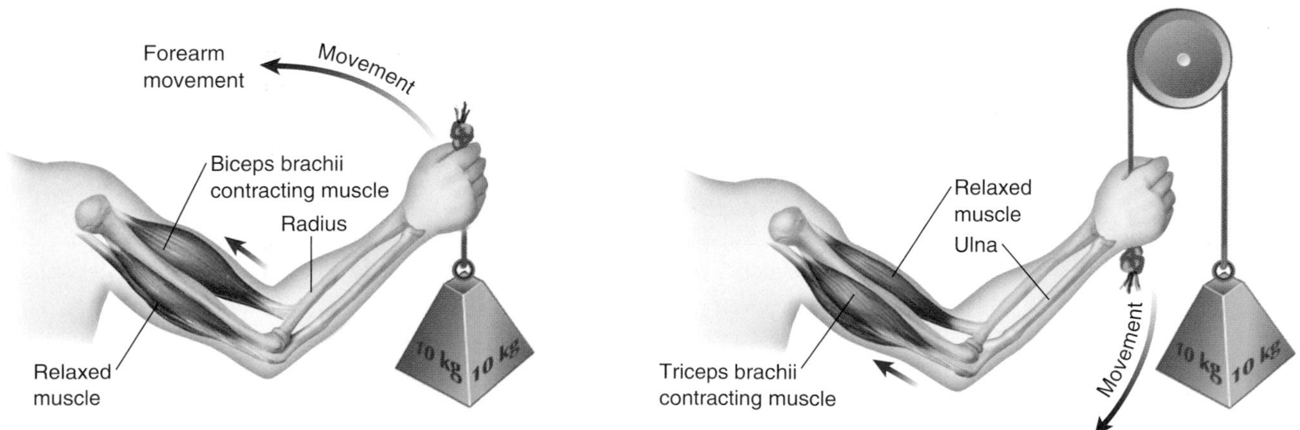

FIGURE 4-14 ▲ When the forearm bends or straightens at the elbow, the bones and muscles function as a lever.

Smooth Muscle

Smooth muscle is found within the walls of tubular structures of the gastrointestinal tract and urinary systems, blood vessels, eye, and bronchi of the respiratory system. Smooth muscle is *involuntary* because you cannot control its movement. Smooth muscle contractions are strong and slow. They respond to stimuli, such as stretching, heat, and cold. In the iris of the eye, smooth muscle regulates pupil size. The contraction of the smooth muscle that surrounds the intestines causes food and feces to move along the digestive tract. In blood vessels, smooth muscle helps maintain blood pressure. In the bronchi, the constriction of smooth muscle may result in breathing problems.

A person has no voluntary control over smooth muscle. The contraction and relaxation of smooth muscle are controlled by the body's needs. For example, when a person eats, he or she does not think about the digestive process. The food is broken down in the stomach and moved forward to the intestinal tract. Nutrients are absorbed and waste is excreted. This process occurs involuntarily with each meal.

Cardiac Muscle

Your heart beats about 100,000 times every day.

Cardiac muscle, found in the walls of the heart, produces the heart's contractions and pumps blood. Cardiac muscle is found *only* in the heart and has its own supply of blood through the coronary arteries. It can tolerate an interruption of its blood supply for only very short periods. Normal cardiac muscle contractions are strong and rhythmic.

Like smooth muscle, cardiac muscle is involuntary. The heart can change its rate, rhythm, and strength of contraction according to the needs of the other muscles and organ systems within the body. The heart is the body's hardest working muscle. The muscles of the heart contract thousands of times a day, without rest, year after year, to move blood through the body.

A comparison of the three muscle types appears in Table 4-2.

Infants and Children

The skulls of infants and children are thin and flexible. When an infant or a child suffers trauma to the head, force is more likely to be transferred to the brain instead of fracturing the skull. In infants and young children, the ligaments of the neck are underdeveloped and the muscles of the neck are relatively weak. The head is also larger and heavier relative to the rest of the body. In addition, young children have less muscle mass and more fat and cartilage than older children.

TABLE 4-2 Comparison of Muscle Types

	Skeletal	Smooth	Cardiac
Location	Attached to bone	Walls of the esophagus, stomach, intestines, bronchi, uterus, blood vessels, glands	Walls of the heart
Function	• Moves the skeleton • Produces heat, which helps maintain a constant body temperature • Maintains posture	• Moves food through the digestive tract • Adjusts the size of blood vessels to control blood flow	• Contraction and relaxation of the heart • Moves blood through the body
Type of Control	Voluntary	Involuntary	Involuntary

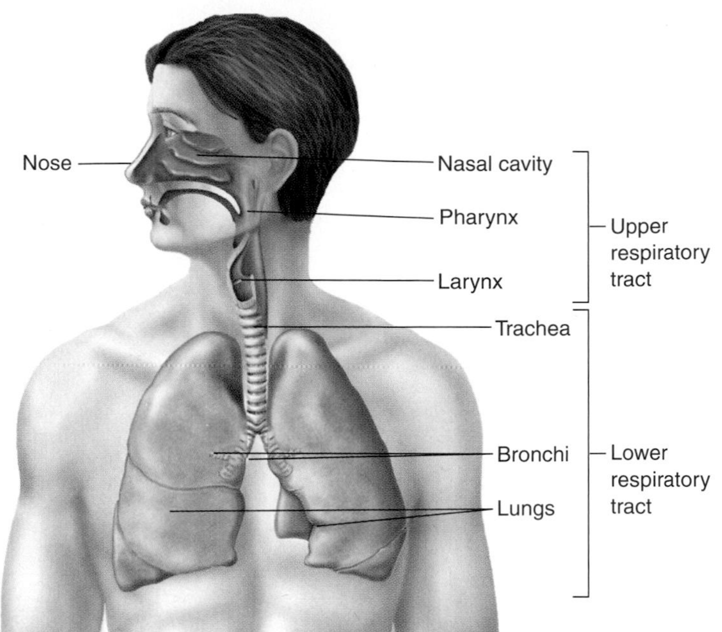

FIGURE 4-15 ▲ The upper and lower respiratory tract.

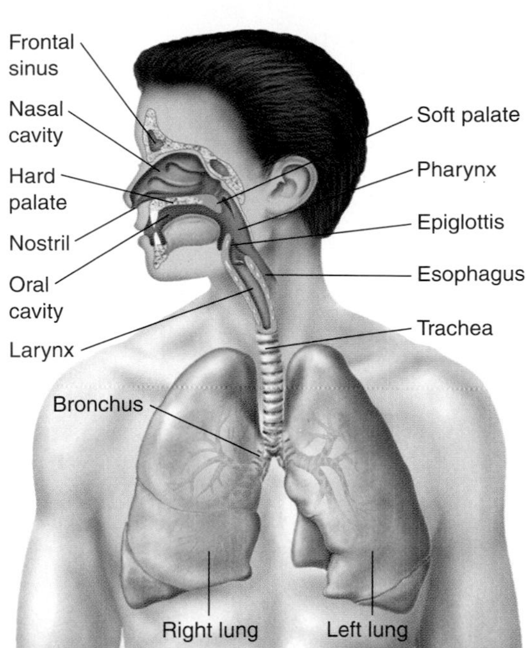

FIGURE 4-16 ▲ The structures of the respiratory system.

Injuries to the spinal cord and spinal column are uncommon in infants and young children. When they do occur, children younger than eight years of age tend to sustain injury to the uppermost area of the cervical spine.

The Respiratory System

Objective 1 ▶

The body's cells need a continuous supply of oxygen to sustain life. Working with the circulatory system, the respiratory system supplies oxygen from the air we breathe to the body's cells. It also transports carbon dioxide (a waste product of the body's cells) to the lungs. Carbon dioxide is removed from the body in the air we exhale.

The uvula is the small piece of tissue that looks like a mini punching bag and hangs down in the back of the throat.

The respiratory system is divided into the upper and lower airways (Figure 4-15). The upper airway is made up of structures outside the chest cavity. These structures include the nose, the **pharynx** (throat), and the **larynx** (voice box). The lower airway consists of parts found almost entirely within the chest cavity, such as the **trachea** (windpipe) and the lungs.

Air enters the body through the nose or the mouth (Figure 4-16). It is warmed, moistened, and filtered as it moves over the damp, sticky lining (mucous membrane) of the nose. Air then travels down the throat through the larynx and the trachea. The throat is common to both the respiratory and the digestive systems. It serves as a passageway for food, liquids, and air. The trachea is located in the front of the neck. In adults, it is about 4 inches long and slightly less than an inch in diameter. It contains rigid, C-shaped rings of cartilage that function to keep the windpipe open. The **esophagus,** which is part of the digestive system, is a muscular tube about 9 inches long. It is located behind the trachea and serves as a passageway for food. The open part of each C-shaped cartilage faces the esophagus, allowing it to expand slightly into the trachea during swallowing. You cannot swallow and breathe at the same time because the **epiglottis,** a special flap of cartilage, covers the trachea when you are eating or drinking so that food or liquids do not enter the lungs (Figure 4-17).

FIGURE 4-17 ▶ The structures involved in swallowing.

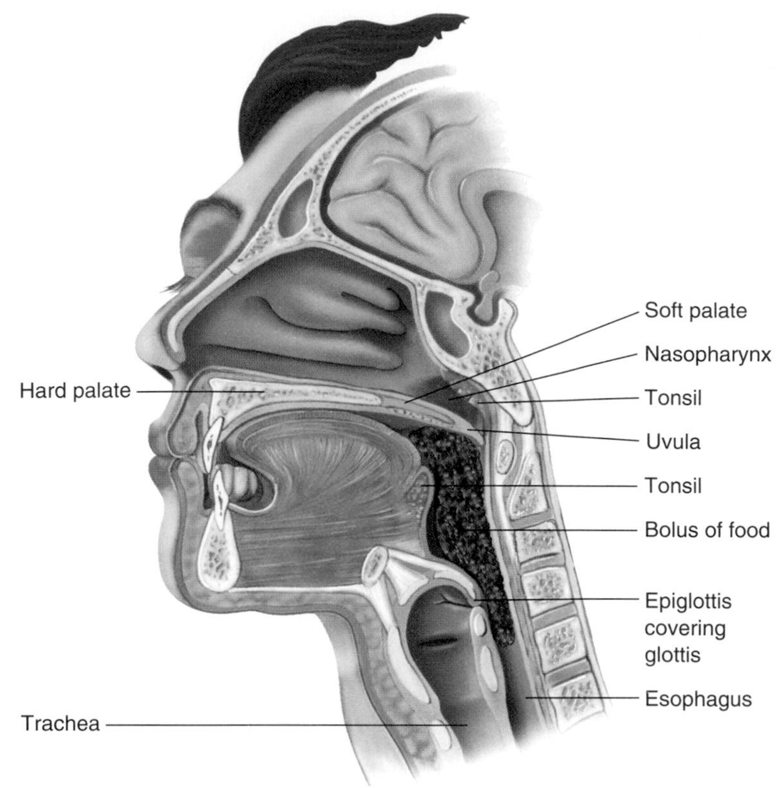

FIGURE 4-18 ▶ The bronchial tree consists of the passageways that connect the trachea and the alveoli.

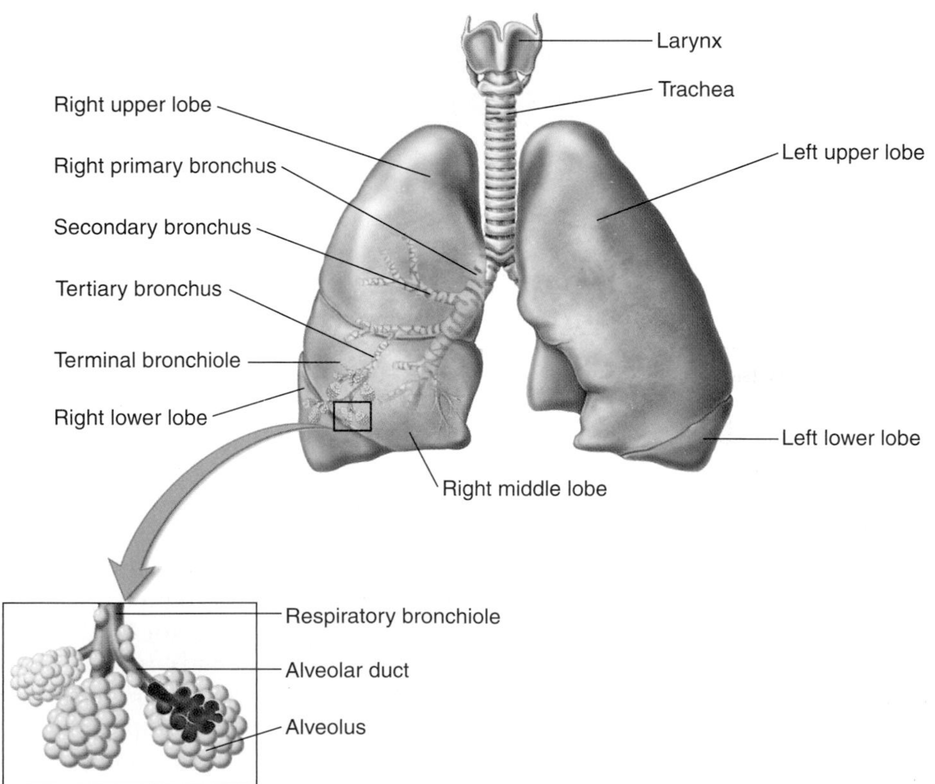

The bronchi and bronchioles serve as passageways for air to and from the alveoli.

The trachea continues into the chest, where it branches into large airway tubes called the right and left mainstem bronchi. The right mainstem bronchus is shorter, wider, and straighter than the left. Each **bronchus** is joined to a lung, so one tube leads to the right lung and the other leads to the left lung. The bronchi are covered with mucus, which traps dirt and germs that get into the lungs. Small, hair-like structures (cilia) work like brooms to get rid of the debris caught in the mucus. The mainstem bronchi branch into smaller and smaller tubes called **bronchioles.** At the ends of the bronchioles are tiny sacs that look like clusters of grapes. These tiny sacs are called **alveoli.** The bronchial tree consists of passageways that connect the trachea and the alveoli (Figure 4-18).

There are about 300 million alveoli in the human body.

The alveoli are the sites where gases—oxygen and carbon dioxide—are exchanged between the air and blood. The wall of an alveolus consists of a single layer of cells. Each alveolus is surrounded by a network of pulmonary capillaries (Figure 4-19). Oxygen-rich air passes over the surface of the alveoli each time you breathe in. Oxygen-poor blood in the capillaries passes over the alveoli. Oxygen enters the capillaries from the alveoli as carbon dioxide passes over the alveoli from the capillaries. A thin film of **surfactant** coats each alveolus and prevents the alveoli from collapsing.

The **lungs** are spongy, air-filled organs. They are bound from above (superiorly) by the clavicles and from below (inferiorly) by the diaphragm

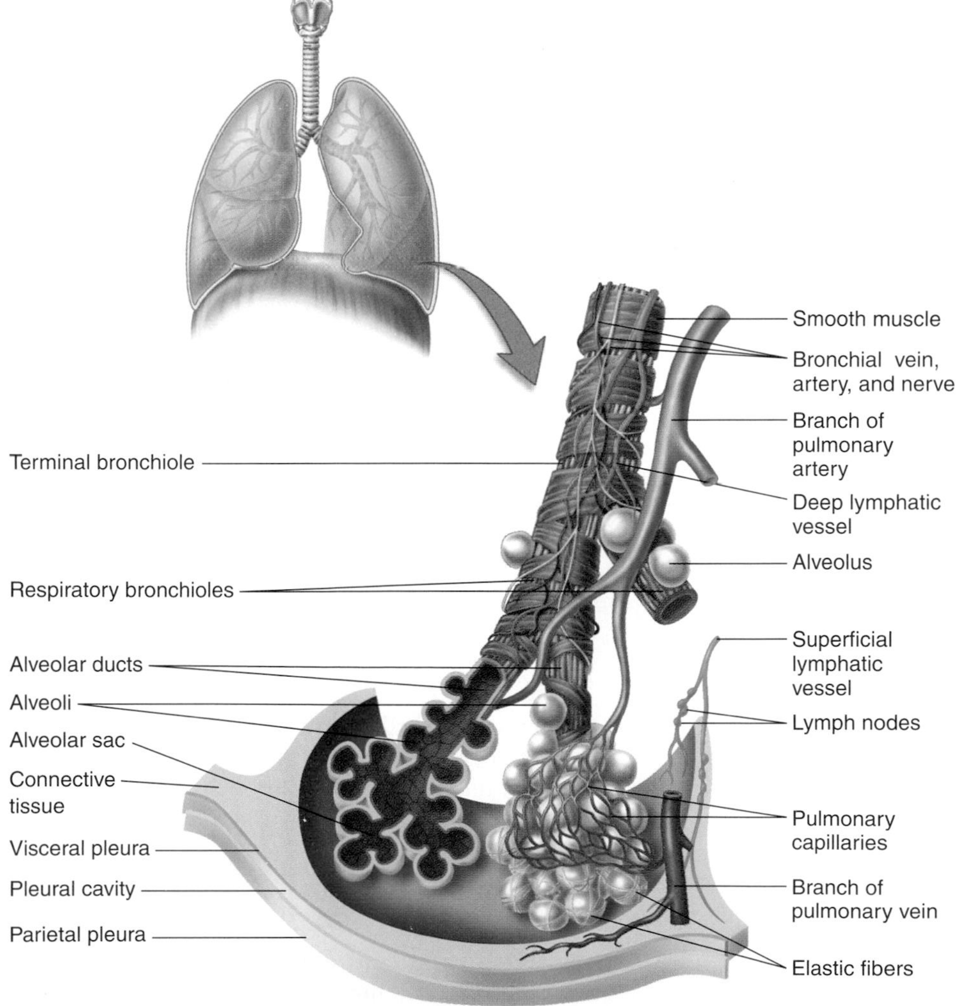

FIGURE 4-19 ► The mainstem bronchi branch into smaller and smaller tubes called bronchioles. At the ends of the bronchioles are tiny sacs that look like clusters of grapes. These tiny sacs are called the alveoli. Alveoli are the sites of gas exchange between the air and blood.

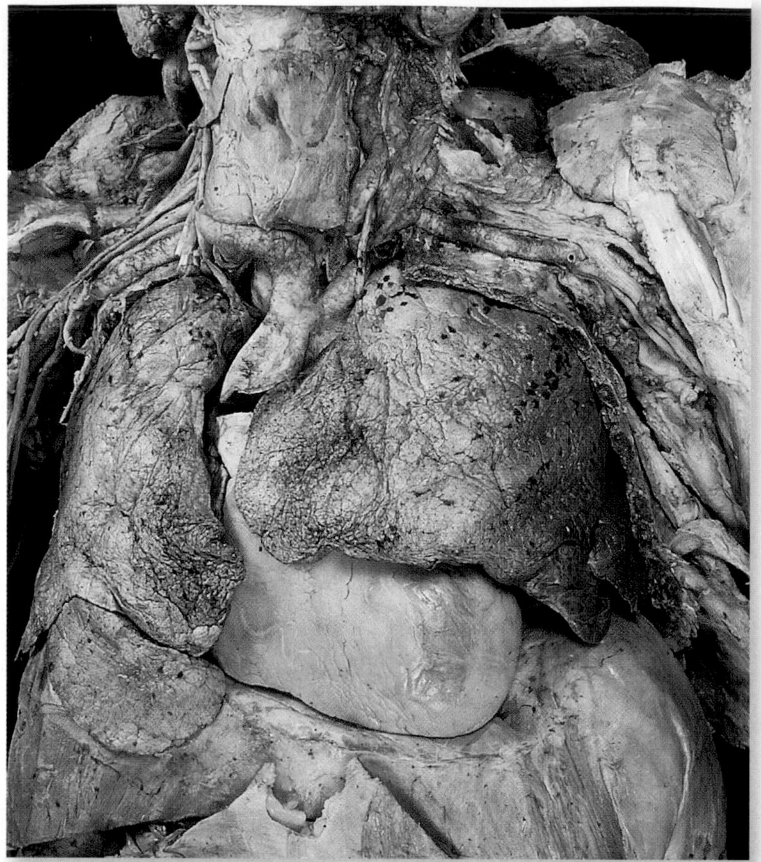

FIGURE 4-20 ▶ Anterior view of the chest. © The McGraw-Hill Companies, Inc./Karl Rubin, photographer

(Figure 4-20). The lungs bring air into contact with the blood so that oxygen and carbon dioxide can be exchanged in the alveoli. The apex of the lung is the uppermost portion of the lung; it reaches above the first rib. The base of the lung is the portion of the lung resting on the diaphragm. The **mediastinum** is part of the space in the middle of the chest, between the lungs. The mediastinum extends from the sternum (breastbone) to the spine. It contains all of the organs of the thorax—the heart, major blood vessels, the esophagus, the trachea, and nerves—except the lungs.

The lungs are divided into lobes. The right lung has three lobes. It is shorter than the left lung, because the diaphragm is higher on the right to make room for the liver, which lies below it. The left lung has two lobes. Because two thirds of the heart lies to the left of the midline of the body, the left lung contains a notch to make room for the heart.

Certain illnesses or injuries can cause air, blood, or both to fill the pleural space. This can collapse the lung on the affected side.

The lungs "float" within separate pleural cavities. They are separated from the chest wall by a space containing pleural fluid. The **pleurae** are the serous (oily), double-walled membranes that enclose each lung (Figure 4-21). The parietal pleura is the outer lining, which lines the wall of the thoracic cavity (the rib cage, diaphragm, and mediastinum). The visceral pleura is the inner layer, which covers the surface of the lungs. The **pleural space** is a space between the visceral and parietal pleurae filled with a small amount of oily fluid. Pleural fluid allows the lungs to glide easily against each other as the lungs fill and empty during breathing.

The Mechanics of Breathing

Breathing (also called pulmonary ventilation) is the mechanical process of moving air into and out of the lungs. **Inspiration** (inhalation) is the process of breathing in and moving air into the lungs. **Expiration** (exhalation) is the process

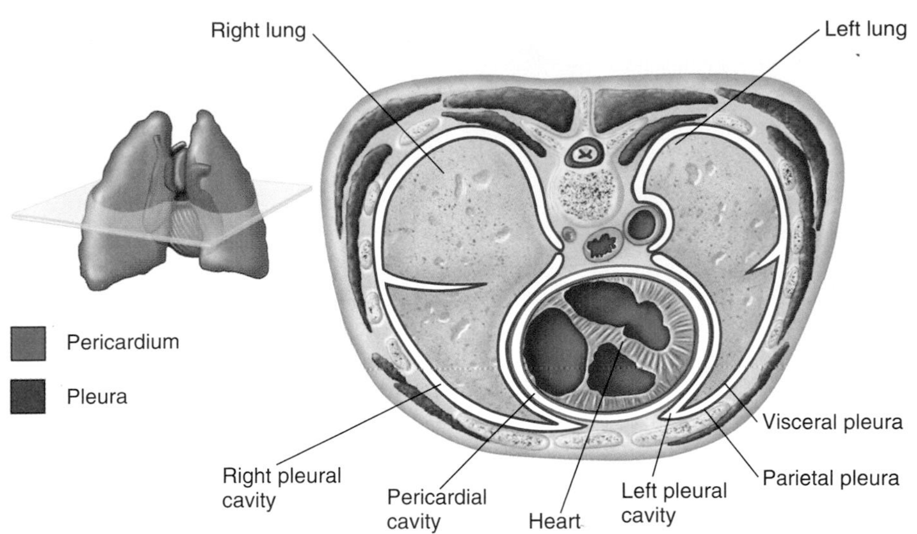

FIGURE 4-21 ► Each lung is surrounded by a pleural cavity. The parietal pleura lines each pleural cavity and the visceral pleura covers the surface of the lungs. The potential spaces between the pleural membranes (the left and right pleural cavities) are shown here as actual spaces.

of breathing out and moving air out of the lungs. **Respiration** is the exchange of gases between a living organism and its environment. Oxygen is an essential "fuel" needed by all body cells for survival. Most cells begin to die if their oxygen supply is interrupted for even a few minutes.

Every three to five seconds, nerve impulses stimulate the breathing process.

The rate and depth of breathing are controlled by the brain. The brain is sensitive to the level of carbon dioxide in the bloodstream. When the level of carbon dioxide in the blood is increased, a person breathes faster and deeper to get rid of the carbon dioxide and bring in more oxygen, which is necessary for cell function.

When the brain senses there is not enough oxygen in the bloodstream, it sends a signal to the diaphragm and intercostal muscles (muscles between the ribs), causing them to contract. The **diaphragm** is the dome-shaped muscle below the lungs. It is the main muscle of respiration; it separates the thoracic cavity from the abdominal cavity. The external intercostal muscles are located between the ribs. The internal intercostal muscles and abdominal muscles may be used during forceful expiration.

The mechanics of breathing can be compared to that of a bellows: When it is opened, air enters; as it closes, air is forced out.

When the diaphragm and external intercostal muscles contract, the chest cavity enlarges and fills with air. Recall that this process is called inspiration. Inspiration is an active process because it requires muscle contraction. When the diaphragm and external intercostal muscles relax, the chest cavity becomes smaller, the lungs are compressed, and air is forced out. Recall that this process is called expiration. Expiration is normally a passive process because the lungs recoil due to their elasticity (Figure 4-22).

Infants and Children

The respiratory anatomy of infants and young children differs from that of older children and adults. In general, all the structures are smaller. Because they are smaller, they are more easily blocked than in adults. The nasal passages are soft and narrow and have little supporting cartilage. It is important to keep the nasal passages clear in infants under six months of age, because they breathe mostly through the nose, not the mouth. If the nasal passages are blocked due to tissue swelling or a buildup of mucus, difficulty breathing and problems with feeding can result.

In infants and young children, the tongue takes up proportionally more space in the mouth. The tracheal rings are softer and more flexible. This puts them at risk for compression if the neck is not positioned properly.

The chest wall of an infant or young child is softer and more elastic than that of an older child or adult. This is because it is made of more cartilage

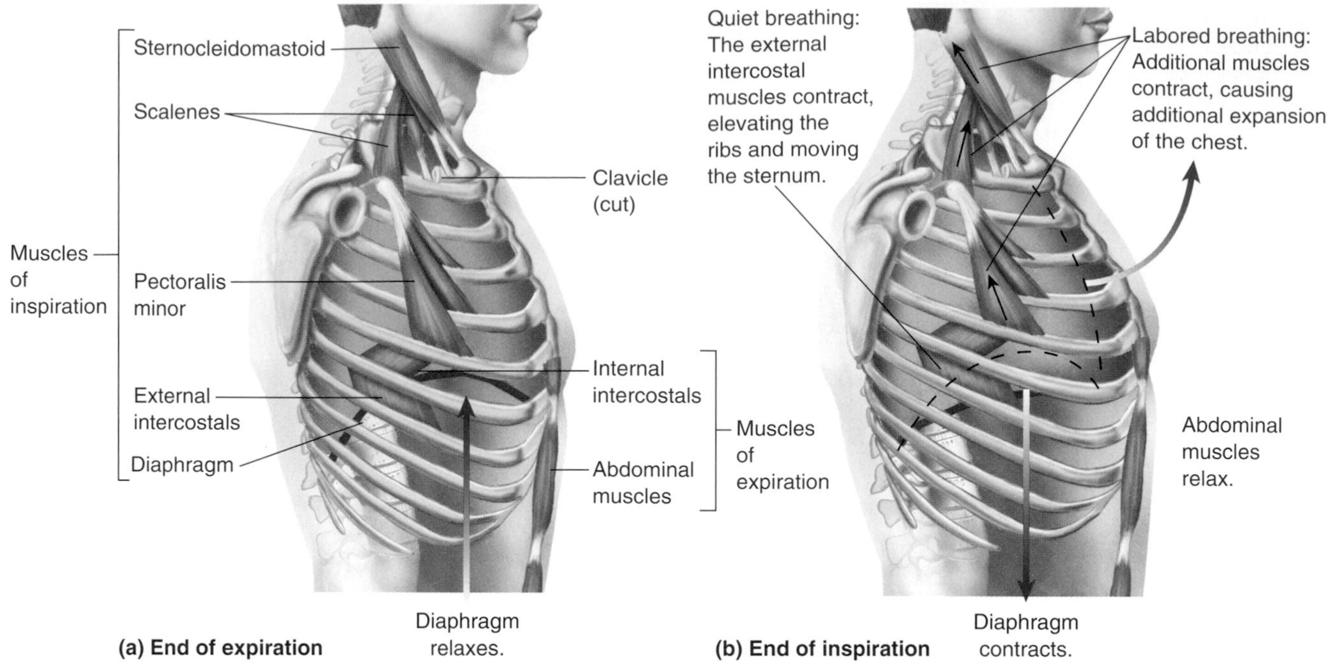

FIGURE 4-22 ▲ (a) The muscles of respiration at the end of expiration. During a normal exhalation, these muscles relax and the chest volume returns to normal. (b) The muscles of respiration at the end of inspiration. During inhalation, the diaphragm and external intercostal muscles between the ribs contract, causing the volume of the chest cavity to increase.

than bone. Children also have fewer and smaller alveoli. Thus, the potential area for exchanging oxygen and carbon dioxide is smaller. Because the chest wall is soft and flexible, rib and sternum fractures are less common in children than in adults. However, the force of the injury is more easily transmitted to the delicate tissues of the underlying lung. This results in bruising of the lung and bleeding in the alveoli, which reduce the number of alveoli available for gas exchange. This type of injury is potentially life threatening.

Infants and young children depend more heavily on the diaphragm for breathing than do adults. Air can build up in the stomach during rescue breathing or when CPR is performed on them due to improper technique. As a result, the stomach swells with air, movement of the diaphragm is limited, and effective breathing is reduced.

You Should Know

The main cause of cardiac arrest in infants and children is an uncorrected respiratory problem.

The Circulatory System

Objective 2 ▶

The circulatory system is made up of the cardiovascular and lymphatic systems. The cardiovascular system is made up of three main parts: a pump (the heart), fluid (blood), and a container (the blood vessels). The lymphatic system consists of lymph, lymph nodes, lymph vessels, tonsils, the spleen, and the thymus gland. The spleen and liver are also associated with the circulatory system because they form and store blood.

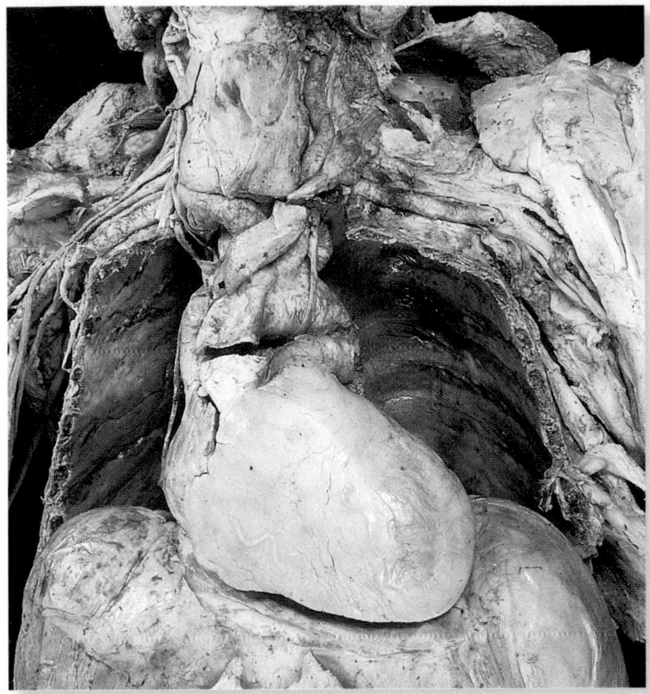

FIGURE 4-23 ► Anterior view of the human heart in the chest (without the lungs).

The functions of the circulatory system are the following:

- Deliver oxygen-rich blood and nutrients to body tissues
- Help maintain body temperature
- Protect the body against infection

The Heart

The heart is located slightly to the left of the center of the chest. It is attached to the chest through the great vessels (pulmonary arteries and veins, the aorta, and the superior and inferior vena cavae). With its thick walls of cardiac muscle, the heart pumps blood through the vessels of the body (Figure 4-23).

The heart has four hollow chambers. The two upper chambers are the right and left **atria.** The job of the atria is to receive blood from the body and lungs. The two lower chambers of the heart are the right and left **ventricles.** The ventricles are larger and have thicker walls than the atria, because their job is to pump blood to the lungs and body.

The right atrium receives blood that is low in oxygen from the body by means of veins. Blood flows from the right atrium through a one-way valve, the tricuspid valve. The tricuspid valve forces the blood to always move in the right direction, into the right ventricle. When the right ventricle contracts, blood is pumped through another one-way valve, the pulmonic valve, into the pulmonary arteries. Blood flows from the pulmonary arteries to the lungs, where it receives a fresh supply of oxygen. From the lungs, the oxygen-rich blood flows along the pulmonary veins to the left upper chamber of the heart, the left atrium. The left atrium pumps the blood through the mitral (bicuspid) valve to the left ventricle. The left ventricle is about three times thicker than the right ventricle because it has to produce enough pressure to push the blood out of the heart, through the aortic valve, and into the aorta, the body's largest artery. The aorta and its branches distribute the oxygen-rich blood throughout the body (Figure 4-24).

FIGURE 4-24 ▶ Blood flow through the heart and lungs.

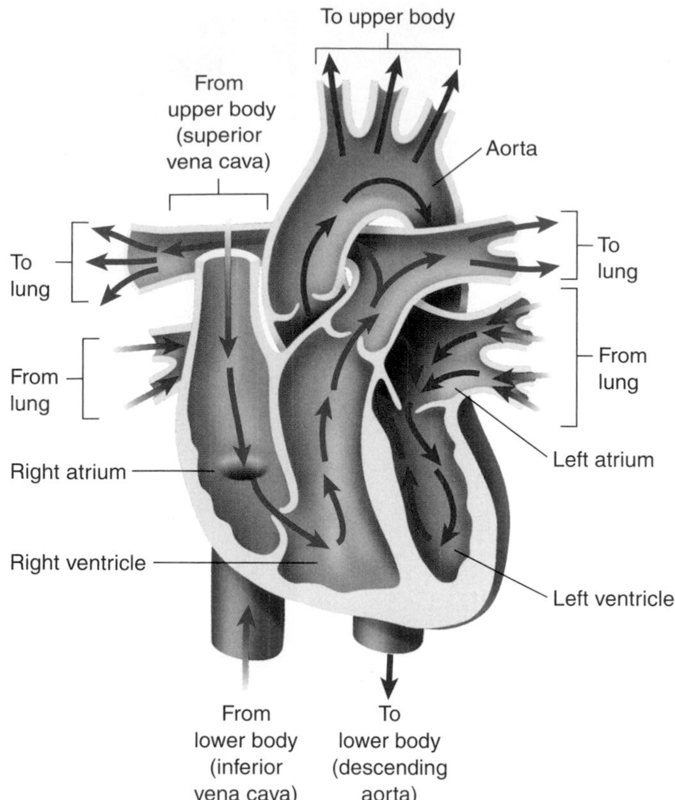

The normal heartbeat begins as an electrical signal in a small area of specialized tissue in the upper right atrium of the heart. The impulse spreads through a system of pathways called the conduction system. A disruption of these pathways can cause the heart to malfunction. For example, a heart attack disrupts the flow of oxygen and nutrients to the heart's cells. This disruption can cause the heart to beat too quickly or too slowly. It can also affect the heart's ability to contract and pump blood to the rest of the body.

Blood

About 5–6 liters of blood flow through an adult's circulatory system.

Blood is a type of transport system. It is the means by which oxygen, food, hormones, minerals, and other essential substances are carried to all parts of the body. Blood carries carbon dioxide and other waste material from the body's cells to the lungs, kidneys, or skin for removal. To help maintain body temperature, blood vessels narrow (constrict) and widen (dilate) as needed to keep or lose heat at the skin's surface. The blood and lymphatic system work together to protect the body against infection.

Each red blood cell has about 250 million hemoglobin molecules.

Blood is made up of liquid and formed elements (Figure 4-25). The liquid portion of the blood is called **plasma.** Plasma carries blood cells, vitamins, proteins, glucose, and many other substances throughout the body. The formed elements of the blood include red blood cells, white blood cells, and platelets. Red blood cells (erythrocytes) contain hemoglobin. **Hemoglobin** is an iron-containing protein that chemically bonds with oxygen. Thus, hemoglobin is the part of the red blood cell that picks up oxygen in the lungs and transports it to the body's cells. Hemoglobin is red, giving blood its red color.

After delivering oxygen to the cells, red blood cells gather up carbon dioxide and transport it to the lungs, where it is removed from the body when we exhale. White blood cells (leukocytes) attack and destroy germs that enter the body.

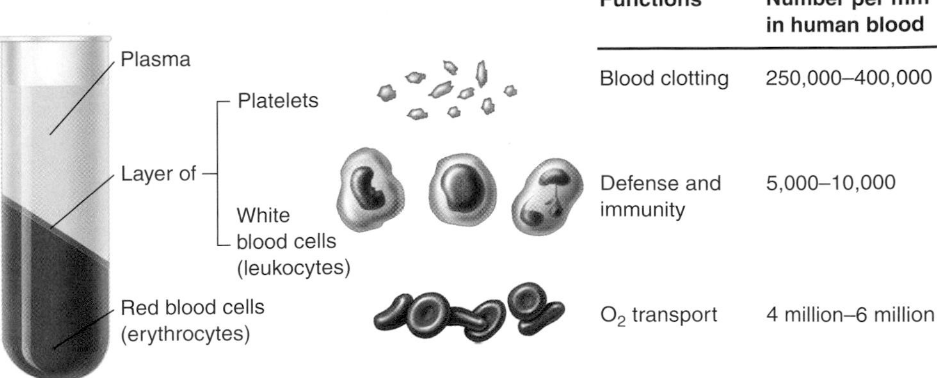

FIGURE 4-25 ► Blood is made up of liquid (plasma) and formed elements (red blood cells, white blood cells, and platelets).

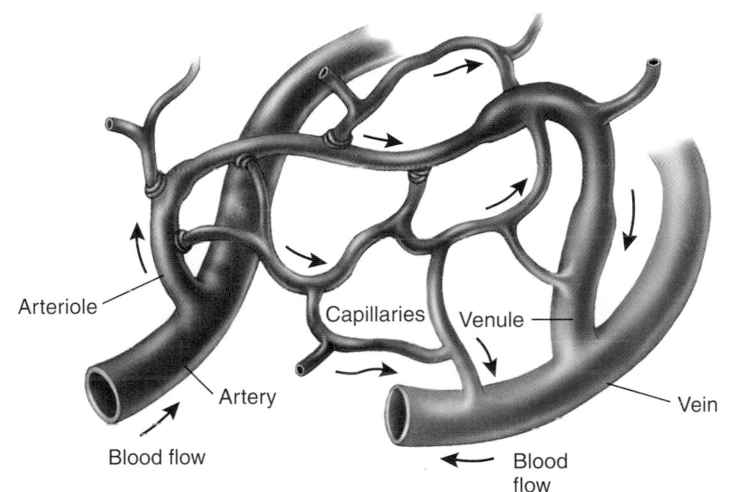

FIGURE 4-26 ► Blood flow from the heart through the body moves through the following vessels: arteries ⟶ arterioles ⟶ capillaries ⟶ venules ⟶ veins.

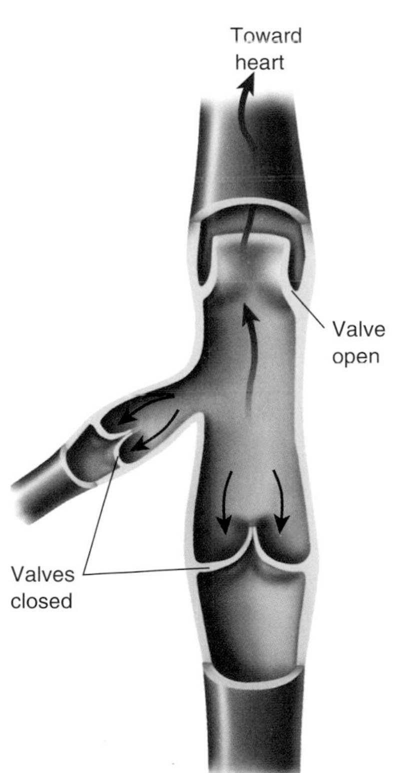

FIGURE 4-27 ▲ Veins contain one-way valves, which keep blood flowing toward the heart.

Platelets are irregularly shaped blood cells that have a sticky surface. When a blood vessel is damaged and starts to bleed, platelets gather at the site of injury. The platelets begin sticking to the opening of the damaged vessel and seal it, stopping the flow of blood.

Blood Vessels

Blood vessels that carry blood away from the heart to the rest of the body are called **arteries** (Figure 4-26). Blood is forced into the arteries when the heart contracts. Arteries have thick walls, because they transport blood under high pressure. Arteries normally carry oxygen-rich blood. However, the pulmonary artery and its two branches, the left and right pulmonary arteries, carry oxygen-poor blood.

Arterioles are the smallest branches of arteries. They connect arteries to capillaries. **Capillaries** are the smallest and most numerous blood vessels. They are very thin (thinner than a human hair). The exchange of oxygen, nutrients, and waste products between blood and body cells occurs through the walls of capillaries. Capillaries connect arterioles and venules. **Venules** are the smallest branches of veins. They connect capillaries and veins. **Veins** are vessels that return blood to the heart. Veins normally carry oxygen-poor blood. However, the pulmonary vein and its two branches (the left and right pulmonary veins) carry oxygen-rich blood. (There are four pulmonary veins, two from each lung.) The walls of veins are thinner than those of arteries. Because the pressure in the veins is low, veins contain one-way valves, which help keep the blood flowing toward the heart (Figure 4-27).

FIGURE 4-28 ► Major arteries and veins.

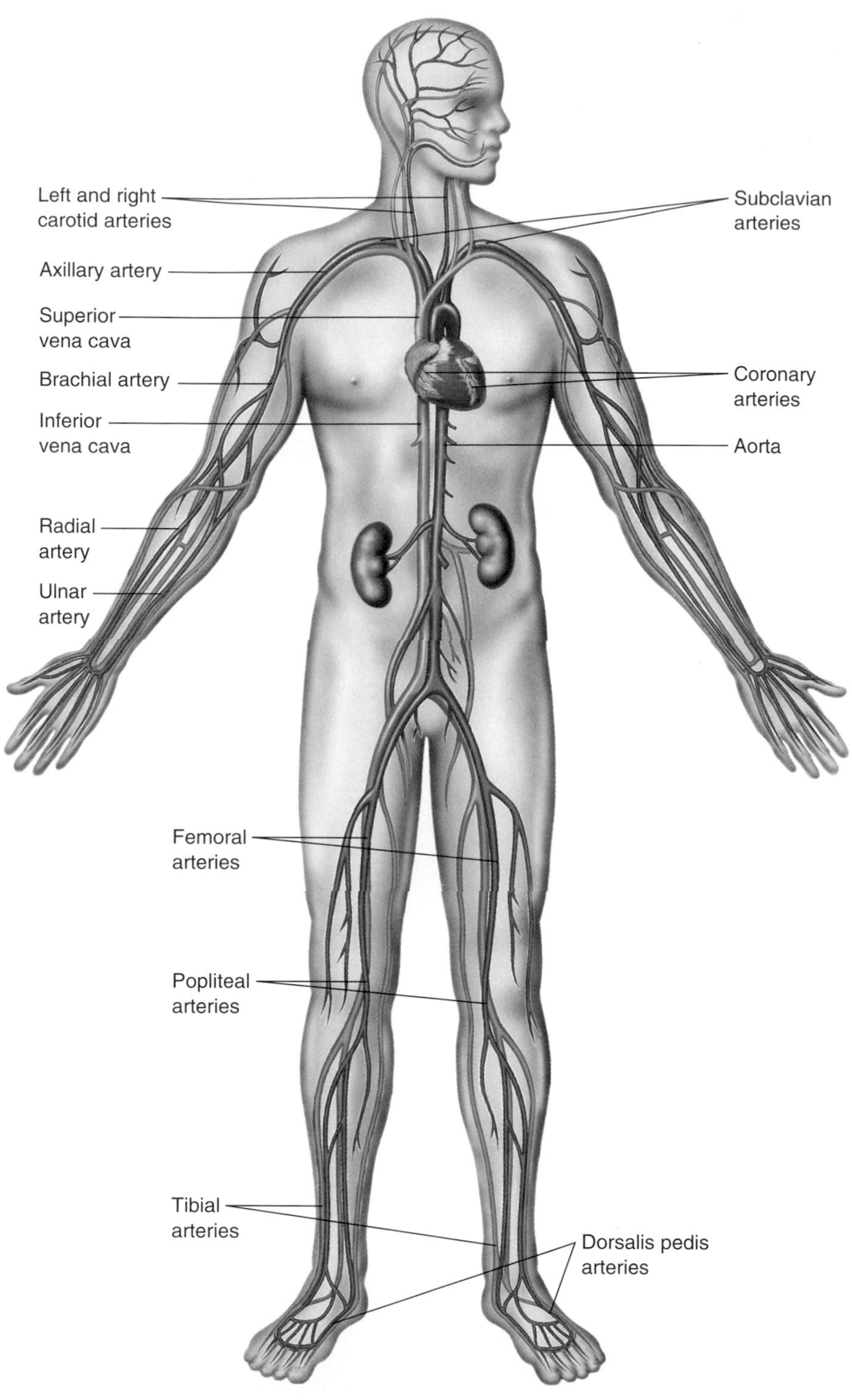

Major Arteries

Remember: *A*rteries = *A*way.

Blood flows from the **aorta,** the largest artery in the body, to all parts of the body. The aorta lies in front of the spine in the thoracic and abdominal cavities (Figure 4-28). The coronary arteries are the first blood vessels that branch off the aorta. Because the heart must have a constant blood supply, it supplies itself with oxygenated blood first through the coronary arteries. When the heart relaxes, the coronary arteries fill with blood and supply the heart muscle with the oxygen it needs.

Branches of the aorta form the carotid and subclavian arteries. The left and right carotid arteries are the major arteries of the neck, supplying the head and neck with blood. A carotid pulse can be felt on each side of the neck. The subclavian arteries run under the clavicles and supply blood to the upper extremities. The subclavian arteries branch into the axillary and brachial arteries in the upper arm. A brachial pulse can be felt on the inside of the arm between the elbow and the shoulder. This artery is used when determining blood pressure (BP) with a blood pressure cuff and stethoscope. The brachial arteries branch into the radial and ulnar arteries. These arteries supply the forearm with blood. The radial artery is the major artery of the lower arm. A radial pulse can be felt on the side of the wrist below the thumb.

The femoral arteries are the major arteries of the thigh, supplying the lower extremities with blood. A femoral pulse can be felt in the groin area (the crease between the abdomen and the thigh). Behind the knees, the femoral arteries become the popliteal arteries. The popliteal arteries supply blood to the lower legs. Slightly below the knee, the popliteal arteries become the tibial arteries. The posterior tibial pulse is located just behind the ankle bone. At the ankle, one of the tibial arteries becomes the dorsalis pedis artery, which supplies blood to the foot. A dorsalis pedis pulse (often called a pedal pulse) can be felt on the top of the foot.

Major Veins

The two largest veins in the human body are the inferior vena cava and the superior vena cava. These two veins empty oxygen-poor blood into the heart's right atrium. The superior vena cava returns blood from the head and upper extremities to the heart. The inferior vena cava returns blood from the trunk and lower extremities to the heart.

You Should Know

Coronary Artery Bypass Graft (CABG)

A coronary artery bypass graft (CABG) is a surgical procedure that may be performed to fix a blocked coronary artery. The bypass graft is usually part of a healthy blood vessel taken from the patient's leg, chest, or arm. The blood vessel is sewn from one healthy area of the heart to another. This newly placed vessel creates a detour around the blocked area. The vessel most often used for the graft is the saphenous vein in the leg. This vessel is used because it is long, reaching from the ankle to the thigh, and is about the same size as a coronary artery.

The Physiology of Circulation

Pulse

When the left ventricle contracts, a wave of blood is sent through the arteries, causing the arteries to expand and recoil. A **pulse** is the regular expansion and recoil of an artery caused by the movement of blood from the heart as it contracts. A pulse can be felt anywhere an artery passes near the skin surface and over a bone. Central pulses are located close to the heart, such as the carotid and femoral pulses. Peripheral pulses are located farther from the heart, such as the radial, brachial, posterior tibial, and dorsalis pedis pulses.

Blood Pressure

Methods used to measure blood pressure are discussed in Chapter 8.

Blood pressure is the force exerted by the blood on the inner walls of the heart and blood vessels. The **systolic blood pressure** is the pressure in an artery when the heart is pumping blood (systole). The **diastolic blood pressure** is the pressure in an artery when the heart is at rest (diastole). A blood pressure measurement is made up of both the systolic and diastolic pressures. It is measured in millimeters of mercury (mm Hg). Blood pressure is written as a fraction (for example, 115/78), with the systolic number first. In an adult, a normal systolic blood pressure ranges from 100 to 119 mm Hg. A normal diastolic blood pressure ranges from 60 to 79 mm Hg. Blood pressure is dependent on the contraction of the heart, the blood volume, and the condition of the blood vessels. A slow or fast heart rate, a loss of blood, or changes in the elasticity of the blood vessels may lead to changes in blood pressure.

Perfusion

Perfusion is the flow of blood through an organ or a part of the body. **Shock** (hypoperfusion) is the inadequate flow of blood through an organ or a part of the body.

The Nervous System

Objective 4 ▶

The nervous system is a collection of specialized cells that conduct information to and from the brain. The functions of the nervous system are to

- Control the voluntary (conscious) and involuntary (unconscious) activities of the body
- Provide for higher mental function (such as thought and emotion)

The nervous system has two divisions: the central nervous system (CNS) and the peripheral nervous system (PNS) (Figure 4-29).

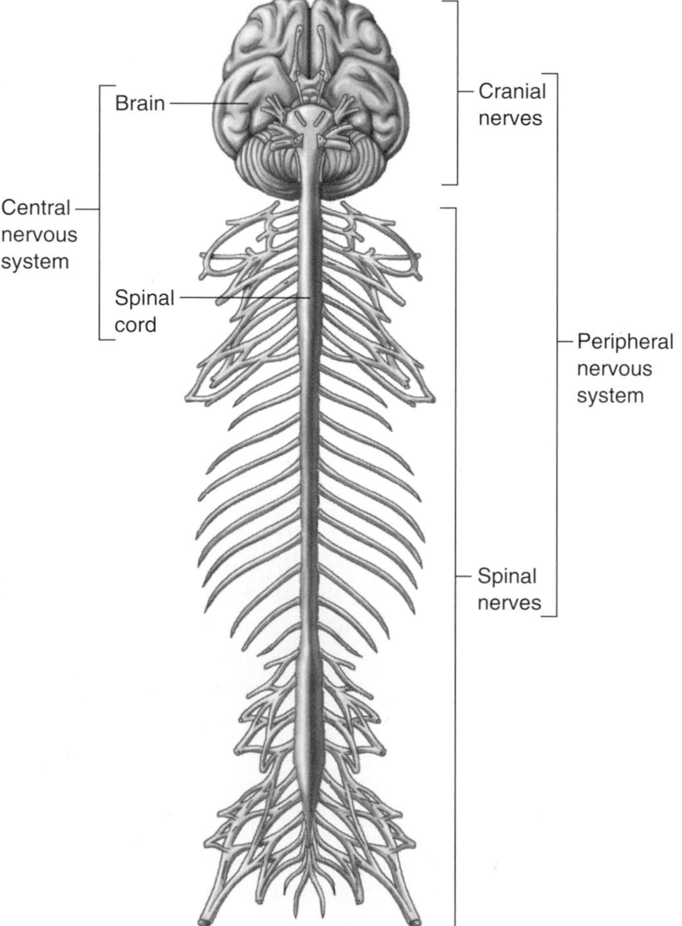

FIGURE 4-29 ▶ The central nervous system consists of the brain and spinal cord. The peripheral nervous system consists of cranial nerves, which arise from the brain, and spinal nerves, which arise from the spinal cord. The nerves actually extend throughout the body.

FIGURE 4-30 ▶ The areas of the brain.

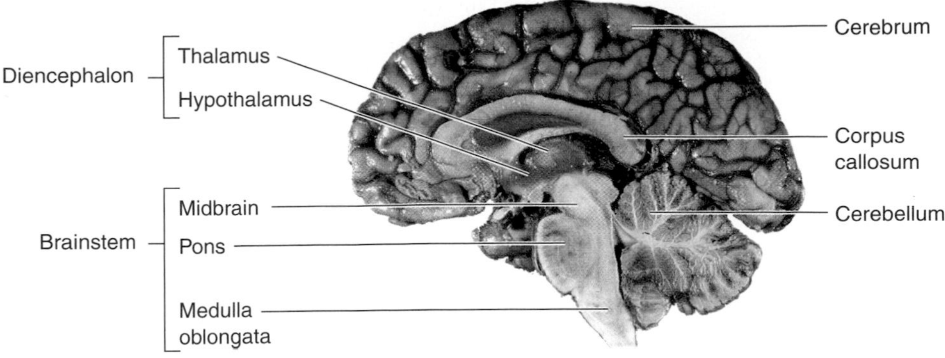

The Central Nervous System

The CNS has been compared to a state-of-the-art computer system. The right and left hemispheres of the brain are two computers in the network. The corpus callosum is the cable that connects (networks) the two computers.

The **central nervous system** consists of the brain and the spinal cord. The brain is made up of many nerve cells that are involved in higher mental function. These higher functions include the ability to think; to perform unconscious motor functions, such as breathing and controlling blood vessel diameter; and to experience and express emotion.

The brain is located in the **cranium** (skull), where it is protected. The spinal cord is protected in the spinal canal, where it travels through the **foramen magnum,** which is the opening in the base of the skull, and down the vertebral column. The central nervous system is also protected by the meninges, a covering over the brain and spinal cord, and **cerebrospinal fluid (CSF),** a clear liquid that is circulated continuously. CSF acts as a shock absorber for the central nervous system. It also provides a means for the exchange of nutrients and wastes among the blood, brain, and spinal cord.

The **cerebrum** is the largest part of the human brain (Figure 4-30). It consists of two cerebral hemispheres, which are joined by the **corpus callosum,** a very thick bundle of nerve fibers. Although no area of the brain functions alone, each cerebral hemisphere is divided into four lobes, named for the bones that lie over them:

- **Frontal.** The frontal lobes control motor activity and integrate muscle activity. They also process speech and thought.
- **Parietal.** The parietal lobes receive and process information about touch, taste, pressure, pain, heat, and cold.
- **Occipital.** The occipital lobes receive and interpret visual information.
- **Temporal.** The temporal lobes receive auditory signals and interpret language. They are also involved in personality, behavior, emotion, and memory storage.

The **cerebellum** is the second largest part of the human brain. It is responsible for the precise control of muscle movements, as well as posture and balance. The **diencephalon** is the part of the brain between the cerebrum and the brainstem. It contains the thalamus and hypothalamus. The thalamus functions as a relay station for impulses going to and from the cerebrum. The hypothalamus plays an important role in the control of thirst, hunger, and body temperature. It also serves as a link between the nervous and endocrine systems.

The **brainstem** is made up of the midbrain, the pons, and the medulla oblongata. The midbrain connects the pons and cerebellum with the cerebrum. It acts as a relay for auditory and visual signals. The pons, whose name means "bridge," connects the parts of the brain with one another by means of tracts. It influences respiration. The medulla oblongata is the lowest part of the brainstem. It joins the brainstem to the spinal cord. The medulla contains nerves that pass from the spinal cord to the brain and nerves that pass from the brain to the spinal cord. The medulla oblongata is involved in controlling blood vessel diameter, respiration, and the centers that control reflexes, such as coughing, swallowing, sneezing, and vomiting.

The spinal cord is continuous with the medulla and is the center for many reflex activities of the body. It relays electrical signals to and from the brain and peripheral nerves.

The Peripheral Nervous System

Even though the cranial nerves exit from the brain, they are still considered a part of the peripheral nervous system.

The cells of the nervous system are called neurons.

The peripheral nervous system (PNS) is made up of nerves that connect the brain and spinal cord to the rest of the body. Twelve pairs of cranial nerves are linked directly to the brain. The cranial nerves are involved in the senses, such as vision, hearing, smell, and taste. They are also involved in eye, face, and tongue movements. Cranial nerves relay signals to and from the brain.

Spinal nerves relay impulses to and from the spinal cord. There are three types of spinal nerves: sensory, motor, and mixed nerves. Sensory nerve cells receive information from the body. They send electrical signals *to* the brain and spinal cord, allowing the body to respond to sensory input. The brain and spinal cord's response is sent along motor nerve cells. Motor nerves send electrical signals *from* the brain and spinal cord. For example, when a person touches hot water, the sensory nerve signal travels up to the brain and then back down via motor nerve cells to the muscles of the involved extremity, causing movement away from the hot water.

The skin is the largest organ system of the human body. In a 150-pound man, the skin weighs about 9 pounds and covers an area of about 18 square feet.

The Integumentary System

The integumentary system is made up of the skin, hair, nails, sweat glands, and oil (sebaceous) glands. The skin protects the body from the environment, bacteria, and other organisms. Blood vessels and the sweat glands in the skin help

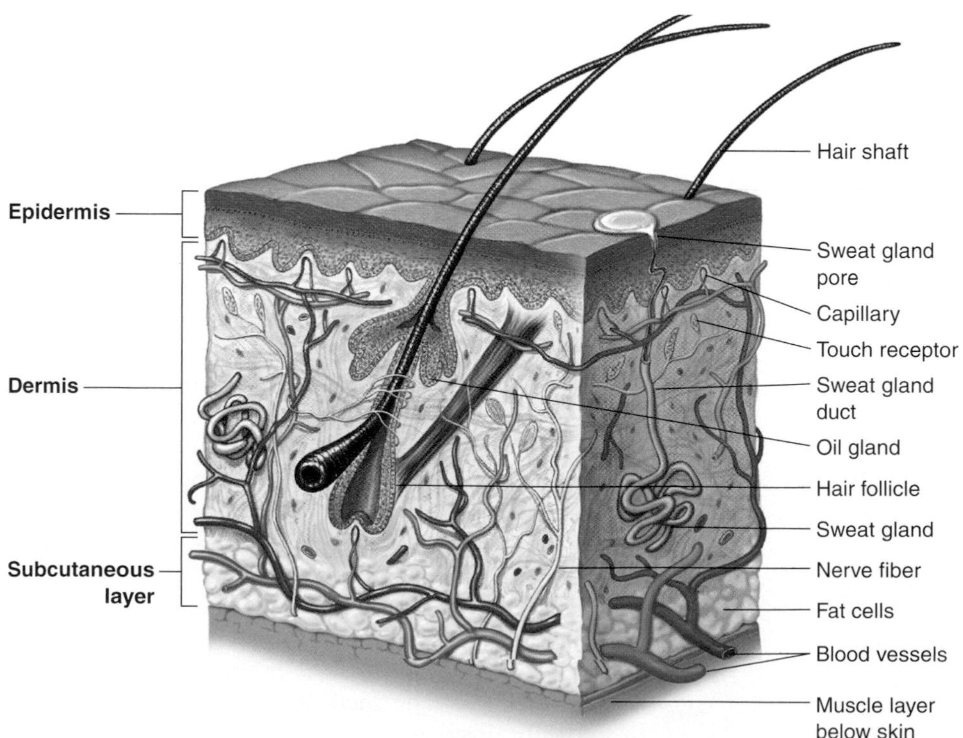

FIGURE 4-31 ► Human skin consists of the epidermis and dermis. The subcutaneous layer is beneath the dermis. Associated structures include hair follicles, sweat glands, and sebaceous (oil) glands.

control and maintain body temperature. The skin acts as a sense organ, detecting sensations such as heat, cold, touch, pressure, and pain. The skin relays this information to the brain and spinal cord.

The skin has multiple layers, including the epidermis, dermis, and subcutaneous tissue, which lie over muscle and bone. Each layer contains different structures. The epidermis is the outer portion of the skin. It does not contain blood vessels and is thickest on the palms of the hands and soles of the feet. The dermis is the thick layer of skin below the epidermis. The dermis contains hair follicles, sweat and oil glands, small nerve endings, and blood vessels (Figure 4-31). The subcutaneous layer is thick and lies below the dermis. It contains fat and insulates the body from changes in temperature. This layer is loosely attached to the muscles and bones of the musculoskeletal system.

The components and functions of all of the organ systems of the human body are summarized in Table 4-3.

TABLE 4-3 Organ Systems

System	Components	Function
Muscular	Skeletal muscle, smooth muscle, and cardiac muscle	Gives the body shape, protects internal organs, provides movement of parts of the skeleton
Skeletal	Ligaments, cartilage, and bones	Gives the body shape, protects vital internal organs
Respiratory	Air passages (mouth, nose, trachea, larynx, bronchi, and bronchioles) and lungs	Delivers oxygen to the body, removes carbon dioxide from the body
Circulatory	Heart, blood, blood vessels, lymph, and lymph vessels	Delivers oxygen and nutrients to the tissues, removes waste products from the tissues
Nervous	Brain, spinal cord, and nerves	Controls the voluntary and involuntary activity of the body, provides for higher mental function (thought, emotion)
Integumentary	Skin, hair, fingernails, toenails, sweat glands, and sebaceous glands	Protects the body from the environment, bacteria, and other organisms; helps regulate the temperature of the body; senses heat, cold, touch, pressure, and pain
Digestive	Mouth, esophagus, stomach, liver, pancreas, and intestines	Ingestion and digestion of food that is absorbed into the body through the membranes of the intestines
Endocrine	Pituitary gland, thyroid gland, parathyroid glands, adrenal glands, ovaries, testes, pineal gland, and the Islets of Langerhans in the pancreas	Interacts with the nervous system to regulate many body activities; secretes chemicals (hormones) to stimulate many body functions
Reproductive	Female: ovaries, uterus, vagina, and mammary glands Male: testes and penis	Manufactures cells (sperm, eggs) that allow continuation of the species
Urinary	Kidneys, urinary bladder, ureters, and urethra	Removes body wastes, assists in regulating blood pressure

On The Scene

Wrap-Up

The Paramedics arrive within 20 minutes. By then, your patient is complaining of difficulty breathing. You note that he is working hard to breathe. His skin is now pale and cool. You have trouble getting him to remain still because he is so anxious. Oxygen is given with no improvement. The patient is rapidly secured to a long spine board. Within 8 minutes, the Paramedics and patient have left the scene. ■

Sum It Up

- ▶ The body's most basic building block is a *cell.* The human body contains billions of cells. Clusters of cells form *tissues.* Specialized types of tissues form *organs,* such as the brain and the liver. An *organ system* (also called a *body system*) consists of tissues and organs that work together to perform a specialized function. The circulatory and respiratory systems are examples of organ systems.
- ▶ Organ systems work together to maintain a state of *homeostasis* (balance). These systems need a constant internal environment to perform the required functions of the body.
- ▶ In your role as an Emergency Medical Responder, it is important to know the terms used to describe body positions and directions. You must be able to use these terms correctly, so that you can describe the position in which a patient is found and transported. You will also need to know body positions so that you can place a patient in a specific position based on the patient's condition.
- ▶ A *body cavity* is a hollow space in the body that contains internal organs. Knowing the body cavities and the organs found within each cavity will help you describe the location of the injury or the symptoms of a sick or injured patient.
- ▶ The musculoskeletal system gives the human body its shape and ability to move, and it protects the major organs of the body. It consists of the skeletal system (bones) and the muscular system (muscles).
- ▶ The respiratory system supplies oxygen from the air we breathe to the body's cells. It also removes carbon dioxide (a waste product of the body's cells) from the lungs when we breathe out. This system is made up of an upper and a lower airway. The upper airway includes the nose, the *pharynx* (throat), and the *larynx* (voice box). The lower airway consists of structures found mostly within the chest cavity, such as the *trachea* (windpipe) and the lungs.
- ▶ The circulatory system is made up of the cardiovascular and lymphatic systems. This system has three main functions: (1) to deliver oxygen-rich blood and nutrients to body tissues, (2) to help maintain body temperature, and (3) to protect the body against infection. The cardiovascular system consists of the heart, blood, and blood vessels. The lymphatic system consists of lymph, lymph nodes, lymph vessels, tonsils, the spleen, and the thymus gland.
- ▶ The nervous system is a collection of specialized cells that transfer information to and from the brain. The two main functions of the nervous system are to control the voluntary (conscious) and involuntary (unconscious) activities of the body and to provide for higher mental function (such as thought and emotion). The nervous system has two divisions: (1) the central nervous system (CNS) and (2) the peripheral nervous system (PNS).
- ▶ The integumentary system is made up of the skin, hair, nails, sweat glands, and oil (sebaceous) glands. The skin is the largest organ of the body. It protects the body from the environment, bacteria, and other organisms.

▶ Tracking Your Progress

After reading this chapter, can you	Page Reference	Objective Met?
• Describe the anatomy and function of the respiratory system?	107–112	☐
• Describe the anatomy and function of the circulatory system?	112–118	☐
• Describe the anatomy and function of the musculoskeletal system?	98–107	☐
• Describe the components and function of the nervous system?	118–120	☐

Chapter Quiz

Multiple Choice

In the space provided, identify the letter of the choice that best completes each statement or answers each question.

_____ **1.** You find a man lying face down in an alley. The medical term for this position is
- **a.** supine.
- **b.** prone.
- **c.** lateral recumbent.
- **d.** shock position.

_____ **2.** Which of the following are bones of the forearm?
- **a.** humerus and femur
- **b.** tibia and radius
- **c.** fibula and humerus
- **d.** radius and ulna

_____ **3.** Select the correct statement about the circulatory system.
- **a.** The upper chambers of the heart are called the ventricles.
- **b.** The heart contains four one-way valves that make sure blood flows in the proper direction.
- **c.** The walls of the heart are made up of skeletal muscle.
- **d.** The lower chambers of the heart are called the atria.

_____ **4.** White blood cells
- **a.** help the body fight infection.
- **b.** are also called erythrocytes.
- **c.** are irregularly shaped blood cells that have a sticky surface.
- **d.** gather at the site of an injured blood vessel and stop the flow of blood.

_____ **5.** Which of the following arteries is found in the upper extremity?
- **a.** brachial artery
- **b.** posterior tibial artery
- **c.** femoral artery
- **d.** carotid artery

_____ **6.** The exchange of oxygen and carbon dioxide between the air and blood occurs in the
- **a.** trachea.
- **b.** alveoli.
- **c.** bronchioles.
- **d.** larynx.

_____ **7.** Which of the following are parts of the upper airway?
- **a.** trachea, bronchioles, lungs
- **b.** nose, bronchioles, pharynx
- **c.** nose, pharynx, larynx
- **d.** lungs, larynx, pharynx

True or False

Decide whether each statement is true or false. In the space provided, write T for true or F for false.

_____ **8.** Hemoglobin is an oxygen-carrying protein in red blood cells.

_____ **9.** The chambers of the heart that have the thickest walls are the ventricles.

Matching

Match the key terms in the left column with the definitions in the right column by placing the letter of each correct answer in the space provided.

_____ **10.** Thoracic cavity
_____ **11.** Abdominal cavity
_____ **12.** Body cavity
_____ **13.** Pelvic cavity
_____ **14.** Pleural cavities
_____ **15.** Spinal cavity
_____ **16.** Cranial cavity
_____ **17.** Pericardial cavity

a. Surrounds the heart
b. Surrounds the lungs
c. Located in the head; contains the brain
d. Extends from the bottom of the skull to the lower back; contains the spinal cord
e. Hollow space in the body that contains internal organs
f. Located below the diaphragm and above the pelvis
g. Body cavity below the abdominal cavity
h. Located below the neck and above the diaphragm; contains the heart, major blood vessels, and lungs

_____ **18.** Pulse
_____ **19.** Appendicular skeleton
_____ **20.** Homeostasis
_____ **21.** Tissue
_____ **22.** Aorta
_____ **23.** Physiology
_____ **24.** Cerebellum
_____ **25.** Systolic blood pressure
_____ **26.** Cells
_____ **27.** Xiphoid process
_____ **28.** Perfusion
_____ **29.** Corpus callosum

a. Largest artery in the body
b. Basic building blocks of the body
c. Upper and lower extremities (arms and legs), shoulder girdle, and pelvic girdle
d. Thick bundle of nerve fibers that joins the two hemispheres of the brain
e. Second largest part of the brain
f. Pressure in an artery when the heart is pumping blood
g. Regular expansion and recoil of an artery caused by the movement of blood from the heart as it contracts
h. "Steady state"
i. Cells that cluster together to perform a specialized function
j. Flow of blood through an organ or a part of the body
k. Study of the normal functions of an organism
l. Piece of cartilage that makes up the inferior portion of the breastbone

_____ **30.** Posterior
_____ **31.** Midline
_____ **32.** Lateral
_____ **33.** Medial
_____ **34.** Distal
_____ **35.** Inferior
_____ **36.** Proximal
_____ **37.** Anterior
_____ **38.** Superior

a. Farthest from the point of attachment to the body
b. Front portion of the body or body part
c. Above or in a higher position than another part of the body
d. In a position lower than another
e. Nearer to the point of attachment to the body
f. Toward the midline of the body
g. Toward the side of the body
h. Line down the center of the body that divides the body into right and left sides
i. Back side of the body or body part

Short Answer

Answer each question in the space provided.

39. List the three formed elements of the blood.

1. ______________________________

2. ______________________________

3. ______________________________

40. List the two parts of the central nervous system.

1. ______________________________

2. ______________________________

CHAPTER

5 Lifting and Moving Patients

By the end of this chapter, you should be able to

Knowledge Objectives ▶

1. Define body mechanics.
2. Discuss the guidelines and safety precautions that need to be followed when lifting a patient.
3. Describe the indications for an emergency move.
4. Describe the indications for assisting in non-urgent moves.
5. Discuss the various devices associated with moving a patient in the out-of-hospital arena.

Attitude Objectives ▶

6. Explain the rationale for properly lifting and moving patients.
7. Explain the rationale for an emergency move.

Skill Objectives ▶

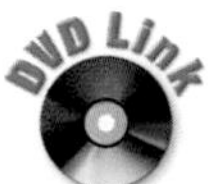

8. Demonstrate an emergency move.
9. Demonstrate a non-urgent move.
10. Demonstrate the use of equipment utilized to move patients in the out-of-hospital arena.

On The Scene

A fire at a nursing home is everyone's nightmare. And here you are, living it. Residents from the wing that is on fire are being evacuated to the recreation area until units can be brought in to evacuate them. A firefighter arrives, carrying an elderly man over his shoulders. The man is confused but pleasant and does not appear injured. Another firefighter appears in the doorway, dragging an approximately 250-pound woman with a blanket. As he turns around to go back, two of his coworkers burst through the fire doors, holding a frightened man in a two-person seat carry.

You quickly begin to sort the new arrivals and assess for any injuries while trying to calm them. Your chief radios that the fire is spreading through the attic. These people will need to be moved outside within the next 10 minutes. You quickly survey your situation. There are eight residents who can walk, four on the floor, two who are unconscious in hospital beds, and three in wheelchairs. You are on the third floor. "Send me the following . . . ," you calmly radio to your chief. ■

THINK ABOUT IT

As you read this chapter, think about the following questions:

- What additional equipment will you need to evacuate the residents?
- What type of carries can be used to move some of these residents?
- What lift can you use to move the patients safely from the floor onto a stretcher?
- What general safety measures should be taken each time you lift one of the residents?

Introduction

Back injuries account for nearly 20% of all injuries and illnesses in the workplace.

Safe Moving and Lifting

Many Emergency Medical Responders are injured every year because they attempt to lift or move patients improperly. Improper lifting and moving techniques can result in muscle strains and tears, ligament sprains, joint and tendon inflammation, pinched nerves, and related conditions. These conditions may develop gradually or may result from a specific event, such as a single, heavy lift. Pain, a loss of work, and disability may result. In most cases, these injuries are preventable.

There is no one best way to move all patients. Many circumstances will affect the method you choose to use. The key is to take a brief moment to analyze the situation and think of all your options. Then choose the method that is safest for you, your coworkers, and the patient.

The Role of the Emergency Medical Responder

You will most often provide care to a patient in the position in which he or she is found. Your responsibility is to distinguish an emergency from a nonemergency situation. You should move only those patients who are in immediate danger. Your role will also include

- Positioning patients to prevent further injury
- Recognizing when to call for more help
- Assisting EMS professionals in lifting and moving patients

Principles of Moving Patients

Objective 3 ▶

Objective 7 ▶

An emergency move is a move used because there is an immediate danger to you or the patient.

THE BIG DECISION . . . What is an emergency that requires immediately moving a patient from the area? In general, a patient should be moved *immediately* (an **emergency move**) when one of the following situations exists:

1. *Scene hazards.* The patient may need to be moved if you are unable to protect the patient from hazards in the area and there is an immediate danger to you or the patient if he or she is not moved. Examples of possible scene hazards include
   - Fire or the danger of fire
   - Uncontrolled traffic
   - Explosives or the danger of an explosion
   - Electrical hazards
   - Rising flood water

- Toxic gases
- Radiation
- Structural collapse or the threat of a structural collapse
- Potentially violent scenes (such as a shooting when the perpetrator has not been caught)

2. *The inability to reach other patients who need lifesaving care.* For example, if there are multiple patients in a vehicle, you may need to move a patient to reach one who is more seriously injured.
3. *The patient's location or position prevents providing immediate, lifesaving care.* For example, a patient in cardiac arrest who is sitting in a chair or lying on a bed must be moved to the floor in order to provide effective CPR.

All of these situations put you at great risk. Always consider your safety first and then make the decision whether to attempt an emergency move or to wait for EMS support.

Never push, pull, or drag a patient sideways.

The greatest danger in moving a patient quickly is the possibility of aggravating a spinal injury. Always drag the patient in the direction of the length (the long axis) of the body. This action will provide as much protection as possible to the patient's spine. In the rare event that you need to perform an emergency move, realize that you will be putting yourself at risk for injury, as well as possibly complicating the patient's injury. For example, if you need to remove a patient from a vehicle using an emergency move, it is impossible to provide the same level of spinal protection that would be accomplished with spine stabilization devices. *Think before you act!* Remember that, in most cases—and except in the situations stated earlier—a patient is better off being treated in place until additional help arrives.

Remember This!

Bystanders are often eager to provide assistance in emergencies. Before asking a bystander to assist you, check your agency's policy regarding these situations. This is particularly important in situations in which there is a risk of injury to you, the patient, or the bystander, such as when lifting or moving a patient. If you are permitted to use bystanders to help you, make sure to provide them with specific instructions to avoid injury.

Objective 4 ▶

If no immediate threat to life exists, when ready for transport, move the patient using a **non-urgent move.** Non-urgent moves are the types of moves you will perform most often. They will be done with the help of other responders. It is important to communicate with each other and the patient before, during, and after the lift. Work as a team for success.

Body Mechanics and Lifting Techniques

Safety Precautions and Preparation

Objective 1 ▶

The term **body mechanics** refers to the way we move our bodies when lifting and moving. Body mechanics includes body alignment, balance, and coordinated body movement. Proper body alignment is synonymous with good posture and is an important part of body mechanics (Figure 5-1). Good posture means that the spine is in a neutral position when standing, sitting, or lying. This position recognizes that the spine has four natural curves. These curves are in the areas of the cervical, thoracic, lumbar, and sacral vertebrae (Figure 5-2). When you use good posture, there is minimal strain on your muscles, ligaments, bones,

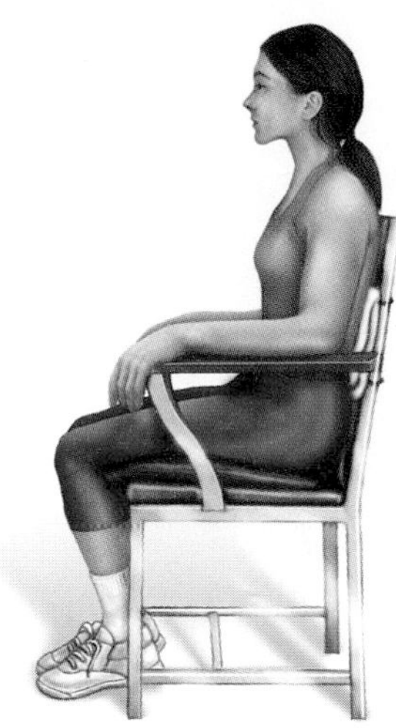

FIGURE 5-1 ▲ Good body mechanics includes good posture.

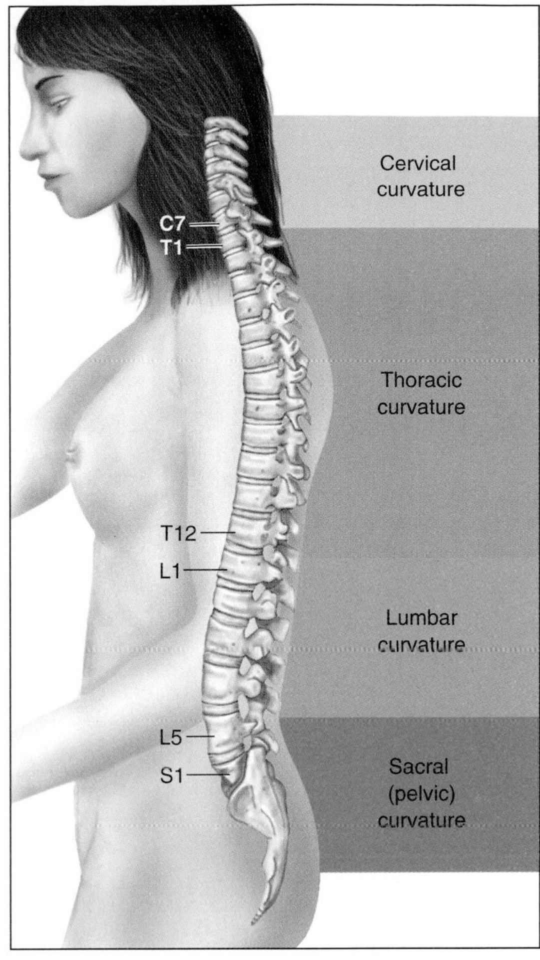

FIGURE 5-2 ► The adult spine has four natural curves in the areas of the cervical, thoracic, lumbar, and sacral (pelvic) vertebrae.

joints, and nerves. By maintaining proper body alignment, you reduce strain on your spine as well as on the muscles and ligaments that support it.

You also improve your balance when you use good posture. Balance can be further improved by

- Separating your feet to a comfortable distance
- Bending your knees
- Flexing your hips to reach a squatting position

These actions broaden your base of support and help reduce your risk of injury.

To protect yourself and the patient, you should prepare and plan *before* you actually move a patient. Important factors to consider include

- The patient's weight
- The patient's condition
- The presence of hazards or potential hazards at the scene
- The terrain
- The distance the patient must be moved
- Your physical abilities and any limitations
- The availability of any equipment or personnel to assist with the move

A patient may be in an awkward position or a tight space. The patient's position or location may require you to bend or move out of balance. In these situations, it is best to call for additional help before moving the patient. In some situations, the *patient* may be able to tell you the best technique to move him or

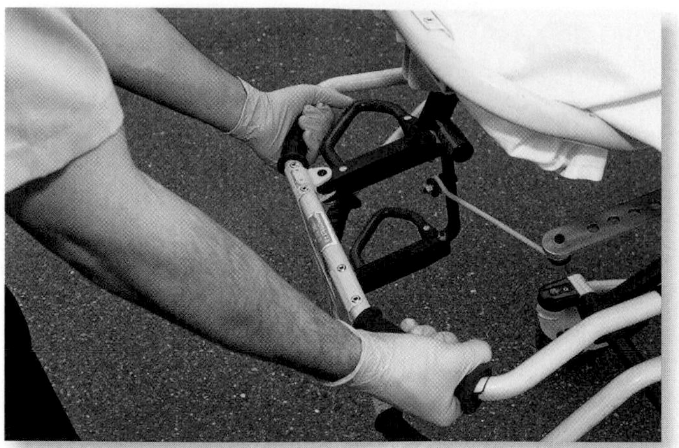

FIGURE 5-3 ▶ The power grip.

her. In all cases, it is very important to communicate clearly and frequently with your partner and the patient throughout the process. Work as a team and remind each other to use proper lifting techniques.

The Power Grip

When lifting, your arms and hands are strongest when positioned with your palms up.

When lifting an object, use the **power grip** (underhand grip) to take full advantage of the strength of your hands, forearms, and biceps. With your palms up, grasp the object you are preparing to lift. Position your hands a comfortable distance apart, usually about 10 inches. Your palms and fingers should be in complete contact with the object, with all fingers bent at the same angle (Figure 5-3).

Guidelines for Safe Lifting

Objective 2 ▶

Safe lifting means keeping your back aligned as vertically as possible, using your leg strength, and maintaining your center of balance while lifting. Follow these important rules to prevent injury when lifting:

Objective 6 ▶

- Consider the weight of the patient and the need for additional help.
- Know your physical ability and limitations.
- Plan how you will move the patient and where you will move him or her. If a commercially made stair chair is available, use it when transporting patients down stairs. If it is not available, use a sturdy chair for this purpose.
- It is often helpful to mentally picture the patient's final position and work backwards to the patient's current position. Working in this way helps prevent arms from getting crossed and bodies from becoming twisted during the actual move.
- Make sure your path is clear of obstructions.
- When working with others, determine in advance who will direct the move. *One* person (usually the person at the patient's head) must assume responsibility for directing the actions of the others: "On my count, lift on three: one, two, three." "On my count, turn on three: one, two, three." Agree in advance that if anyone involved in the move says "No," the move is stopped and the patient is immediately returned to the starting position.
- Position your feet a comfortable distance apart (usually a shoulder's width) on a firm surface. Wear proper footwear to protect your feet and maintain a firm footing.
- Tense the muscles of your abdomen and buttocks before lifting. This tensing helps relieve the stress on your back muscles.
- Bend at your knees and hips, not at your waist, and keep your back straight. All movement in the lift comes from your *legs*.

You must think about these guidelines before *every* lift.

"Hug the load."

- Use your legs to lift, not your back. Your legs are much stronger than your back.
- Lift using a smooth, continuous motion. *Do not jerk or twist* when lifting. Jerking or twisting increases your risk of injury.
- Keep the patient's weight as close to you as possible. Doing so moves your center of gravity closer to the patient, helps you maintain balance, and reduces muscle strain.
- When possible, move forward rather than backward.
- Walk slowly, using short steps.
- Look where you are going.
- Move slowly, communicating clearly and frequently with other EMS personnel and the patient throughout the move.

The **power lift** is a way to lift heavy objects using the proper body mechanics just described. Skill Drill 5-1 shows a two-person power lift being used to lift a wheeled stretcher.

Stop and Think!

Always practice proper lifting techniques. Learning to lift using proper body mechanics takes training and practice. When practicing, use "spotters" to alert you when you are performing a technique incorrectly. Practice and practice again until using correct lifting techniques becomes a habit. One bad lift can damage your back for the rest of your life!

Guidelines for Safe Reaching

To avoid injury when reaching, follow these important rules:

- Keep your back straight.
- Avoid stretching or leaning back from your waist (hyperextending) when reaching overhead. Lean from your hips.
- Avoid twisting while reaching.
- Avoid reaching more than 15–20 inches in front of your body to grasp an object.
- Avoid situations in which prolonged strenuous effort (more than a minute) is needed.

Guidelines for Safe Pushing and Pulling

To avoid injury when pushing and pulling, follow these guidelines:

- Push, rather than pull, whenever possible.
- Keep your back straight.
- Avoid twisting or jerking when pushing or pulling an object.
- Push at a level between your waist and shoulders.
- When the patient or object is below your waist, kneel to push or pull.
- When pulling, avoid reaching more than 15–20 inches in front of your body. Change your position (move back another 15–20 inches) when your hands have reached the front of your body.
- Keep the line of the pull through the center of your body by bending your knees.
- Keep the weight close to your body.
- Keep your elbows bent and your arms close to your sides.
- If possible, avoid pushing or pulling from an overhead position.

Skill Drill 5-1

Two-Person Power Lift

STEP 1 ▶ Position your feet a shoulder's width apart on a firm surface. Wear proper footwear to protect your feet and maintain a firm footing.

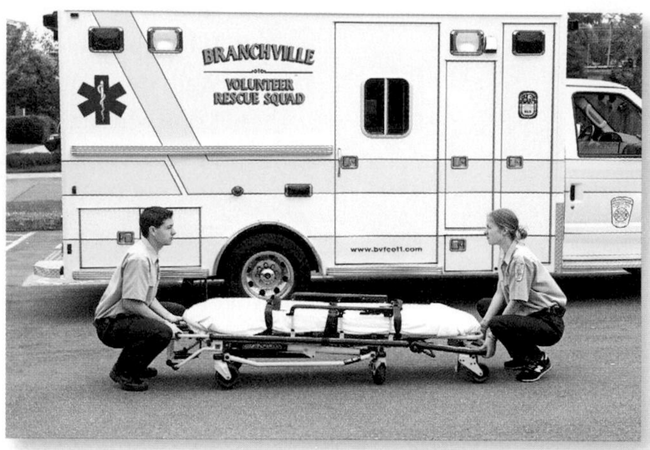

STEP 2 ▶ Use the power grip to grasp the stretcher. Tense the muscles of your abdomen and buttocks. Bend at your knees and hips, not at your waist, and keep your back straight.

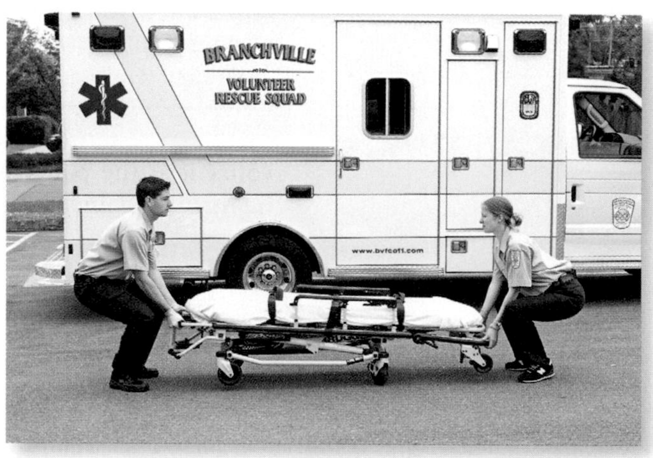

STEP 3 ▶ Communicating with each other and the patient, lift at the same time with your legs, not your back. Use a smooth, continuous motion.

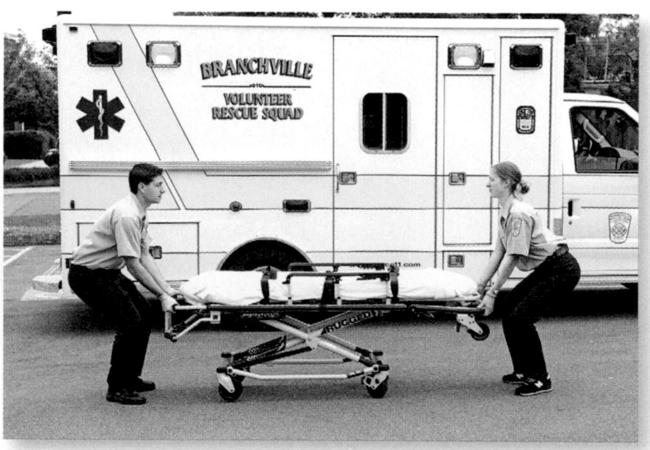

Emergency Moves

Drags

Drags are a good way to move patients already on the ground.

Dragging or pulling is more difficult than pushing. You will be surprised by how tired you become in a short time. Stabilize the patient's head and neck as much as possible before beginning the move. The clothes drag and blanket drag may be used when the patient must be moved quickly and an injury to the head or spine is suspected. Although it is not ideal material to stabilize the spine, the patient's clothing or a blanket provides material against which the patient's head and neck is cradled during the move.

When dragging a patient, always pull along the length of the spine from either the patient's shoulders or the patient's feet and legs. *Never* pull the patient's head away from his or her neck and shoulders. Broaden your base of support by moving your rear leg back (if you are facing the patient) or by moving your front foot forward (if you are facing away from the patient).

Stop and Think!

Before performing an emergency move, make sure your path is clear of obstructions. Doing so will protect the patient from being dragged through broken glass, metal fragments, or other sharp objects that can cause additional injury.

Clothes Drag

To perform a clothes drag (also called the *clothing pull* or *shirt drag*), position yourself at the patient's head (Figure 5-4). To prevent the patient's arms from being pulled upward during the move, consider securing the patient's wrists together or tucking his hands into his waistband. Gather the shoulders of the patient's shirt and pull him toward you so that a cradle is formed for the patient's head and neck. Make sure you have a firm grasp on the patient's clothing and begin pulling the patient to safety. When using this move, check often to make sure you are not choking the patient as his clothes slide up around his neck.

Always use the part of the blanket under the patient's head as a handle. Doing so will keep his head and shoulders slightly raised, so that his head will not strike the ground.

Blanket Drag

To perform a blanket drag, lay a blanket, sleeping bag, tarp, bed sheet, bedspread, or similar material lengthwise beside the patient. Make sure there is approximately 2 feet of the blanket above the patient's head. The uppermost section of the blanket will provide a cradle for the patient's head. It will also be used as the handle with which you will drag the patient. Kneel on the opposite

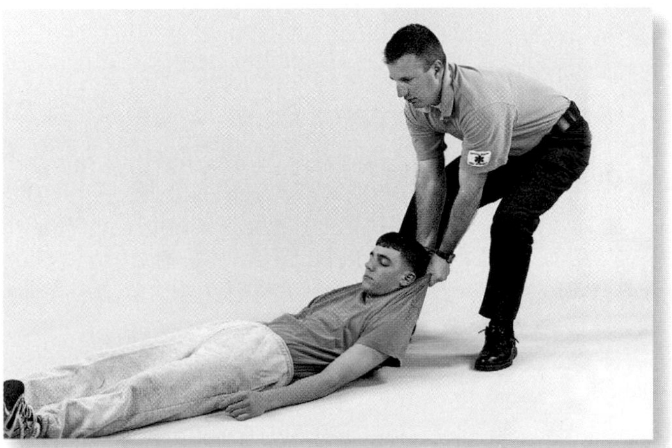

FIGURE 5-4 ▶ The clothes drag.

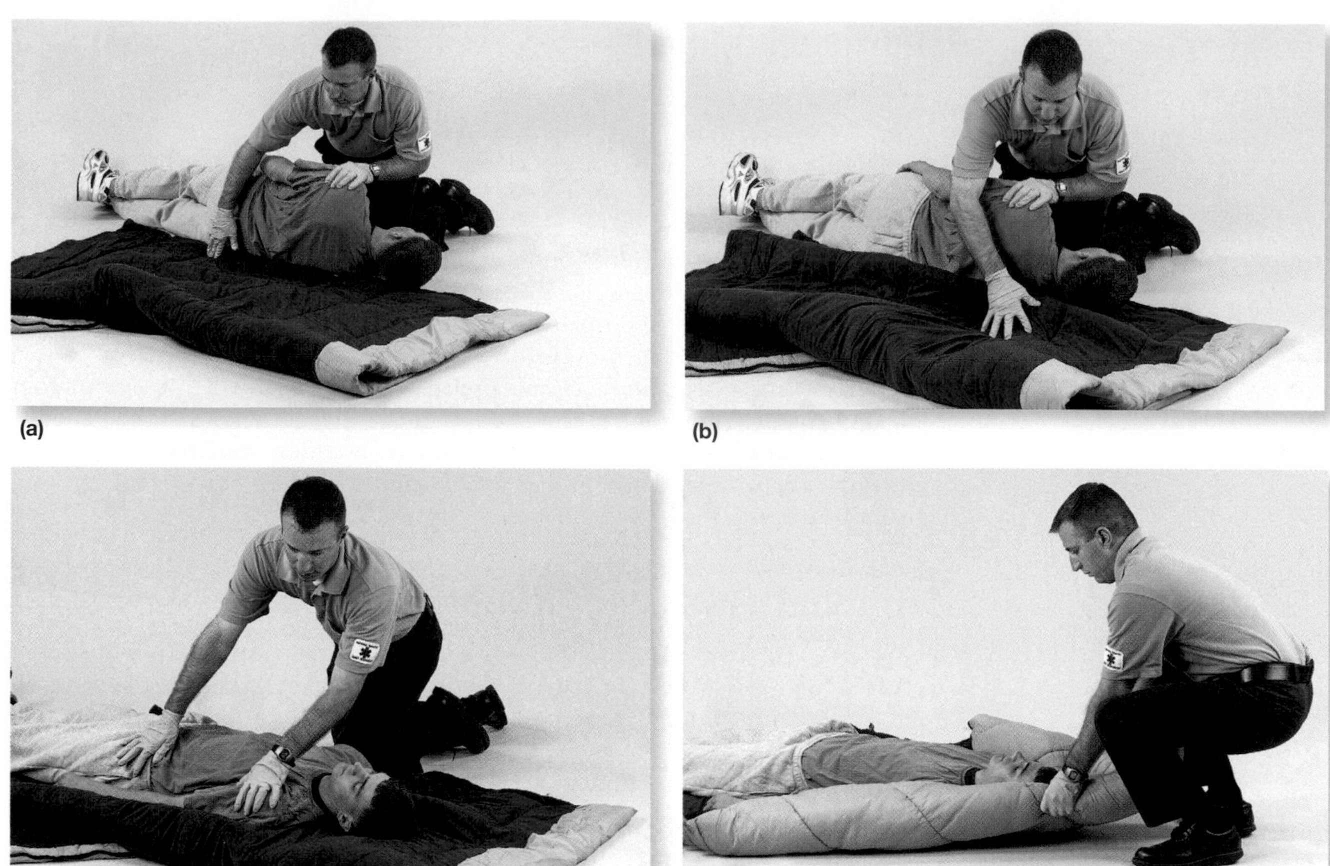

FIGURE 5-5 ▲ The blanket drag.

side of the patient and roll him toward you (Figure 5-5a). Grasp the blanket and tuck half of the blanket under the patient. Leave the remainder of the blanket lying flat (Figure 5-5b). Quickly but gently, roll the patient onto his back. Pull the tucked portion of the blanket out from under the patient. Wrap the corners of the blanket securely around the patient (Figure 5-5c). Using the blanket "handle" that you created above the patient's head, keep the pull as straight and as in-line as possible and drag the patient to safety. Remember to use your legs, not your back, and keep your back as straight as possible (Figure 5-5d).

Shoulder Drag

This emergency move is often used because it does not require any additional materials.

To perform a shoulder drag, position yourself behind the patient and prop her up into a sitting position. From your position behind the patient, slide your hands under her armpits and drag her to safety (Figure 5-6).

Forearm Drag

To perform a forearm drag (also called a *bent-arm drag*), position yourself as you would in a shoulder drag. After sliding your hands under the patient's armpits, grasp her forearms and drag (Figure 5-7). Note that the forearm drag provides *no* protection for the patient's spine.

Ankle Drag

To perform an ankle drag, grasp the patient's ankles or pant cuffs (Figure 5-8). This emergency move is not recommended because the patient's head is not supported and it may bounce if the patient is not pulled over a smooth surface.

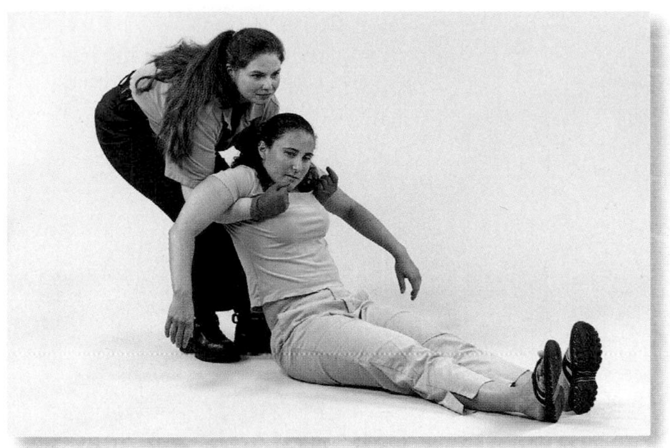

FIGURE 5-6 ▲ The shoulder drag.

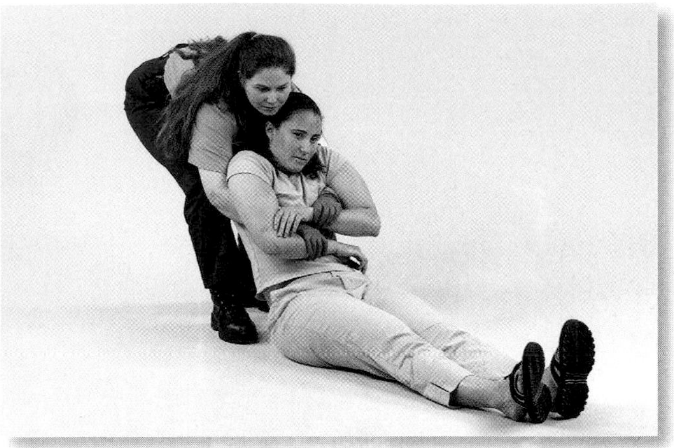

FIGURE 5-7 ▲ The forearm drag.

FIGURE 5-8 ▶ The ankle drag.

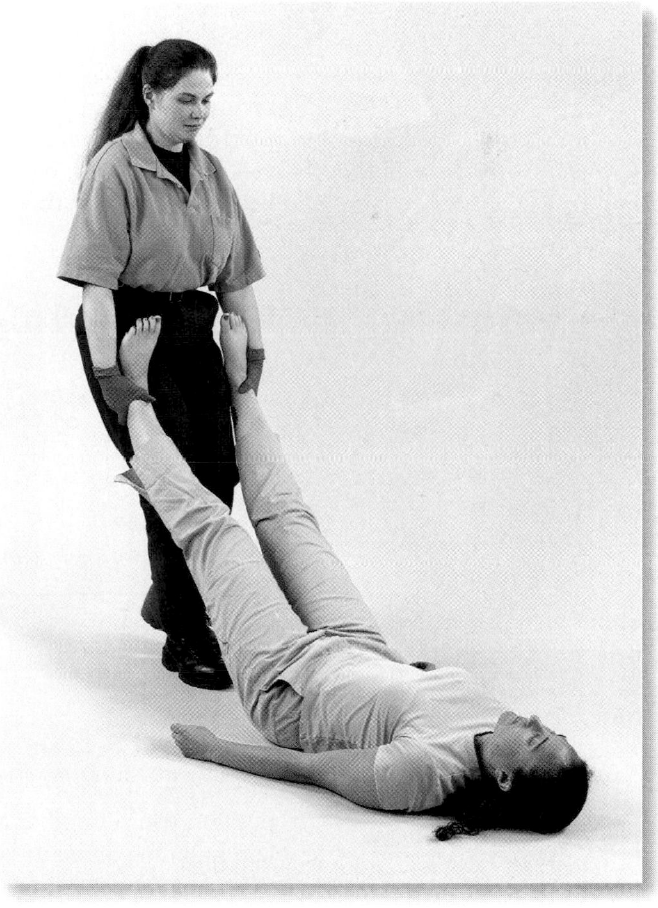

However, you may encounter a situation in which you have no other means of moving the patient.

Firefighter's Drag

The firefighter's drag is particularly useful when you must crawl underneath a low structure for a short distance or move a patient from a smoke-filled area. To perform a firefighter's drag, place the patient on his back (Figure 5-9). Cross his wrists and

FIGURE 5-9 ▶ The firefighter's drag.

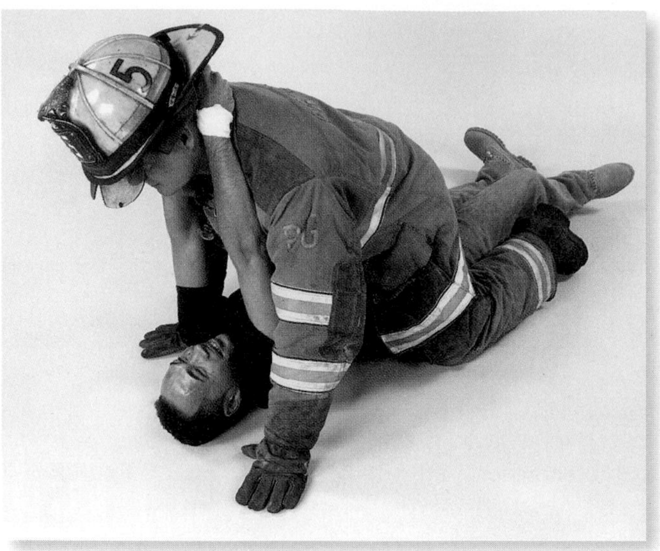

secure them together with gauze, a triangular bandage, or a necktie. Straddle the patient and lift his arms over your head so that his wrists are behind your neck. As you crawl forward, be sure to raise your shoulders high enough so that the patient's head does not hit the ground.

Remember This!

Dragging Tips

Remember:

- Always drag the patient along the length (long axis) of the spine.
- Never push, pull, or drag a patient sideways.
- Never pull the patient's head away from his or her neck and shoulders.

Carries

Firefighter's Carry

The patient's abdomen bears the weight with this move.

The firefighter's carry can be used to move a patient quickly. To perform this move, position yourself toe to toe with the patient. Crouch down, grasp the patient's wrists, and pull the patient to a sitting position (Figure 5-10a). Step on the patient's toes with the tip of your shoes. While grasping the patient's wrists, pull the patient to a standing position (Figure 5-10b). Quickly place your shoulder into the patient's abdomen and pull the patient lengthwise across your shoulders (Figure 5-10c). Place one arm through the patient's legs. Use your other hand to grasp one of the patient's arms, secure the patient in position on your shoulders, and then stand up (Figure 5-10d). Remember to lift with your legs, not your back.

Cradle Carry

The cradle carry (also called the *one-person arm carry*) may be used if the patient is a child or a small adult. To perform a cradle carry, kneel next to the patient.

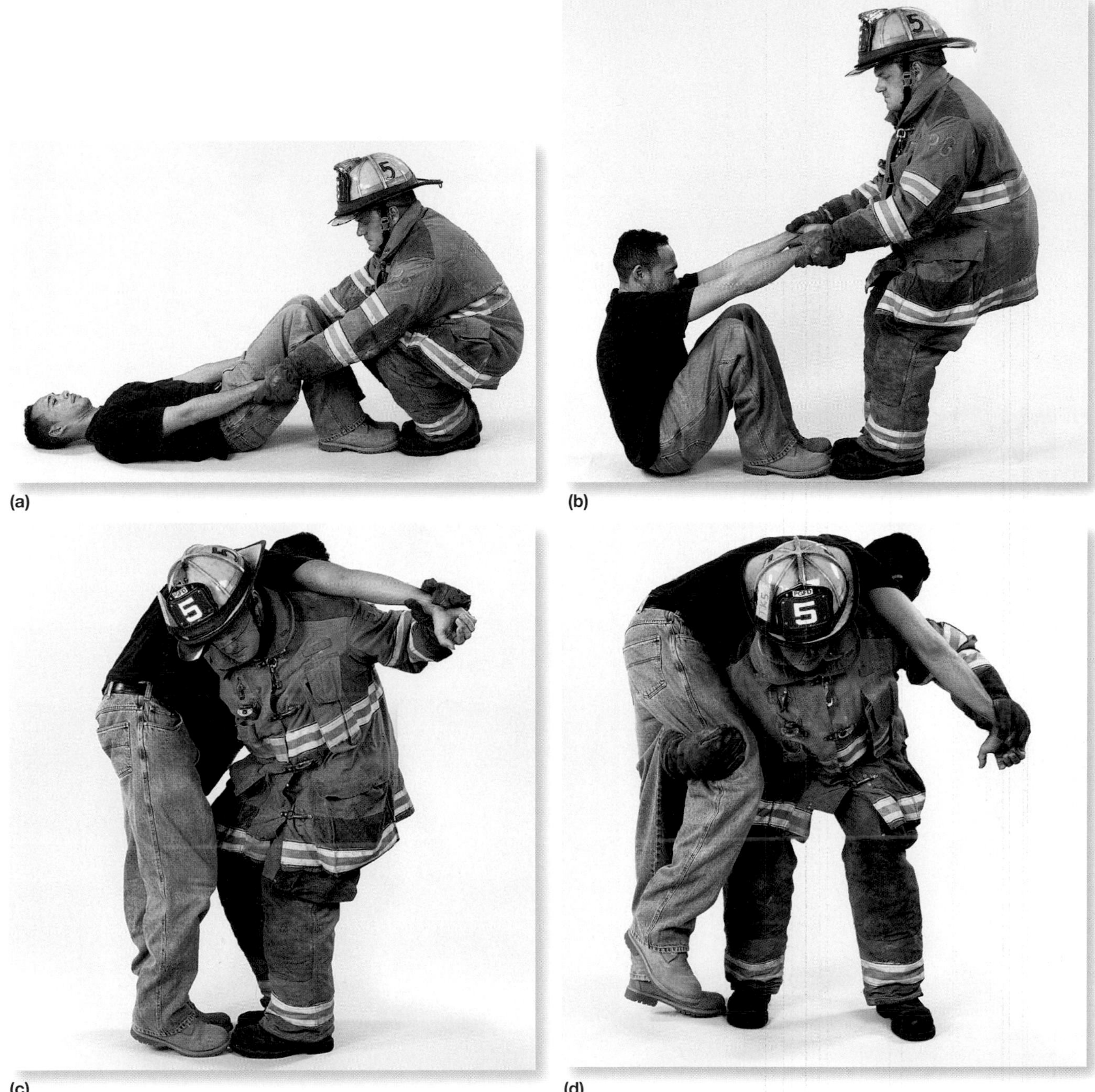

FIGURE 5-10 ▲ The firefighter's carry.

Place one hand under the patient's shoulders and the other under her knees; then stand up, using the strength of your legs (Figure 5-11).

Pack-Strap Carry

This move requires no equipment.

The pack-strap carry is best used with a conscious patient, unless someone is available to help you position the patient. To perform the pack-strap carry, kneel in front of a seated patient with your back to her. Have the patient place her arms over your shoulders so that they cross your chest. Be sure the patient's armpits are over your shoulders. Cross the patient's wrists in front of you and grasp her wrists. While holding her wrists, lean forward, rise up on your knees, and pull the patient up onto your back. Hold both of the patient's wrists close

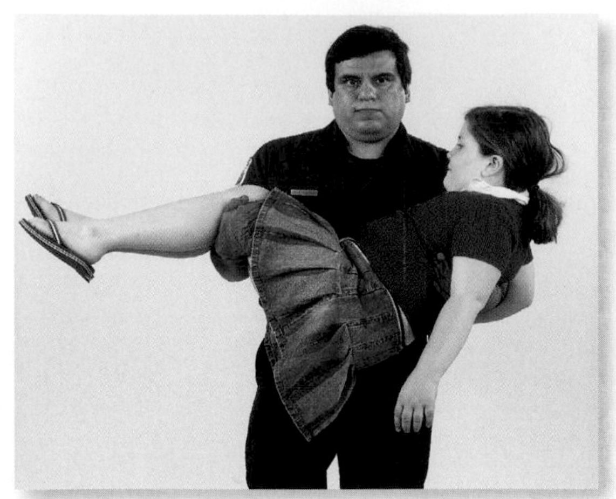

FIGURE 5-11 ► The cradle carry.

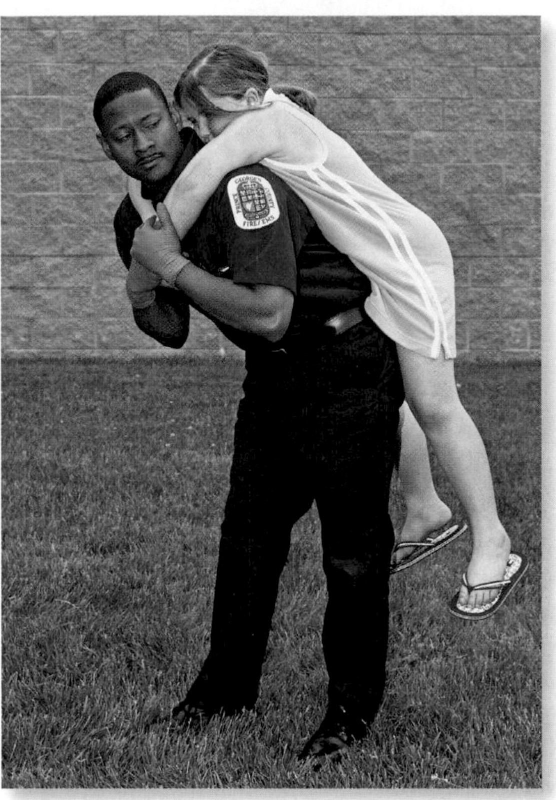

FIGURE 5-12 ► The pack-strap carry.

to your chest as you stand up (Figure 5-12). If the patient is small, it may be possible to grasp both of her wrists with one hand. This action leaves your other hand free to open doors and move obstructions.

Piggyback Carry

The piggyback carry is used when the patient cannot walk but can use her arms to hold onto you. To perform this move, kneel in front of a seated patient with your back to her. Have the patient place her arms over your shoulders, so that they cross your chest. Cross the patient's wrists in front of you and grasp her wrists. While holding her wrists, lean forward, rise up on your knees, and pull the patient up onto your back. Hold both of the patient's wrists close to your chest as you stand up (Figure 5-13a). As you prepare to reposition your arms and hands, instruct the patient to hold onto you with her arms. Position your forearms under the patient's knees and grasp her thighs (Figure 5-13b).

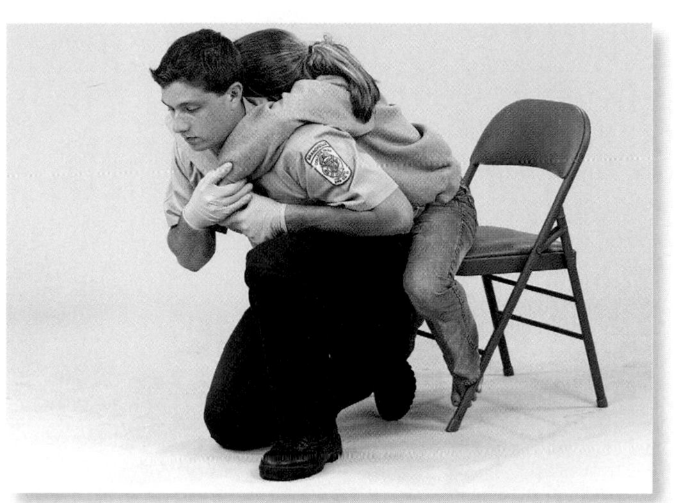

(a)

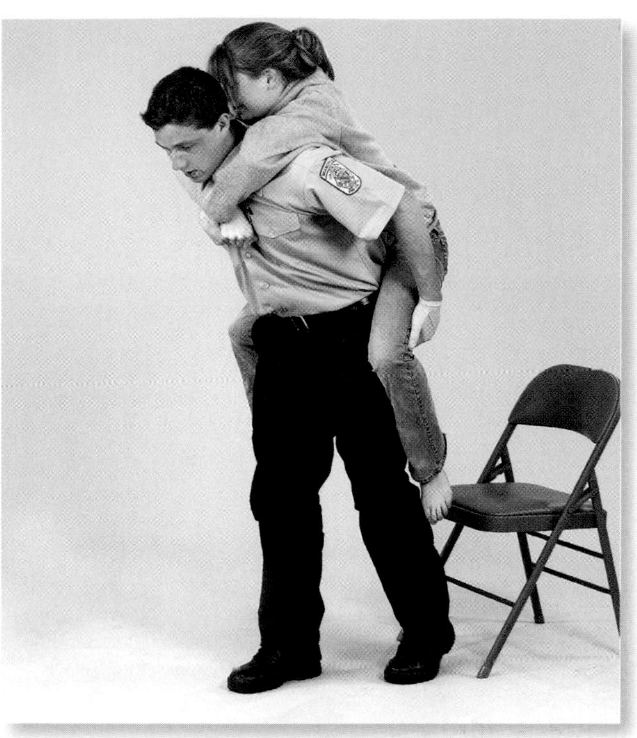

(b)

FIGURE 5-13 ▲ The piggyback carry.

Two-Person Carry

It is best to have two rescuers of about the same height and size perform this move.

If the patient is unable to walk, two people can make a "seat" for the patient. To perform the two-person carry (also called the *two-person seat carry*), place one arm under the patient's thighs and the other across the patient's back. Grasp the arms of the other rescuer and lock them in position at the elbows, forming a seat. Both rescuers then rise slowly to a standing position (Figure 5-14).

Human Crutch Move

One or two rescuers may be used for this move.

In some situations, the patient may be able to walk but requires assistance. You can assist him to safety by acting as a crutch. To perform the human crutch move (also called the *rescuer assist* or *walking assist*), place the patient's arm across your shoulders and hold his wrist with one hand. Place your other hand around his waist and help him to safety (Figure 5-15).

Non-Urgent Moves

Direct Ground Lift

If the patient is going to be transferred to a stretcher, place the stretcher as close to the patient as possible.

The **direct ground lift** is used to lift and carry a patient with no suspected spinal injury from the ground to a bed or a stretcher. While this lift can be performed with two rescuers, three is the safest method. A lot of communication and teamwork is necessary to lift and move patients safely. Skill Drill 5-2 shows the steps for a three-person direct ground lift.

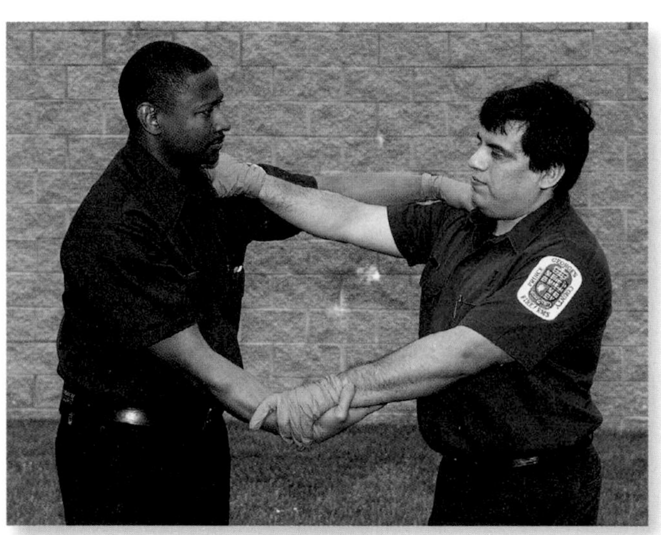

FIGURE 5-14 ▲ The two-person carry.

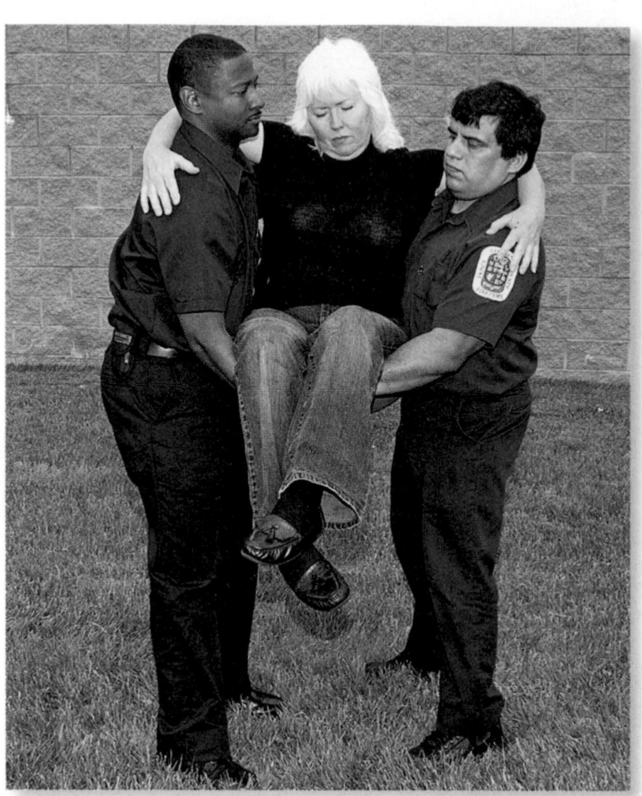

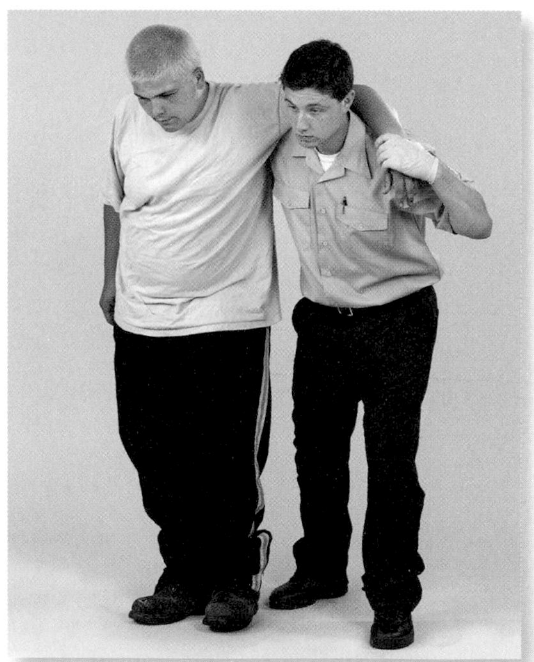

FIGURE 5-15 ▲ The human crutch move.

Remember This!

Do *not* perform a direct ground lift or an extremity lift if trauma to the patient's head, neck, or back is suspected because the head is not stabilized during these moves. The extremity lift must also be avoided if an extremity is injured.

Three-Person Direct Ground Lift

STEP 1

- Three rescuers line up on the same side of a supine patient. If three rescuers are available, position one at the patient's head, the second at the patient's waist, and the third at the patient's knees.
- To maintain balance throughout the move, all rescuers should kneel on one knee. The same knee should be used by all rescuers. If possible, place the patient's arms across his or her chest.
- If only two rescuers are available, position one at the patient's chest and the other at the patient's thighs.

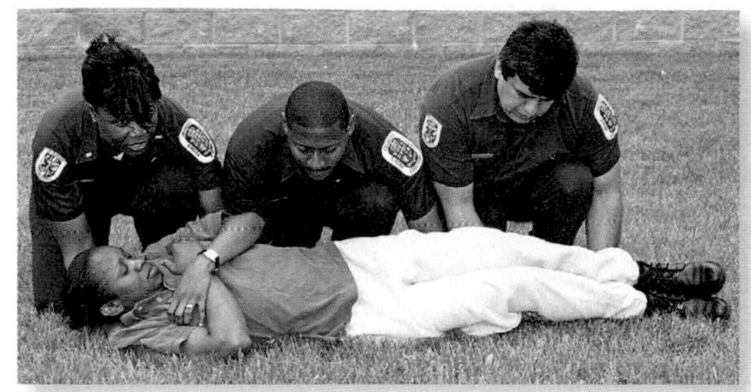

STEP 2

- The rescuer at the head places one arm under the patient's neck and shoulders, cradling the patient's head. The first rescuer's other arm is placed under the patient's lower back. The second rescuer places one arm above and one arm below the patient's waist. The third rescuer places one arm under the patient's knees and the other under the patient's ankles.
- If only two rescuers are available, the first rescuer places one arm under the patient's head and neck and cradles the patient's head. He or she places the other hand under the patient's shoulders. The second rescuer places his or her arms under the patient's lower back and buttocks.

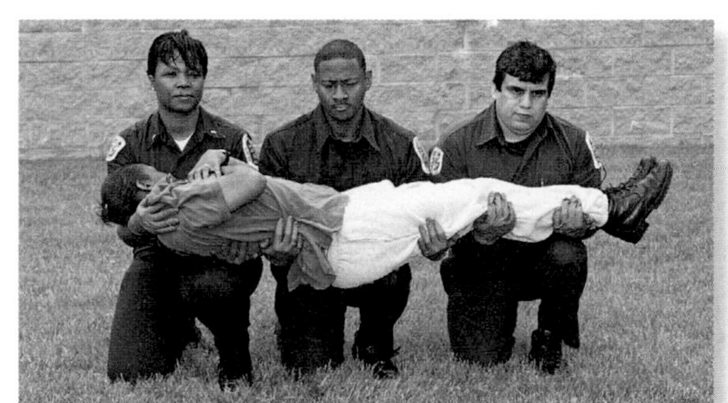

STEP 3

- On the command of the rescuer at the patient's head, all the rescuers should lift the patient to their knees.
- Once everyone is balanced, the patient is rolled toward the rescuers' chests. This action keeps the weight of the patient close to the rescuers' bodies, reducing the risk of back injury to the rescuers.

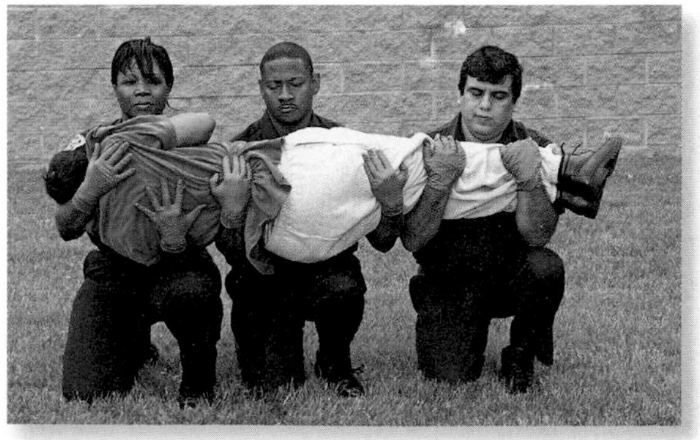

Continued on next page

Skill Drill 5-2

Three-Person Direct Ground Lift *(continued)*

STEP 4 ▶
- On the command of the rescuer at the patient's head, all the rescuers should stand and move the patient to the desired location.
- To lower the patient, simply reverse the steps.

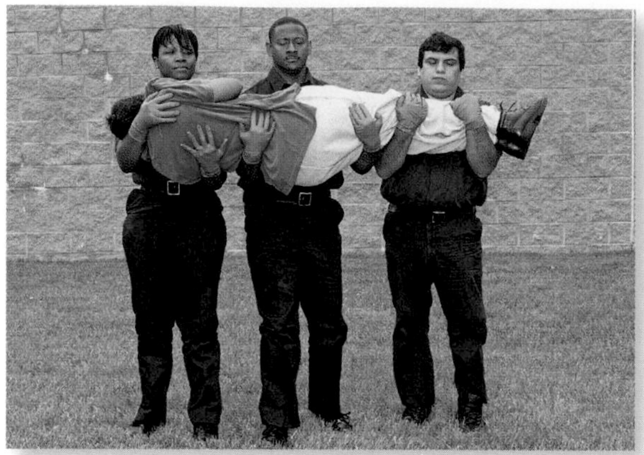

Extremity Lift

The extremity lift is used to lift a patient onto a carrying device, such as a stretcher. Two rescuers are needed to perform an extremity lift. This lift should *not* be used on a patient with a suspected head, neck, back, or extremity injury. Skill Drill 5-3 shows a two-person extremity lift.

Transfer of a Supine Patient from a Bed to a Stretcher

There are two common methods used to transfer a supine patient from a bed to a stretcher. The first method is the direct carry. It is used when you are required to move a patient to a stretcher that cannot be placed parallel to the bed. The second, the draw sheet transfer, is by far the most common. This method requires the stretcher to be placed parallel to the patient's bed. In both cases, you will be assisting hospital personnel or another EMS professional. As with previous moves, teamwork and coordination are essential.

Direct Carry

The direct carry is used to move a patient with no suspected spinal injury from a bed to a stretcher. Skill Drill 5-4 illustrates a direct carry.

Stop and Think!

Use the following tips when performing a direct carry:

- Some older stretchers do not have brakes. If there is no brake, ask someone to stabilize the stretcher for you.
- Remember to lift with your legs.
- Be careful not to jerk or twist when lifting the patient.

Two-Person Extremity Lift

STEP 1 ▶ One rescuer kneels at the patient's head. The second rescuer kneels between the patient's bent knees with his or her back to the patient.

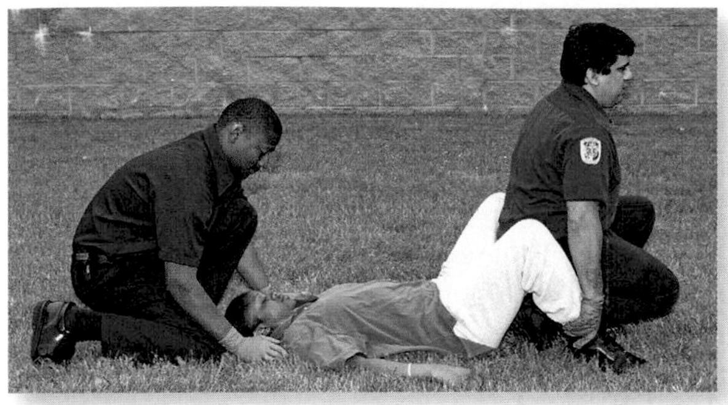

STEP 2 ▶ The rescuer at the patient's head places one hand under each of the patient's armpits and grasps the patient's wrists. The second rescuer slips his or her hands behind the patient's knees.

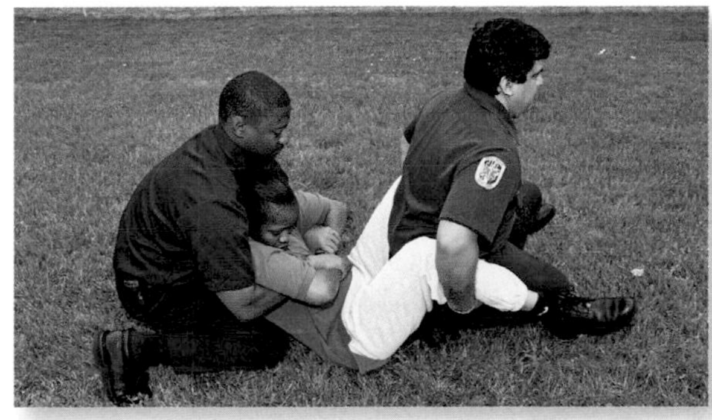

STEP 3 ▶ On a signal from the rescuer at the patient's head, both rescuers move up to a crouching position.

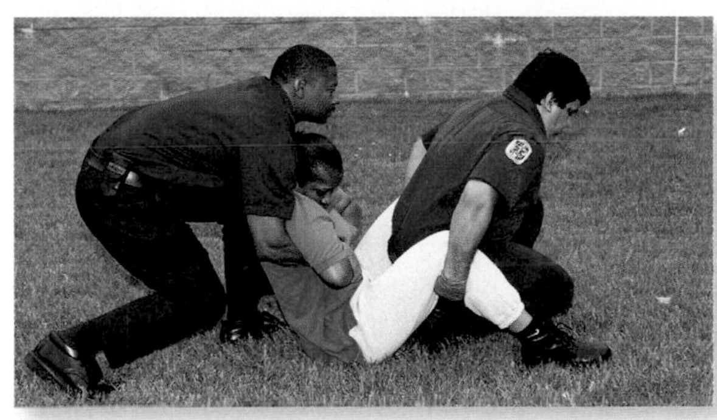

STEP 4 ▶ On a signal from the rescuer at the patient's head, both rescuers stand at the same time and move with the patient.

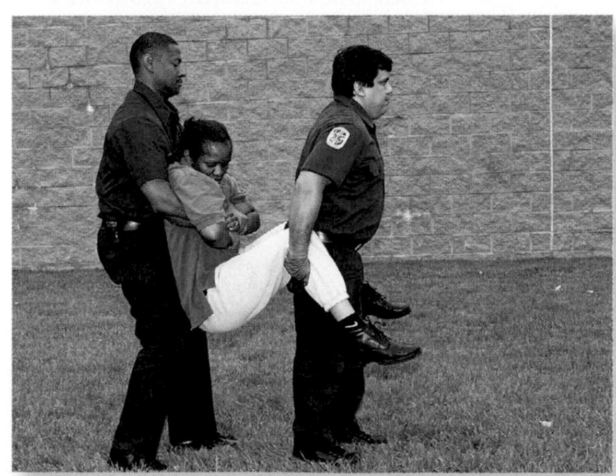

Skill Drill 5-4

Direct Carry

STEP 1 ▶

- Place the stretcher at a 90-degree angle to the bed, with the head end of the stretcher at the foot of the bed. Prepare the stretcher by unbuckling the straps, adjusting the height of the stretcher to be even with the bed, and lowering the side rails. Set the brakes on the stretcher (if so equipped) to the "on" position.
- Both rescuers should stand between the bed and the stretcher and face the patient.

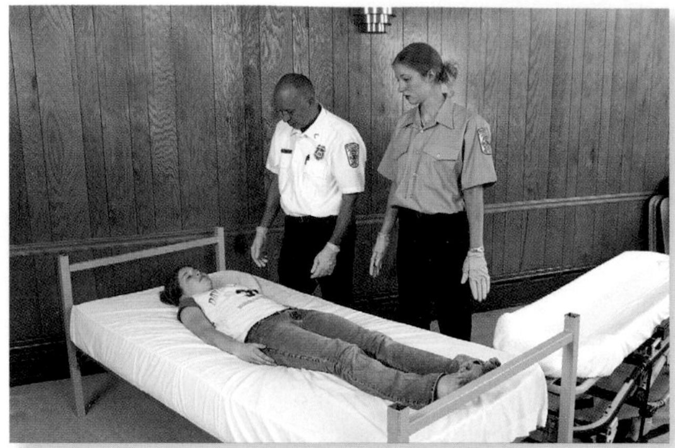

STEP 2 ▶

- The rescuer at the head slides one arm under the patient's neck, cupping the patient's far shoulder with his hand and cradling the patient's head. The rescuer then slides his other arm under the patient's lower back.
- The second rescuer slides one hand under the patient's hip and lifts slightly. The rescuer then places her other arm under the patient's hips and calves.

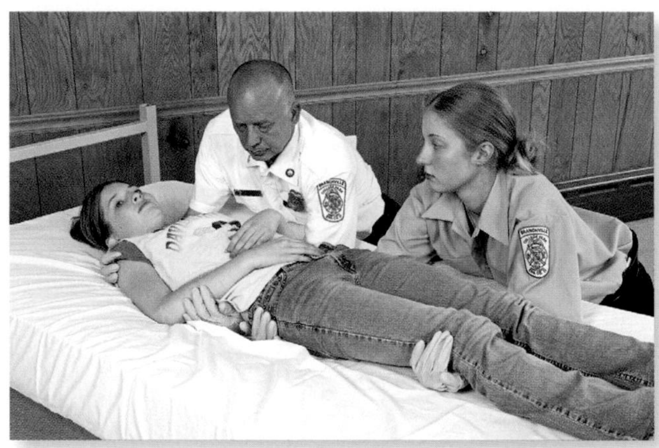

STEP 3 ▶

- On a signal from the rescuer at the patient's head, both rescuers slide the patient toward them to the edge of the bed. Both rescuers should lift with their legs.

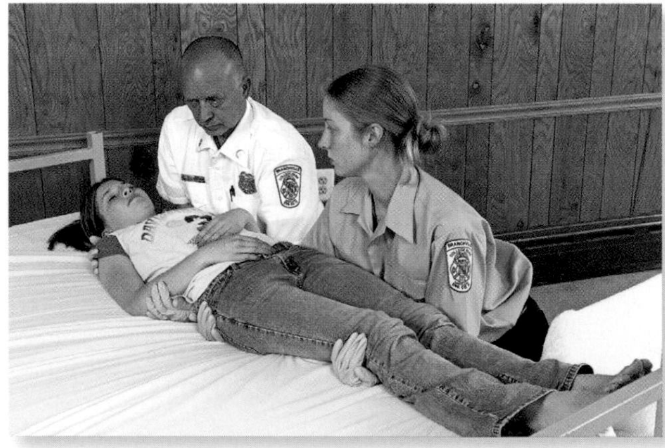

STEP 4 ▶ • On a signal from the rescuer at the patient's head, the patient is lifted and curled toward the rescuers' chests. Both rescuers should be careful not to jerk or twist.

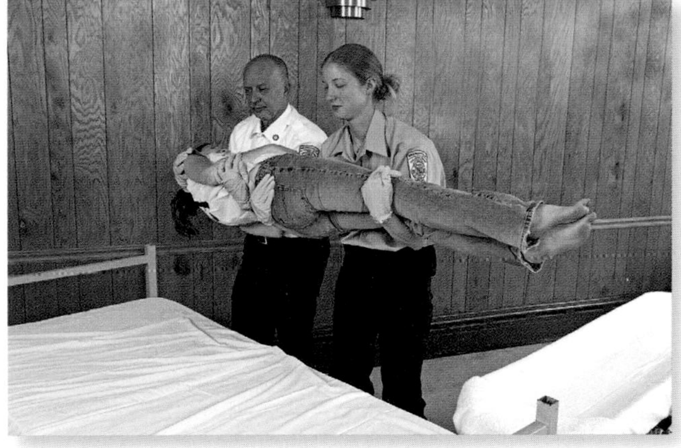

STEP 5 ▶ • On a signal from the rescuer at the patient's head, both rescuers then rotate together, lining up with the stretcher, and gently place the patient onto the stretcher.

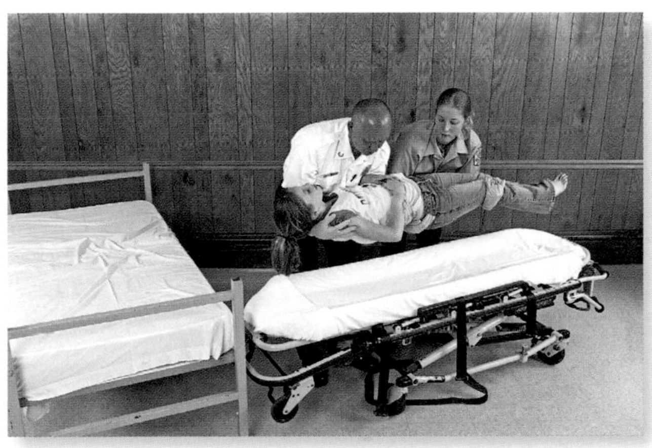

Draw Sheet Transfer

A **draw sheet** is a narrow sheet placed crosswise on a bed under the patient. It is used to assist in moving a patient or when changing soiled bed sheets. The draw sheet transfer requires a minimum of two people to perform; however, the use of four rescuers is preferred. To move a patient using a draw sheet, follow the steps outlined in Skill Drill 5-5.

Patient Positioning

The left side is preferred so that the patient faces the EMS professional during ambulance transport. This position also allows secretions to drain from the patient's nose and mouth.

Although patient positioning is often overlooked, it is an essential part of your patient care. In some cases, simply changing the patient's position can improve his or her condition. Consider the following situations:

- Your patient was golfing when he suddenly felt hot and lightheaded. He sat down in the grass to rest. As you approach, he lies down. Your patient is now unresponsive without a possible head, neck, or back injury. He is breathing and a pulse is present. This patient should be placed in the

Draw Sheet Transfer

STEP 1
- Loosen the draw sheet on the bed and form a long roll to grasp.
- Prepare the stretcher by unbuckling the straps, adjusting the height of the stretcher to be even with the bed, and lowering the side rails.
- Set the brakes on the stretcher (if so equipped) to the "on" position.
- Position the stretcher next to and touching the patient's bed.

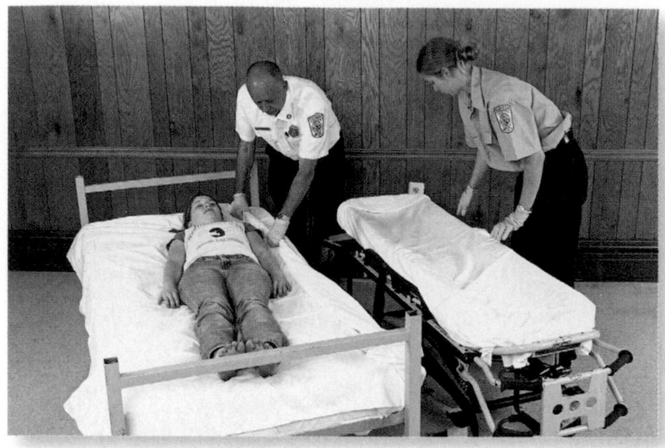

STEP 2 Both rescuers should stand on the same side of the stretcher and then reach across it to grasp the draw sheet firmly at the patient's head and hips.

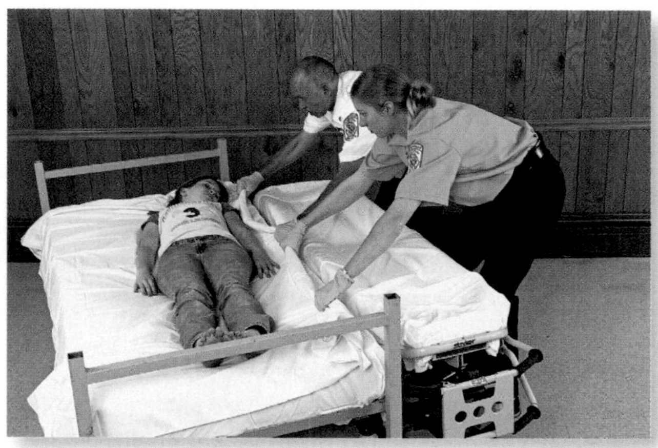

STEP 3 On a signal from the rescuer at the patient's head, gently slide the patient from the bed to the stretcher.

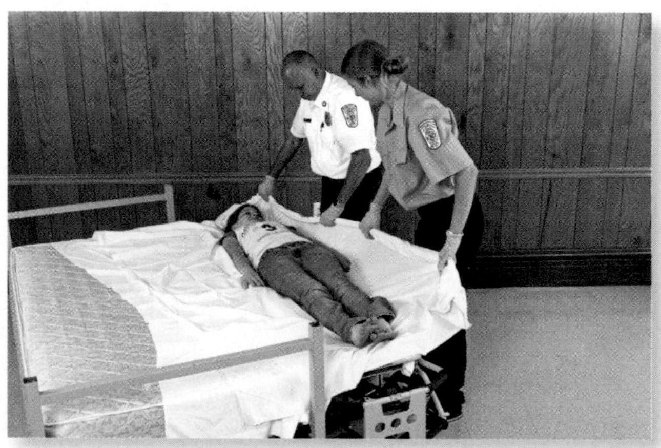

recovery position (Figure 5-16). To place a patient in the recovery position, raise the patient's left arm above his head, so that his head will rest on his arm once he is log-rolled onto his left side. Kneel on the left side of the patient. Grasp the patient's leg and shoulder and roll him toward you, onto his left side. This positioning allows the patient's head to rest on his raised left arm with his face in a slightly downward position. It also helps secretions drain from the patient's nose and mouth, reducing the risk of a blocked airway. If the patient stops breathing or no longer has a pulse, roll him onto his back and begin CPR.

Any patient with a suspected spinal injury should be fully stabilized on a long backboard.

Do not permit a patient complaining of chest pain or difficulty breathing to walk to the stretcher or ambulance.

- Your patient has fallen from a ladder while trimming tree branches. You suspect a head, neck, or back injury. This patient should *not* be moved until additional EMS resources can evaluate and stabilize the patient. Be sure to have suction readily available should vomiting occur.
- Your patient was running at the track and is now experiencing difficulty breathing. This patient should be allowed to assume a position of comfort. Most often, this will be a seated position. In a **Fowler's position,** the patient is lying on his back with his upper body elevated at a 45- to 60-degree angle (Figure 5-17). In a **semi-Fowler's position,** the patient is sitting up with his head at a 45-degree angle and his legs out straight (Figure 5-18). In a **high-Fowler's position,** the patient is sitting upright at a 90-degree angle (Figure 5-19).

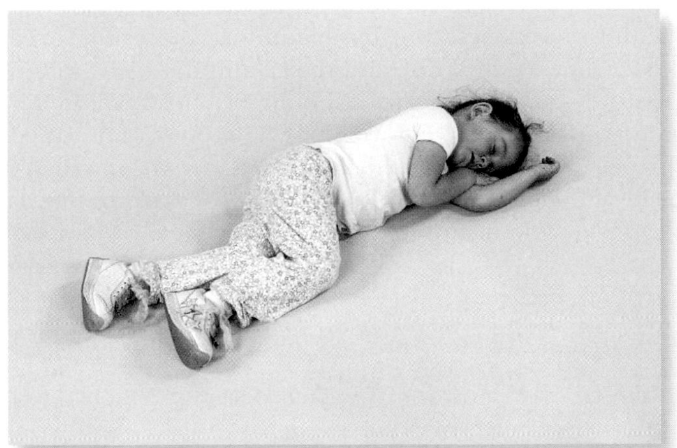

FIGURE 5-16 ▲ The recovery position.

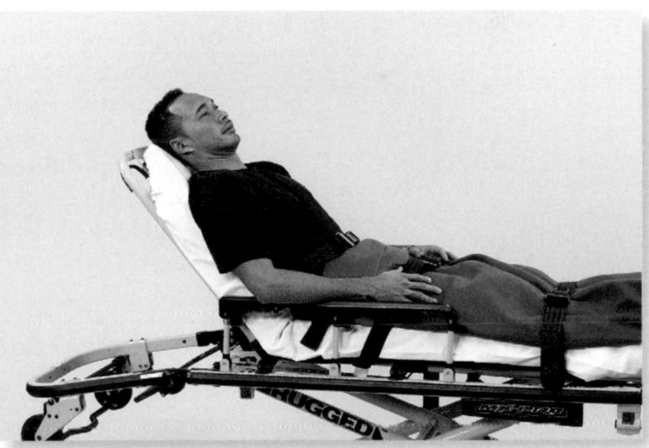

FIGURE 5-17 ▲ The Fowler's position.

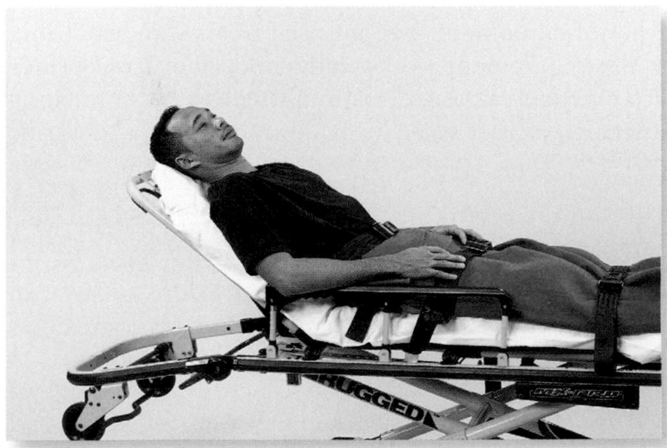

FIGURE 5-18 ▲ The semi-Fowler's position.

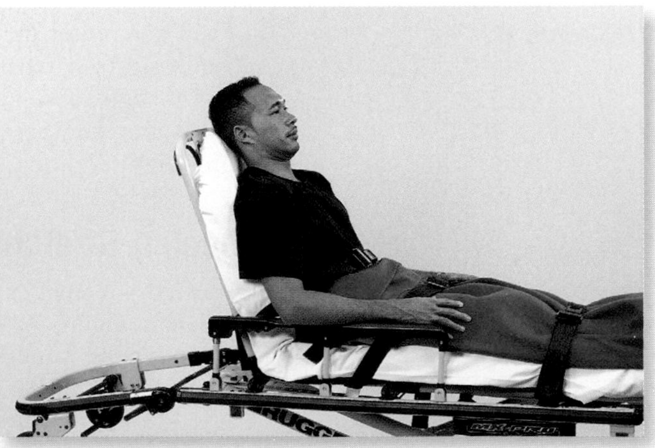

FIGURE 5-19 ▲ The high-Fowler's position.

FIGURE 5-20 ▶ The shock position.

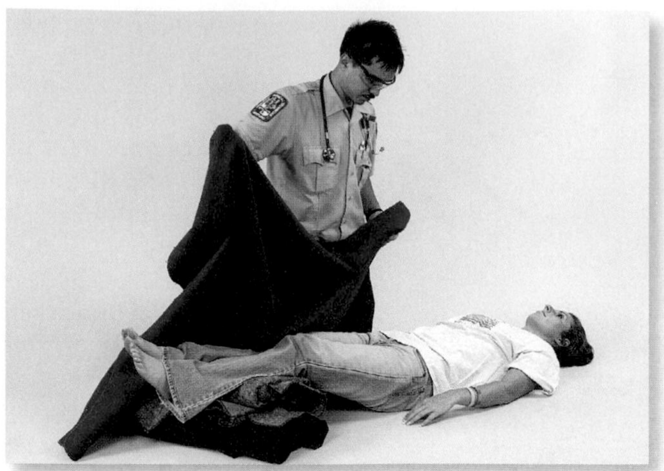

- Your patient is experiencing a sudden onset of severe abdominal pain or non-traumatic back pain. Patients with this complaint are often most comfortable on their back or side with their knees slightly bent.
- Your patient is vomiting. He is awake and alert with a strong pulse. There is no history or evidence of trauma. This patient should be allowed to assume a position of comfort. Be prepared to manage his airway and place him in the recovery position if his level of consciousness decreases.
- Your patient is complaining of weakness. She has had flu symptoms for three days. She is confused. Her skin is pale, cool, and moist, and her heart rate is fast. A patient with signs and symptoms of shock should be placed flat on her back with her feet elevated 8–12 inches (Figure 5-20). This position is called the **shock position.** This position should *not* be used if the patient has an injury to her head or neck, chest, abdomen, pelvis, spine, or lower extremities. It should also *not* be used if the patient shows signs or symptoms of respiratory distress.

Remember This!

Do not place a patient in the recovery position if you suspect the patient has experienced an injury to his or her head, neck, or spine.

Equipment

Objective 5 ▶

You will encounter many types of equipment that are used to assist in stabilizing and moving your patients. Most equipment works under the same basic principle, with slight design and cosmetic variations. It is important to become familiar with the equipment used in your area. The following sections describe commonly used equipment.

Wheeled Stretcher

A wheeled stretcher is a rolling bed that is commonly found in the back of an ambulance (Figure 5-21). There are many manufacturers, but all wheeled stretchers work under the same basic premise. Most wheeled stretchers can be adjusted to various heights to ease patient transfers. The head of the stretcher can be adjusted to several different angles. Wheeled stretchers have handles used for lifting and rolling. If you are lifting a wheeled stretcher with someone who does not operate it often, take the control end so that you can make sure the wheels will drop properly.

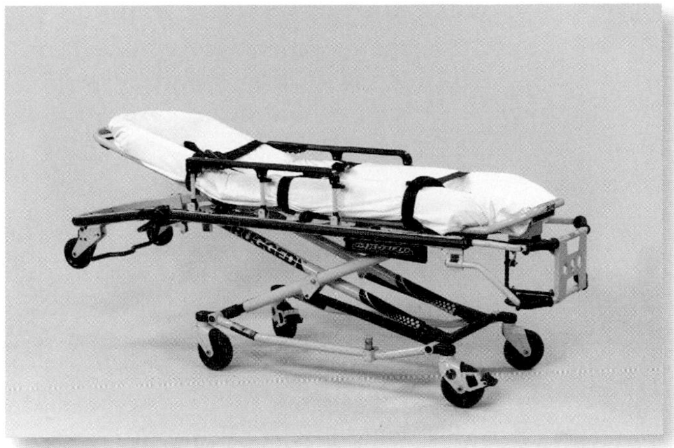

FIGURE 5-21 ▲ A wheeled stretcher.

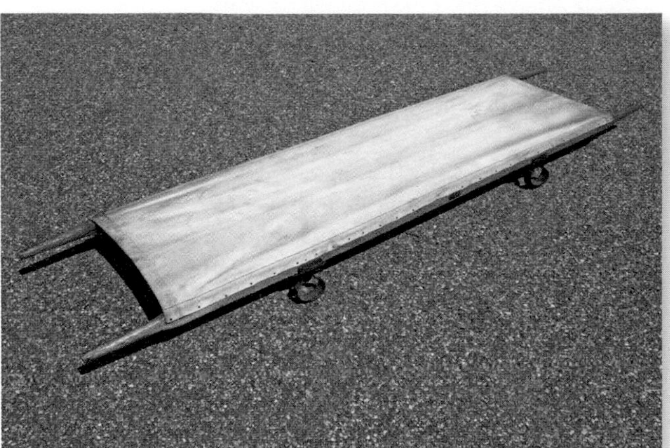

FIGURE 5-22 ▲ A portable stretcher.

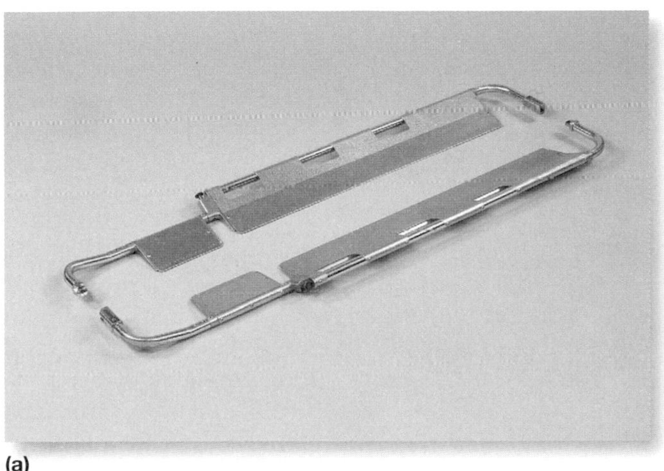

(a)

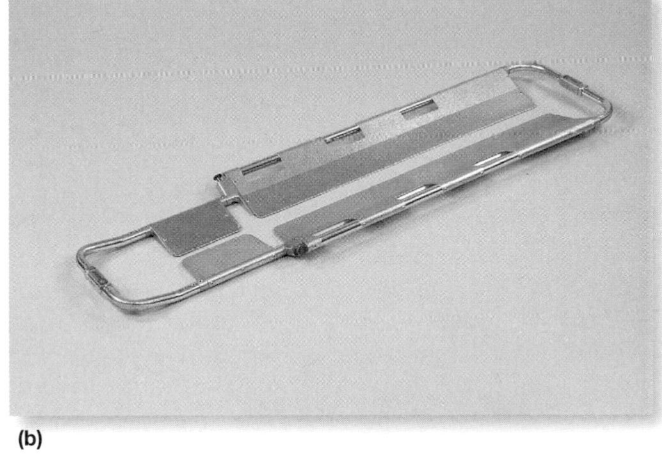

(b)

FIGURE 5-23 ▲ A scoop stretcher. **(a)** sides separated; **(b)** sides together.

Be sure you know the weight limitations of the stretcher you are using. Exceeding them could cause injury to the patient, the crew, or both.

Portable Stretcher

A portable stretcher usually folds or collapses when it is not in use. Many are made of heavy canvas or heavy plastic (Figure 5-22). It may be used in the following situations:

- To carry patients down stairs, downhill, or over rough terrain
- To remove patients from spaces too confined or narrow for a wheeled stretcher
- In incidents in which you need to transfer a large number of people quickly from one place to another

The scoop stretcher is also called a split litter. To use this device, both sides of the patient must be accessible.

Scoop Stretcher

A scoop (orthopedic) stretcher is unique in that it is hinged and opens at the head and feet to fit around and under the patient (Figure 5-23). The two halves of the stretcher are adjusted to the patient's length. Each piece is then slid under the patient and reconnected, effectively scooping the patient onto the device. The scoop stretcher may be used to carry a supine patient up or down stairs. However, a scoop stretcher does not adequately stabilize the spine. If a spinal injury is suspected, the patient and scoop stretcher should be secured to a long backboard for stabilization.

Remember This!

To decrease your patients' anxiety, always carry patients head first up the stairs and feet first down the stairs.

Basket Stretcher

A basket stretcher is also called a basket litter or Stokes basket.

A basket stretcher (Figure 5-24) is shaped like a long basket and can hold a scoop stretcher or a long backboard. Some basket stretchers are too narrow to hold all widths of backboards. If you will be using a basket stretcher, be sure to check how wide it is to make certain your backboard will fit.

The basket is made of fiberglass-plastic composites, plastic with an aluminum frame, or a steel frame with wire or plastic mesh. Some basket stretchers have holes in the bottom to allow for water drainage. A basket stretcher is used for moving patients over rough terrain, in water rescues, or in high-angle rescues. It can also be pulled over snow and ice, much like a sled.

Flexible Stretcher

A flexible stretcher can be rolled up for easy storage and carrying, but it forms a rigid surface that conforms to the sides of the patient when in use. Examples of flexible stretchers include the Reeves stretcher (Figure 5-25), the SKED, and the Navy stretcher. Flexible stretchers are made of canvas or flexible, synthetic material with carrying handles. Straps are used to secure the patient. This type of stretcher is particularly useful when space is limited to access the patient. It can be used in narrow hallways, stairs, cramped corners, high-angle rescues, and hazardous materials situations. Because the flexible stretcher conforms around the patient, it may not be possible to access all areas of the patient when giving emergency care. Also, flexible stretchers do not provide the kind of impact

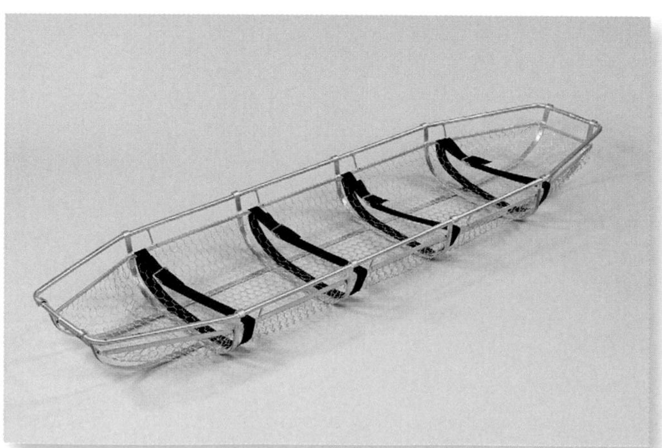

FIGURE 5-24 ▲ A basket stretcher.

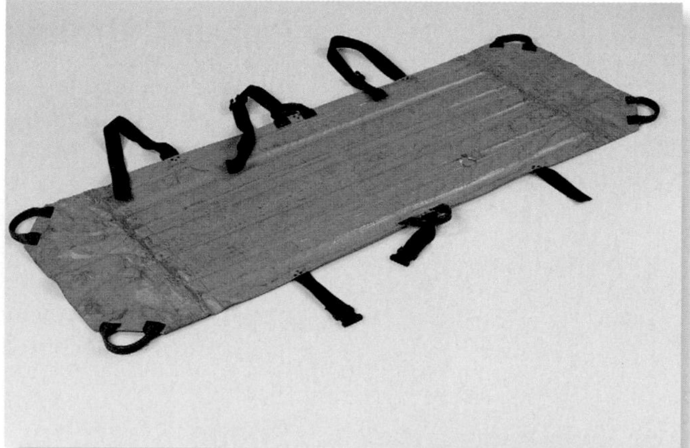

FIGURE 5-25 ▲ A flexible stretcher.

protection for the patient as do many basket stretchers. You will need to exercise greater care when moving your patient in a flexible stretcher.

Stair Chair

At least two rescuers are required to move a patient in a stair chair.

A stair chair is a commercially made chair (Figure 5-26). It is used to transfer patients up or down stairways, through narrow hallways and doorways, into small elevators, or in narrow aisles in aircraft and buses. It is a very helpful device when a patient does not need to lie flat. The stair chair has belts and straps with which to secure the patient. It also has handles for lifting.

Backboard

Backboards (also called spine boards) come in many shapes, sizes, and colors. The long backboard has holes spaced along the head and foot ends, as well as the sides (Figure 5-27). These holes are made for handholds and inserting straps. The long backboard is used in the following situations:

- Securing a patient who is either lying or standing and needs to be immobilized to prevent worsening a potential spinal injury
- Lifting and moving patients
- Providing secondary support when a short backboard or scoop stretcher is used
- Providing a firm surface on which to perform CPR

A vest-type device can be used in place of a short backboard.

The short backboard is used to secure the head, neck, and back of a stable patient seated in a vehicle (Figure 5-28). Once secured, the patient can then be transferred to a long backboard for full stabilization that includes the hips and legs.

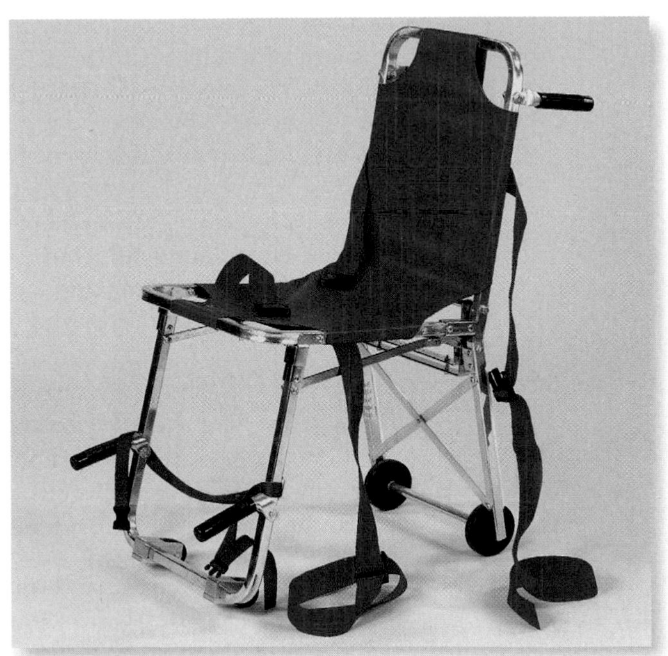

FIGURE 5-26 ▲ A stair chair.

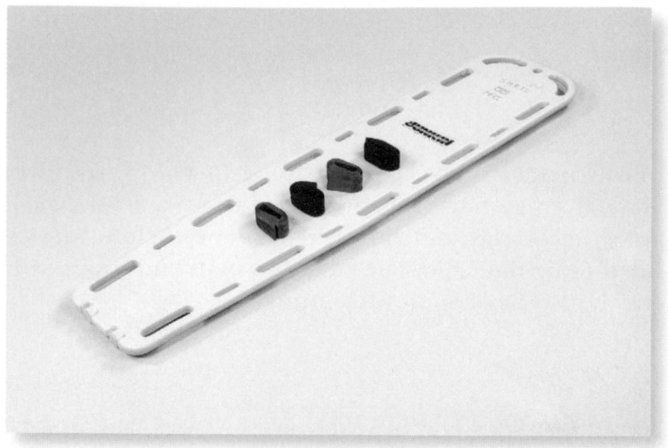

FIGURE 5-27 ▲ A long backboard.

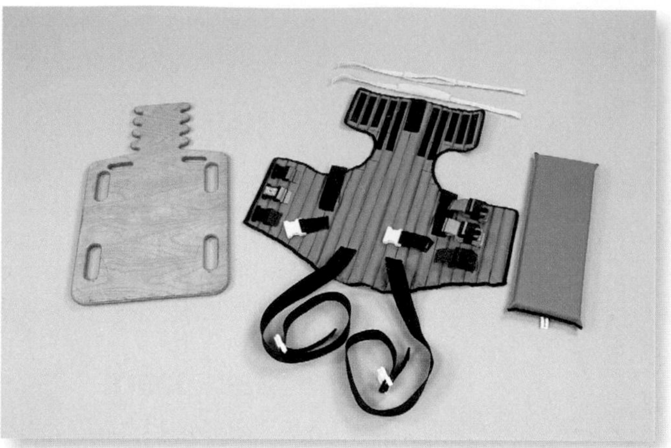

FIGURE 5-28 ▲ A short backboard and vest-type device.

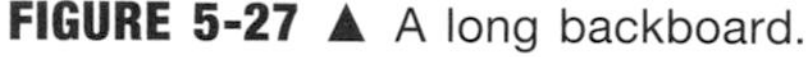

On The Scene

Wrap-Up

Equipment and personnel begin to arrive quickly. You direct them to take the unconscious patients using available stretchers. Stair chairs are used to evacuate others who are too large and too weak to walk. One elderly woman is able to walk with a firefighter who uses the human crutch move to assist her. As you wait for the equipment to return, your aide reports that the fire doors are becoming very hot. You can see a wisp of smoke curling around them at the ceiling. You pick up the last, tiny woman in a cradle carry and evacuate the building. Thirty minutes later, the ceiling collapses, crushing the room you and your patients were in. ■

Sum It Up

- As an Emergency Medical Responder, you will most often give care to a patient in the position in which he or she is found. You should move only patients who are in immediate danger. Therefore, you will need to be able to recognize an emergency from a nonemergency situation. Your role will also include positioning patients to prevent further injury and assisting other EMS professionals in lifting and moving patients.
- An *emergency move* is used when there is an immediate danger to you or the patient. These dangers include scene hazards, the inability to reach patients who need lifesaving care, and a patient location or position that prevents your giving immediate and lifesaving care.
- *Body mechanics* is the way we move our bodies when lifting and moving. Body mechanics includes body alignment, balance, and coordinated body movement. Good posture is key to proper body alignment.
- In order to lift safely, you should use the *power grip* (underhand grip). To perform this grip, you should position your hands a comfortable distance apart (about 10 inches). With your palms up, grasp the object you are preparing to lift. The power grip allows you to take full advantage of the strength of your hands, forearms, and biceps.
- Safely lifting patients requires you to use good posture and good body mechanics. You should consider the weight of the patient and call for help if needed. Plan how you will move the patient and where you will move him or her. It is also important to remember to lift with your legs, not your back. When lifting with other EMS professionals, communication and planning are key.

- *Drags* are one type of emergency move. When dragging a patient, remember to stabilize the patient's head and neck as much as possible before beginning the move. Also, always remember to pull along the length of the spine. *Never* restore pull the patient's head away from his or her neck and shoulders. You should also never drag a patient sideways. *Carries* are the second major type of emergency move. As an Emergency Medical Responder, you should become familiar with the types of carries.
- *Non-urgent moves* are used to move, lift, or carry patients with *no* known or suspected injury to the head, neck, spine, or extremity. The *direct ground lift* and the *extremity lift* are the two main types of non-urgent moves.
- The *direct carry* and the *draw sheet transfer* are the two primary methods used to transfer a supine patient to a bed or stretcher. In both transfer types, you will assist hospital personnel or another EMS professional. Therefore, teamwork and coordination are essential.
- Patient positioning is an important part of the patient care you provide. In some cases, simply changing a patient's position can improve his or her condition. As an Emergency Medical Responder, you should become familiar with the types of positions and when to use them.
- Many types of equipment are used to assist in stabilizing and moving patients. In your role as an emergency care provider, it is important to become familiar with the equipment used in your area. Commonly used equipment includes various types of stretchers and backboards, as well as the stair chair.

▶ Tracking Your Progress

After reading this chapter, can you:	Page Reference	Objective Met?
• Define body mechanics?	128	☐
• Discuss the guidelines and safety precautions that need to be followed when lifting a patient?	130–131	☐
• Describe the indications for an emergency move?	127–128	☐
• Describe the indications for assisting in non-urgent moves?	128	☐
• Discuss the various devices associated with moving a patient in the out-of-hospital arena?	148–152	☐
• Explain the rationale for properly lifting and moving patients?	130–131	☐
• Explain the rationale for an emergency move?	127–128	☐

Chapter Quiz

Multiple Choice

In the space provided, identify the letter of the choice that best completes each statement or answers each question.

_____ 1. Which of the following is an example of a situation that requires an emergency move?
  a. an 88-year-old man who is sitting in a chair in his home and is confused
  b. a 57-year-old woman who is in a supermarket, complaining of difficulty breathing
  c. a 72-year-old woman who is sitting in a chair and is unresponsive, is not breathing, and has no pulse
  d. a 5-year-old boy who is sitting on a bench in a park, complaining of stomach pain

_____ 2. Which of the following is an emergency move?

a. direct ground lift
b. extremity lift
c. direct carry
d. blanket drag

_____ 3. Which of the following may be used in a high-angle rescue?

a. wheeled stretcher, basket stretcher
b. basket stretcher, flexible stretcher
c. portable stretcher, wheeled stretcher
d. flexible stretcher, scoop stretcher

_____ 4. Which of the following statements about safe lifting techniques is true?

a. Place your feet close together.
b. Know your physical abilities and limitations.
c. Use the large muscles of your back to lift.
d. Keep the weight at least 20–30 inches from your body.

True or False

Decide whether the statement is true or false. In the space provided, write T for true or F for false.

_____ 5. Both sides of the patient must be accessible when using a scoop stretcher.

Matching

Match the key terms in the left column with the definitions in the right column by placing the letter of each correct answer in the space provided.

_____ 6. Emergency move
_____ 7. High-Fowler's position
_____ 8. Semi-Fowler's position
_____ 9. Power grip
_____ 10. Draw sheet
_____ 11. Fowler's position
_____ 12. Recovery position
_____ 13. Wheeled stretcher
_____ 14. Shock position
_____ 15. Non-urgent move

a. Patient move used when no immediate threat to life exists and the patient's safety is the primary concern
b. Narrow sheet placed crosswise on a bed under a patient
c. Lying on the back with the upper body elevated at a 45- to 60-degree angle
d. Placing an unresponsive patient who is breathing and in no need of CPR (and in whom trauma is not suspected) on his or her side to help keep his or her airway open
e. Sitting upright at a 90-degree angle
f. Move used because there is an immediate danger to the patient or rescuer
g. Method of placing your hands, before a lift, that is designed to take full advantage of the strength of your hands and forearms
h. Sitting up with the head at a 45-degree angle and the legs out straight
i. Rolling bed commonly found in the back of an ambulance
j. Flat on the back with the feet elevated 8–12 inches

Short Answer

Answer each question in the space provided.

16. A 62-year-old man was the driver of a vehicle that struck a power pole at approximately 80 miles per hour. He was not wearing his seatbelt. What is the greatest danger in moving this patient, if you determine that an emergency move is necessary?

____

____

____

17. You are preparing to transfer a patient from a stretcher to a bed using a direct carry. Where should you place the stretcher?

____

____

____

Sentence Completion

In the blanks provided, write the words that best complete the sentence.

18. When dragging a patient, avoid reaching more than ____________ ____________ in front of your body.

Module 2

Airway

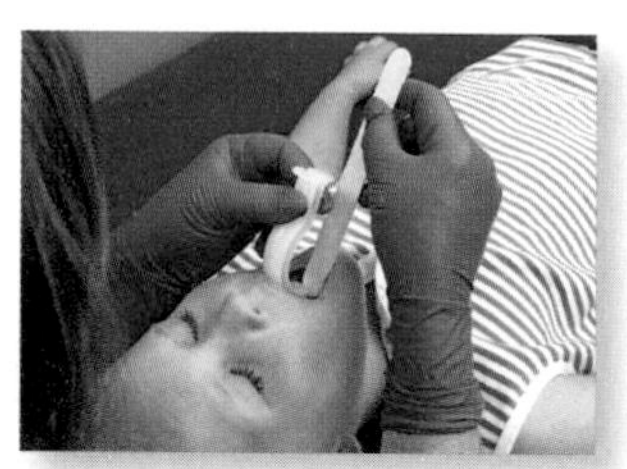

CHAPTER

6 Airway and Breathing

By the end of this chapter, you should be able to

Knowledge Objectives ▶

1. Name and label the major structures of the respiratory system on a diagram.
2. List the signs of inadequate breathing.
3. Describe the steps in the head tilt–chin lift.
4. Relate mechanism of injury to opening the airway.
5. Describe the steps in the jaw thrust.
6. State the importance of having a suction unit ready for immediate use when providing emergency medical care.
7. Describe the techniques of suctioning.
8. Describe how to ventilate a patient with a resuscitation mask or barrier device.
9. Describe how ventilating an infant or child is different from an adult.
10. List the steps in providing mouth-to-mouth and mouth-to-stoma ventilation.
11. Describe how to measure and insert an oropharyngeal (oral) airway.
12. Describe how to measure and insert a nasopharyngeal (nasal) airway.
13. Describe how to clear a foreign body airway obstruction in a responsive adult.
14. Describe how to clear a foreign body airway obstruction in a responsive child with complete obstruction or partial airway obstruction and poor air exchange.
15. Describe how to clear a foreign body airway obstruction in a responsive infant with complete obstruction or partial airway obstruction and poor air exchange.
16. Describe how to clear a foreign body airway obstruction in an unresponsive adult.
17. Describe how to clear a foreign body airway obstruction in an unresponsive child.
18. Describe how to clear a foreign body airway obstruction in an unresponsive infant.

Attitude Objectives ▶

19. Explain why Basic Life Support ventilation and airway protective skills take priority over most other Basic Life Support skills.
20. Demonstrate a caring attitude toward patients with airway problems who request emergency medical services.

21. Place the interests of the patient with airway problems as the foremost consideration when making any and all patient care decisions.
22. Communicate with empathy to patients with airway problems, as well as with family members and friends of the patient.

Skill Objectives ▶ DVD Link

23. Demonstrate the steps in the head tilt–chin lift.
24. Demonstrate the steps in the jaw thrust.
25. Demonstrate the techniques of suctioning.
26. Demonstrate the steps in mouth-to-mouth ventilation with body substance isolation (barrier shields).
27. Demonstrate how to use a resuscitation mask to ventilate a patient.
28. Demonstrate how to ventilate a patient with a stoma.
29. Demonstrate how to measure and insert an oropharyngeal airway.
30. Demonstrate how to measure and insert a nasopharyngeal airway.
31. Demonstrate how to ventilate infant and child patients.
32. Demonstrate how to clear a foreign body airway obstruction in a responsive adult.
33. Demonstrate how to clear a foreign body airway obstruction in a responsive child.
34. Demonstrate how to clear a foreign body airway obstruction in a responsive infant.
35. Demonstrate how to clear a foreign body airway obstruction in an unresponsive adult.
36. Demonstrate how to clear a foreign body airway obstruction in an unresponsive child.
37. Demonstrate how to clear a foreign body airway obstruction in an unresponsive infant.

On The Scene

You know the ambulance will be at least 10 minutes behind you when you pull up to a house for "an unconscious person." As you grab your emergency kit and approach the door, a tearful woman directs you to the bathroom. She tells you, "I think he's taken a heroin overdose." A 21-year-old man is seated limply on the toilet, taking an occasional weak gasp. His skin is gray, cool, and wet. "Let's get him out of here," you tell the police officer. You struggle to drag him to the next room, aware that he is deeply unconscious. As you lay him on his back, you perform a head tilt–chin lift. You listen carefully for airway movement from his nose or mouth. As you look at his chest, you can see that he is taking only three or four breaths each minute. You deliver two breaths with your pocket mask and then slide your fingers into the groove in his neck. You can feel a strong pulse. ■

THINK ABOUT IT

As you read this chapter, think about the following questions:

- What findings suggest that he is not breathing adequately?
- Are there other measures that are needed to open his airway?
- How can you assist his breathing?

Introduction

Airway Emergencies

All living cells of the body require oxygen and produce carbon dioxide. Oxygen is particularly important to the cells of the nervous system because, without it, brain cells begin to die within four to six minutes. The most stressful and chaotic scene usually involves a difficult airway. A nonbreathing patient or a patient with difficulty breathing is a true emergency. To prevent death, you must be able to recognize early signs of breathing difficulty and know what to do.

The Respiratory System

The Functions of the Respiratory System

One of the major functions of the respiratory system is to deliver oxygen-rich blood from the atmosphere to body cells. Another major function is to transport carbon dioxide produced by body cells to the atmosphere. As an Emergency Medical Responder, you must make sure these functions happen by maintaining an open airway. Maintaining an open airway allows a free flow of air into and out of the lungs.

When we breathe in, the air entering the body from the atmosphere is rich in oxygen and contains little carbon dioxide. Carbon dioxide is the waste product we produce in breathing. The oxygen-rich air enters the alveoli in the lungs and passes through the walls of capillaries into the bloodstream. Carbon dioxide passes from the blood through the capillary walls into the alveoli. It leaves the body in the air we breathe out.

Anatomy Review

The Nose and Nasal Cavity

Objective 1 ▶

The nose warms, humidifies, and filters the air before it enters the lungs (Figure 6-1). A wall of tissue, called the **septum,** separates the right and left nostrils. The nose is lined with a mucous membrane that is fragile. When the nose is subjected to trauma, it is prone to bleeding and inflammation, which can cause an airway obstruction. The nose is prone to trauma because of its location on the face. The nasal cavity is separated from the cranium by a thin bone that can become fractured as a result of head trauma.

Do not insert an airway adjunct into the nose of a patient with trauma to the nose or midface.

The Mouth and Oral Cavity

Air entering the mouth is not filtered or warmed as efficiently as air entering the nostrils.

The mouth and its structures serve many functions. The most important is its ability to move fresh air in and out of the lungs. Air enters the body through the mouth or nose and passes down the pharynx (throat), past the epiglottis, down the trachea, and into the lungs.

The upper airway is the most common place for an airway obstruction to occur. When a patient becomes unresponsive, the tongue falls back into the posterior oropharynx (the back of the mouth). This can cause a complete airway obstruction. Other common causes of upper airway obstruction are dislodged teeth or dentures, blood, body secretions, and foreign objects.

You must be able to recognize signs of an airway obstruction and act quickly to remove it in order for the patient to survive.

The **epiglottis** is a piece of cartilage that protects the lower airway from **aspiration.** When we swallow, the epiglottis closes off the trachea and prevents food from entering it. Choking may result if the epiglottis fails to close, allowing food or liquids to enter the airway. When a patient becomes unresponsive, she loses her gag reflex and this protective response. Placing an unresponsive, uninjured patient on her side (recovery position) while suctioning out the airway will allow material to flow from the mouth by gravity and reduce the risk of aspiration.

FIGURE 6-1 ► The anatomy of the respiratory system.

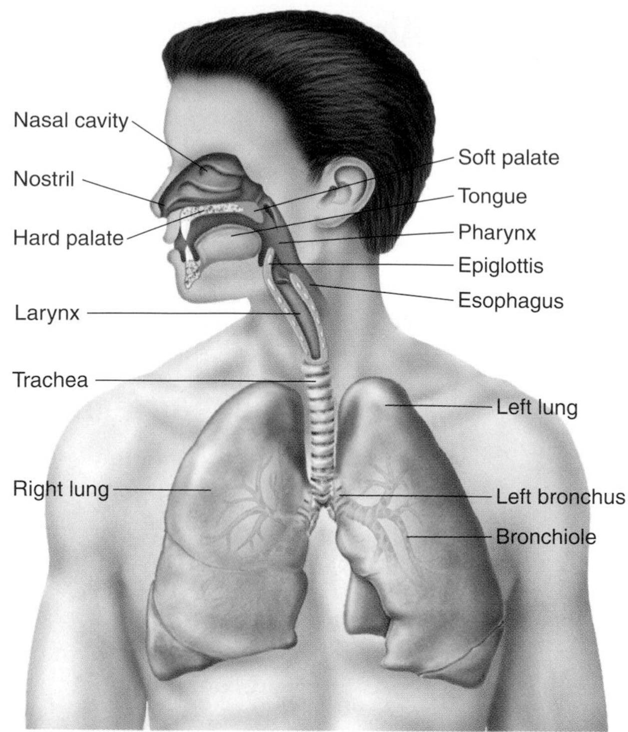

The Trachea and Lower Airway

The larynx contains the vocal cords. This area is the narrowest part of an adult's airway. The vocal cords are responsible for sound production. An airway obstruction at or below this level will affect the ability to produce sound. The space between the vocal cords is called the **glottis.** The largest cartilage of the larynx is the thyroid cartilage, also called the Adam's apple. The cricoid cartilage is the most inferior (lowest) of the cartilages of the larynx. The narrowest part of a child's airway is at the level of the cricoid cartilage.

Continuing down the windpipe, the trachea extends to the level of the upper and middle portion of the breastbone (sternum). The trachea is protected and supported by C-shaped rings of cartilage. This allows for some expansion during breathing and coughing. At about the middle of the breastbone, the trachea divides into two main branches. One branch, the right mainstem bronchus, allows air into and out of the right lung. The other, the left mainstem bronchus, allows air into and out of the left lung.

The Lungs

The lungs are very elastic and are made up of many tiny air sacs (alveoli). The lungs are divided into three separate lobes on the right and two lobes on the left. Even a tiny blockage in the lower airways can completely collapse a segment of the lung, making breathing much more difficult. This situation can also occur because of a penetrating injury to the lung, as in a stabbing or gunshot wounds. If an opening occurs between the outside atmosphere and the lung, it will collapse the lung and require emergency treatment.

The Diaphragm

At the bottom of the lungs is the diaphragm, a dome-shaped muscle used for breathing. The diaphragm divides the chest cavity from the abdominal cavity.

The Mechanics of Breathing

The Muscles of Breathing

The diaphragm is the primary muscle of breathing. External intercostal muscles are located between the ribs. The internal intercostal muscles and abdominal muscles may be used during forceful exhalation.

As the diaphragm moves down, abdominal pressure increases and the chest moves outward. The pressure within the lungs decreases to allow for inspiration. After inhalation, the alveoli are inflated while oxygen and carbon dioxide cross a membrane. Oxygen enters the circulation, while carbon dioxide enters the alveoli. Carbon dioxide is exhaled into the atmosphere as the diaphragm returns to its resting state, pushing air from the lungs.

A Is for *Airway*

You must perform an initial assessment on *every* patient. The initial assessment begins after the scene or situation has been found or made safe and you have gained access to the patient. The purpose of the initial assessment is to find and care for immediate, life-threatening problems.

As you approach the patient, you will first form a general impression of him to determine if he appears "sick" or "not sick." You will also determine the urgency of further assessment and care. Using your senses of sight and hearing (look and listen), quickly determine if the patient is ill (a medical patient) or injured (a trauma patient). Look at the patient and determine if he has a life- threatening problem. If a life-threatening condition is found, you must treat it immediately. Examples of life-threatening conditions include

- Unresponsiveness
- An obstructed airway
- Absent breathing (respiratory arrest)
- Severe bleeding

After forming a general impression of your patient, you must assess the patient's level of responsiveness. Begin by speaking to him. If the patient appears to be awake, tell the patient your first name and identify yourself as an Emergency Medical Responder. Explain that you are there to help. You may ask, "Why did you call 9-1-1 today?" If the patient appears to be asleep, gently rub his shoulder and ask, "Are you okay?" or "Can you hear me?" Do not move the patient.

A patient who is alert and talking clearly or crying without difficulty has a **patent** (open) airway. If the patient is unable to speak, cry, cough, or make any other sound, his airway is completely obstructed. If the patient has noisy breathing, such as snoring or gurgling, he has a partial airway obstruction.

Remember This!

When resuscitating a patient, it is important to know the definitions of an infant, a child, and an adult:

- Infant: less than one year of age
- Child: one to 12 to 14 years of age
- Adult: greater than 12 to 14 years of age

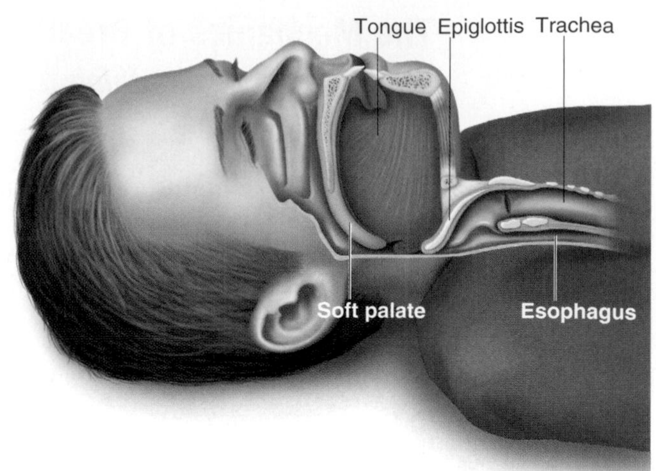

FIGURE 6-2 ▶ An unresponsive patient loses the ability to keep his own airway open because he loses muscle tone. The tongue falls into the back of the throat, blocking the airway.

Opening the Airway

Objective 19 ▶

A patient without an open airway has no chance of survival. If the airway is not open, there is no breathing. Without breathing, the patient's heart will stop beating unless you open the airway and begin breathing for him. Therefore, one of the most important actions you can perform is to open the airway of an unresponsive patient. An unresponsive patient loses the ability to keep his own airway open because he loses muscle tone. This loss of muscle tone causes the soft tissues of the throat and the base of the tongue to relax. If the patient is lying on his back, his tongue falls into the back of his throat, blocking the airway (Figure 6-2). Because the tongue is attached to the lower jaw, moving the jaw forward will lift the tongue away from the back of the throat.

Stop and Think!

Because the risk of exposure to blood, vomitus, or potentially infectious material is high, you must remember to take appropriate body substance isolation precautions when managing a patient's airway.

Head Tilt–Chin Lift

The head tilt–chin lift maneuver is the most effective method for opening the airway in a patient with no known or suspected trauma to the head or neck. It requires no equipment and is simple to perform. When the procedure is done correctly, the base of the tongue will be displaced from blocking the back of the throat (Figure 6-3). Patients who are likely to need the head tilt–chin lift maneuver include

- An unresponsive patient with no known or suspected trauma to the head or neck
- A patient who is not breathing with no known or suspected trauma to the head or neck
- A patient who is not breathing and has no pulse (cardiac arrest) with no known or suspected trauma to the head or neck

Remember This!

Never use the head tilt–chin lift maneuver to open the airway if trauma to the head or neck is suspected. Damage to the patient's spinal cord can result.

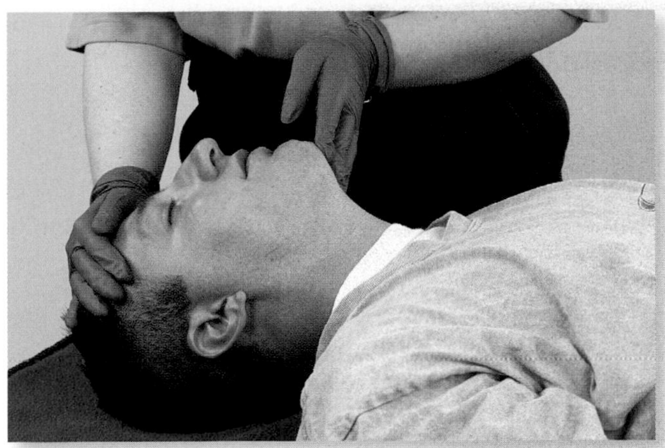

FIGURE 6-3 ▲ The head tilt–chin lift.

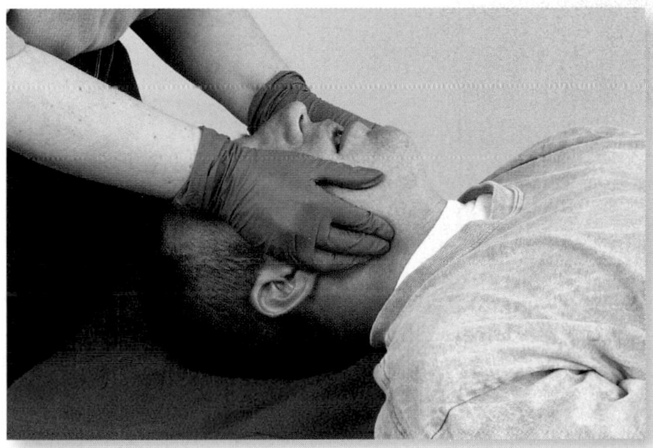

FIGURE 6-4 ▲ The jaw thrust without head tilt.

Follow these steps to perform a head tilt–chin lift:

Objective 3 ▶

1. Position the patient on his back.
2. Place your hand closest to the patient's head on his forehead. Apply back pressure with your palm, gently tilting the patient's head backward.
3. Place the fingers of your hand that is closest to the patient's feet under the bony part of his chin. Do not compress the soft tissues under the chin; doing so can result in an airway obstruction.
4. Lift the chin forward and support the jaw.
5. Make sure the patient's mouth is open. If the patient is wearing dentures and they fit well, leave them in place. If the dentures are loose or do not fit well, remove them.
6. Look, listen, and feel for breathing.

Jaw Thrust Without Head Tilt

Objective 4 ▶

Use the jaw-thrust without head tilt maneuver to open the airway of an unresponsive patient when trauma to the head or neck is suspected (Figure 6-4). Although this method of opening the airway is effective, it is less effective than the head tilt–chin lift and is more tiring. Because this technique requires the use of both hands, a second rescuer will be needed if the patient requires ventilation. Patients who are likely to need the jaw-thrust without head tilt maneuver include

- An unresponsive trauma patient
- An unresponsive patient with an unknown mechanism of injury

Follow these steps to perform a jaw-thrust without head tilt maneuver:

Objective 5 ▶

1. Position the patient on his back and kneel at the top of the patient's head.
2. While keeping the patient's head and neck in line with the rest of his body, place your hands on each side of the patient's lower jaw. It may be helpful to rest your elbows on the surface on which the patient is lying.
3. Gently grasp the angles of the patient's lower jaw. Lift with both hands, gently moving the lower jaw forward. Make sure the patient's mouth is open. If the patient's lips close, gently pull back the lower lip with your gloved thumb.
4. Look, listen, and feel for breathing.

Inspecting the Airway

After opening the airway, look in the mouth of every unresponsive patient and any responsive patient who cannot protect his or her airway. This can be done by opening the patient's mouth with your gloved hand. Look inside the patient's mouth for an actual or a potential airway obstruction, such as a foreign body, blood, vomitus, teeth, or the patient's tongue. If you see a foreign body in the patient's mouth, attempt to remove it with your gloved fingers. If there is blood, vomitus, or other fluid in the patient's airway, clear it with suctioning.

Clearing the Airway.

There are three methods you can use to clear a patient's airway: the recovery position, finger sweeps, and suctioning. The patient's situation will dictate which technique is most appropriate.

The Recovery Position

Reverse these directions if it is necessary to place the patient on his or her right side.

The recovery position involves positioning a patient on his side (Figure 6-5). This position is used as the first step in maintaining an open airway in an unresponsive and uninjured patient who is breathing adequately. In this position, gravity allows fluid to flow from the mouth and helps keep the airway clear. Follow these steps to place a patient in the recovery position:

1. Raise the patient's left arm above his head and then cross the patient's right leg over his left leg.
2. While supporting the patient's face, grasp his right shoulder and roll him toward you onto his left side. The patient's head should be in as close to a

FIGURE 6-5 ► The recovery position.

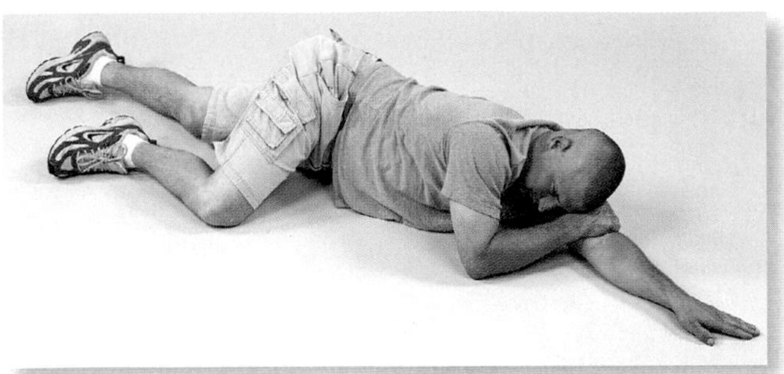

midline position as possible. The patient's head, torso, and shoulders should move at the same time without twisting.

3. Place the patient's right hand under the side of his face.
4. Continue to monitor the patient until additional EMS personnel arrive and assume care.

Remember This!

Do *not* place a patient with a known or suspected spinal injury in the recovery position.

Finger Sweeps

The removal of foreign material from the airway is critical for patient survival.

A finger sweep is not performed on responsive patients or on unresponsive patients who have a gag reflex.

Finger sweeps are used to remove material from an unresponsive patient's upper airway. If you see foreign material in the patient's mouth, remove it immediately.

Follow these steps to perform a finger sweep:

1. If the patient is uninjured, roll him to his side.
2. Wipe out liquids from the airway using your index and middle fingers covered with a cloth.
3. Remove solid objects using your gloved index finger positioned like a hook. Use your little finger when performing a finger sweep in an infant or a child.

Remember This!

A "blind" finger sweep is performed without first seeing foreign material in the airway. Blind finger sweeps should *never* be performed on an infant or a child. Doing so may cause the object to become further lodged in the patient's throat.

Suctioning

Objective 6 ►

Suctioning may be needed if the recovery position and finger sweeps are not effective in clearing the patient's airway. It may also be needed if trauma is suspected and the patient cannot be placed in the recovery position. **Suctioning** is a procedure used to vacuum vomitus, saliva, blood, food particles, and other material from the patient's airway. It requires the use of a device that creates negative pressure. Suction units can be powered manually, electrically, or by air

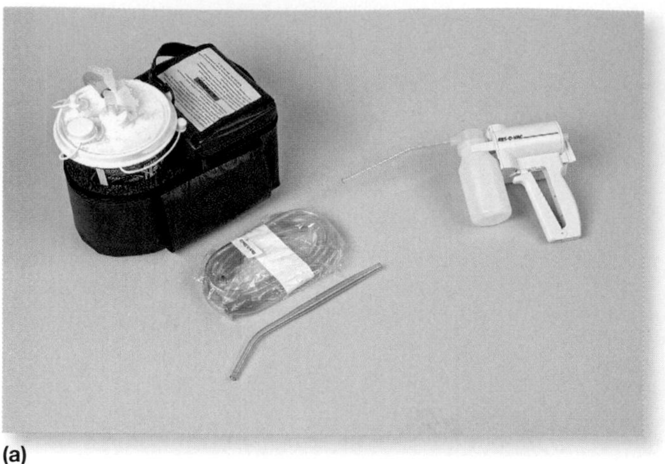
(a)

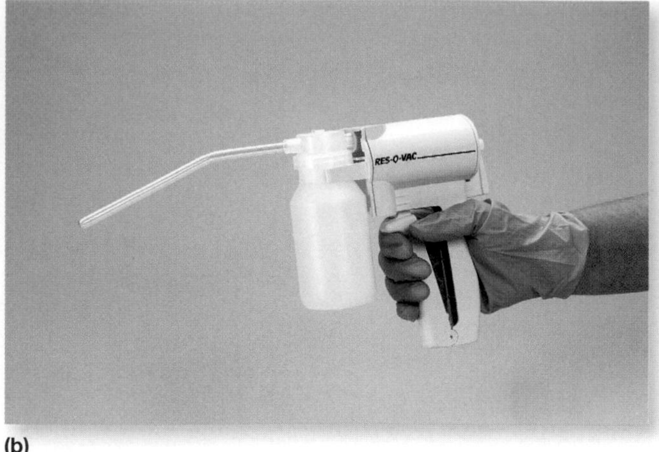

(b)

FIGURE 6-6 ▲ (a) A battery-powered and a manual suction unit. (b) Close-up of a manual suction unit.

FIGURE 6-7 ► A rigid suction catheter can be used to remove secretions from a patient's mouth. This type of catheter should be inserted no deeper than to the base of the tongue.

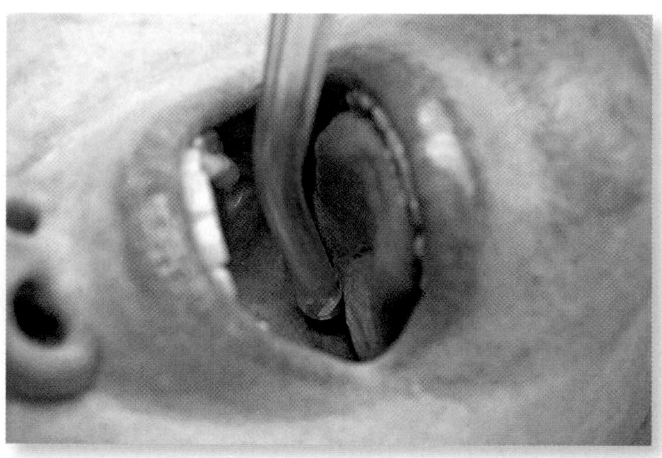

(Figure 6-6). Most suction units are inadequate for removing solid objects, such as teeth, foreign bodies, and food.

You should always have suction equipment available when you are managing a patient's airway or assisting a patient's breathing. If you hear a gurgling sound as a patient breathes, he or she needs to be suctioned immediately.

Use a rigid suction catheter to remove secretions from a patient's mouth. When suctioning a patient with this type of catheter, insert it into the patient's mouth no deeper than to the base of the tongue (Figure 6-7).

You Should Know

A rigid suction catheter is also called a *hard suction catheter,* a *tonsil tip catheter,* and a *tonsil sucker.*

Objective 7 ►

Follow these steps to suction a patient's mouth:

1. Turn on the power of the suction unit and make sure it is working.
2. Attach the suction catheter.
3. *Without applying suction,* place the tip of the catheter into the patient's mouth. Gently advance the catheter tip along one side of the mouth. Insert the catheter tip no deeper than the measured distance.

4. Apply suction while moving the tip of the catheter from side to side as you withdraw it from the patient's mouth. Because you are removing air (oxygen) from the patient when suctioning, do not suction an adult for more than 15 seconds at a time. When suctioning an infant or a child, do not apply suction for more than 10 seconds at a time.

Because suctioning can cause serious changes in your patient's heart rate, you must watch your patient closely when you perform this procedure. The patient's heart rate may slow or become irregular due to a lack of oxygen or if the tip of the catheter stimulates the back of the tongue or throat. These changes in the heart rate can occur in any patient. However, they are particularly common in infants and children. If the patient's heart rate slows, stop suctioning and provide ventilation.

Keeping the Airway Open: Airway Adjuncts

The use of an airway adjunct does not eliminate the need for maintaining proper head positioning.

Airway adjuncts are devices used to help keep a patient's airway open. When using an airway adjunct, the patient's airway must first be opened using one of the techniques already described. The airway adjunct is then inserted and the proper head position maintained while the device is in place.

Oropharyngeal Airway (OPA)

An oropharyngeal airway is also called an *oral airway.*

An **oropharyngeal airway (OPA)** is a curved device made of rigid plastic. An OPA is inserted into the patient's mouth and used to keep the tongue away from the back of the throat. It may only be used in unresponsive patients without a gag reflex. If you attempt to use an OPA in a patient with a gag reflex, he or she may vomit and aspirate the vomitus into the lungs.

Objective 11 ▶

OPAs are available in a variety of sizes. Before inserting an OPA, you must determine the correct size for your patient. To select the correct size, hold the OPA against the side of the patient's face. Select an OPA that extends from the corner of the patient's mouth to the tip of the ear lobe, or from the center of the patient's mouth to the angle of the jaw. If you select an OPA of the wrong size, you can *cause* an airway obstruction. An OPA that is too long can press the epiglottis against the entrance of the larynx, resulting in a complete airway obstruction. An OPA that is too short may come out of the mouth or may push the tongue into the back of the throat, causing an airway obstruction. Skill Drill 6-1 shows the steps for sizing and inserting an oropharyngeal airway.

Nasopharyngeal Airway (NPA)

Objective 12 ▶

A **nasopharyngeal airway (NPA)** is a soft, rubbery tube with a hole in it that is placed in the patient's nose. The NPA allows air to flow from the hole in the NPA down into the lower airway. When an NPA of the proper size is correctly positioned, the tip rests in the back of the throat. This positioning helps keep the tongue from blocking the upper airway. It can be placed in either nostril to help maintain an open airway. Remember that the bevel of the NPA needs to be kept against the nasal septum.

This airway can be used in an unresponsive patient. A nasopharyngeal airway may be useful in semi-responsive patients who have a gag reflex. Situations in which a semi-responsive patient may need this type of airway include the following:

- Intoxicated patient
- Drug overdose
- Stroke
- After a seizure
- Low blood sugar

Skill Drill 6-2 shows the steps for sizing and inserting a nasopharyngeal airway.

Skill Drill 6-1

Sizing and Inserting an Oropharyngeal Airway

STEP 1 ▶ Use Steps 1–4 to insert an OPA in an unresponsive adult.

- Place the patient on his back. Position yourself at the patient's head.
- Open the patient's airway with a head tilt–chin lift maneuver. If trauma is suspected, use the jaw-thrust without head tilt maneuver to open the airway.
- Select the correct size OPA. An OPA is the correct size if it extends from the corner of the patient's mouth to the tip of the earlobe, or from the center of the mouth to the angle of the jaw.

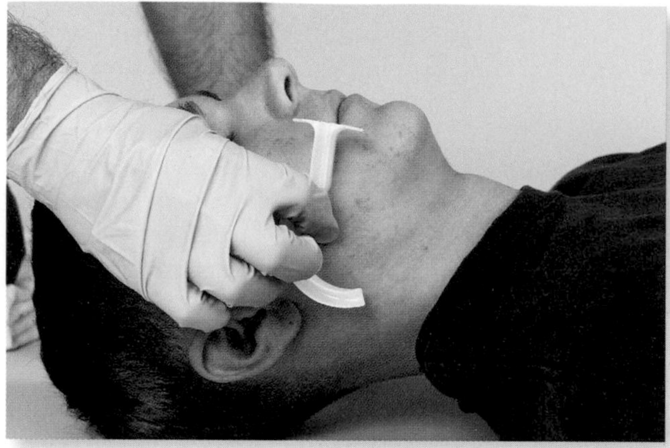

STEP 2 ▶

- Open the patient's mouth. Suction any secretions from the mouth.
- Insert the airway upside down, with the tip pointing toward the roof of the patient's mouth. Advance the airway gently along the roof of the mouth.

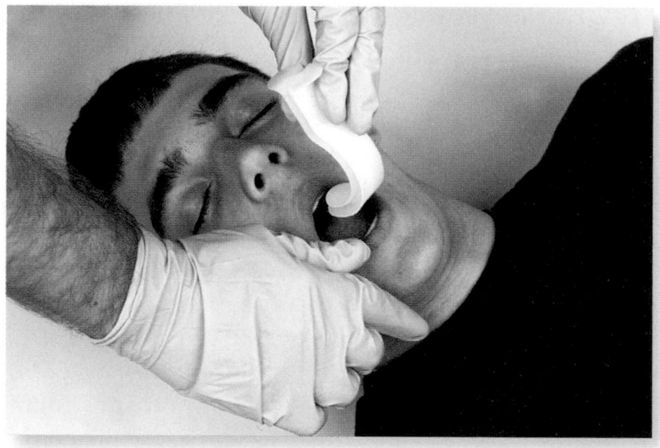

STEP 3 ▶ When the tip of the airway approaches the back of the throat, rotate the airway 180 degrees, so that it is positioned over the tongue. Be careful not to push the tongue into the back of the throat.

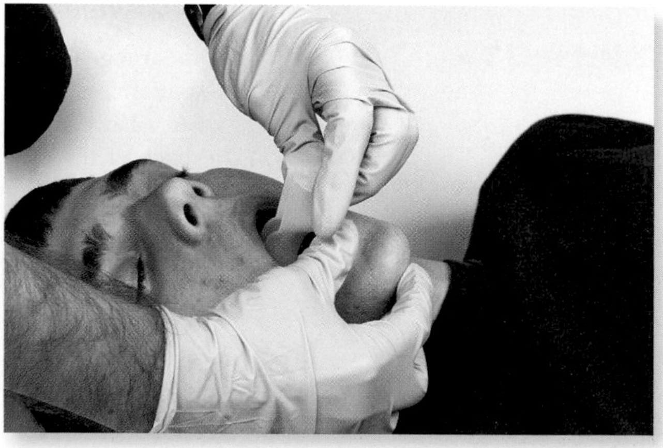

STEP 4 ▶

- When the OPA is correctly positioned, the flange end should rest on the patient's lips or teeth. Remove the OPA *immediately* if the patient begins gagging as you slide it between the tongue and the back of the throat.
- Ventilate the patient.

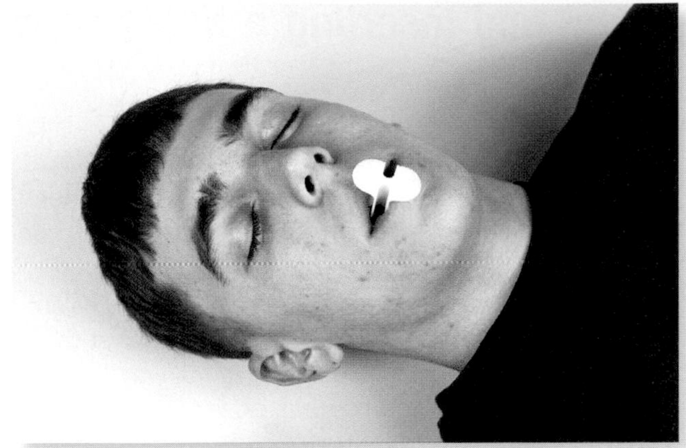

STEP 5 ▶

Use the following steps to insert an OPA in an unresponsive infant or child:

- Place the patient on his or her back. Position yourself at the patient's head.
- Open the patient's airway with a head tilt–chin lift maneuver. If trauma is suspected, use the jaw-thrust without head tilt maneuver to open the airway.
- Select the correct size OPA.
- Open the patient's mouth. Suction any secretions from the patient's mouth.
- Use a tongue blade to press the tongue down.
- Insert the OPA with the tip following the base of the tongue.
- Advance the OPA until the flange rests on the patient's lips or teeth.
- Remove the OPA *immediately* if the patient begins gagging as you slide it between the tongue and the back of the throat.
- Ventilate the patient.

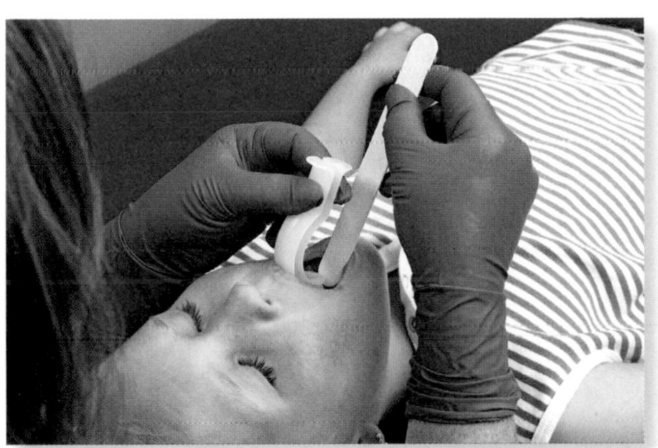

Skill Drill 6-2

Sizing and Inserting a Nasopharyngeal Airway

STEP 1 ▶
- Place the patient on his back. Position yourself at the patient's head.
- Open the patient's airway with a head tilt–chin lift maneuver. If trauma is suspected, use the jaw-thrust without head tilt maneuver to open the airway.
- Choose the proper size NPA. To select an NPA of proper size, hold the NPA against the side of the patient's face. Select an airway that extends from the tip of the patient's nose to the earlobe.

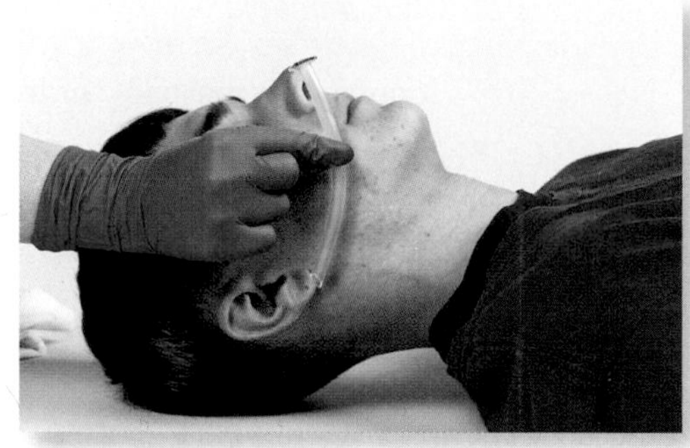

STEP 2 ▶ Lubricate the outside of the NPA with a water-soluble lubricant, if available.

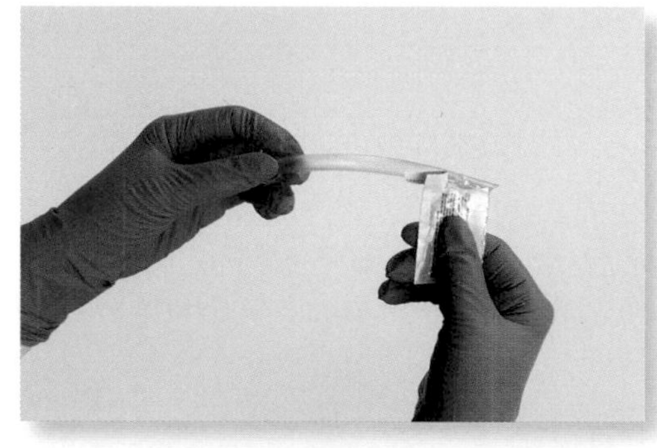

STEP 3 ▶
- Gently push the tip of the patient's nose back slightly.
- Gently insert the NPA with the bevel pointing toward the nasal septum. During insertion, do not direct the airway upward. Do not force the NPA into position. Serious bleeding that is hard to control can result.

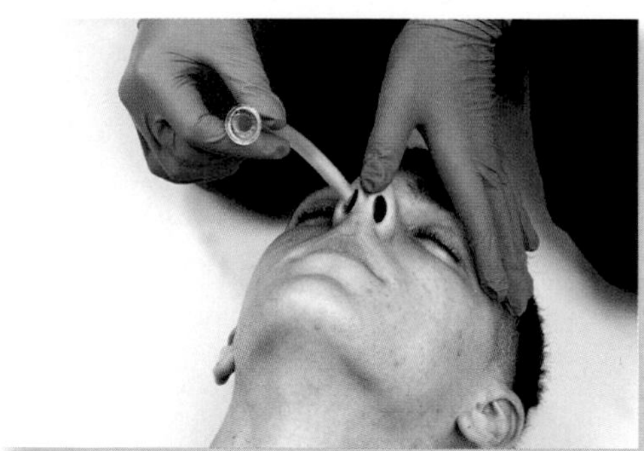

STEP 4 ▶
- Stop advancing the NPA when the bevel of the device is flush against the opening of the nostril.
- Assess placement by feeling for air coming from the device.

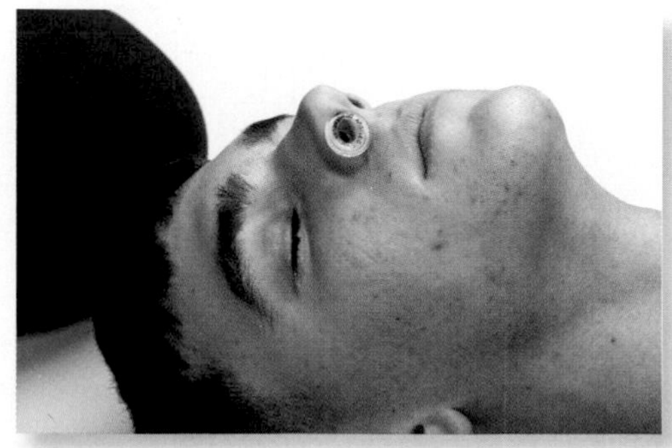

Remember This!

If a nasal airway cannot be inserted into one nostril, try the other nostril.

B Is for *Breathing*

Is the Patient Breathing?

Breathing assessment is described in more detail in Chapter 8.

After making sure that the patient's airway is open, check for breathing. Normal breathing is quiet and painless, and it occurs at a regular rate. Both sides of the chest rise and fall equally. Normal breathing does not require excessive use of the muscles between the ribs, above the collarbones, or in the abdomen during inhalation or exhalation. These muscles are called **accessory muscles** for breathing.

Remember This!

The best way to learn how to assess a patient's normal work of breathing is to watch a person without medical problems breathe while he or she is asleep. This is a good baseline to see comfortable breathing without signs of respiratory distress. It is also a good picture to recall when you have to ventilate a patient.

Is Breathing Adequate or Inadequate?

If the patient is breathing, quickly determine if breathing is adequate or inadequate. A patient who is breathing adequately

- Does not appear to be in distress
- Speaks in full sentences without pausing to catch his or her breath
- Breathes at a regular rate and within normal limits for his or her age
- Has an equal rise and fall of the chest with each breath
- Has an adequate depth of breathing (tidal volume)
- Has normal skin color

A patient who is having difficulty breathing is working hard (laboring) to breathe. She may be gasping for air. You may see her use the muscles in her neck to assist with inhalation. She may use her abdominal muscles and the muscles between the ribs to assist with exhalation. You may see **retractions** (a "sinking in") of the soft tissues between and around the ribs or above the collarbones.

Normal breathing is quiet.

Noisy breathing is usually abnormal breathing and a sign that the patient is in distress. **Stridor** is a sound usually heard during inhalation that suggests the upper airway is partially obstructed. Stridor sounds like the bark of a seal. The sound of **snoring** suggests the upper airway is partially obstructed by the tongue. **Gurgling** is a wet sound that suggests fluid is collecting in the patient's upper airway. **Wheezing** is a whistling sound that is usually heard on exhalation. Wheezing suggests that the lower airways are partially obstructed with fluid or mucus.

Objective 2 ▶

The signs of inadequate breathing include the following:

- An anxious appearance and concentration on breathing
- Confusion and restlessness
- A breathing rate that is too fast or slow for the patient's age
- An irregular breathing pattern
- A depth of breathing that is unusually deep or shallow
- Noisy breathing (snoring, gurgling, wheezing)

Inadequate breathing must be treated aggressively before it becomes absent breathing.

- A patient who is sitting upright and leaning forward to breathe
- An inability to speak in complete sentences
- Pain with breathing
- Skin that looks flushed, pale, gray, or blue or that feels cold or sweaty

If your patient is awake but appears to have trouble breathing, ask," Can you speak?" or "Are you choking?" If he is able to speak or make noise, air is moving past his vocal cords. If he is unresponsive, open his airway. Place your ear close to the patient's mouth and nose. Look, listen, and feel for breathing:

- Look for a rise and fall of the chest.
- Listen for air escaping during exhalation.
- Feel for air coming from the mouth or nose.

If a complete airway obstruction is present, you may initially see a rise and fall of the chest, but you will not hear or feel air movement. If the patient's heart stops, you may see irregular, gasping breaths (agonal respirations) just after this occurs. Do not confuse gasping respirations with adequate breathing.

How to Ventilate

If your patient's breathing is inadequate or absent, you will need to begin breathing for her immediately. When a patient is not breathing, she has only the oxygen-rich blood remaining in her lungs and bloodstream to survive on. You can assist breathing by forcing air into the patient's lungs. This action is called positive-pressure ventilation. Mouth-to-mask ventilation, mouth-to-barrier device ventilation, mouth-to-mouth ventilation, and bag-valve-mask ventilation are methods used to deliver positive-pressure ventilation.

Applying Cricoid Pressure (the Sellick Maneuver)

If positive-pressure ventilation is performed too rapidly or with too much volume, air can enter the stomach. The cricoid cartilage is the most inferior cartilage of the larynx. It is the only ring in the larynx that is completely made of cartilage (Figure 6-8). When pressure is applied to the cricoid cartilage, the trachea is pushed backward and the esophagus is compressed (closed) against the cervical vertebrae. This compression helps decrease the amount of air entering the stomach during positive-pressure ventilation, which reduces the likelihood of vomiting and aspiration. Cricoid pressure (also called the Sellick

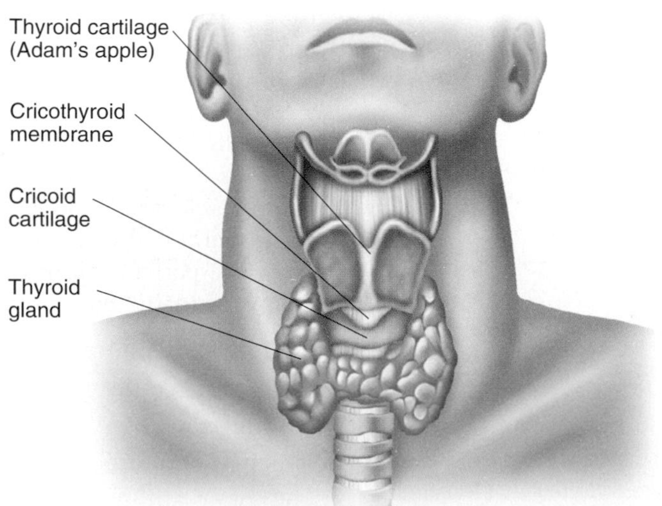

FIGURE 6-8 ► The cricoid cartilage is the most inferior of the laryngeal cartilages.

FIGURE 6-9 ► Applying cricoid pressure.

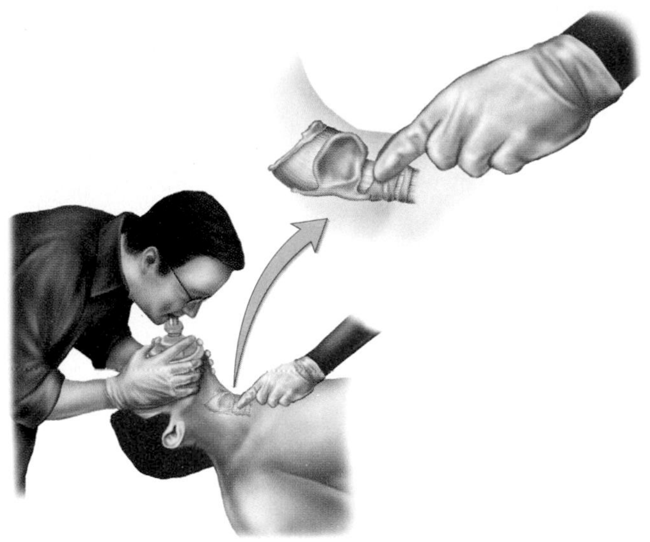

maneuver) should only be used in unresponsive patients. It is usually applied by a third person during positive-pressure ventilation.

Follow these steps to apply cricoid pressure:

The cricoid cartilage may be difficult to find in women, obese patients, and patients with thick necks.

Too much pressure can cause an airway obstruction.

1. Using your index finger, locate the patient's Adam's apple on the front of the neck (Figure 6-9). Slowly move your finger downward until you feel a depression. Just below this depression is a firm ring of cartilage. This is the cricoid cartilage.
2. Make sure the cricoid cartilage is between your thumb and index finger and apply firm backward pressure. The cricoid cartilage should remain in the midline position; it should not move to either side.
3. Maintain pressure until the patient begins breathing on his own, a tube has been inserted in the patient's trachea by Advanced Life Support personnel, or the patient becomes responsive by moving, coughing, or gagging.

Mouth-to-Mask Ventilation (Pocket Mask)

The piece of equipment used for mouth-to-mask ventilation is called a *pocket mask, pocket facemask, ventilation facemask,* or *resuscitation mask.* The mask provides a physical barrier between you and the patient's nose, mouth, and secretions. The mask should have a one-way valve, which directs the patient's exhaled breath away from you (Figure 6-10). This helps prevent exposure to infectious disease. The mask should also have a disposable high-efficiency particulate air (HEPA) filter. A HEPA filter snaps inside the mask and is used to trap respiratory particles from patients with diseases such as tuberculosis. All masks should be transparent so that vomiting can be seen and suctioned from the airway. Some pocket masks have an oxygen inlet that allows delivery of supplemental oxygen.

Mouth-to-mask ventilation is very effective because you can use two hands to hold the mask in place on the patient's face and maintain proper head positioning at the same time. It also allows you to get a better face-to-mask seal, reducing the likelihood that air will leak from the mask. With a pocket mask, you can also adjust the volume of air to meet the patient's needs. You can do this by increasing or decreasing your own breath. When ventilating the patient through the mask, watch the rise and fall of his or her chest to determine if you need to adjust the volume of your breath.

The rates for positive-pressure ventilation are listed in Table 6-1.

FIGURE 6-10 ▶ A pocket facemask. (a) The mask. (b) HEPA filter. (c) One-way valve. (d) Pocket facemask assembled with mask, HEPA filter, and one-way valve.

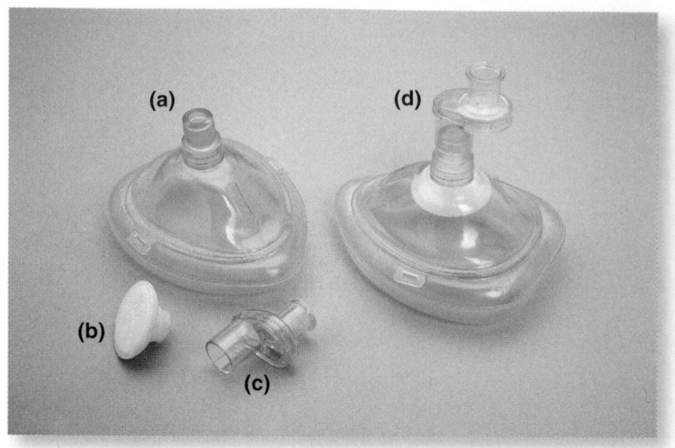

Skill Drill 6-3 shows the steps in mouth-to-mask ventilation.

TABLE 6-1 Rates for Positive-Pressure Ventilation

Patient	Breaths per Minute	Length of Each Breath
Adult	10 to 12 (1 breath every 5 to 6 seconds)	1 second
Infant/child	12 to 20 (1 breath every 3 to 5 seconds)	1 second
Newborn	40 to 60 (1 breath every 1 to 1.5 seconds)	1 second

Making a Difference

Use the following guidelines when providing mouth-to-mask ventilation:

- Position the narrow portion of the mask over the bridge of the patient's nose. The wide portion of the mask should rest in the groove between the patient's lower lip and chin.
- You are providing adequate ventilation if you see the patient's chest gently rise and fall with each breath.

Remember This!

The position of the mask is critical. If you use the wrong size, air will leak from the mask. A small leak can be overcome by increasing the volume of the breath you deliver. If the mask is too large, you can turn it upside down and place the patient's nose in the chin piece of the mask.

Mouth-to-Barrier Device Ventilation

Use a barrier device if a pocket mask is not available.

A barrier device is a thin film of plastic or silicone that is placed on the patient's face. It is used to reduce direct contact between the patient and rescuer. Face shields, a type of barrier device, are compact and portable. Some face shields are equipped with a short tube (1–2 inches long) that is inserted in the patient's mouth.

Mouth-to-Mask Ventilation

STEP 1

- Connect a one-way valve and HEPA filter to the mask. Place the patient on his or her back. Open the airway with a head tilt–chin lift maneuver. If trauma is suspected, use the jaw thrust without head tilt to open the airway.
- Position yourself at the top of the patient's head. Lower the mask over the patient's nose and mouth. Create a face-to-mask seal by forming a *C* around the ventilation port with your thumb and index finger. Place the third, fourth, and fifth fingers of the same hand along the bony portion of the lower jaw. (These fingers form an *E*.) Lift up slightly on the jaw using these fingers.

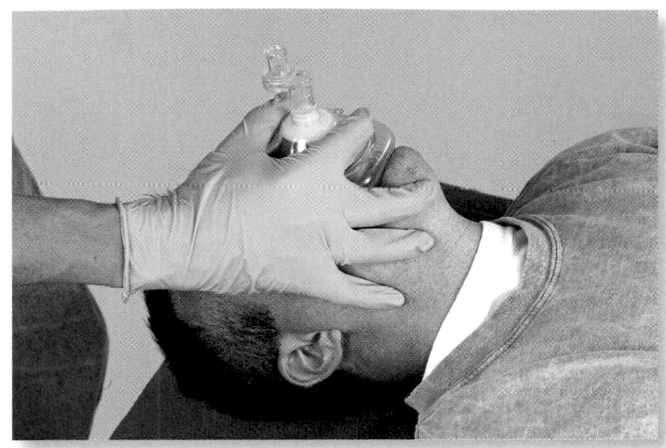

STEP 2

- Take a regular breath and place your mouth around the one-way valve. Exhale slowly with just enough volume to make the chest rise. Deliver each breath over 1 second. (See Table 6-1.)
- Watch for a gentle rise and fall of the patient's chest with each ventilation. Stop ventilation when adequate chest rise is observed. Remove your mouth from the one-way valve and allow the patient to exhale between breaths.
- If air does not go in or the chest does not rise, reposition the patient's head. Reapply the mask to the patient's face and try again to ventilate. If the air still does not go in, suspect an airway obstruction.
- Ventilate once every 3 to 5 seconds for an infant or child and once every 5 to 6 seconds for an adult.

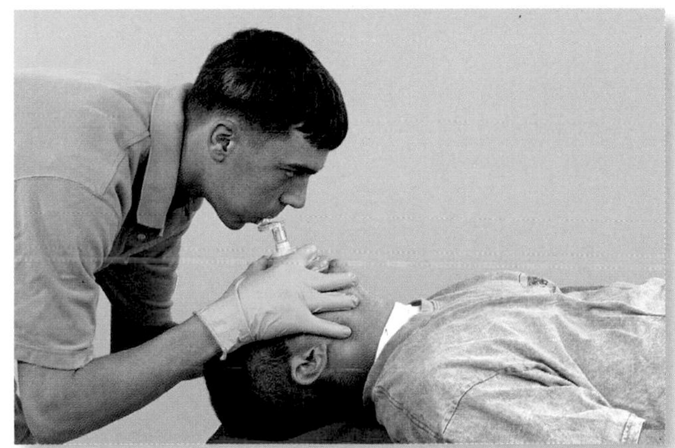

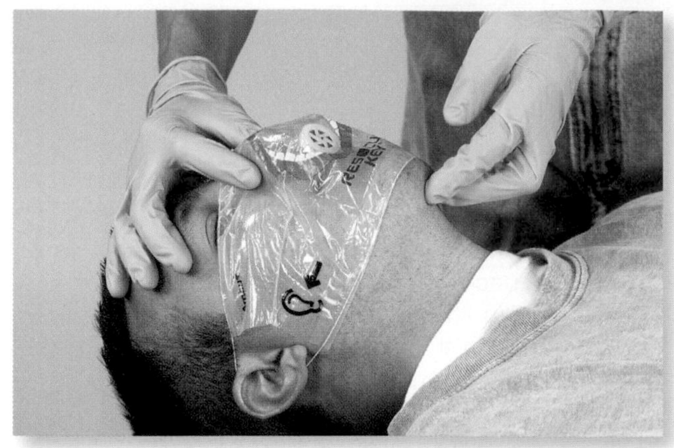

FIGURE 6-11 ▶ Mouth-to-barrier device ventilation.

Air leaks are common when using a barrier device.

Although their features vary, most barrier devices have a one-way valve or filter in the center of the face shield. This allows the patient's exhaled air to escape between the shield and the patient's face when you lift your mouth off the shield between breaths.

Follow these steps for mouth-to-barrier ventilation:

Objective 8 ▶

1. Place the patient on his back. Open his airway with a head tilt–chin lift maneuver. If trauma is suspected, use the jaw thrust without head tilt to open the airway.
2. Position yourself at the patient's head. Place the barrier device over the patient's mouth and nose. The opening at the center of the device should be placed over the patient's mouth (Figure 6-11). If the device has a tube, insert the tube into the patient's mouth, over the tongue.
3. Gently close the patient's nostrils with your thumb and index finger. Take a regular (not a deep) breath and place your mouth over the mouthpiece on the barrier device. Give a breath over 1 second with enough volume to make the chest rise.
4. Watch for the rise and fall of the patient's chest with each ventilation. Stop ventilation when an adequate chest rise is observed. Remove your mouth from the one-way valve and allow the patient to exhale between breaths. Continue ventilation at the proper rate.
5. If the patient's chest does not rise, ventilation is not effective. In this case, the airway is obstructed or more volume or pressure is needed to provide effective ventilation. Readjust the position of the patient's head, make sure the mouth is open, and try again to ventilate. If the chest still does not rise, suspect an airway obstruction.

Too large a volume of air or a breath given too fast will cause the air to enter the stomach.

Mouth-to-Mouth Ventilation

Objective 10 ▶

Mouth-to-mouth ventilation is the delivery of your exhaled air to a patient while making mouth-to-mouth contact. Your exhaled air contains enough oxygen to support life. Mouth-to-mouth ventilation is a quick and effective method of delivering oxygen to a nonbreathing patient. Should you choose to ventilate a patient using the mouth-to-mouth technique, you must be aware of the risks. The most significant risk is being exposed to the patient's body fluids, including blood, vomit, and exhaled air. The decision to perform mouth-to-mouth ventilation is not recommended but will be your personal choice. Whenever possible, you should use a barrier device or a pocket mask.

Room air contains 21% oxygen. Your exhaled air contains 16% to 17% oxygen.

Follow these steps for mouth-to-mouth ventilation:

1. Place the patient on her back. Position yourself at the patient's head. Open her airway with a head tilt–chin lift maneuver. If trauma is suspected, use the jaw thrust without head tilt to open the airway.
2. If the patient is an adult or a child, gently close the patient's nostrils with your thumb and index finger. Take a deep breath and place your mouth over the patient's mouth, creating an airtight seal. If the patient is an infant, place your mouth over the infant's mouth and nose.
3. Give a breath over 1 second with enough volume to make the chest rise.
4. Remove your mouth and release the patient's nose to allow the patient to exhale.
5. Ventilation is adequate if there is adequate rise and fall of the chest and escaping air is heard or felt during exhalation. Continue ventilation at the proper rate.
6. If the chest does not rise, either the airway is obstructed or more volume or pressure is needed to provide effective ventilation. Readjust the position of the patient's head, make sure the patient's mouth is open, and try again to ventilate. If the chest still does not rise, suspect an airway obstruction.

Objective 9 ▶

Bag-Valve-Mask Ventilation

A bag-valve-mask (BVM) device is a self-inflating bag with a one-way valve and an oxygen reservoir. A soft, transparent mask with an air-filled cuff is attached to the bag (Figure 6-12). The one-way valve prevents the patient's exhaled air from reentering the bag. The reservoir is an oxygen collector, allowing the delivery of a higher concentration of oxygen to the patient.

Ventilation performed using a BVM is often referred to as "bagging."

Although BVM ventilation can be done using one person, it is best performed with two rescuers. It is difficult for one person to maintain the proper position of the patient's head, make sure the mask is sealed tightly on the patient's face, and compress the bag at the same time. When two people are available, one takes responsibility for compressing the bag. The other is responsible for maintaining the patient's head in the proper position and making sure the mask is sealed tightly on the patient's face.

Although a BVM can be used to assist ventilations in a patient with inadequate breathing, it is more commonly used to ventilate a nonbreathing patient. When a BVM is not connected to supplemental oxygen, 21% oxygen (room air) is delivered to the patient. If the BVM is connected to supplemental oxygen and a reservoir is present on the bag, between 90% and 100% oxygen can be delivered to the patient if there is a good face-to-mask seal.

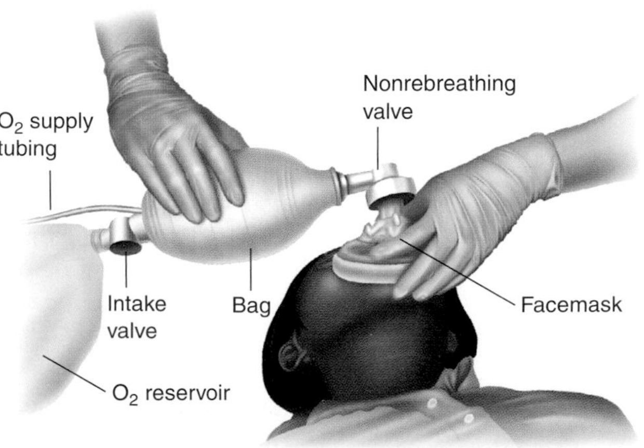

FIGURE 6-12 ▶ The components of a bag-valve-mask device.

Making a Difference

Blow-By Oxygen

Some patients will not tolerate oxygen delivered by means of a nasal cannula (an oxygen delivery device) or facemask. If you are faced with a situation like this, consider blow-by oxygen. When oxygen is delivered using this method, the device used to deliver the oxygen does not make actual contact with the patient. For example, oxygen tubing can be attached to a toy or inside a paper cup. Oxygen is then "blown-by" when the toy or cup is held near the patient's face. Although this method is not ideal for delivering oxygen, it is better than breathing room air.

Follow these steps if you are by yourself and are using a BVM to ventilate a patient who is not breathing:

1. Connect the bag to the mask.
2. Place the patient on her back. Open her airway with a head tilt–chin lift maneuver. If trauma is suspected, use the jaw thrust without head tilt to open the airway. Size and insert an oropharyngeal or a nasopharyngeal airway.
3. Position the narrow portion of the mask over the bridge of the patient's nose. Position the wide portion of the mask between the patient's lower lip and chin. Lower the mask over the patient's nose and mouth.
4. Create a face-to-mask seal by forming a *C* around the ventilation port with your thumb and index finger. Place the third, fourth, and fifth fingers of the same hand along the bony portion of the lower jaw. (These fingers form an *E*.) Lift up slightly on the jaw using these fingers, bringing the patient's jaw up to the mask.
5. With your other hand, squeeze the bag until you see a gentle chest rise (Figure 6-13a). Deliver each ventilation over 1 second. Watch for the rise and fall of the patient's chest with each ventilation. Stop ventilation when you see adequate chest rise. Allow the patient to exhale between breaths.
6. Ventilate at an age-appropriate rate: once every 3 to 5 seconds for an infant or a child and once every 5 to 6 seconds for an adult.
7. If oxygen is available and you have been trained to use it, connect the bag to oxygen at 15 liters per minute (LPM) and attach the reservoir.

Follow these steps if two rescuers are present and are using a BVM:

1. Connect the bag to the mask.
2. Place the patient on his back. Open his airway with a head tilt–chin lift maneuver. If trauma is suspected, use the jaw thrust without head tilt to open the airway. Size and insert an oropharyngeal or a nasopharyngeal airway.
3. Position the narrow portion of the mask over the bridge of the patient's nose. Position the wide portion of the mask between the patient's lower lip and chin. Lower the mask over the patient's nose and mouth.
4. Create a face-to-mask seal by forming a *C* around the ventilation port with your thumb and index finger. Place the third, fourth, and fifth fingers of the same hand along the bony portion of the lower jaw. (These fingers form an *E*.) Lift up slightly on the jaw using these fingers, bringing the patient's jaw up to the mask.
5. Have an assistant squeeze the bag with two hands until you see gentle chest rise (Figure 6-13b). Deliver each ventilation over 1 second. Watch for the

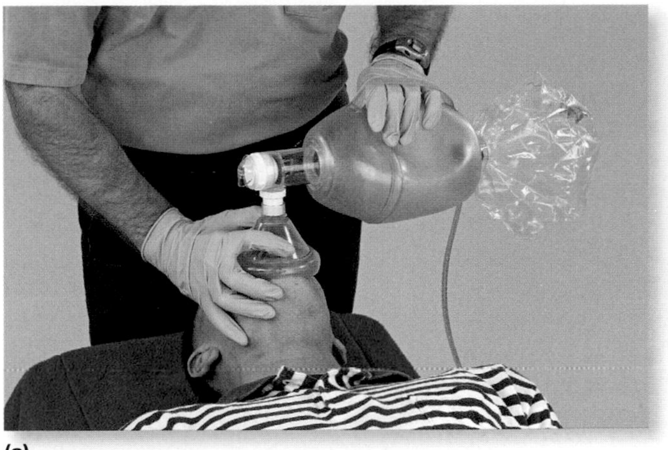
(a)

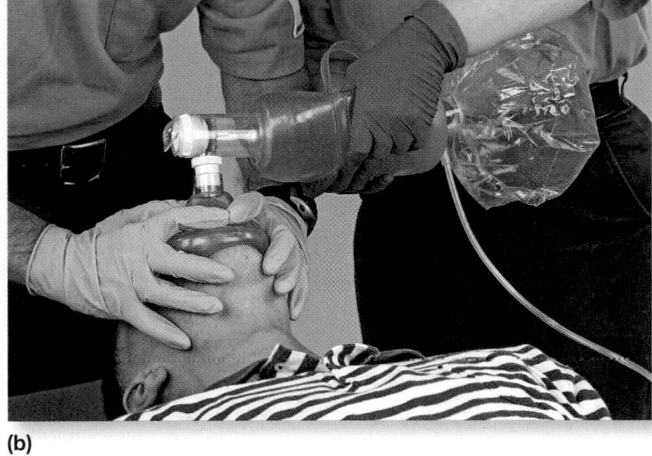
(b)

FIGURE 6-13 ▲ Bag-valve-mask ventilation. (a) One-person technique. (b) Two-person

rise and fall of the patient's chest with each ventilation. Stop ventilation when you see adequate chest rise. Allow the patient to exhale between breaths.

6. Ventilate once every 3 to 5 seconds for an infant or a child and once every 5 to 6 seconds for an adult.
7. If oxygen is available and you have been trained to use it, connect the bag to oxygen at 15 LPM and attach the reservoir.

Airway Obstruction

A choking adult or child may hold his or her neck with the thumb and fingers. This sign is the universal distress signal for choking.

A foreign body airway obstruction (FBAO) is one reason a person's heart may stop beating. For example, a piece of food, bleeding into the airway, or vomitus can block the airway. If the obstruction is not cleared, the heart, brain, and other organs of the body will be deprived of oxygen. When the heart stops, a patient is said to be in **cardiac arrest.** The longer the heart goes without oxygen, the greater the likelihood of cardiac arrest. Brain damage begins four to six minutes after the patient suffers a cardiac arrest. The longer a patient is in cardiac arrest, the lower the patient's chance of survival. In addition to cardiac arrest, the patient can suffer irreversible brain damage due to a lack of oxygen.

The tongue is the most common cause of upper airway obstruction in an unresponsive patient.

A foreign body airway obstruction can also result *from* a cardiac arrest. When a person becomes unresponsive, the jaw and tongue relax. The tongue falls into the back of the throat, obstructing the airway. In a breathing patient, snoring respirations can be heard when the upper airway is partially obstructed by the tongue. Loose dentures, vomitus, or trauma to the head, face, or neck can also block the airway. You may be able to correct an airway obstruction caused by the patient's tongue by properly positioning the patient's head and neck to open the airway.

The signs and symptoms of an airway obstruction caused by a foreign body depend on the following:

- The size of the foreign body
- What the foreign body is made of
- Where the foreign body is located (for example, in the patient's esophagus, upper airway, or lower airway)
- How long the foreign body has been present
- If the obstruction produced by the foreign body is partial or complete

In adults, an FBAO most often occurs during eating. Meat is the most common cause of obstruction. Elderly patients who have difficulty swallowing are at risk for an FBAO. Choking in adults is often associated with the following:

- Attempts to swallow large, poorly chewed pieces of food
- Alcohol use
- Loose or poorly fitting dentures

Remember This!

- Infants and children are at risk of an FBAO because they are like little vacuum cleaners. *Everything* goes in the mouth.
- Infants and children six months to five years of age are at the highest risk for an FBAO.

Most episodes of choking in infants and children occur during eating or play. An FBAO in children is often caused by the following:

- Small foods, such as nuts, raisins, sunflower seeds, and popcorn
- Poorly chewed pieces of meat, grapes, hot dogs, raw carrots, or sausages
- Items commonly found in the home, including disc batteries, pins, rings, nails, buttons, coins, plastic or metal toy objects, and marbles (Figure 6-14)

Suspect an obstruction caused by infection when an infant or a child presents with fever and congestion.

Other causes of airway obstruction in children include infection, such as croup and pneumonia. If you suspect an infection is the cause of an airway obstruction in an infant or a child, arrange for rapid transport of the child to the closest appropriate medical facility. Do not waste time on the scene in a useless and possibly dangerous attempt to relieve this type of obstruction.

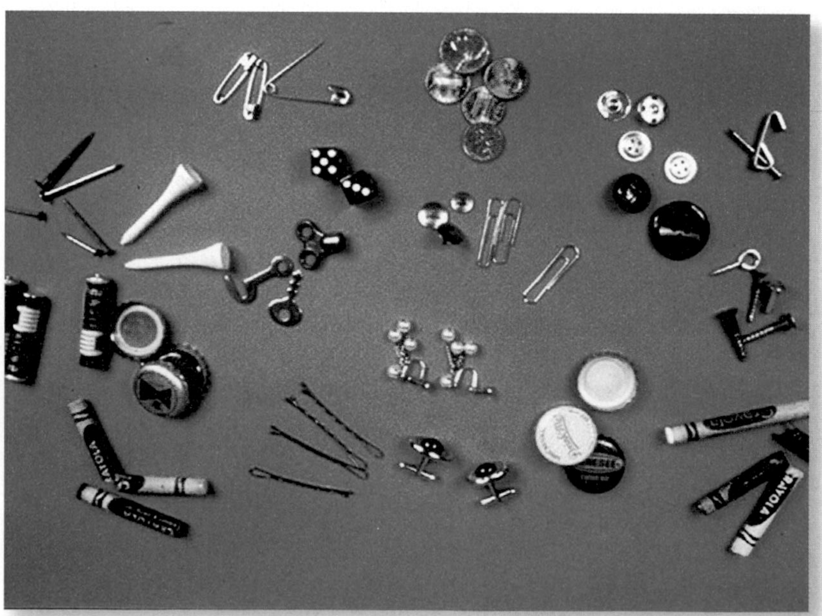

FIGURE 6-14 ▶ Items commonly found in the home may cause a foreign body airway obstruction.

Airway obstructions can be divided into three categories. As an Emergency Medical Responder, you should be able to tell the difference among the three and rapidly determine the action that must be taken. The three categories of airway obstruction are

1. Partial airway obstruction with good air exchange
2. Partial airway obstruction with poor air exchange
3. Complete airway obstruction with no air exchange

Treat a partial airway obstruction with poor air exchange as a complete airway obstruction.

A person who has a partial airway obstruction with good air exchange remains responsive, can speak or make sounds, and can cough forcefully. You may hear wheezing between coughs. Signs of a partial obstruction with poor air exchange include

- A weak, ineffective cough that sounds like gasping
- A high-pitched noise on inhalation (stridor)
- Difficulty breathing or speaking
- Blue skin (cyanosis)

You should attempt to clear only a complete or partial airway obstruction with poor air exchange.

A person who has a complete airway obstruction cannot speak, cough, or breathe. If the patient's airway is completely obstructed, there is no air exchange. Death due to suffocation will follow rapidly if you do not take prompt action.

Objective 20 ▶

Objective 22 ▶

When caring for a conscious patient who is choking, it is important to remember that the patient's level of responsiveness will change as the amount of oxygen in the patient's blood decreases. The patient will usually be very anxious and restless and may even be combative. Reassure the patient and any family members who are present that you are going to help him or her. If the obstruction is not quickly relieved and the patient remains conscious (as in a partial airway obstruction with poor air exchange), remember to remain calm and continue to provide reassurance while providing emergency care.

You Should Know

Signs of a Partial Airway Obstruction

Good Air Exchange

- Responsive
- Able to speak or make sounds
- Can cough forcefully
- Wheezing may be present between coughs

Poor Air Exchange

- Weak, ineffective cough
- High-pitched noise on inhalation
- Difficulty breathing, speaking
- Turning blue (cyanosis)

Signs of a Complete Airway Obstruction

- No air exchange
- Patient cannot speak, breathe, or cough

Objective 21 ▶

If your patient is having difficulty breathing, contact your dispatcher right away to request additional EMS resources. If more than one EMR is present, one should attend to the patient while the other contacts the dispatcher and requests EMS assistance.

Foreign Body Airway Obstruction – Adults

Performance Guidelines for a Conscious Choking Adult

Objective 13 ▶

Skill Drill 6-4 shows the steps used to care for a conscious choking adult.

Skill Drill 6-4

Clearing a Foreign Body Airway Obstruction in a Conscious Adult

STEP 1 ▶
- Find out if the patient can speak or cough. Ask, "Are you choking?"
- If the patient can cough or speak, encourage him or her to cough out the obstruction. Watch the patient closely to make sure the object is expelled.

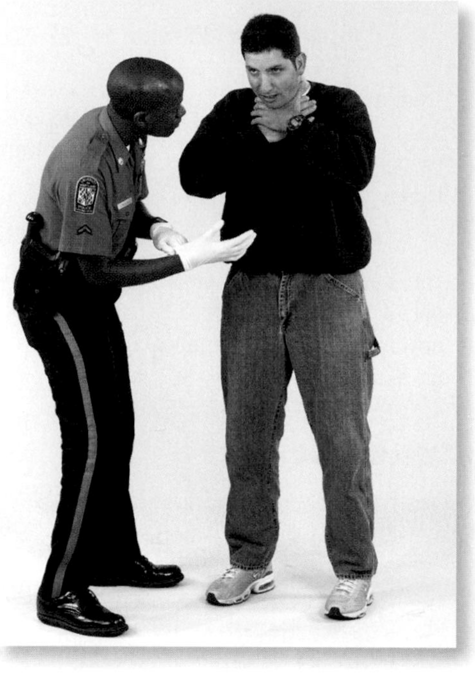

STEP 2 ▶
- If the patient cannot cough or speak, perform abdominal thrusts (the Heimlich maneuver).
- Stand behind the patient and wrap your arms around his or her waist.
- Make a fist with one hand. Place your fist, thumb side in, just above the patient's navel.

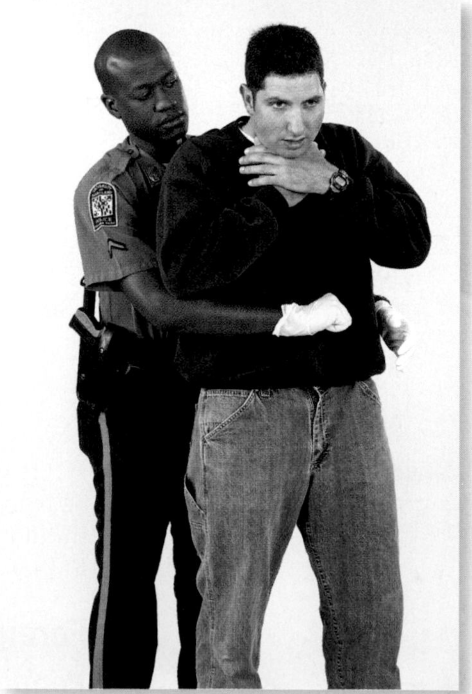

STEP 3 ▶

- Grab your fist tightly with your other hand. Pull your fist quickly inward and upward.
- Continue performing abdominal thrusts until the foreign body is expelled or the patient becomes unresponsive. Perform each abdominal thrust with the intent of relieving the obstruction. If abdominal thrusts are not effective, consider the use of chest thrusts to relieve the obstruction.

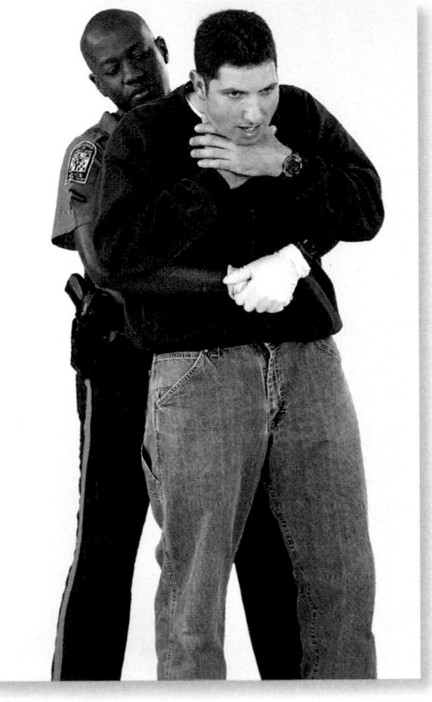

STEP 4 ▶ If your patient is obese or in the later stages of pregnancy, perform chest thrusts instead of abdominal thrusts:

- Place your arms around the patient's chest, directly under the armpits. Do not place your hands on the patient's ribs or on the bottom of the breastbone (xiphoid process). Press your hands backward, giving quick thrusts into the middle of the breastbone. The xiphoid process can easily be broken off the breastbone and cut underlying organs, such as the liver.

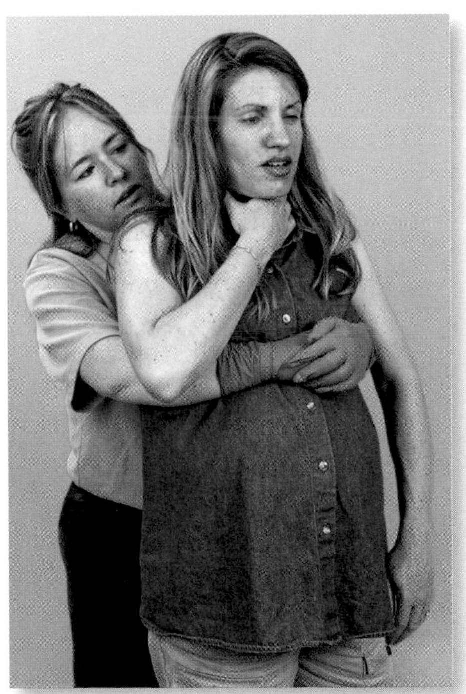

You Should Know

If you are choking and no one is around to help you, perform abdominal thrusts on yourself to try to clear the obstruction. Make a fist with one hand. Place your fist, thumb side in, above your navel. (Make sure your hands are below the lowest part of your breastbone). Grab your fist tightly with your other hand. Pull your fist quickly inward and upward. You may need to do this several times to relieve the obstruction. If this action is unsuccessful, bend over the back of a chair or the side of a table, countertop, or railing. Press your upper abdomen against the edge with a quick thrust. Repeat this movement until the object is expelled.

Performance Guidelines for an Unconscious Choking Adult

Objective 16 ▶

Skill Drill 6-5 shows the steps used to care for an unconscious choking adult.

If the obstruction is removed,

- Assess breathing. If the patient is not breathing, give 2 rescue breaths.
- Assess circulation. If there is no pulse or other signs of circulation, begin chest compressions.
- If breathing is absent but a pulse is present, deliver 1 breath every 5 to 6 seconds (10 to 12 breaths/minute). Recheck the patient's pulse frequently.
- If the patient is breathing and breathing is adequate, place the patient in the recovery position if he or she is not injured. Reassess the patient frequently.

Foreign Body Airway Obstruction – Infants and Children

Remember This!

Suspect an FBAO in any person, particularly an infant or a child, who suddenly has difficulty breathing, who is coughing, gagging, or who is breathing noisily.

Performance Guidelines for a Conscious Choking Child

Objective 14 ▶

Skill Drill 6-6 shows the steps used to care for a conscious choking child.

Performance Guidelines for an Unconscious Choking Child

Objective 17 ▶

Skill Drill 6-7 shows the steps used to care for an unconscious choking child.

If the obstruction is removed,

- Assess breathing. If the child is not breathing, give 2 rescue breaths.
- Assess circulation and perfusion. If there is no pulse or other signs of circulation, or if the heart rate is < 60 beats per minute with signs of poor perfusion, begin chest compressions.
- If breathing is absent but a pulse is present, deliver 1 breath every 3 to 5 seconds (12 to 20 breaths/minute) and monitor the child's pulse.
- If the child is breathing and breathing is adequate, place him or her in the recovery position if uninjured. Reassess the child frequently.

Performance Guidelines for a Conscious Choking Infant

Objective 15 ▶

Assess the infant. If the infant can cough or cry, watch him or her closely to make sure the object is expelled. If the infant is unable to cough or cry, provide care. Skill Drill 6-8 shows the steps used to care for a conscious choking infant.

Clearing a Foreign Body Airway Obstruction in an Unconscious Adult

STEP 1 ▶
- Make sure that the patient is unresponsive. Tap the patient's shoulder and ask, "Are you okay?"
- Place the patient on his back on a hard surface. Using a head tilt-chin lift (or jaw thrust without head tilt if trauma is suspected), open the airway.
- Check the nose and mouth for secretions, vomitus, a foreign body, or other obstruction. Suction fluids from the airway as needed. If you can see the object, perform a finger sweep to remove it.

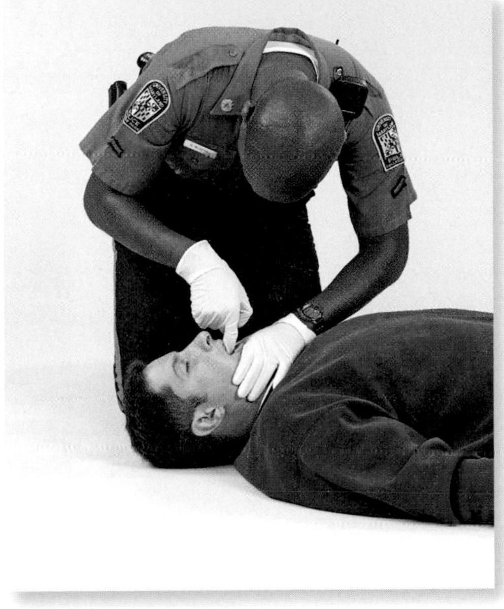

STEP 2 ▶ Try to ventilate the patient. If the chest does not rise, reposition the patient's head, reopen the airway, and try again to ventilate.

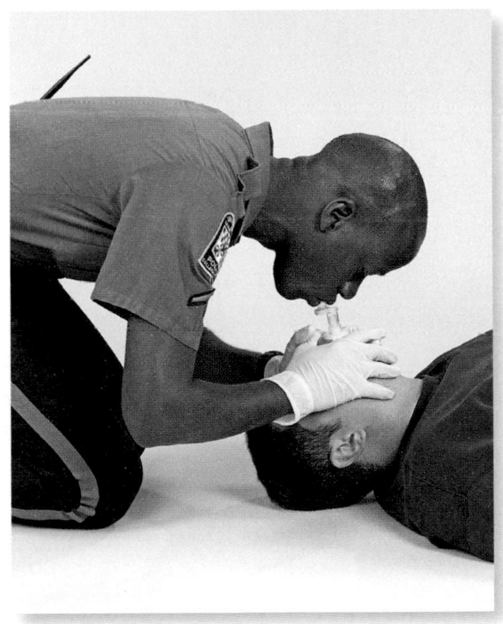

Continued on next page

Skill Drill 6-5

Clearing a Foreign Body Airway Obstruction in an Unconscious Adult *(continued)*

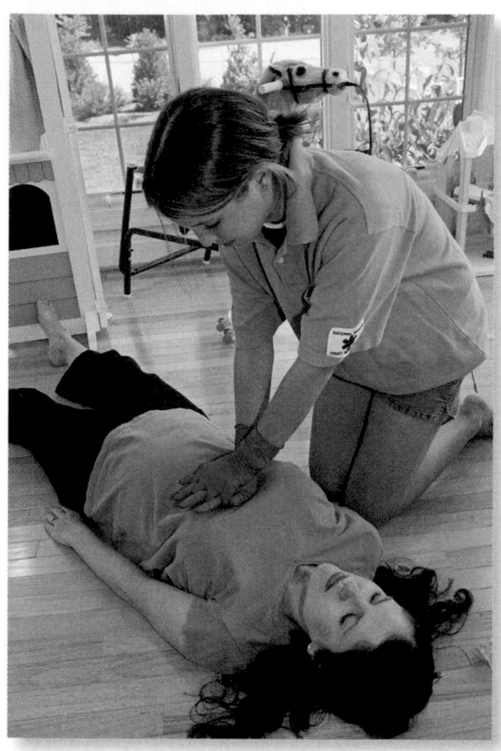

STEP 3 ▲ If the chest does not rise, begin CPR.

- Place the heel of your hand in the middle of the patient's breastbone. Be sure not to place your hand on the patient's ribs or on the bottom of the breastbone (xiphoid process). Place your other hand on top of the first. Press your hands downward, compressing the chest 30 times.
- Look into the mouth. Perform a finger sweep to remove visible objects. Attempt to ventilate the patient. If the chest does not rise, reposition the patient's head, reopen the airway, and try again to ventilate.
- If the rescue breaths do not result in chest rise, continue the sequence of attempts to ventilate, performing chest compressions, looking in the mouth, and performing a finger sweep (if the object is seen) until the obstruction is relieved.

Clearing a Foreign Body Airway Obstruction in a Conscious Child

STEP 1 ▶
- Find out if the child can speak or cough. Ask, "Are you choking?"
- If the child can cough or speak, encourage the child to cough. Watch her closely to make sure the object is expelled.

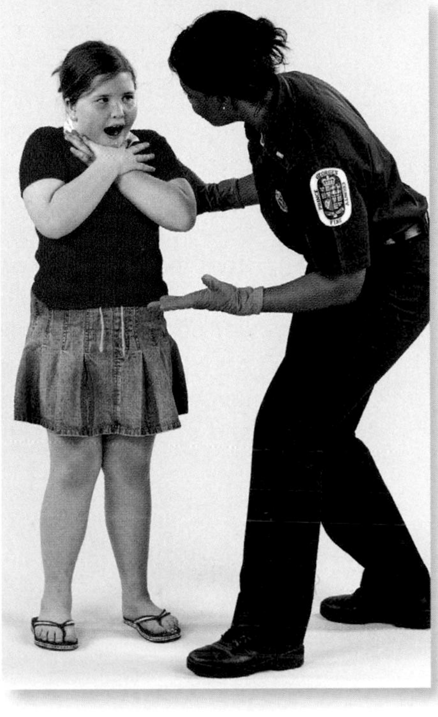

STEP 2 ▶ If the child cannot cough or speak, perform abdominal thrusts:
- Stand behind the child and wrap your arms around her waist.
- Make a fist with one hand. Place your fist, thumb side in, just above the patient's navel. Grab your fist tightly with your other hand. Pull your fist quickly inward and upward.
- Continue performing abdominal thrusts until the object is expelled or the child becomes unresponsive.

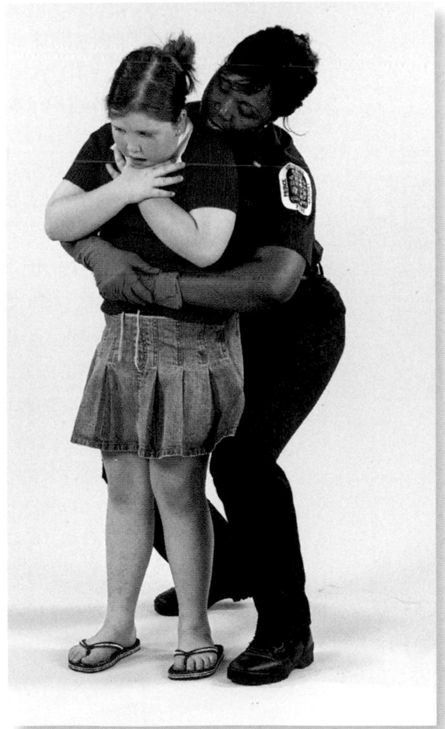

Skill Drill 6-7

Clearing a Foreign Body Airway Obstruction in an Unconscious Child

STEP 1 ▶

- Make sure that the child is unresponsive. Tap the patient's shoulder and ask, "Are you okay?"
- Place the child on her back on a hard surface. Using a head tilt–chin lift or tongue-jaw lift (or jaw thrust without head tilt if trauma is suspected), open the airway.
- Check the nose and mouth for secretions, vomit, a foreign body, and other obstructions. Suction fluids from the airway as needed. If a foreign body is visible, remove it using a finger sweep. However, do *not* perform a blind finger sweep.
- Attempt to ventilate the child. If the chest does not rise, reposition the child's head, reopen the airway, and try again to ventilate.

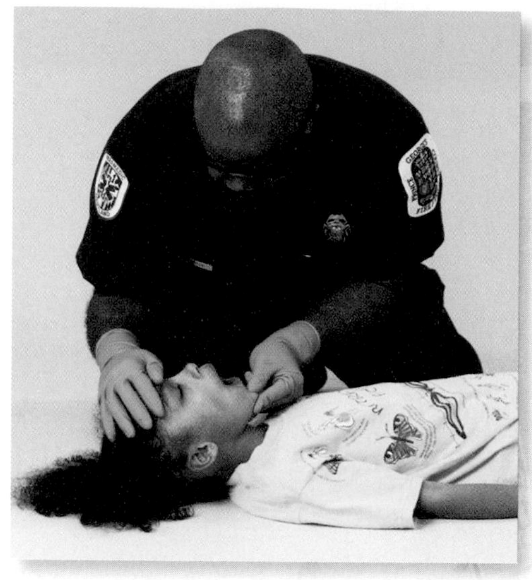

STEP 2 ▶ If the chest does not rise, begin CPR.

- Position yourself directly over the child's chest. Place the heel of one hand on the lower half of the breastbone. With your arms straight and your elbows locked, press down on the child's chest with the heel of one hand. Be sure not to place your hand on the patient's ribs or on the bottom of the breastbone (xiphoid process). Compress the chest 30 times.
- Look into the mouth. If you see the foreign body, remove it using a finger sweep.
- Attempt to ventilate the patient. If the chest does not rise, reposition the patient's head, reopen the airway, and try again to ventilate.
- If the rescue breaths do not result in chest rise, continue the sequence of attempts to ventilate, performing chest compressions, looking in the mouth, and performing a finger sweep (if the object is seen) until the obstruction is relieved.

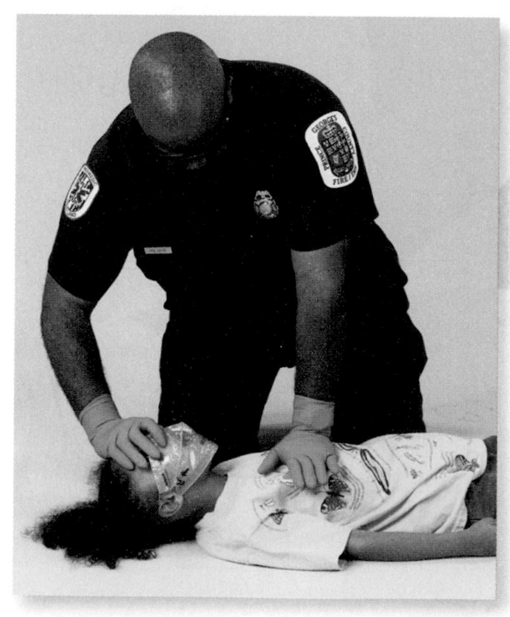

Clearing a Foreign Body Airway Obstruction in a Conscious Infant

STEP 1 ▶ While supporting the infant's head, place the infant face down over your forearm. You may find it helpful to rest your forearm on your thigh to support the weight of the infant. Keep the infant's head slightly lower than the rest of the body.

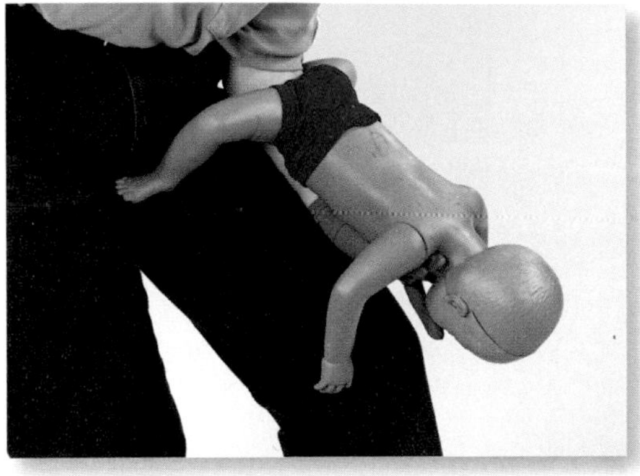

STEP 2 ▶ Using the heel of one hand, forcefully deliver up to five back blows between the infant's shoulder blades.

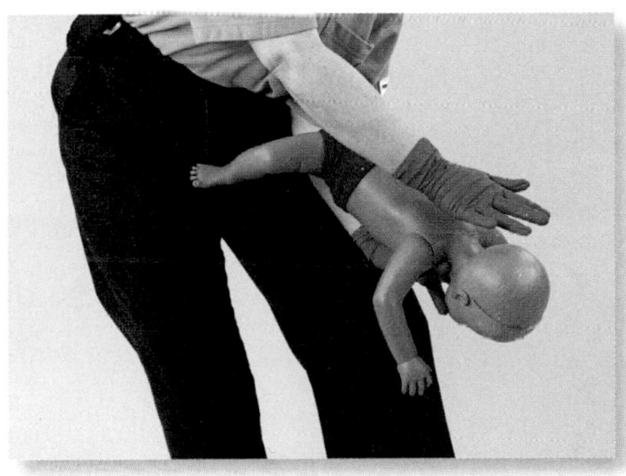

STEP 3 ▶

- If the foreign body is not expelled, deliver chest thrusts. Place your free hand on the infant's back. Turn the infant over onto his or her back while supporting the back of the head with the palm of your hand. Imagine a line between the infant's nipples. Place the flat part of one finger about one finger width below this imaginary line. Place a second finger next to the first on the infant's sternum. Deliver up to five quick downward chest thrusts.
- Check the infant's mouth. If you see the foreign body, remove it.
- Continue alternating up to five back blows and up to five chest thrusts, attempting to visualize the object until the object is expelled or the infant becomes unresponsive.

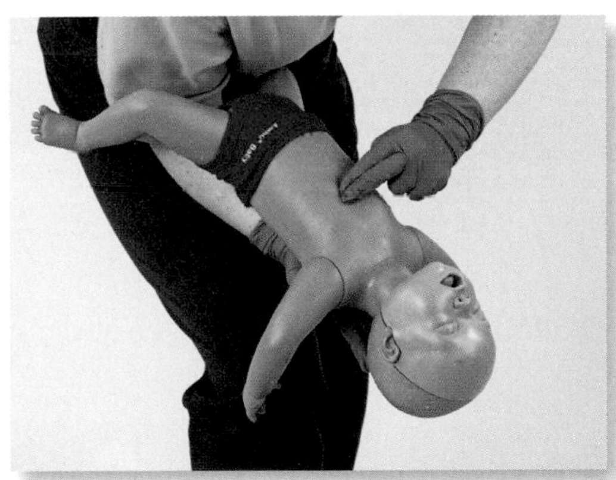

Making a Difference

Use the following guidelines when clearing an FBAO in a conscious infant:

- Support the infant's head by firmly holding his or her jaw. Do not compress the soft tissues of the infant's throat.
- Keep the head lower than the trunk. Deliver chest thrusts at a rate of approximately one per second.

Performance Guidelines for an Unconscious Choking Infant

Objective 18 ▶

Skill Drill 6-9 shows the steps used to care for an unconscious choking infant.

If the obstruction is removed,

- Assess breathing. Suction fluids and particulate matter if necessary. If the infant is not breathing, give 2 rescue breaths.
- Assess circulation and perfusion. If there is no pulse or other signs of circulation, or if the heart rate is < 60 beats per minute with signs of poor perfusion, begin chest compressions.
- If breathing is absent but a pulse is present, perform rescue breathing by giving 1 breath every 3 to 5 seconds (12 to 20 breaths/minute). Reassess the infant's pulse frequently.
- If the infant is breathing and breathing is adequate, reassess frequently.

Special Considerations

Tracheal Stomas

A tracheal stoma is a permanent opening at the front of the neck that extends from the skin surface into the trachea. There are many reasons a person may have a stoma:

- A throat tumor or infection
- A severe injury to the neck or mouth
- A disease or an infection that affects swallowing
- The need for long-term breathing assistance with a mechanical ventilator

Patients who have a stoma breathe through this opening in the neck because it is their airway. If artificial ventilation is required, it should be delivered through the stoma; Figure 6-15.

FIGURE 6-15 ▶ Mask-to-stoma breathing.

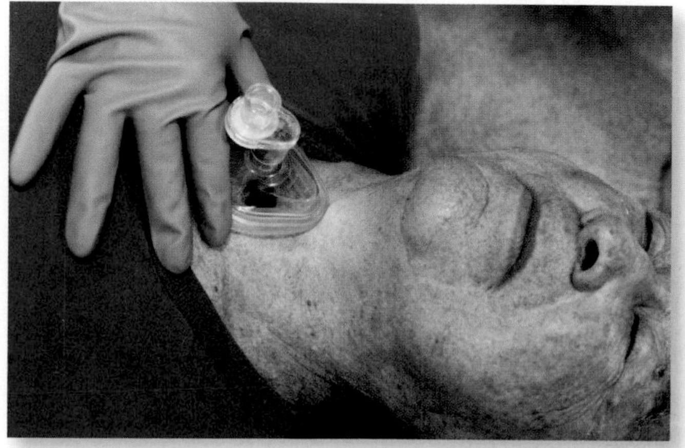

Clearing a Foreign Body Airway Obstruction in an Unconscious Infant

STEP 1 ▶
- Confirm that the infant is unresponsive.
- Place the infant on his or her back on a flat surface or on your forearm. Support the infant's head.
- Open the airway using a head tilt–chin lift or tongue-jaw lift (or jaw thrust without head tilt if trauma is suspected).

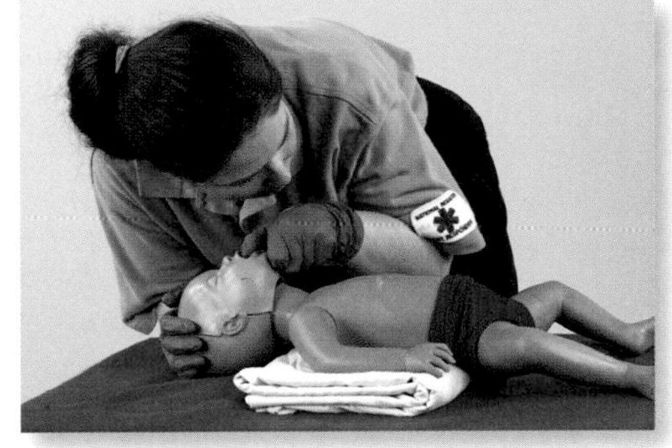

STEP 2 ▶
- Check the nose and mouth for secretions, vomitus, a foreign body, or other obstruction. Suction fluids from the airway as needed. If you can see a foreign body, remove it using a finger sweep. However, do *not* perform a blind finger sweep.
- Try to ventilate the infant. If the chest does not rise, reposition the infant's head, reopen the airway, and try to ventilate again.

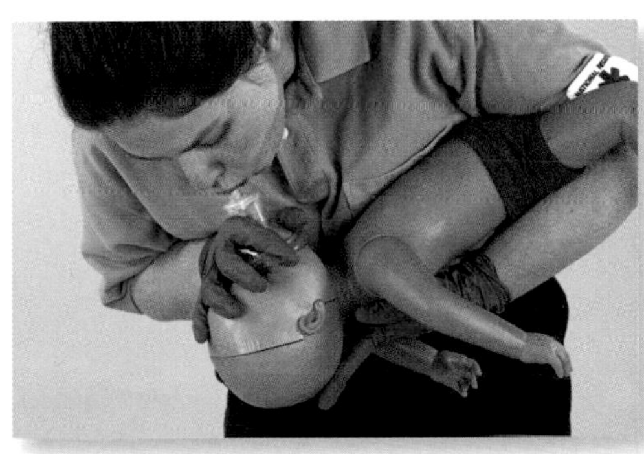

STEP 3 ▶ If the chest does not rise, begin CPR.
- Place your free hand on the infant's back. Turn the infant over onto his or her back while supporting the back of the head with the palm of your hand. Imagine a line between the infant's nipples. Place the flat part of one finger about one finger width below this imaginary line. Place a second finger next to the first on the infant's sternum.
- Give 30 compressions. Depress the breastbone 1/3 to 1/2 the depth of the chest with each compression. After 30 chest compressions, look into the mouth. If you see the foreign body, remove it using a finger sweep. Do NOT perform a blind finger sweep. Attempt to ventilate the infant.
- If the chest does not rise, reposition the baby's head, reopen the airway, and try again to ventilate. If the rescue breaths do not result in chest rise, continue the sequence of attempts to ventilate, performing chest compressions, looking in the mouth, and performing a finger sweep (if the object is seen) until the obstruction is relieved.

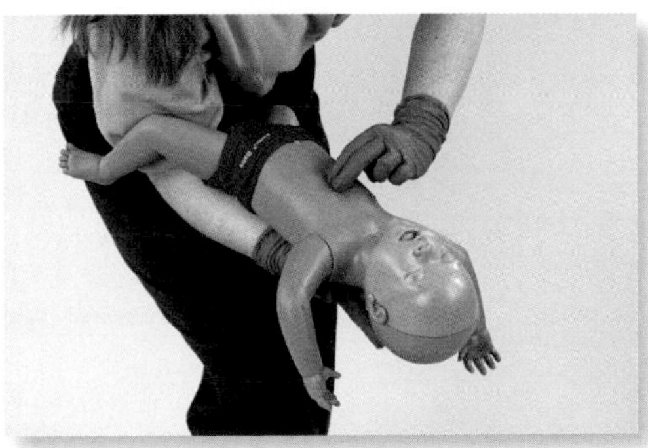

Follow these steps to perform mask-to-stoma breathing (the use of a mask over the stoma is preferred; Figure 6-15):

Objective 10 ▶

- If present, remove any garment (scarf, necktie) covering the stoma.
- Place a pediatric facemask or barrier device on the patient's neck over the stoma. Make an airtight seal around the stoma.
- Slowly blow into the one-way valve on the mask until the chest rises.
- Remove your mouth from the mask to allow the patient to exhale.

Dental Appliances

Dentures that fit well in the patient's mouth should be left in place. If they become loose or dislodged, remove them from the mouth because they can become a foreign body obstruction. Note that when you ventilate a patient with dentures removed, it is more difficult to obtain a seal.

Infants and Children

Objective 9 ▶

The airway of infants and young children differs from that of older children and adults. Infants less than six months of age breathe primarily through their nose, not their mouth. Their airway is much smaller, allowing a greater opportunity for obstruction. One such obstruction is their tongue, which is large compared with the size of their mouth.

The primary cause of cardiac arrest in infants and children is an uncorrected respiratory problem.

The supporting cartilage of a child's trachea is less developed than an adult's, making it prone to compression with improper neck positioning. Be sure to place an infant's head in a neutral position. The narrowest part of a child's airway is at the cricoid cartilage, which is lower in the airway than it is in an adult. These differences allow for easier airway obstruction in an infant or a child.

Gastric distention (swelling) is common when ventilating infants and children. When providing positive-pressure ventilation, avoid using excessive volume. Use only enough volume to cause a gentle chest rise.

Supplemental Oxygen

Some EMS agencies permit Emergency Medical Responders to give oxygen. Check with your instructor and medical oversight authority to find out if you are allowed to use oxygen.

Oxygen Cylinders

Oxygen is stored in steel or aluminum cylinders (Figure 6-16). Oxygen cylinders may be green, or they may be silver or chrome with green around the valve stem. The tank pressure of a fully pressurized cylinder is approximately 2,000 pounds per

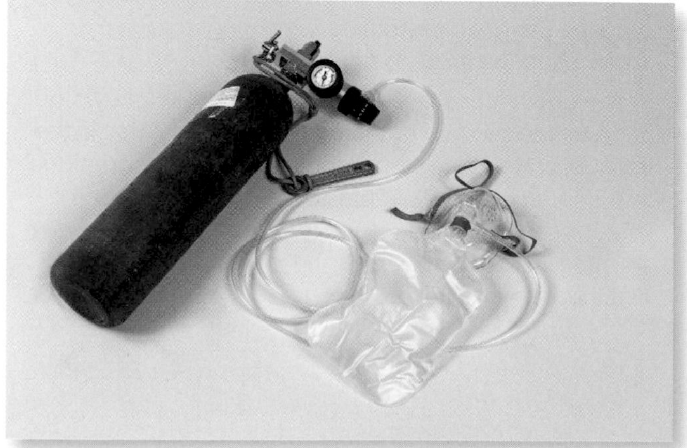

FIGURE 6-16 ▶ An oxygen delivery system.

square inch (psi), but tank pressure varies with the temperature. Tank pressure increases with increased temperature and decreases with decreased temperature. The amount of oxygen in various sizes of cylinders is noted in Table 6-2.

Safety Considerations

Oxygen cylinders should be handled carefully because their contents are under pressure. Tanks should be positioned to prevent falling and blows to the valve-gauge assembly. Be sure to secure the tanks during transport. Always keep combustible materials away from oxygen equipment and never position any part of your body in front of the cylinder's valve.

Pressure Regulators

A pressure regulator reduces pressure in the oxygen cylinder to a safe range. A flow meter controls the liters of oxygen delivered per minute.

Operating Procedures

Place the cylinder in an upright position and position yourself to the side of the cylinder. Remove the protective seal. Quickly open and then shut the valve to remove dust and debris. Attach the pressure regulator to the tank with an appropriate O-ring seal. Attach the oxygen device to the flow meter. Open the valve with one-half to one full turn to pressurize the flow meter. Open the flow meter to the desired setting. Apply the oxygen delivery device, such as a nonrebreather mask, to the patient. When oxygen delivery is complete, remove the device from the patient, turn off the cylinder valve and remove all pressure from the regulator.

Oxygen Delivery Devices

Nonrebreather Mask

A nonrebreather mask is the preferred method of oxygen delivery in the field for a patient who is breathing adequately (Figure 6-17). It allows the delivery of high-concentration oxygen to a breathing patient. At 15 LPM, the oxygen concentration delivered is approximately 90%. A one-way valve allows exhaled air to escape the mask but prevents room air from being breathed in.

When using a nonrebreather mask, be sure to fill the reservoir bag with oxygen before placing the mask on the patient. After placing the mask on the patient, adjust the flow rate so that the bag does not completely deflate when the patient inhales, usually 15 LPM. Enough supplemental oxygen must be available for each breath.

TABLE 6-2 Oxygen Cylinders

Cylinder Type	Amount of Oxygen in Liters
D	350
E	625
M	3,000
G	5,300
H	6,900

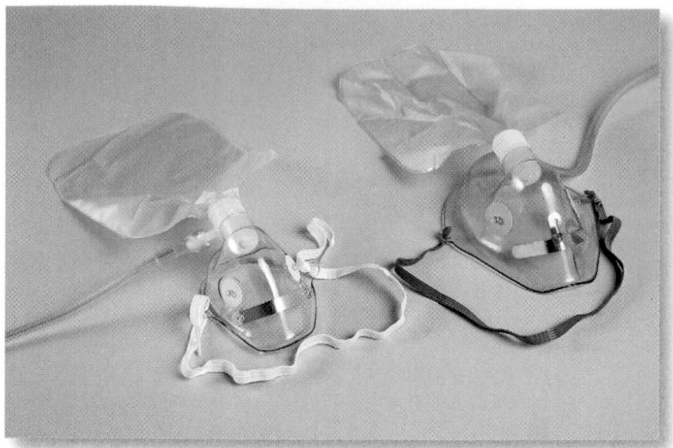

FIGURE 6-17 ▲ A pediatric and adult nonrebreather mask.

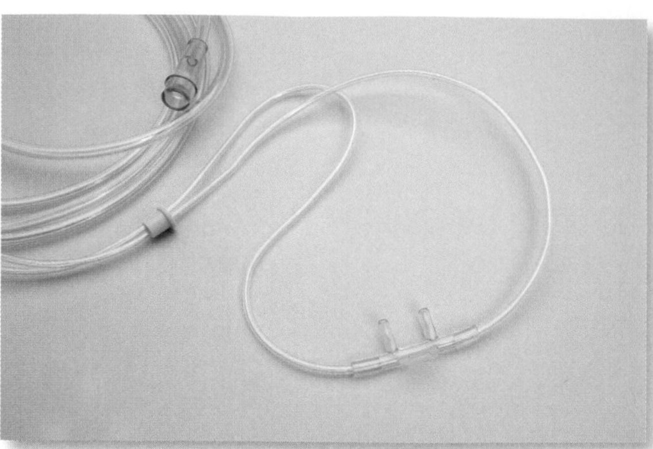

FIGURE 6-18 ▲ A nasal cannula.

Nasal Cannula

The use of a nasal cannula requires a breathing patient.

A nasal cannula is a piece of plastic tubing with two soft prongs that stick out from the tubing (Figure 6-18). The prongs are inserted into the patient's nostrils and the tubing is secured to the patient's face. This oxygen delivery device is rarely the best method of delivering adequate oxygen in the field. It should be used only when patients will not tolerate a nonrebreather mask despite coaching. A nasal cannula can deliver an oxygen concentration of 25–45% at 1–6 LPM. Flow rates of more than 6 LPM are irritating to the nasal passages.

On The Scene

Wrap-Up

You carefully slide an oropharyngeal airway into the patient's mouth. Positioning your pocket mask over his nose and mouth, you deliver rescue breaths at the proper rate, pausing to let him exhale each time you see his chest rise. When the ambulance crew arrives, they note that his pupils are very small. They connect a BVM to oxygen and you continue to ventilate him. A paramedic quickly starts an IV. As she begins giving the patient an IV medication, you can feel your patient's breathing rate increase between the breaths you are giving. Within minutes his eyes are open, he is breathing on his own, and he is trying to sit up. As the ambulance pulls away, his sister tearfully tells you she thought he had quit taking drugs and was trying to get clean. You realize that if she had waited a few more minutes to call, he would have been in cardiac arrest. ■

Sum It Up

- As an Emergency Medical Responder, you must maintain an open airway to allow a free flow of air into and out of the patient's lungs. You must be familiar with the structures of the upper and lower airways. You must also understand the mechanisms of breathing.
- One of the most important actions you can perform is to open the airway of an unresponsive patient. You must become familiar with the two main methods of opening an airway: (1) the head tilt–chin lift, and (2) the jaw-thrust without head tilt maneuver.

- Remember that you must *never* use the *head tilt–chin lift maneuver* to open the airway if trauma to the head or neck is suspected. Damage to the patient's spinal cord can result.
- When trauma to the head or neck of an unresponsive patient is suspected, use the *jaw thrust without head tilt* to open the patient's airway. This method of opening the airway is effective, but it is less effective than the head tilt–chin lift and is more tiring. Because this technique requires the use of both hands, a second rescuer will be needed if the patient requires ventilation.

▶ If a patient's airway is obstructed, you must clear it. The three primary ways of clearing the airway of an unresponsive, injured patient are with the recovery position, finger sweeps, and suctioning.

- You can use the *recovery position* as the first step in maintaining an open airway in an unresponsive patient. This position involves positioning a patient on his or her side. As an Emergency Medical Responder, you must become familiar with placing a patient in this position. You must also remember *never* to place a patient with a known or suspected spinal injury in the recovery position.
- If you see foreign material in the patient's mouth, you must remove it immediately. *Finger sweeps* are used to remove material from an unresponsive patient's upper airway. A blind finger sweep is performed without first seeing foreign material in the airway. Remember that blind finger sweeps should *never* be performed on an infant or a child as they may cause the object to become further lodged in the patient's throat.
- You should always have suction equipment available when you are managing a patient's airway or assisting a patient's breathing. *Suctioning* is a procedure used to vacuum vomitus, saliva, blood, food particles, and other material from the patient's airway. Suctioning may be needed if the recovery position and finger sweeps are not effective in clearing the patient's airway. It may also be needed if trauma is suspected and the patient cannot be placed in the recovery position.

▶ After you have opened a patient's airway, you may need to use an *airway adjunct* to keep it open. After the airway adjunct is inserted, the proper head position must be maintained while the device is in place.

- An *oropharyngeal airway (OPA)* is a device that is used only in unresponsive patients without a gag reflex. An OPA is inserted into the patient's mouth and used to keep the tongue away from the back of the throat.
- A *nasopharyngeal airway (NPA)* is a device that is placed in the patient's nose. An NPA keeps the patient's tongue from blocking the upper airway. It also allows air to flow from the hole in the NPA down into the patient's lower airway.

▶ After making sure that the patient's airway is open, you must check for breathing. If the patient is breathing, you must determine if the patient is breathing adequately or inadequately. You must also learn the sounds of noisy breathing, which include *stridor, snoring, gurgling,* and *wheezing.*

▶ If your patient's breathing is inadequate or absent, you will need to assist the patient by forcing air into the patient's lungs. This action is called *positive-pressure ventilation* and includes the following: *mouth-to-mask ventilation, mouth-to-barrier ventilation, mouth-to-mouth ventilation,* and *bag-valve-mask ventilation.* As an Emergency Medical Responder, you will need to become familiar with performing all of these ventilation methods. You must also learn how to remove foreign body airway obstructions in patients of every age.

▶ You may need to give patients supplemental oxygen. Become familiar with the features and functioning of oxygen cylinders. Remember always to keep combustible materials away from oxygen equipment and never position any part of your body over the cylinder.

- The two most common oxygen delivery devices are the *nonrebreather mask* and the *nasal cannula.* In the field, the nonrebreather mask is the preferred method of oxygen delivery. It allows the delivery of high-concentration oxygen to a breathing patient. The nasal cannula is rarely the best method of delivering adequate oxygen in the field. It should be used only when patients will not tolerate a nonrebreather mask despite coaching.

▶ Tracking Your Progress

After reading this chapter, can you	Page Reference	Objective Met?
• Name and label the major structures of the respiratory system on a diagram?	159–160	☐
• List the signs of inadequate breathing?	171–172	☐
• Describe the steps in the head tilt–chin lift?	163	☐
• Relate mechanism of injury to opening the airway?	163	☐
• Describe the steps in the jaw thrust?	163	☐
• State the importance of having a suction unit ready for immediate use when providing emergency medical care?	165–166	☐
• Describe the techniques of suctioning?	166–167	☐
• Describe how to ventilate a patient with a resuscitation mask or barrier device?	176	☐
• Describe how ventilating an infant or child is different from an adult?	177	☐
• List the steps in providing mouth-to-mouth and mouth-to-stoma ventilation?	176–177, 192	☐
• Describe how to measure and insert an oropharyngeal (oral) airway?	167–169	☐
• Describe how to measure and insert a nasopharyngeal (nasal) airway?	167, 170	☐
• Describe how to clear a foreign body airway obstruction in a responsive adult?	182–183	☐
• Describe how to clear a foreign body airway obstruction in a responsive child with complete obstruction or partial airway obstruction and poor air exchange?	187	☐
• Describe how to clear a foreign body airway obstruction in a responsive infant with complete obstruction or partial airway obstruction and poor air exchange?	189	☐
• Describe how to clear a foreign body airway obstruction in an unresponsive adult?	184–185	☐
• Describe how to clear a foreign body airway obstruction in an unresponsive child?	184, 188	☐
• Describe how to clear a foreign body airway obstruction in an unresponsive infant?	190–191	☐
• Explain why Basic Life Support ventilation and airway protective skills take priority over most other Basic Life Support skills?	162	☐

• Demonstrate a caring attitude toward patients with airway problems who request emergency medical services?	181	☐
• Place the interests of the patient with airway problems as the foremost consideration when making any and all patient care decisions?	181	☐
• Communicate with empathy to patients with airway problems, as well as with family members and friends of the patient?	181	☐

Chapter Quiz

Multiple Choice

In the space provided, identify the letter of the choice that best completes each statement or answers each question.

_____ **1.** Do not suction an adult for more than

a. 3 seconds.
b. 5 seconds.
c. 10 seconds.
d. 15 seconds.

_____ **2.** Which of the following signs indicate a complete airway obstruction?

a. absence of cough, speech, or breathing
b. weak, ineffective cough and a high-pitched noise on inhalation
c. wheezing between coughs
d. the ability to speak and to cough forcefully

_____ **3.** A six-year-old child is found unresponsive in the living room by his mother. No spinal injury is suspected. Which of the following maneuvers should you use to open the child's airway?

a. head tilt–chin lift maneuver
b. jaw-thrust without head tilt maneuver
c. tongue-jaw lift maneuver
d. Sellick maneuver

_____ **4.** Select the correct statement regarding the airway of an infant or a child.

a. The narrowest part of a child's airway is at the vocal cords.
b. The tongue of an infant or a child is large relative to the size of the mouth.
c. The supporting cartilage of a child's trachea is more developed than that of an adult.
d. An infant less than six months of age breathes primarily through the mouth.

_____ **5.** A 92-year-old man has a tracheal stoma. If it is necessary to provide positive-pressure ventilation for this patient, which of the following methods is preferred?

a. placing your mouth directly over the stoma
b. aiming a nasal cannula at the stoma
c. placing a nonrebreather mask over the stoma
d. placing a pediatric pocket mask over stoma

_____ **6.** A 35-year-old woman is choking in a restaurant. She is awake but is unable to cough or speak. She is quickly turning blue. Your first action should be to

a. tell her you are going to help her and perform abdominal thrusts.
b. place her on the floor and perform a jaw thrust without head tilt.
c. apply a pocket mask to her face and begin rescue breathing.
d. check for a pulse and prepare to perform chest compressions.

True or False

Decide whether each statement is true or false. In the space provided, write T for true or F for false.

_____ **7.** An oropharyngeal airway can be used in responsive, semi-responsive, and unresponsive patients.

_____ **8.** A finger sweep may be used on responsive patients or unresponsive patients who have a gag reflex.

Matching

Match the key terms in the left column with the definitions in the right column by placing the letter of each correct answer in the space provided.

_____ **9.** Nasal septum

_____ **10.** Aspiration

_____ **11.** Patent

_____ **12.** Airway adjuncts

_____ **13.** Glottis

_____ **14.** Diaphragm

_____ **15.** Epiglottis

_____ **16.** Suctioning

a. Piece of cartilage that closes off the trachea during swallowing
b. Primary muscle of respiration
c. Breathing a foreign substance into the lungs
d. Space between the vocal cords
e. Wall of tissue that separates the right and left nostrils
f. Open
g. Procedure used to vacuum material from the patient's airway
h. Devices used to help keep a patient's airway open

Short Answer

Answer each question in the space provided.

17. Describe how to select an oropharyngeal airway of the correct size for a patient.

____

____

____

18. List five signs of inadequate breathing.

1. ______________________
2. ______________________
3. ______________________
4. ______________________
5. ______________________

19. List three types of patients for which chest thrusts may be used to relieve an upper airway obstruction.

1. ______________________
2. ______________________
3. ______________________

20. List the three categories of upper airway obstruction.

1. ______________________________

2. ______________________________

3. ______________________________

21. List three methods that may be used to open an airway.

1. ______________________________

2. ______________________________

3. ______________________________

22. List three ways to deliver positive-pressure ventilation.

1. ______________________________

2. ______________________________

3. ______________________________

23. What is the most common cause of upper airway obstruction in an unresponsive patient?

____

____

____

24. What gases are exchanged during the process of breathing?

____

____

____

Sentence Completion

In the blanks provided, write the words that best complete each sentence.

25. The largest cartilage of the larynx is the thyroid cartilage, also called the ______________ ______________.

26. OPA stands for ______________ ______________ ______________.

27. When providing rescue breathing for an infant or child, give 1 breath every ______________ seconds, which is ______________ breaths/minute.

28. When providing rescue breathing for an adult, give 1 breath every ______________ seconds, which is ______________ breaths/minute.

Module 3

Circulation

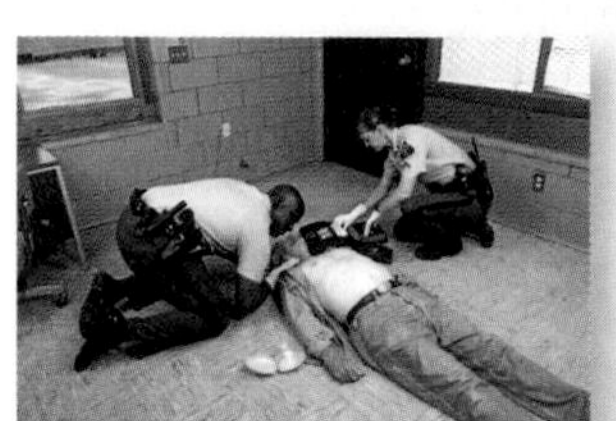

CHAPTER

7 Circulation

By the end of this chapter, you should be able to

Knowledge Objectives ▶

1. List the reasons for the heart to stop beating.
2. Define the components of cardiopulmonary resuscitation.
3. Describe each link in the Chain of Survival and how it relates to the EMS system.
4. List the steps of one-rescuer adult CPR.
5. Describe the technique of external chest compressions on an adult patient.
6. Describe the technique of external chest compressions on an infant.
7. Describe the technique of external chest compressions on a child.
8. Explain when the Emergency Medical Responder is able to stop CPR.
9. List the steps of two-rescuer adult CPR.
10. List the steps of infant CPR.
11. List the steps of child CPR.

Attitude Objectives ▶

12. Respond to the feelings that the family of a patient may be having during a cardiac event.
13. Demonstrate a caring attitude toward patients with cardiac events who request Emergency Medical Services.
14. Place the interests of the patient with a cardiac event as the foremost consideration when making any and all patient care decisions.
15. Communicate with empathy with family members and friends of the patient with a cardiac event.

Skill Objectives ▶

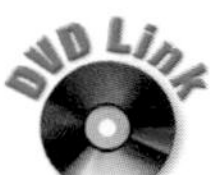

16. Demonstrate the proper technique of chest compressions on an adult.
17. Demonstrate the proper technique of chest compressions on a child.
18. Demonstrate the proper technique of chest compressions on an infant.
19. Demonstrate the steps of adult one-rescuer CPR.
20. Demonstrate the steps of adult two-rescuer CPR.
21. Demonstrate child CPR.
22. Demonstrate infant CPR.

On The Scene

Your quiet shift at the casino ends abruptly when you see an elderly woman slump forward onto a nickel slot machine. "Code 99, slot machines," you radio to the other security officers. Donning your gloves, you move quickly to the patient. She doesn't respond to your voice or a shoulder shake, so you lower her limp body gently onto her back on the floor. "Call 9-1-1," you tell the next arriving officer. Carefully tilting her head back, you lower your ear above her nose and mouth and look to see if her chest rises. She is not breathing so you deliver two slow breaths, just enough to make her chest rise. Then, sliding your fingers into the groove beside her trachea, you feel for a carotid pulse. There is none, so you place your hands over her breastbone and begin chest compressions. You scan the room, hoping the other officer will arrive quickly with the AED. ■

THINK ABOUT IT

As you read this chapter, think about the following questions:

- What could have caused the patient's heart to stop beating?
- What ratio of compressions to breaths will you provide?
- Why is it important for the AED to arrive quickly?
- How will you know if her circulation resumes?

Introduction

Circulatory Emergencies

Emergencies involving the circulatory system are very common. Bleeding, heart attack, and cardiac arrest are just a few of the types of emergencies you may encounter. As an Emergency Medical Responder, you must be able to recognize the emergency and know what to do. In situations like these, your actions can make a difference until more advanced help arrives.

The Circulatory System

The Functions of the Circulatory System

The circulatory system is responsible for transporting oxygen, water, and nutrients (such as sugar and vitamins) throughout the body. It also carries away wastes (such as carbon dioxide) produced by body cells to the lungs, kidneys, or skin for removal from the body.

The Components of the Circulatory System

PFC = pump (the heart), fluid (blood), container (blood vessels)

The circulatory system consists of the cardiovascular and lymphatic systems. The cardiovascular system is made up of three main parts: (1) a pump (the heart), (2) fluid (blood), and (3) a container (blood vessels) (Figure 7-1). The lymphatic system consists of lymph, lymph nodes, lymph vessels, the tonsils, the spleen, and the thymus gland.

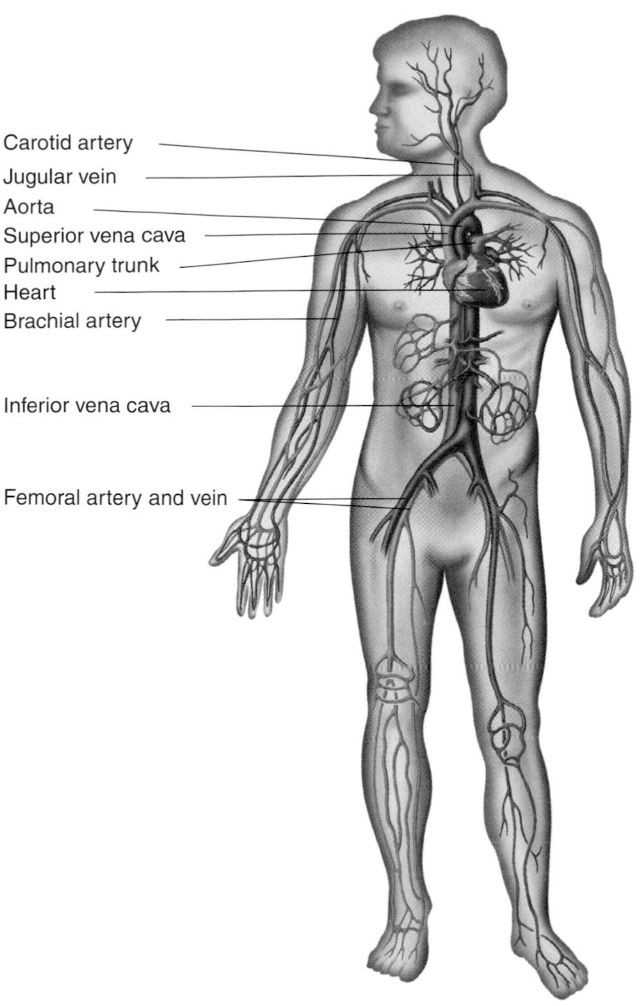

FIGURE 7-1 ▶ The heart, blood, and blood vessels are the major components of the cardiovascular system.

The Heart

The heart is located slightly to the left of the center of the chest. Its job is to pump blood through the vessels of the body (Figure 7-2). The heart is divided into four chambers. The two upper chambers are the right and left **atria.** The job of the atria is to receive blood from the body and lungs. The right atrium receives blood that is low in oxygen from the body. The left atrium receives blood rich in oxygen from the lungs. The two lower chambers of the heart are the right and left **ventricles.** The ventricles are larger and have thicker walls than the atria because their job is to pump blood to the lungs and body. The right ventricle pumps blood to the lungs. The left ventricle pumps blood to the body. Valves in the heart prevent the backflow of blood and keep the blood moving in one direction (Figure 7-3).

Blood

Blood carries oxygen and nutrients to body cells. It also removes waste products, such as carbon dioxide, from body cells. Blood is made up of liquid and formed elements. The liquid portion of the blood is called **plasma** (Figure 7-4). Plasma carries blood cells throughout the body. The formed elements of the blood include red blood cells, white blood cells, and platelets. Red blood cells pick up oxygen in the lungs and transport it to body cells. After delivering oxygen to the cells, red blood cells gather up carbon dioxide and transport it to the lungs, where it is removed from the body when we exhale. White blood cells attack and

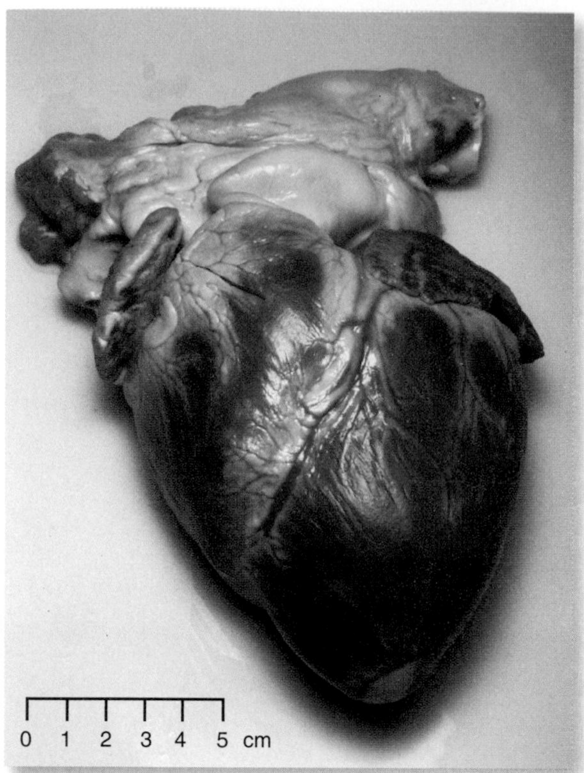

FIGURE 7-2 ▲ Front (anterior) view of a human heart. © A. F. Michler/Peter Arnold, Inc.

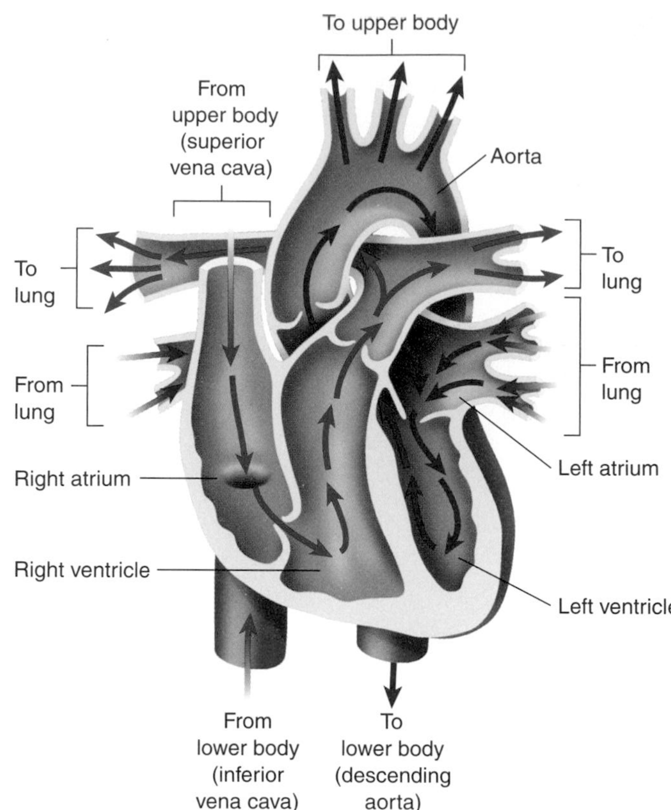

FIGURE 7-3 ▲ Blood flow through the heart. The right atrium receives blood that is low in oxygen from the body. Blood passes through the tricuspid valve into the right ventricle. The right ventricle pumps blood through the pulmonary valve to the lungs. The left atrium receives blood rich in oxygen from the lungs. Blood passes through the mitral valve into the left ventricle. The left ventricle pumps blood through the aortic valve to the aorta and out to the body.

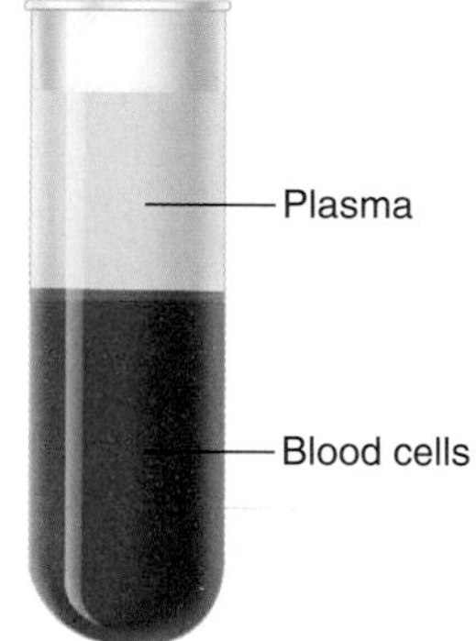

FIGURE 7-4 ▲ Blood is made up of liquid (plasma) and formed elements (red blood cells, white blood cells, and platelets).

Remember: *A*rteries = *A*way.

destroy germs that enter the body (Figure 7-5). Platelets are irregularly shaped blood cells that have a sticky surface. When a blood vessel is damaged and starts to bleed, platelets gather at the site of the injury. The platelets begin to stick to the opening of the damaged vessel and seal the vessel, stopping the flow of blood.

Blood Vessels

The blood vessels that carry blood away from the heart to the rest of the body are called **arteries.** Blood is forced into the arteries when the heart contracts. Arteries have thick walls because they transport blood under high pressure (Figure 7-6). A **pulse** is the rhythmic contraction and expansion of the arteries with each beat of the heart. A pulse can be felt anywhere an artery passes near the skin surface and can be pressed against firm tissue, such as a bone.

Vessels that return blood to the heart are called **veins.** The walls of veins are much thinner than the walls of arteries (see Figure 7-6). Because the pressure in veins is low, veins contain one-way valves that help keep the blood flowing toward the heart (Figure 7-7). **Capillaries** are the smallest and most numerous

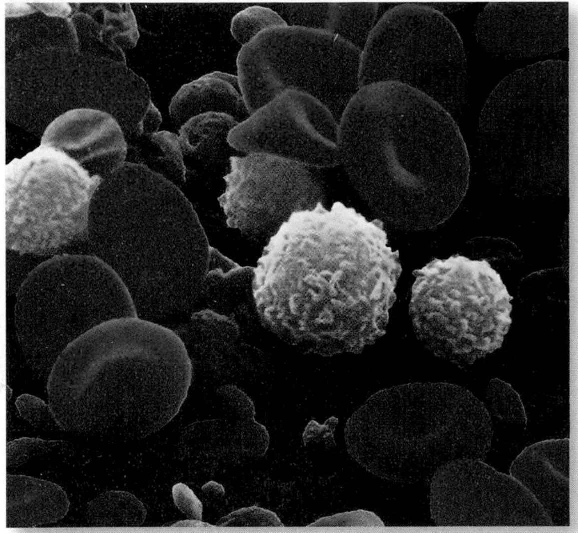

FIGURE 7-5 ▲ Human red and white blood cells.

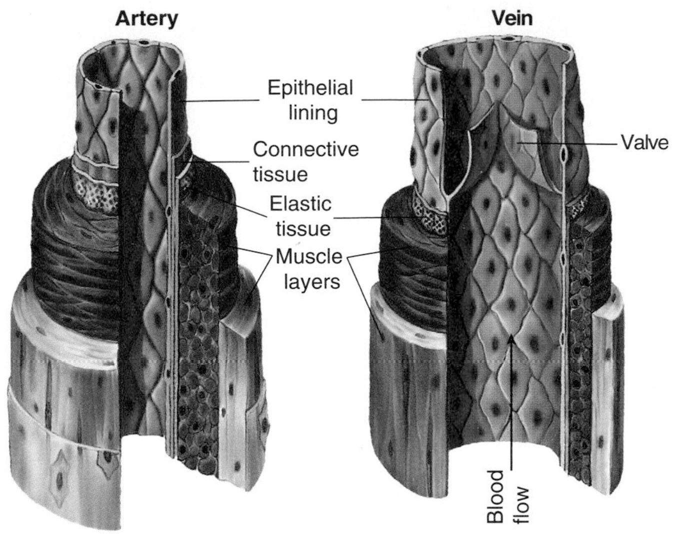

FIGURE 7-6 ▲ The walls of arteries are much thicker than the walls of veins.

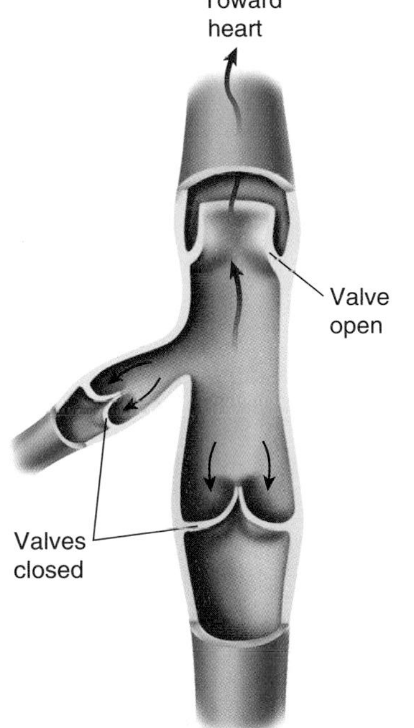

FIGURE 7-7 ▲ The valves in veins are shaped such that blood moving forward (toward the heart) opens each valve. As blood starts to move backward, it closes the valve, maintaining a one-way flow.

All arteries are direct or indirect branches of the aorta.

of the blood vessels. They are very thin and connect arteries and veins. The exchange of oxygen, nutrients, and waste products between blood and body cells occurs through the walls of capillaries.

You Should Know

If you were to cut an artery, a vein, and a capillary, the differences in the vessels would be obvious. Because the pressure in a capillary is low, blood would ooze from the vessel. The pressure within a vein is more than that in a capillary, but less than that in an artery. Blood would flow smoothly and freely from a cut vein. Blood would spurt from a cut artery because an artery transports blood under high pressure.

Major Blood Vessels

The aorta is the largest artery of the body. It is the major artery originating from the heart (Figure 7-8). Like the other organs of the body, the heart must have its own source of oxygen-rich blood. The heart depends on two coronary arteries and their branches for its supply of oxygenated blood. When the left ventricle relaxes, blood flows into the coronary arteries, supplying oxygen and nutrients to the heart. During times of stress, the heart needs more oxygen and depends on widening (dilation) of the arteries to increase blood flow through the coronary arteries.

The carotid artery is the major artery of the neck. It supplies the head and neck with blood. A carotid pulse can be felt on either side of the neck in the soft, hollow area just to the side of the windpipe (Figure 7-9a). The pulmonary arteries begin at the right ventricle of the heart. They carry blood low in oxygen from the right ventricle to the lungs. The brachial artery supplies the upper arm with blood. A brachial pulse can be felt on the inside of the arm between the elbow and the shoulder. This artery is used when assessing a blood pressure (BP) using a blood pressure cuff and stethoscope (Figure 7-9b). The radial artery is the major artery of the lower arm. A radial pulse can be felt on the thumb side of the wrist (Figure 7-9c).

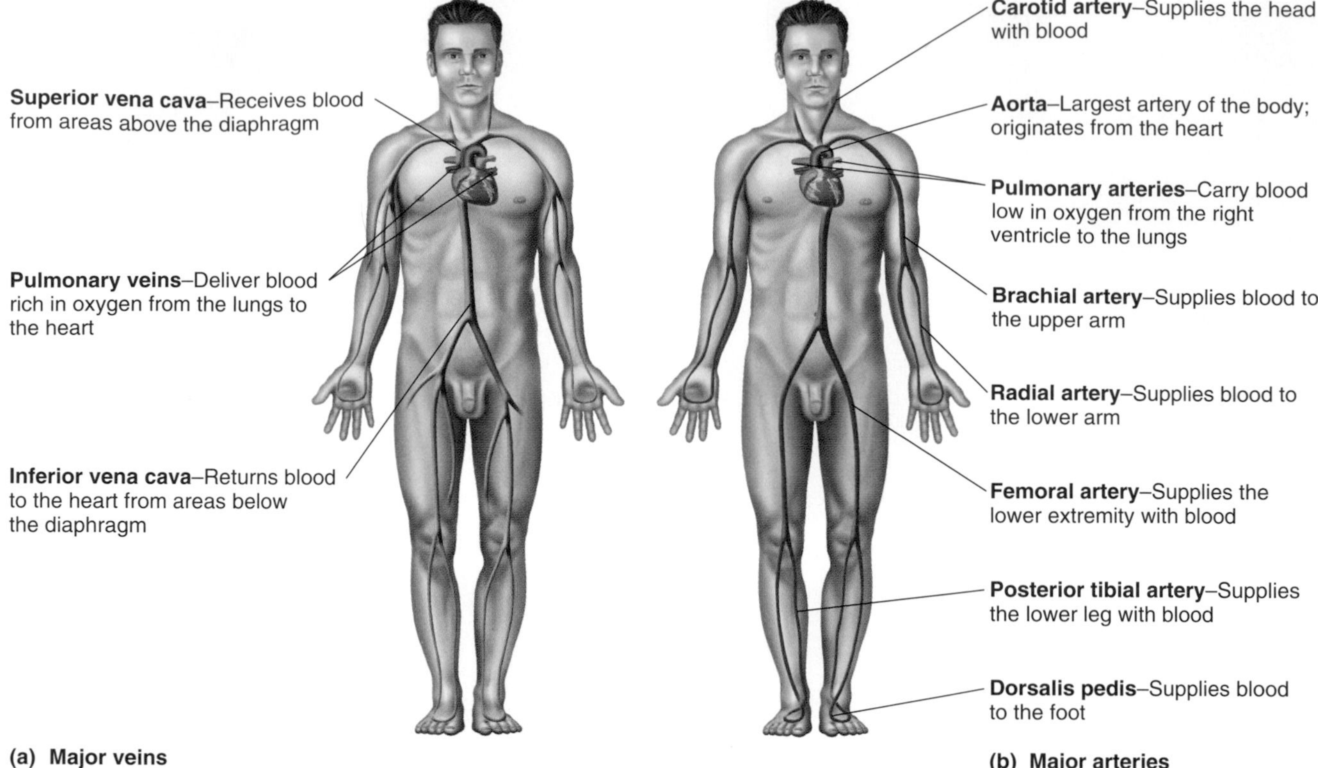

Superior vena cava–Receives blood from areas above the diaphragm
Pulmonary veins–Deliver blood rich in oxygen from the lungs to the heart
Inferior vena cava–Returns blood to the heart from areas below the diaphragm
(a) Major veins
Carotid artery–Supplies the head with blood
Aorta–Largest artery of the body; originates from the heart
Pulmonary arteries–Carry blood low in oxygen from the right ventricle to the lungs
Brachial artery–Supplies blood to the upper arm
Radial artery–Supplies blood to the lower arm
Femoral artery–Supplies the lower extremity with blood
Posterior tibial artery–Supplies the lower leg with blood
Dorsalis pedis–Supplies blood to the foot
(b) Major arteries

FIGURE 7-8 ▲ (a) Major veins and (b) major arteries.

FIGURE 7-9 ► Major arteries and pulses:
(a) Neck, or carotid, pulse.
(b) Arm, or brachial, pulse.
(c) Wrist, or radial, pulse.
(d) Groin, or femoral, pulse.

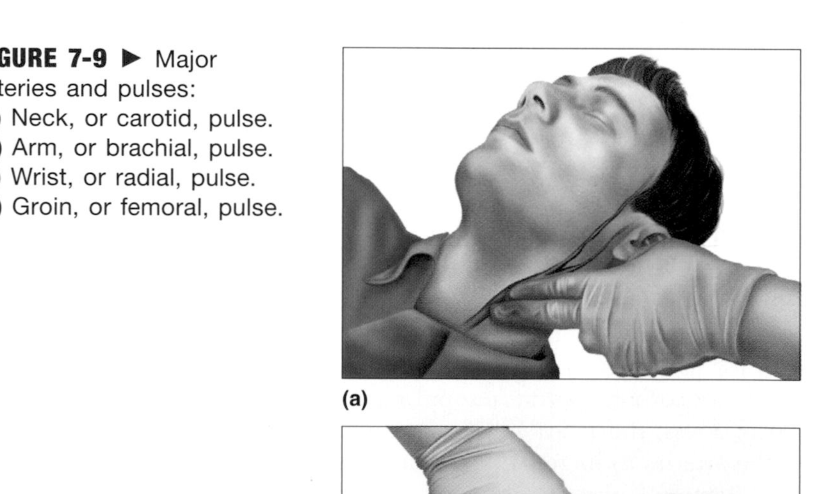

(a)
(c)

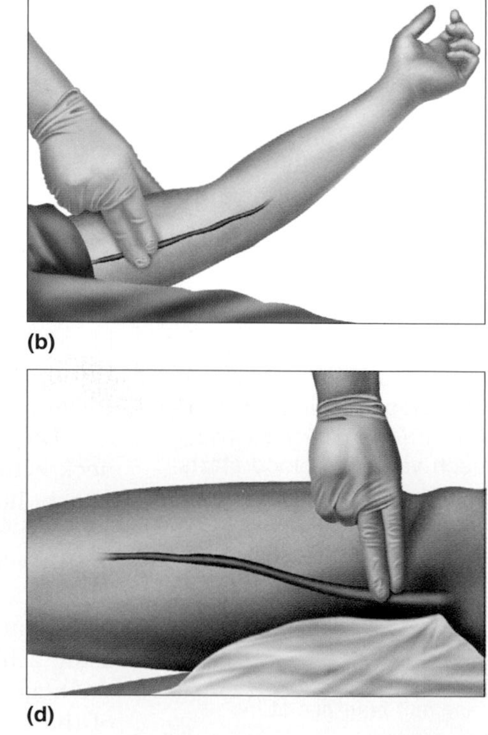

(b)
(d)

Remember This!

Never assess the carotid pulse on both sides of the neck at the same time.

The femoral artery is the major artery of the thigh. It supplies the upper leg with blood. A femoral pulse can be felt in the groin area (the crease between the abdomen and thigh; Figure 7-9d). The posterior tibial artery supplies the lower leg with blood. The posterior tibial pulse is located just behind the ankle bone. The dorsalis pedis artery is an artery in the foot. A pedal pulse can be felt on the top surface of the foot.

The major veins of the body include the pulmonary veins and the superior and inferior vena cavae (see Figure 7-8). The pulmonary veins deliver blood rich in oxygen from the lungs to the left atrium of the heart. The superior vena cava receives blood from areas above the diaphragm, such as the head and upper extremities. The inferior vena cava returns blood to the heart from areas below the diaphragm, such as the torso and lower extremities. Both the superior and inferior vena cavae drain into the right atrium of the heart.

The Physiology of the Circulatory System

The heart has two very important jobs. It must pump blood low in oxygen to the lungs, where the blood gives up carbon dioxide and takes on oxygen. It must also pump oxygen-rich blood to all of the body's cells. To understand how the heart achieves these tasks, think of the heart as a double pump. The pumps are the right heart (lung or pulmonary circuit) and the left heart (body or systemic circuit; Figure 7-10).

Blood low in oxygen leaves the right heart (pulmonary circuit) through the pulmonary arteries. From there, blood goes to the lungs and returns to the left atrium of the heart through the pulmonary veins. Blood rich in oxygen leaves the left heart (systemic circuit) through the aorta. It is then pumped through the arteries to the organs of the body. Cells use the oxygen, along with nutrients from food, to make energy. Then veins carry the blood (now low in oxygen) from the body cells back to the right heart.

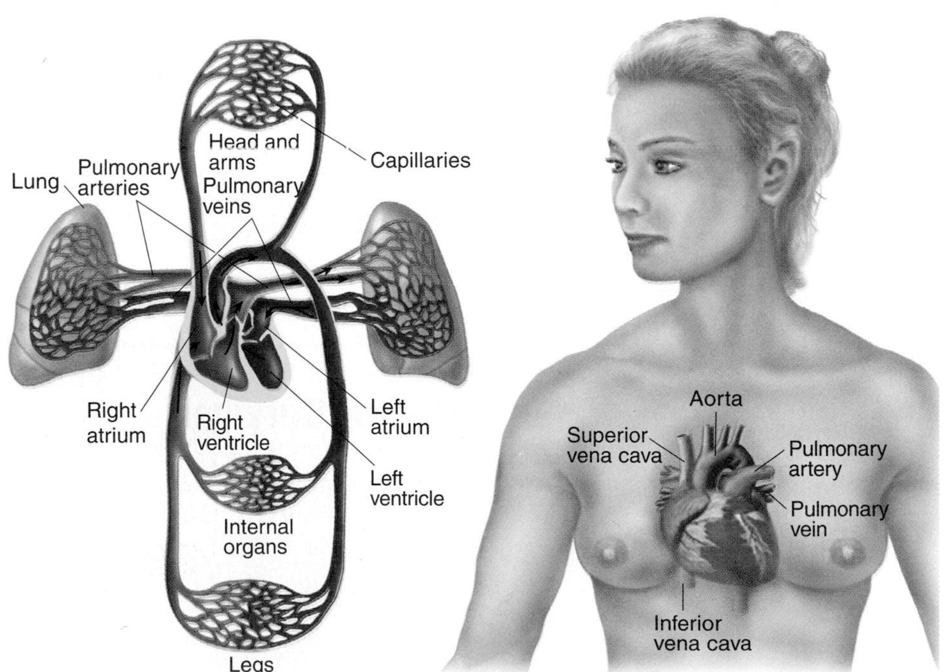

FIGURE 7-10 ▶ The heart works as a double pump. The right heart (pulmonary circuit) pumps blood to the lungs. The left heart (systemic circuit) pumps blood to the cells of the body. Red represents oxygen-rich blood and blue oxygen-poor blood.

Cardiac Arrest

If the heart stops beating, no blood will flow. If no blood flows, oxygen cannot be delivered to the body's cells. When the heart stops, the patient is said to be in **cardiac arrest.** The signs of cardiac arrest include sudden unresponsiveness, absent breathing, and no signs of circulation.

Sudden cardiac death can strike anyone, anywhere, and at any time.

Because the organs of the body must have oxygen, organ damage begins quickly after the heart stops. **Sudden cardiac death** is the unexpected loss of life occurring either immediately or within 1 hour of the onset of cardiac symptoms. Brain damage begins 4–6 minutes after the patient suffers a cardiac arrest. Brain damage becomes irreversible in 8–10 minutes. Chest compressions are used to circulate blood anytime that the heart is not beating. Chest compressions are combined with rescue breathing to oxygenate the blood. The combination of rescue breathing and external chest compressions is called **cardiopulmonary resuscitation (CPR).**

You Should Know

Approximately two thirds of sudden cardiac deaths take place outside the hospital. Most patients who suffer sudden cardiac death have no warning symptoms immediately before collapse.

Objective 1 ▶

There are many possible causes of a cardiac arrest:

- Heart and blood vessel diseases, such as heart attack and stroke
- Choking or respiratory arrest
- Seizures
- Diabetic emergency
- Severe allergic reaction
- Severe electrical shock
- Poisoning or drug overdose
- Drowning
- Suffocation
- Trauma
- Severe bleeding
- Abnormalities present at birth

Regardless of the cause, your initial emergency medical care for the victim of a cardiac arrest is CPR.

Remember This!

The signs of cardiac arrest include sudden unresponsiveness, absent breathing, and no signs of circulation.

The Chain of Survival

Objective 3 ▶

The **Chain of Survival** is the ideal series of events that should take place immediately after recognizing an injury or the onset of sudden illness. The chain consists of four crucial steps (Figure 7-11):

1. Early access (recognition of an emergency and calling 9-1-1)
2. Early CPR

FIGURE 7-11 ▶ The Chain of Survival.

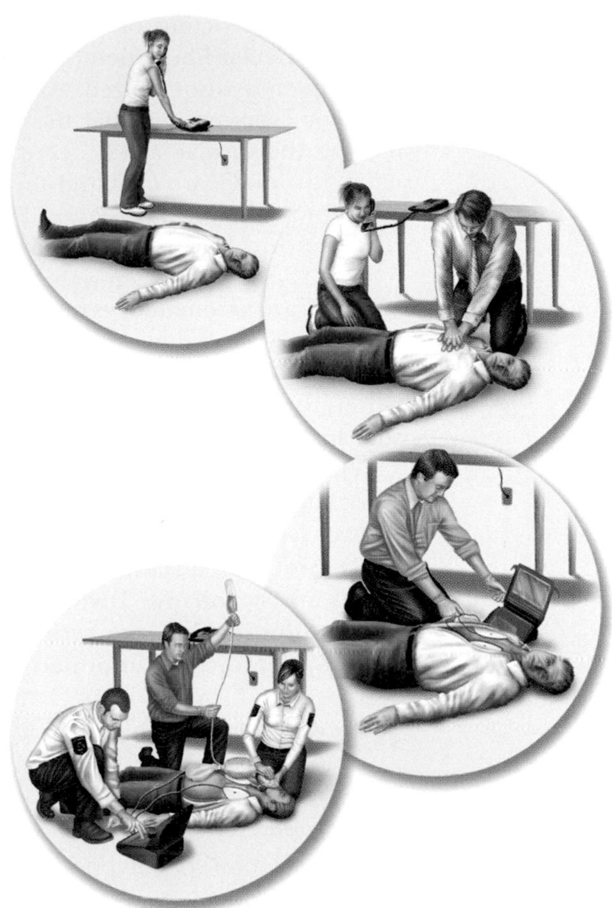

3. Early **defibrillation** (the delivery of an electrical shock to the heart)
4. Early advanced cardiac life support (ACLS)

Time is critical when dealing with a victim of cardiac arrest. A break in any of the links in the chain can reduce the patient's chance of survival.

Cardiopulmonary Resuscitation (CPR)

The Components of CPR

Objective 2 ▶

The components of CPR are

1. Checking the patient's level of responsiveness
2. *A* = *Airway*
3. *B* = *Breathing*
4. *C* = *Circulation*
5. *D* = *Defibrillation,* if necessary

When a cardiac arrest occurs, CPR must be started as early as possible. However, even with the best CPR, CPR provides only about one-third of the normal blood flow to the heart and brain. By itself, CPR is not enough to help someone survive a cardiac arrest.

If you were able to look at the heart while it is in VF, you would see it quivering like a bowl of gelatin.

Most adult victims of cardiac arrest experience an abnormal heart rhythm called **ventricular fibrillation (VF).** When the heart is in VF, the electrical impulses are completely disorganized. As a result, the heart cannot pump blood effectively. For every minute that the patient's heart is in VF, his or her chances of surviving the cardiac arrest decrease by approximately 10%. The only effective treatments for VF are CPR and the delivery of electrical shocks to the heart with a machine called a *defibrillator.* The shock attempts to stop VF and allow the patient's normal heart rhythm to start again.

CPR can keep oxygen-rich blood flowing to the heart and brain until the arrival of an **automated external defibrillator (AED)** and advanced care. An AED is a machine that analyzes the patient's heart rhythm for any abnormalities. If the AED recognizes a heart rhythm that should be shocked, it tells the rescuer to deliver an electrical shock to the patient by means of vocal and visual instructions.

When you arrive at the scene of a cardiac arrest, you should start CPR immediately if the patient is unresponsive, breathless, and without a pulse. However, you should not perform CPR if there is a valid Do Not Resuscitate (DNR) order or in cases of obvious death. If you arrive on the scene of a cardiac arrest and the DNR paperwork is unclear, the validity of the DNR order is questionable, or a written DNR order is not present, begin resuscitation efforts and call additional medical help to the scene.

You Should Know

Signs of Obvious Death

- Decapitation or other obvious mortal injury
- Putrefaction (decomposition)
- Extreme dependent lividity
- Rigor mortis

CPR Techniques

When forming a general impression, look at the patient's appearance, breathing, and circulation.

After determining that the scene is safe, form a general impression of the patient. A patient in cardiac arrest appears unresponsive and does not appear to be breathing. His or her skin color is usually pale, gray, or blue.

Assess Responsiveness

Objective 14 ▶

Use the AVPU scale to quickly check the patient's level of responsiveness (mental status) (Table 7-1). Gently squeeze the patient's shoulders and shout, "Are you all right?" If the patient is an adult, there is no response, and you are alone, phone for help right away. If the patient is an unresponsive infant or child and you are by yourself, shout for help and start CPR. Continue CPR for 5 cycles of chest compressions and breaths (about 2 minutes). Then briefly leave the patient to phone for help and get an AED. If the patient is small and you do not suspect trauma, consider moving the child near a telephone, so that you can call for help more quickly. If you are not alone, ask someone to call for help right away.

TABLE 7-1

Levels of Responsiveness – The AVPU Scale
A = ***A***lert
V = Responds to ***V***erbal stimuli
P = Responds to ***P***ainful stimuli
U = ***U***nresponsive

For chest compressions to be effective, the patient must be positioned on a firm, level surface. If you find the patient in bed, move him to the floor. Place his arms at his sides. If the patient is found face down, ask someone to help you carefully roll the patient, so that his head, shoulders, and chest move together as a unit without twisting. Once the patient is lying face up, position yourself at the patient's side so that you can provide rescue breathing and chest compressions if necessary.

Remember This!

If you know or suspect the patient has experienced trauma to the head or neck, move the patient only if absolutely necessary. Improperly moving a patient with an injury to the spine or spinal cord may cause paralysis.

A = Airway

If the patient is unresponsive and you do not suspect trauma, open his airway using the head tilt–chin lift maneuver. If you suspect trauma, open the airway using the jaw thrust without head tilt. If the patient is an unresponsive infant or child, do not hyperextend the neck when opening the airway.

Look for an actual or a potential airway obstruction, such as a foreign body, blood, vomitus, teeth, or the patient's tongue. If there is blood, vomitus, or other fluid in the patient's airway, remove it with your fingers, a cloth, or any other available material.

B = Breathing

The assessment of breathing should take no more than 10 seconds.

After you have made sure that the patient's airway is open, assess his breathing. Look for the rise and fall of the chest. Listen and feel for air movement from the patient's nose or mouth. If the patient is not breathing, begin rescue breathing using a pocket mask or mouth-to-barrier device. If the patient has dentures, leave them in place to help provide a good mask seal. If the dentures are loose, remove them so they do not fall back into the throat and obstruct the airway.

Making a Difference

If the patient is breathing very slowly or has occasional, gasping breaths, his or her breathing is inadequate. Provide emergency care as if the patient were not breathing at all.

Give slow breaths (each breath over 1 second) with just enough force to make the chest rise with each breath.

Watch the patient's chest while you breathe slowly into the patient. If your breaths are going in, you should see the chest rise with each breath. Be sure to pause between breaths. This pause allows you to take another breath. It also allows the patient's lungs to relax and air to escape. If the patient is unresponsive and an oral airway is available, insert it to maintain an open airway. Continue breathing for the patient until he begins to breathe adequately on his own or another trained rescuer takes over.

Remember This!

Give slow breaths with just enough pressure to make the chest rise with each breath. If you give breaths too quickly or too forcefully, you will push air into the stomach. This causes the stomach to distend (swell) and the patient may vomit. If the patient vomits, roll the patient onto his or her side until the vomiting stops. Clear the vomitus from the patient's mouth using your gloved fingers. Roll the patient onto his or her back and resume rescue breathing if needed.

The tongue is the most common airway obstruction in an unresponsive person.

If your breaths do not go in, gently reposition the patient's head and breathe for him again. If the breaths still do not go in, you must assume the airway is blocked. Attempt to clear the airway using the obstructed airway maneuvers discussed in Chapter 6. Use abdominal thrusts for children and adults. Use chest thrusts and back blows for infants.

C = Circulation

Assess the carotid pulse on the side of the patient's neck nearest you.

Once you have made sure that the patient's airway is open and have started rescue breathing, assess circulation. Use the carotid artery to check the pulse of an unresponsive adult or child older than 1 year of age. Feel for a brachial pulse in an unresponsive infant. Feel for a pulse for about 10 seconds and look for other signs of circulation, such as coughing or movement in response to your rescue breaths. If there is no pulse or signs of circulation, you must begin chest compressions.

Remember This!

Rescue breathing moves oxygen into the blood. Chest compressions move the oxygenated blood throughout the body.

Chest Compressions—Adult

Objective 5 ▶

Kneel beside the patient's chest. To find the correct hand position, place two fingers at the notch at the lower end of the patient's breastbone (the place where the lower ribs meet). Place the heel of your other hand next to your fingers on the patient's breastbone. Place your other hand on top of the first. Interlock the fingers of both hands to keep your fingers off the patient's ribs. If you have arthritis in your hands or wrists, give compressions by grasping the wrist of the hand that is on the patient's chest with your other hand and push down with both.

Remember This!

For children older than 12 to 14 years of age, CPR is performed as it is for an adult.

Position yourself directly above the patient's chest so that your shoulders are directly over your hands. With your arms straight and your elbows locked, press down approximately 1½ to 2 inches on the patient's breastbone with the heels of your hands. Release pressure (let up) after each compression without letting your hands lose contact with the patient's chest. Releasing pressure on the patient's chest allows blood to flow into the chest and heart.

Stop and Think!

Never practice CPR skills on another person.

Objective 4 ▶

Deliver 30 compressions at a rate of about 100 compressions per minute. After 30 compressions, open the patient's airway and deliver 2 breaths. Find the proper hand position and begin 30 more compressions at a rate of about 100 per minute. One cycle consists of 30 chest compressions and 2 rescue breaths. After 5 cycles (which is about 2 minutes), check for a pulse and other signs of circulation. If the patient has a pulse, check her breathing. If the patient has a pulse but is not breathing, give rescue breaths at a rate of 1 breath every 5 to 6 seconds. If there is still no pulse, continue CPR. Check for a pulse again every few minutes. Skill Drill 7-1 shows the steps for one-rescuer adult CPR.

Objective 9 ▶

If another person trained to perform CPR is available to help, follow the steps for two-rescuer CPR. Skill Drill 7-2 shows the steps for two-rescuer adult CPR.

One-Rescuer Adult CPR

STEP 1 ▶
- Quickly check the patient's level of responsiveness. Gently squeeze the patient's shoulders and shout, "Are you all right?"
- If there is no response and you are alone, phone for help right away.

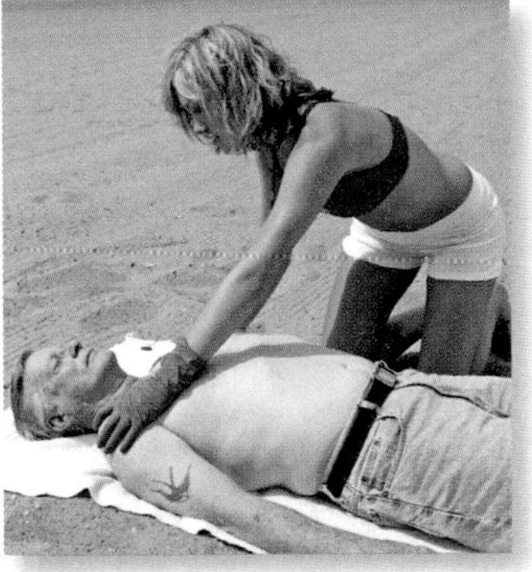

STEP 2 ▶
- If the patient is unresponsive and you do not suspect trauma, open the airway using the head tilt–chin lift maneuver.
- Look for an actual or a potential airway obstruction, such as a foreign body, blood, vomitus, teeth, or the patient's tongue. Clear the airway if necessary.

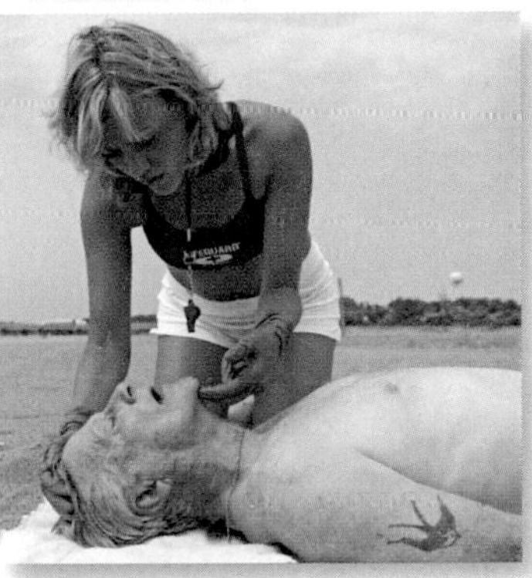

STEP 3 ▶ Look, listen, and feel for breathing for up to 10 seconds.

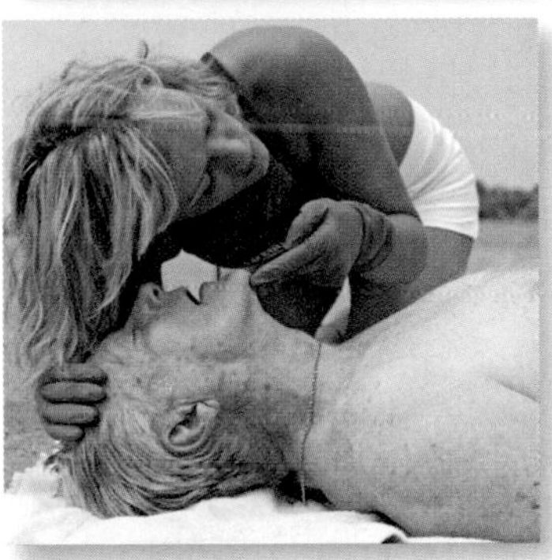

STEP 4 ▶ If the patient is not breathing, begin rescue breathing using a pocket mask or mouth-to-barrier device. Give 2 breaths (each breath over 1 second) with just enough pressure to make the chest rise with each breath.

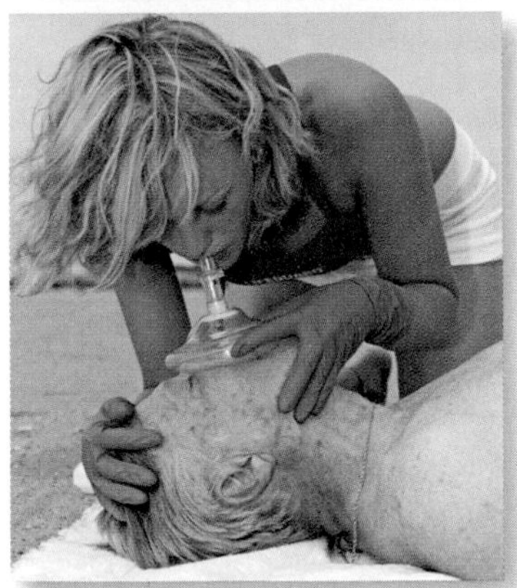

Continued on next page

Skill Drill 7-1

One-Rescuer Adult CPR *(continued)*

STEP 5 ▶ Assess the carotid pulse on the side of the patient's neck nearest you. Feel for a pulse for about 10 seconds and look for other signs of circulation, such as coughing or movement in response to your rescue breaths.

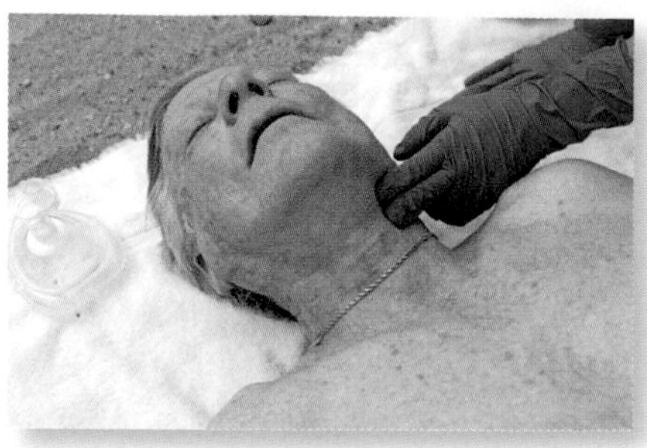

STEP 6 ▶ If there is no pulse, kneel beside the patient's chest. To find the correct hand position, place two fingers at the notch at the lower end of the patient's breastbone (the place where the lower ribs meet). Place the heel of your other hand next to your fingers.

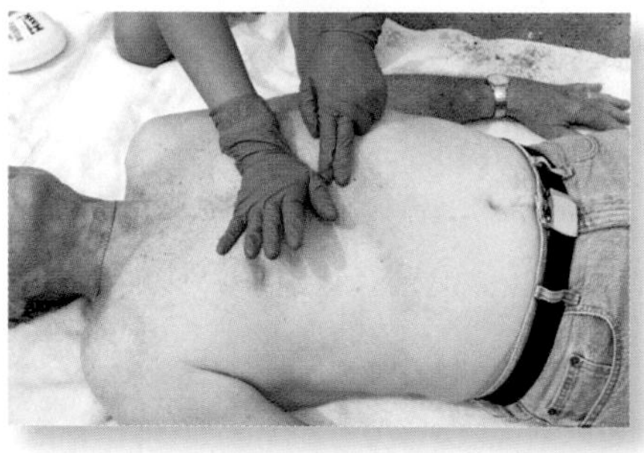

STEP 7 ▶ Place your other hand on top of the first. Interlock the fingers of both hands to keep your fingers off the patient's ribs.

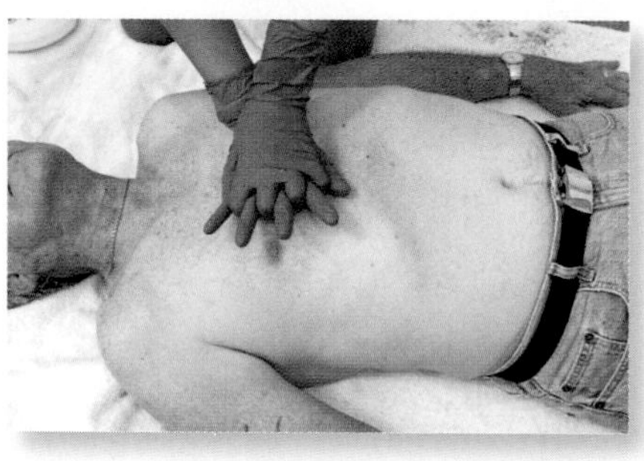

STEP 8 ▶ Position yourself directly above the patient's chest so that your shoulders are directly over your hands.

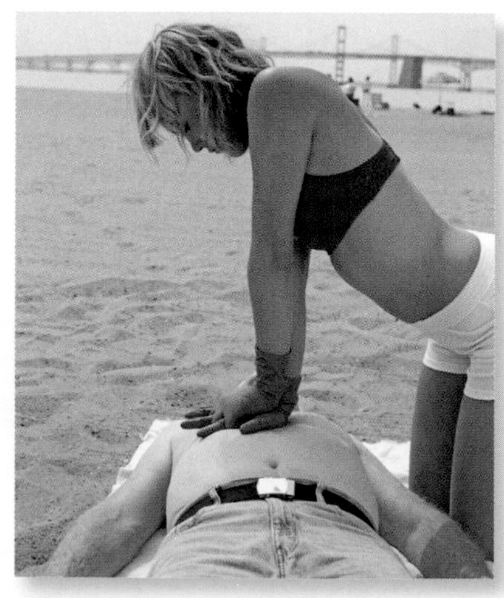

STEP 9 ▸

- With your arms straight and your elbows locked, press down approximately 1½ to 2 inches on the patient's breastbone with the heels of your hands.
- Deliver 30 compressions at a rate of about 100 compressions per minute. Release pressure (let up) after each compression without letting your hands lose contact with the patient's chest.

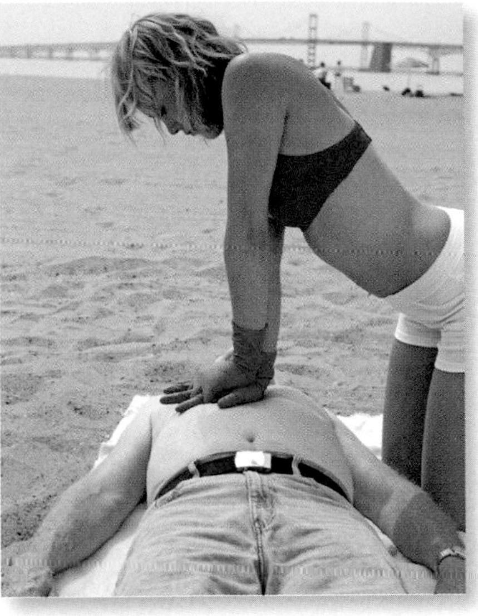

STEP 10 ▸ After 30 compressions, open the patient's airway and deliver 2 breaths.

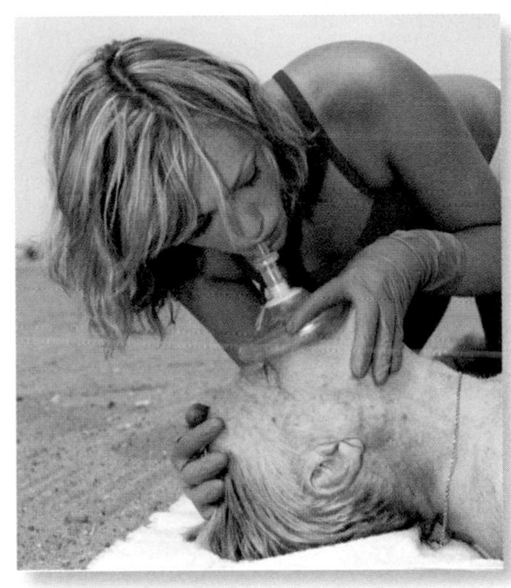

STEP 11 ▸

- After 5 cycles of 30 compressions and 2 rescue breaths, check for a pulse and other signs of circulation.
  - If the patient has a pulse, check his or her breathing.
  - If the patient has a pulse but is not breathing, give rescue breaths at a rate of 1 breath every 5 to 6 seconds.
  - If there is no pulse, continue CPR. Check for a pulse and other signs of circulation every few minutes.

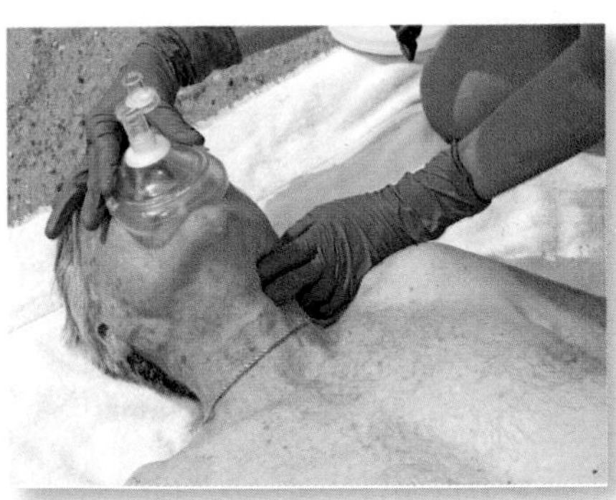

Skill Drill 7-2

Two-Rescuer Adult CPR

STEP 1 ▶
- Quickly check the patient's level of responsiveness. Gently squeeze the patient's shoulders and shout, "Are you all right?"
- If the patient does not respond, one rescuer should call for help.

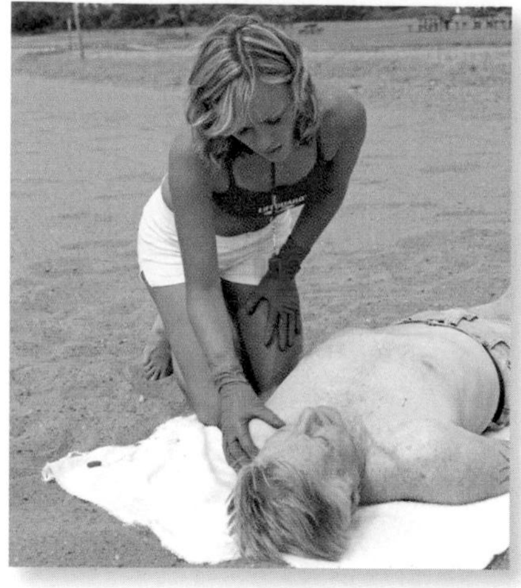

STEP 2 ▶
- If the patient is unresponsive and you do not suspect trauma, open the airway using the head tilt–chin lift maneuver.
- Look for an actual or a potential airway obstruction, such as a foreign body, blood, vomitus, teeth, or the patient's tongue. Clear the airway if necessary.

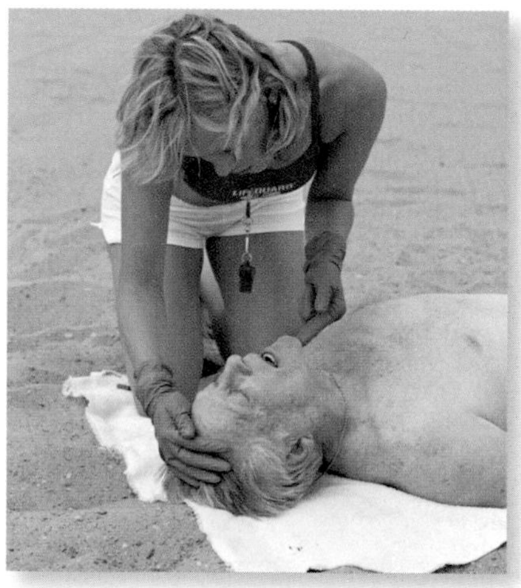

STEP 3 ▶ Look, listen, and feel for breathing for up to 10 seconds.

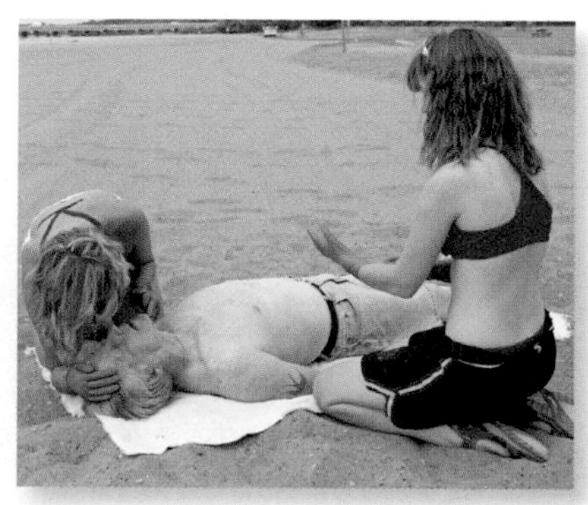

STEP 4 ▶ If the patient is not breathing, the first rescuer should begin rescue breathing using a pocket mask or mouth-to-barrier device. Give 2 breaths with just enough force to make the chest rise with each breath.

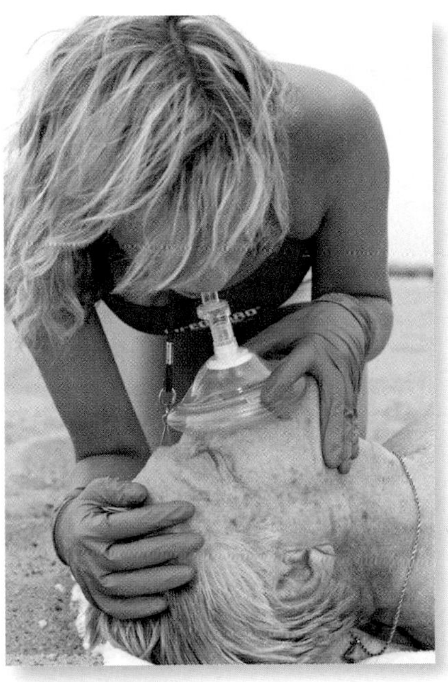

STEP 5 ▶ The first rescuer should assess the carotid pulse on the side of the patient's neck nearest the rescuer. Feel for a pulse for about 10 seconds and look for other signs of circulation, such as coughing or movement in response to the rescue breaths.

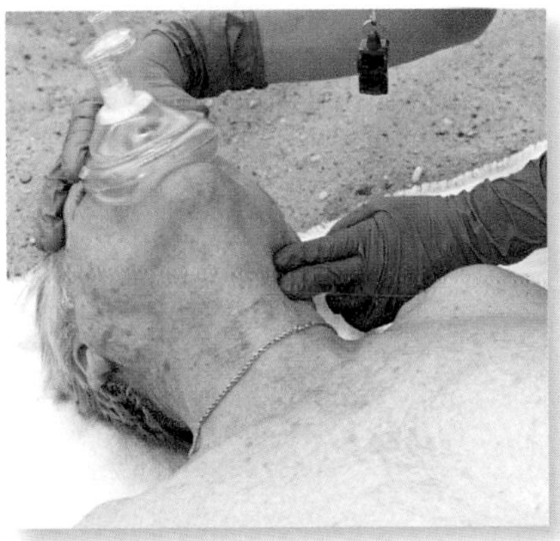

STEP 6 ▶ If there is no pulse, the second rescuer should kneel beside the patient's chest. To find the correct hand position, place two fingers at the notch at the lower end of the patient's breastbone (the place where the lower ribs meet). Place the heel of your other hand next to your fingers.

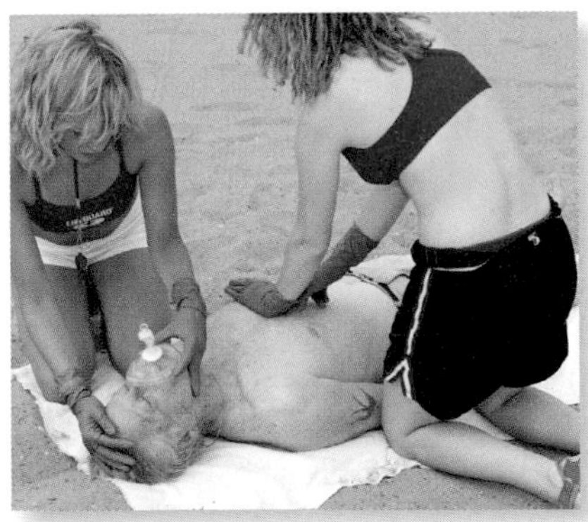

Continued on next page

Two-Rescuer Adult CPR *(continued)*

STEP 7 ▶ Place your other hand on top of the first. Interlock the fingers of both hands to keep your fingers off the patient's ribs.

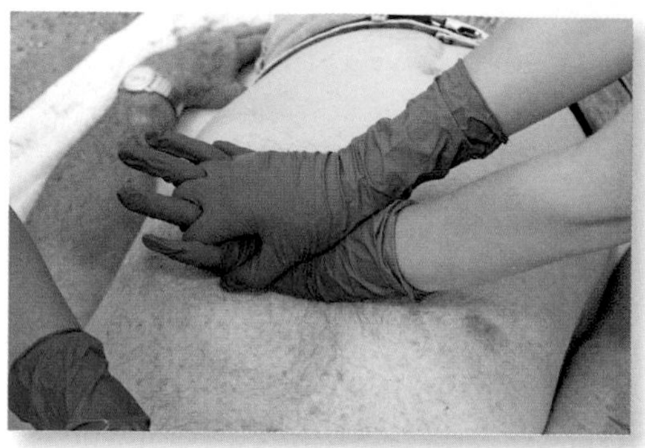

STEP 8 ▶ Position yourself directly above the patient's chest so that your shoulders are directly over your hands.

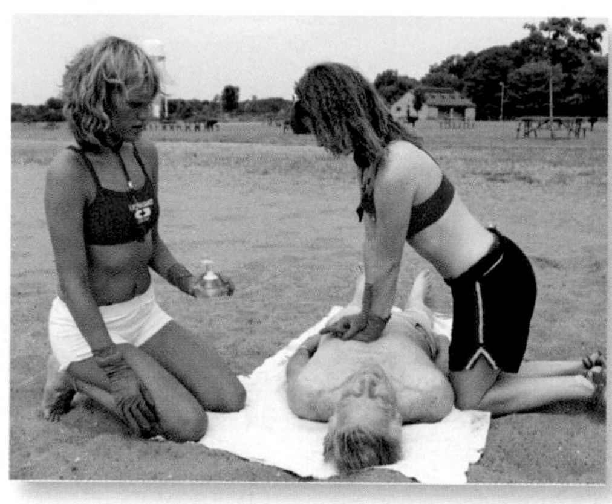

STEP 9 ▶

- With your arms straight and your elbows locked, press down approximately 1½ to 2 inches on the patient's breastbone with the heels of your hands.
- Give compressions at a rate of about 100 compressions per minute.
- Release pressure (let up) after each compression without letting your hands lose contact with the patient's chest.

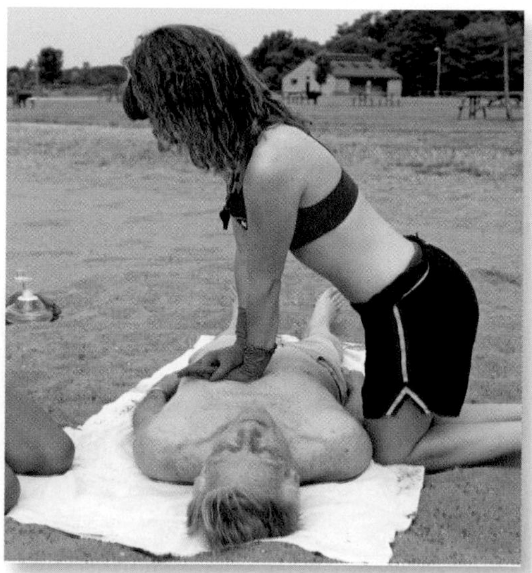

STEP 10 ▶ After 15 compressions, the first rescuer should open the patient's airway and deliver 2 breaths.

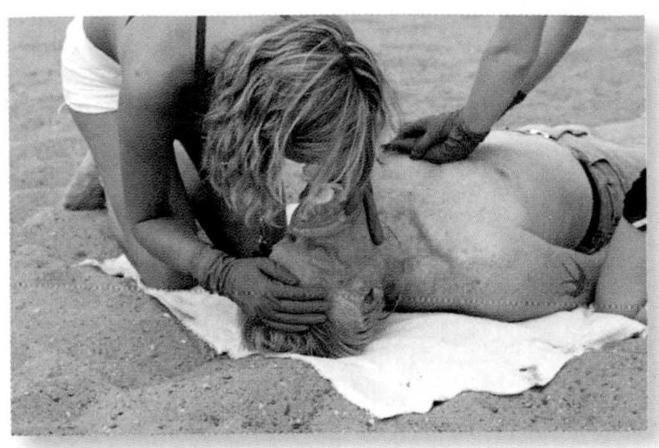

STEP 11 ▶
- After 5 cycles of 15 compressions and 2 rescue breaths, stop chest compressions for no more than 10 seconds to check for a pulse and other signs of circulation. If there is still no pulse, continue CPR with cycles of 15 compressions to 2 breaths.
- Because performing chest compressions is tiring, rescuers should switch roles about every 2 minutes or 5 cycles of CPR. The "switch" should ideally take place in 5 seconds or less.

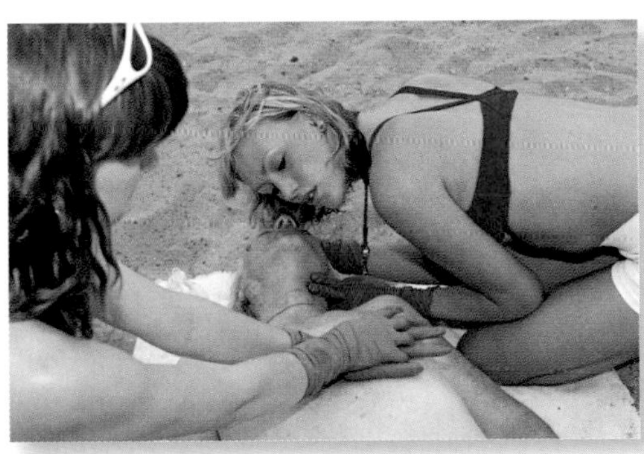

Remember This!

Performing chest compressions is tiring. If either rescuer becomes tired, quickly change positions.

Chest Compressions—Child

Objective 7 ▶

Objective 11 ▶

For the general public, CPR guidelines for a child pertain to a child from 1 to about 8 years of age. For healthcare professionals, a child is considered 1 year to about the start of puberty (about 12 to 14 years of age). For children between the ages of 1 and 12 to 14, perform chest compressions if there is no pulse. You should also perform compressions if a pulse is present but the heart rate is less than 60 beats per minute with signs of poor perfusion (pale, cool, mottled skin). Compress the child's chest with the heel of only one hand. Press down on the breastbone 1 to 1½ inches (about ⅓ to ½ the depth of the chest). Give chest compressions at a rate of about 100 compressions per minute. After every 30 compressions, give 2 rescue breaths. Skill Drill 7-3 shows the steps for one-rescuer child CPR.

Skill Drill 7-3

One-Rescuer Child CPR

STEP 1 ▶
- Quickly check the child's level of responsiveness. Gently squeeze the patient's shoulders and shout, "Are you okay?"
- If the patient does not respond you are alone, and you saw the child collapse, phone for help and get an AED, then begin CPR.
- If the child does not respond, you are alone and you did not witness the child's collapse, begin CPR. After about 2 minutes of CPR, phone for help, and get an AED.

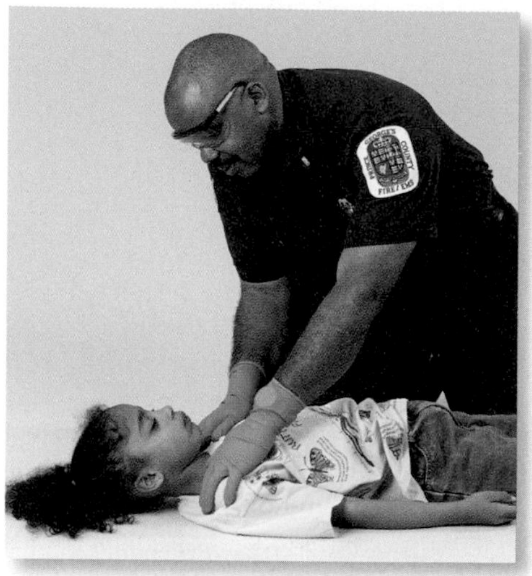

STEP 2 ▶
- If the patient is unresponsive and you do not suspect trauma, open the airway using the head tilt–chin lift maneuver. Push down on the child's forehead with one hand. Place the fingers of your other hand on the bony part of the chin. Gently lift the chin.
- Look for an actual or a potential airway obstruction, such as a foreign body, blood, vomitus, teeth, or the patient's tongue. Clear the airway if necessary.

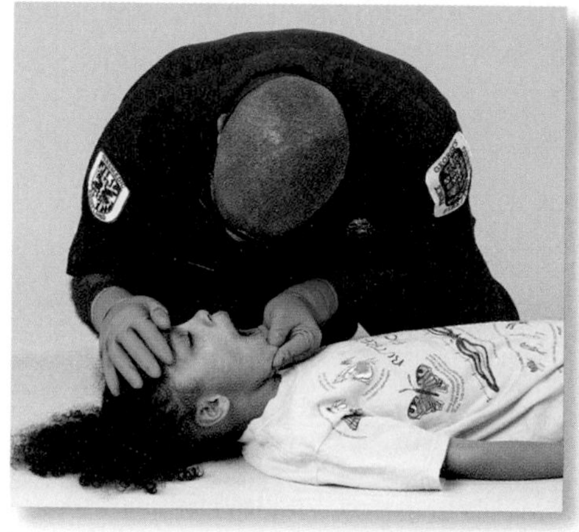

STEP 3 ▶ Hold the airway open and look, listen, and feel for breathing for up to 10 seconds.

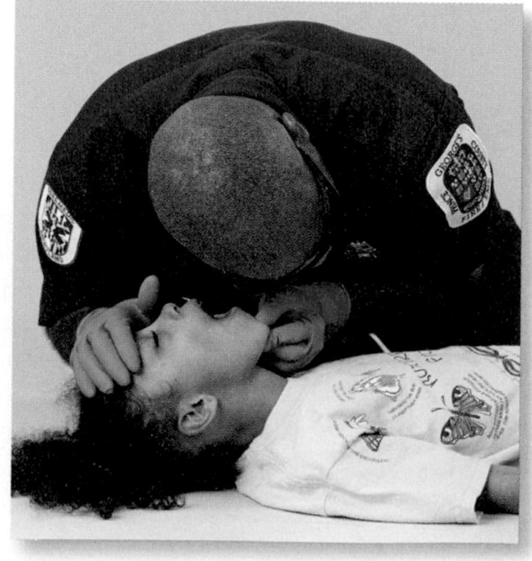

STEP 4 ▶ If the child is not breathing, begin rescue breathing using a pocket mask or mouth-to-barrier device. Give 2 breaths (each breath over 1 second) with just enough pressure to make the chest rise with each breath.

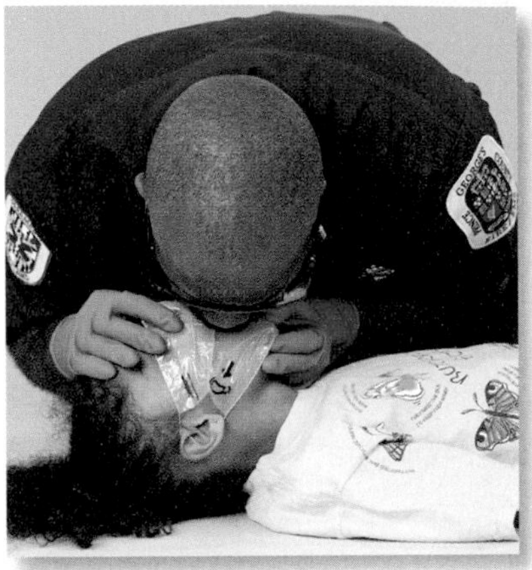

STEP 5 ▶ Assess the carotid pulse on the side of the patient's neck nearest you. Feel for a pulse for about 10 seconds and look for other signs of circulation, such as coughing or movement in response to your rescue breaths.

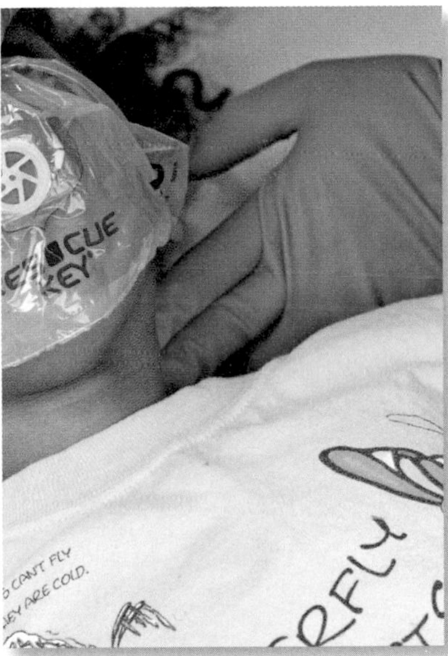

STEP 6 ▶ If there is no pulse or if a pulse is present but the heart rate is less than 60 beats per minute with signs of poor perfusion (pale, cool, mottled skin), begin chest compressions. Kneel beside the patient's chest. Find the lower half of the breastbone (the center of the chest between the nipples).

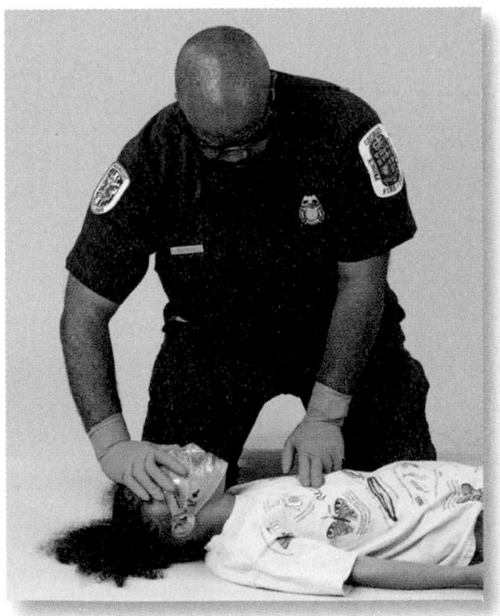

Continued on next page

One-Rescuer Child CPR *(continued)*

STEP 7
- Place the heel of one hand on the lower half of the breastbone.
- Position yourself directly over the child's chest. With your arms straight and your elbows locked, press down on the child's chest with the heel of one hand.
- Give compressions at a rate of about 100 per minute. Apply firm pressure, depressing the breastbone ⅓ to ½ the depth of the chest.
- Release pressure (let up) after each compression without letting your hand lose contact with the child's chest.

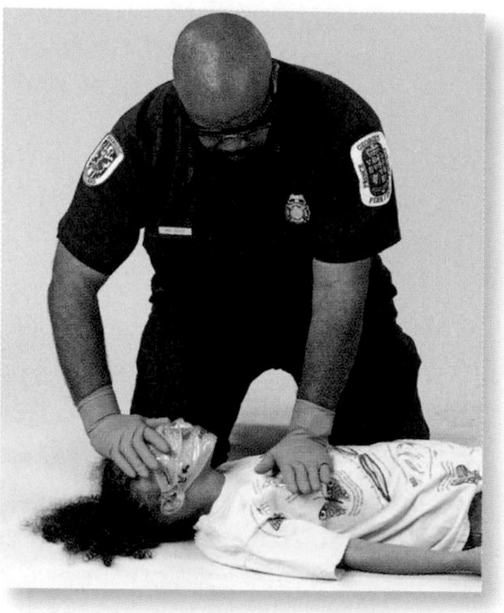

STEP 8 After 30 compressions, open the airway and deliver 2 breaths. If trauma is suspected, use the jaw-thrust without head tilt maneuver.

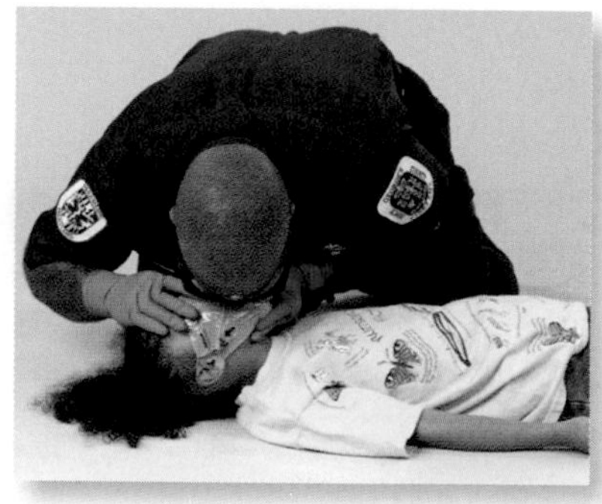

STEP 9
- After 2 minutes of CPR (about 5 cycles of 30 compressions and 2 rescue breaths), stop chest compressions for approximately 10 seconds to check the carotid pulse and look for other signs of circulation.
  - If no signs of circulation are present and no one has called for help, leave the child and phone for help. If the child is small and uninjured, take the child with you.
  - Resume CPR after phoning for help.
  - If a pulse returns, stop chest compressions and continue rescue breathing if needed (1 breath every 3 to 5 seconds).

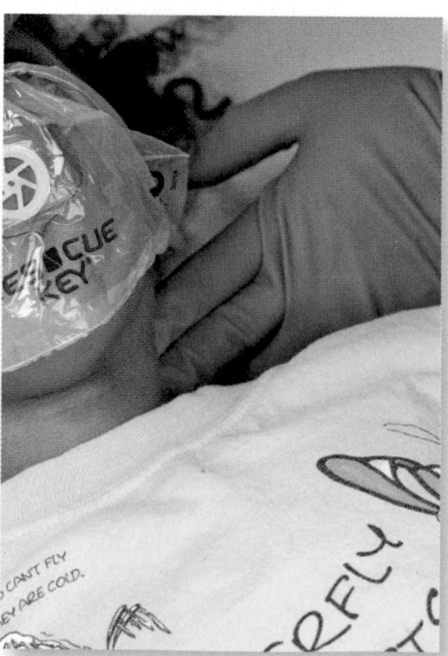

Remember This!

Tips for Performing CPR on a Child

- Chest compressions on a child may be performed using the heel of one hand. It is also acceptable to use the heel of one hand with the other hand on top to compress the chest (the same technique used for adults).
- If trauma is suspected, use the jaw-thrust without head tilt maneuver to open the airway.
- Do not apply pressure over the bottom tip of the breastbone or over the upper abdomen.

Chest Compressions—Infant

Objective 6 ▶

Objective 10 ▶

For an infant, perform chest compressions if there is no pulse. You should also perform compressions if a pulse is present but the heart rate is less than 60 beats per minute with signs of poor perfusion (pale, cool, mottled skin). Compress the infant's chest with two fingers. Press down on the breastbone ½ to 1 inch (about ⅓ to ½ the depth of the chest). Give chest compressions at a rate of about 100 compressions per minute. After every 30 compressions, give 2 rescue breaths. Skill Drill 7-4 shows the steps for one-rescuer infant CPR.

CPR guidelines for adults, children, and infants are presented in Table 7-2.

TABLE 7-2 CPR Guidelines

	Adult	Child	Infant
Patient Age	More than 12 to 14 years	1 to 12 to 14 years	Under 1 year
Rescue Breaths	1 breath every 5 to 6 seconds (10 to 12 breaths/minute)	1 breath every 3 to 5 seconds (12 to 20 breaths/minute)	1 breath every 3 to 5 seconds (12 to 20 breaths/minute)
Location of Pulse Check	Carotid	Carotid	Brachial
Method of Chest Compressions	Heels of 2 hands	Heel of 1 hand or same as for adult	2 fingers (1 rescuer) *or* 2 thumbs with the fingers of both hands encircling the chest (2 rescuers)
Depth of Chest Compressions	1½ to 2 inches	1 to 1½ inches (⅓ to ½ the chest depth)	½ to 1 inch (⅓ to ½ the chest depth)
Rate of Chest Compressions	About 100/minute		
Ratio of Chest Compressions to Rescue Breaths (One Cycle)	1 or 2 rescuers: 30 compressions to 2 breaths (30:2)	1 rescuer: 30 compressions to 2 breaths (30:2) 2 rescuers: 15 compressions to 2 breaths (15:2)	1 rescuer: 30 compressions to 2 breaths (30:2) 2 rescuers: 15 compressions to 2 breaths (15:2)
Pulse Check	After 5 cycles (about 2 minutes)		

Skill Drill 7-4

One-Rescuer Infant CPR

STEP 1 ▶
- Quickly check the infant's level of responsiveness. Gently tap the infant's feet and shout, "Are you okay?"
- If the patient does not respond, you are alone, and you saw the infant collapse, phone for help and then begin CPR.
- If the infant does not respond, you are alone, and you did not witness the infant's collapse, begin CPR. After about 2 minutes of CPR, phone for help, then resume CPR.

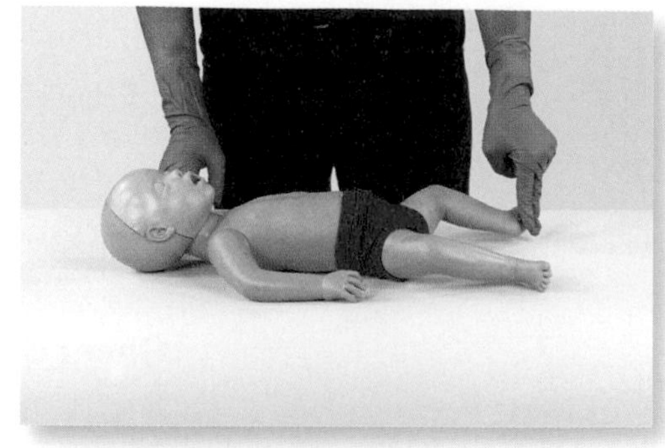

STEP 2 ▶
- If the infant is unresponsive and you do not suspect trauma, open the airway using the head tilt–chin lift maneuver. Push down on the infant's forehead with one hand. Place the fingers of your other hand on the bony part of the chin. Gently lift the chin.
- Look for an actual or a potential airway obstruction, such as a foreign body, blood, vomitus, teeth, or the patient's tongue. Clear the airway if necessary.

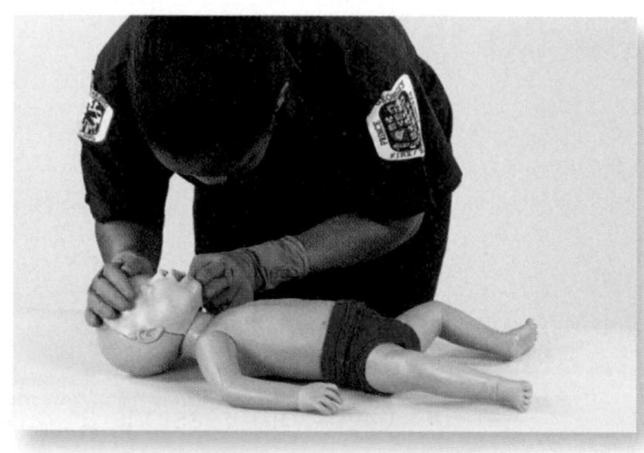

STEP 3 ▶ Hold the airway open and look, listen, and feel for breathing for up to 10 seconds.

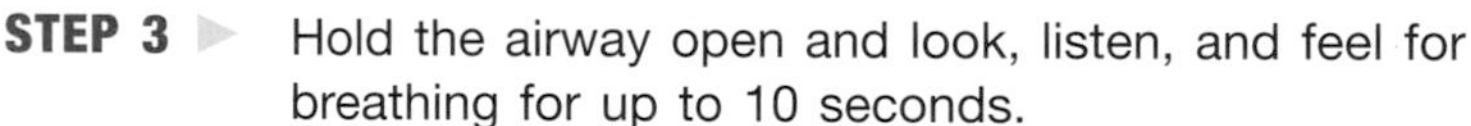

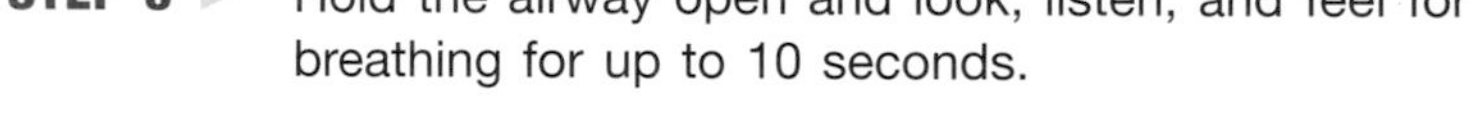

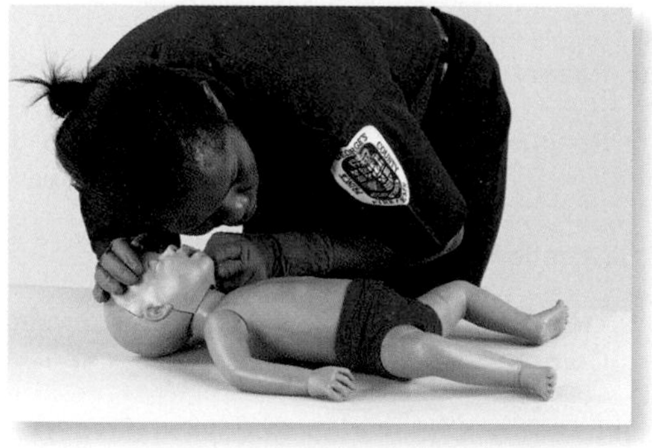

STEP 4 ▶ If the infant is not breathing, begin rescue breathing using a pocket mask or mouth-to-barrier device. Give 2 breaths with just enough pressure to make the chest rise with each breath.

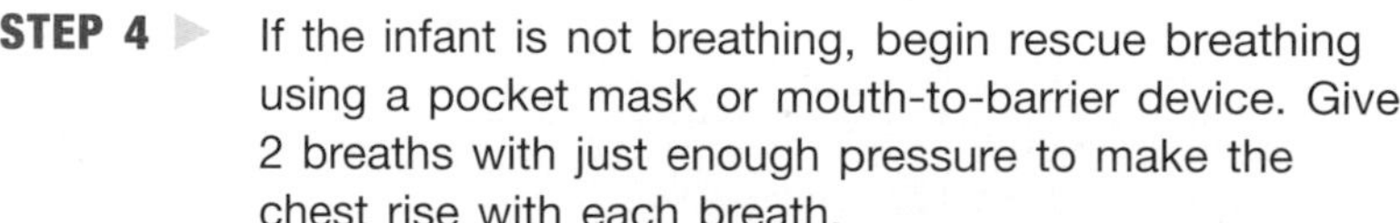

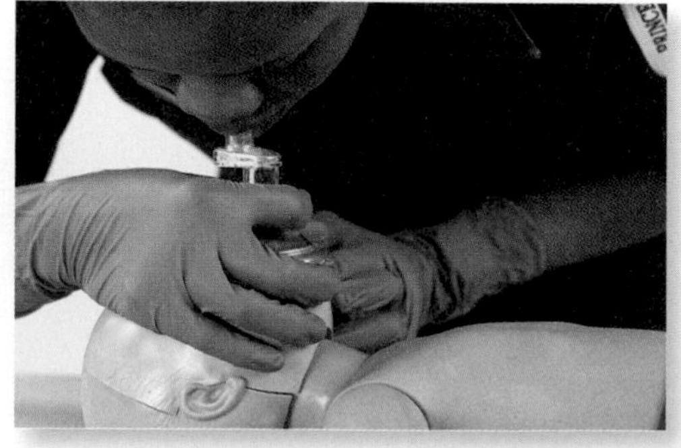

STEP 5 ▶

- Feel for a brachial pulse on the inside of the upper arm. Feel for a pulse for about 10 seconds and look for other signs of circulation, such as coughing or movement in response to your rescue breaths.
- If there is no pulse or if a pulse is present but the heart rate is less than 60 beats per minute with signs of poor perfusion (pale, cool, mottled skin), begin chest compressions.

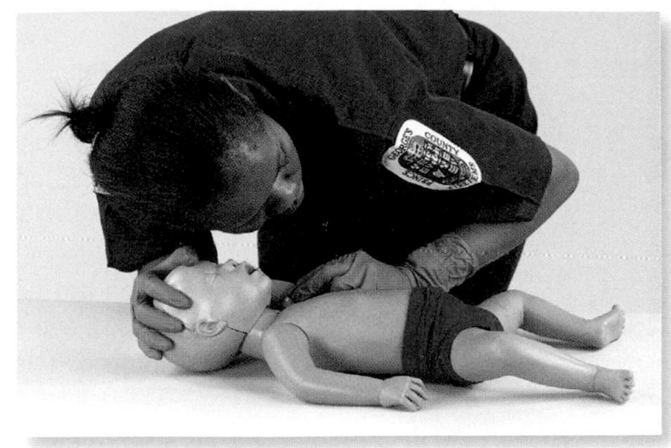

STEP 6 ▶

- Imagine a line between the nipples. Place the flat part of your middle and ring fingers about one finger's width below this imaginary line. Use your other hand to hold the infant's head in a position that keeps the airway open.
- Give compressions at a rate of about 100 per minute. Depress the breastbone ⅓ to ½ the depth of the chest.
- Release pressure (let up) after each compression without letting your fingers lose contact with the infant's chest.

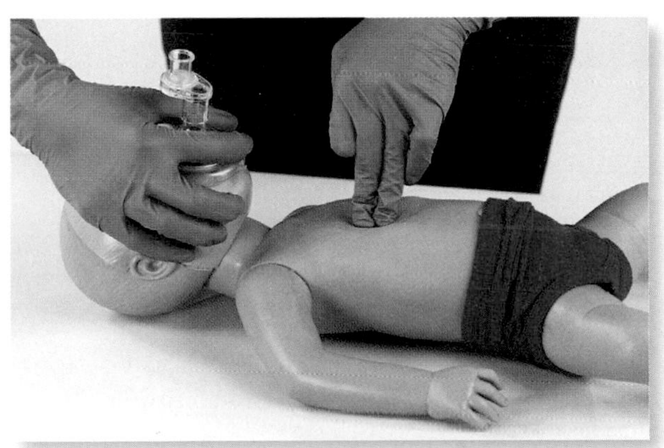

STEP 7 ▶ After 30 compressions, open the airway and deliver 2 breaths.

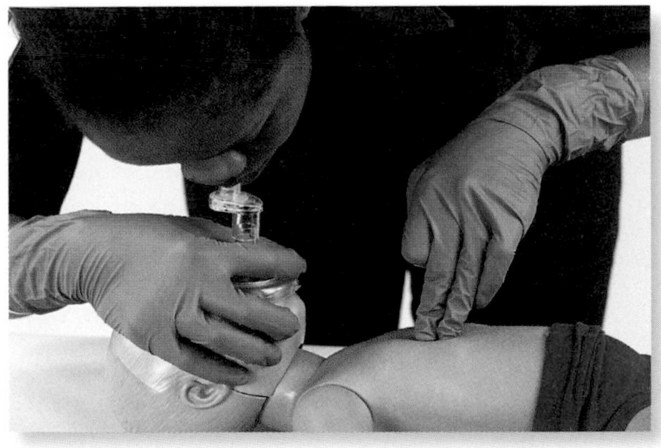

Continued on next page

Skill Drill 7-4

One-Rescuer Infant CPR *(continued)*

STEP 8 ▶ • After about 2 minutes of CPR, stop chest compressions for approximately 10 seconds to check the brachial pulse and look for other signs of circulation. You should check this pulse and look for other signs of circulation every few minutes.

- If no signs of circulation are present and no one has called for help, leave the infant and phone for help. Resume CPR after phoning for help.
- If a pulse returns, stop chest compressions and continue rescue breathing (1 breath every 3 to 5 seconds) if needed.

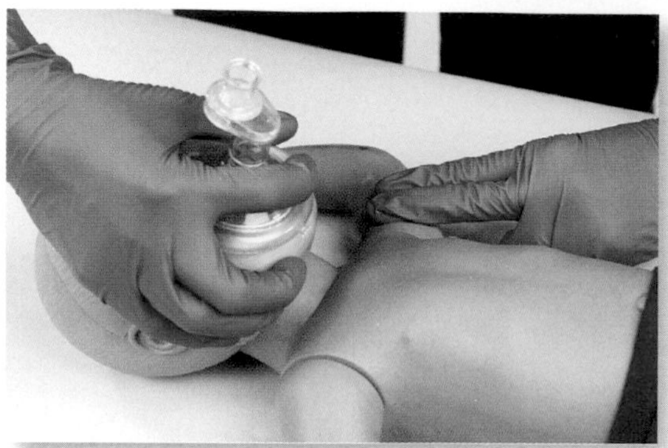

Remember This!

Tips for Performing CPR on an Infant

- Do not apply pressure over the bottom tip of the breastbone or over the upper abdomen.
- If trauma is suspected, use the jaw-thrust without head tilt maneuver to open the airway.

If two healthcare professionals are available to perform CPR on an infant, the two-thumb technique is preferred when performing chest compressions. Place your thumbs side by side or one on top of the other over the lower half of the infant's breastbone. Your thumbs should be placed about one finger's width below the nipple line (Figure 7-12). Encircle the infant's chest with the fingers of both hands. Use your thumbs to compress the chest about ⅓ to ½ the depth of the chest.

D = Defibrillation

You may need to use an automated external defibrillator (AED) during CPR. Recall that an AED is a machine that administers an electric shock through the patient's chest to the heart (Figure 7-13). When special pads are placed on the patient's bare chest, the AED looks at the patient's heart rhythm. The machine contains a computer programmed to recognize heart rhythms that should be shocked, such as ventricular fibrillation. If a shockable rhythm is present, the AED will advise you. It will then talk you through some very simple steps to defibrillate the patient.

FIGURE 7-12 ► The two-thumb method of performing CPR on an infant. This method is used when two rescuers are available.

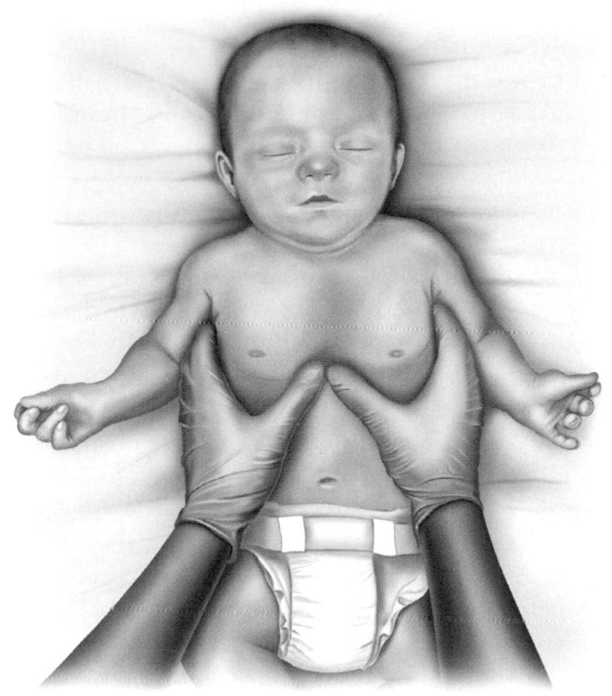

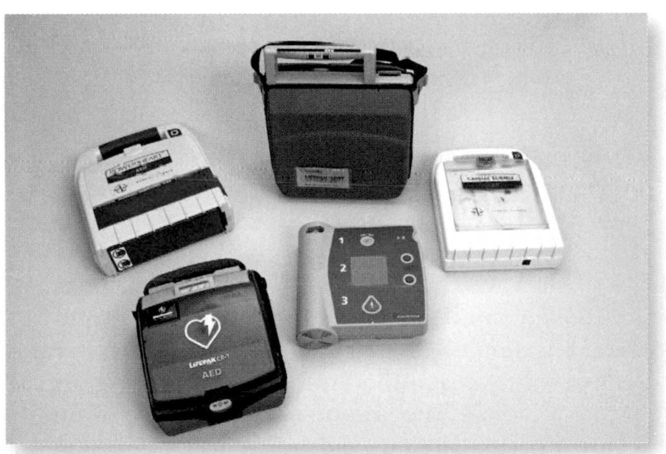

FIGURE 7-13 ▲ Automated external defibrillators (AEDs).

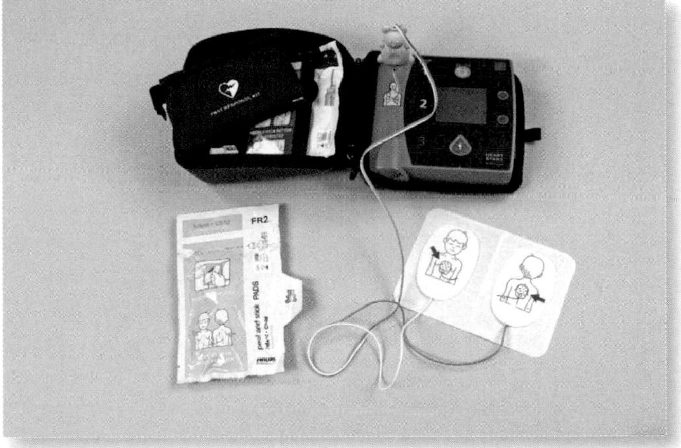

FIGURE 7-14 ▲ Special pads and cables are available for some AEDs for use on children younger than age eight.

Children who weigh more than 55 pounds (25 kg) or are older than 8 years of age are defibrillated as adults. A special key or pad cable system is available for some AEDs so that the machine can be used on children younger than 8 years of age. The key or pad-cable system decreases the amount of energy delivered to a dose appropriate for a child (Figure 7-14). If a child is in cardiac arrest and a key or pad-cable system is not available, use a standard AED.

If the patient has a medication patch on his or her chest, remove it and dry the area with a cloth or towel before applying the AED pads.

Follow these steps to operate an AED:

1. *Power.* Be sure the patient is lying, face up, on a firm, flat surface. Start CPR if the AED is not immediately available. If possible, place the AED next to the patient's left ear. Turn on the power. Depending on the brand of AED, this is done by either pressing the "on" button or lifting up the AED screen or lid.
2. *Pads.* Open the package containing the AED pads. Connect the pads to the AED cables (if not preconnected). Then apply the pads to the patient's chest. The correct position for the pads is usually shown on the package containing the pads. Alternately, it may be shown in a diagram on the AED itself. If the patient's chest is wet, quickly dry it before applying the pads. Briefly stop CPR to allow pad placement on the patient's chest.
3. *Analyze.* Analyze the patient's heart rhythm. Some AEDs require you to press an "analyze" button. Other defibrillators automatically start to analyze when the pads are attached to the patient's chest. Do not touch the patient while the AED is analyzing the rhythm.
4. *Shock.* If the AED advises that a shock is indicated, check the patient from head to toe to make sure no one is touching the patient (including you) before pressing the shock control. Shout, "Stand clear!" Press the shock control once it is illuminated and the machine indicates it is ready to deliver the shock. Resume CPR, beginning with chest compressions, immediately after delivery of the shock.

The adult AED sequence is shown in Skill Drill 7-5.

CPR Complications

Complications can occur during CPR. These include broken bones, injury to internal organs, and vomiting.

You may hear or feel a cracking sound when performing chest compressions. Do not stop CPR! Check your hand position and move your hands to the proper position if necessary. If your hand position is too low, you could injure the patient's internal organs, such as the liver. Check how hard you are pressing down on the patient's chest. If you have been compressing the chest too hard, apply less pressure as you continue compressions.

Vomiting is a common complication of CPR. It usually occurs when breaths are given too quickly or too forcefully. Air is pushed into the stomach and causes the stomach to swell. You can minimize the frequency with which vomiting occurs if you are careful to provide slow breaths with just enough force to see the chest rise. If the patient vomits, roll him onto his side until the vomiting stops. Clear the vomitus from the patient's mouth using your gloved fingers. Roll the patient onto his back and resume CPR if needed.

Supporting the Family

Objective 12 ▶

Any emergency involving a cardiac arrest is a stressful situation, regardless of the cause of the arrest. Family members, friends, and bystanders at the scene may be anxious, angry, sad, hysterical, demanding, or impatient. Allow them to have and express their emotions. However, do not let others distract you from treating the patient. Accept their concerns and recognize that their behavior stems from grief.

Adult AED Sequence

STEP 1 ▶
- Be sure the patient is lying, face up, on a firm, flat surface.
- If possible, place the AED next to the patient's left ear. Turn on the power of the AED.
- If more than one rescuer is present, one rescuer should continue CPR while the other readies the AED for use.
- One rescuer should apply the AED pads to the patient's chest.

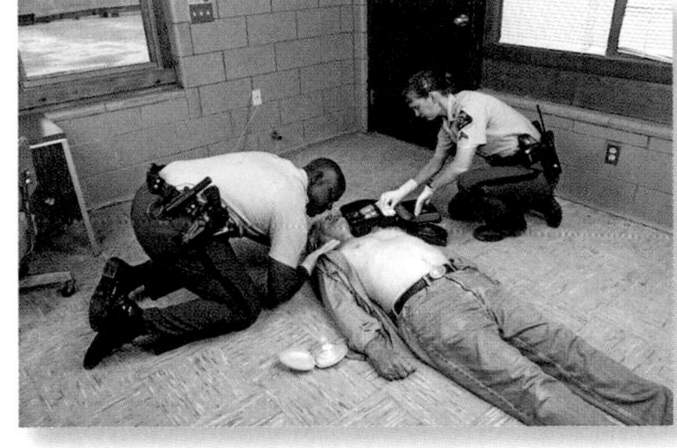

STEP 2 ▶ Analyze the patient's heart rhythm. Do not touch the patient while the AED is analyzing the rhythm.
- If the AED advises that a shock is indicated, check the patient from head to toe to make sure no one is touching the patient (including you) before pressing the shock control.
- Shout, "Stand clear!"

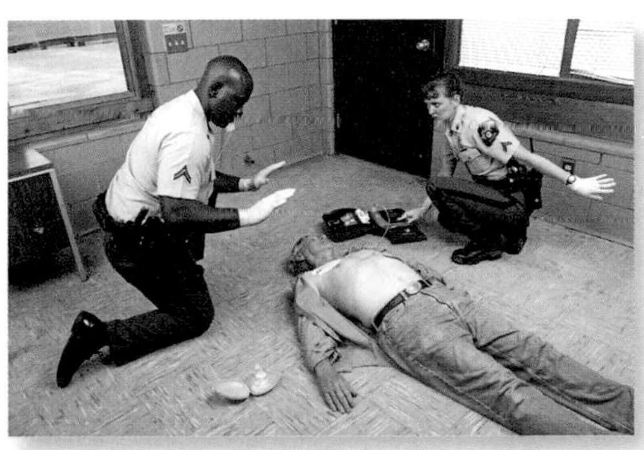

STEP 3 ▶ Press the shock control once it is illuminated and the machine indicates it is ready to deliver the shock.

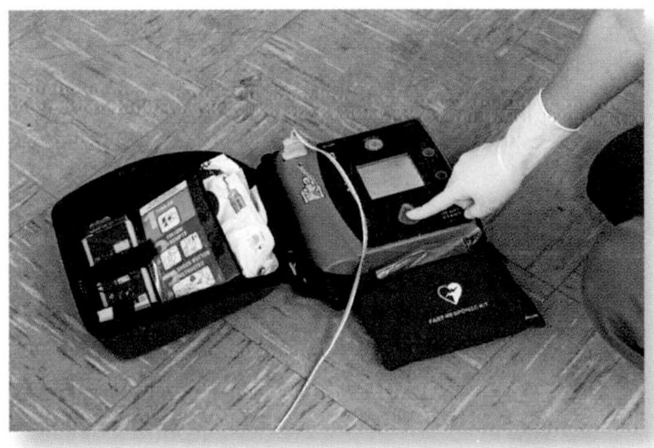

STEP 4 ▶
- After delivery of the shock, quickly resume CPR, beginning with chest compressions. After about 2 minutes of CPR, reanalyze the rhythm.

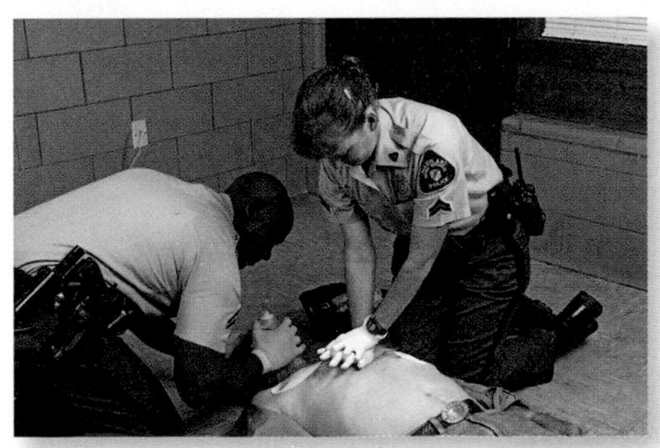

Objective 13 ▶

Identify yourself and, using a gentle but firm tone of voice, let them know that everything that can be done to help will be done. Allow family members to be present, unless they are emotionally distraught and interfere with your efforts to resuscitate the patient. Comfort them by being sympathetic and listening with empathy, but do not give false hope or reassurance.

When to Stop CPR

Objective 15 ▶

You should stop CPR only if

- Effective breathing and circulation have returned
- The scene becomes unsafe
- You are too exhausted to continue
- You transfer patient care to a healthcare professional with equal or higher certification
- A physician assumes responsibility for the patient

Objective 8 ▶

On The Scene

Wrap-Up

Another officer arrives with the AED and turns it on. After the large electrode patches are applied, he tells you to stop CPR so that the machine can analyze the patient's heart rhythm. The machine's monotone voice states, "Shock advised; stand clear." The other officer commands "Stand clear!" and scans the patient to be sure no one is touching her as he depresses the flashing shock button. You see her body twitch as the electric shock travels through the patient's heart. After the shock, you resume CPR for about 2 minutes and then wait anxiously as the machine again analyzes her heart rhythm. As the machine says, "No shock advised," you see her chest heave with a sudden intake of breath. You can feel a carotid pulse, weak at first, but stronger with each beat.

You carefully roll the patient onto her side. Your partner then takes a moment to explain the situation to the patient's husband. When the Paramedics arrive, you give a brief report. The patient is trying to sit up, embarrassed and confused about what has happened. You cannot believe how exhilarated you feel as they wheel her out to the ambulance. ■

Sum It Up

- The circulatory system consists of the *cardiovascular* and *lymphatic systems.* The cardiovascular system is made up of the heart, blood, and blood vessels. The lymphatic system consists of lymph, lymph nodes, lymph vessels, the tonsils, the spleen, and the thymus gland. The circulatory system is responsible for transporting oxygen, water, and nutrients (such as sugar and vitamins) throughout the body. It also carries away wastes (such as carbon dioxide) produced by body cells to the lungs, kidneys, or skin for removal from the body.
- The heart is divided into four chambers. The two upper chambers are the right and left *atria.* The atria receive blood from the body and lungs. The right atrium receives blood that is low in oxygen from the body. The left atrium receives blood rich in oxygen from the lungs. The two lower chambers of the heart are the right and left *ventricles.* The ventricles are larger and have thicker walls than the atria because their function is to pump blood to the lungs and body. The right ventricle pumps blood to the lungs. The left ventricle pumps blood to the body.
- The liquid portion of the blood is called *plasma.* Plasma carries blood cells throughout the body. The formed elements of the blood are the *red blood cells, white blood cells,* and *platelets.* Red blood cells pick up oxygen in the lungs and transport it to body cells. The red blood cells then gather up carbon dioxide and transport it to the lungs, where it is removed from the body when we exhale. White blood cells attack and destroy germs that enter the body. Platelets are irregularly shaped blood cells that have a sticky surface. When a blood vessel is damaged and starts to bleed, platelets gather at the site of the injury. They begin to stick to the opening of the damaged vessel and seal the vessel, stopping the flow of blood.
- Blood vessels that carry blood away from the heart to the rest of the body are called *arteries.* Arteries have thick walls because they transport blood under high pressure. Vessels that return blood to the heart are called *veins.* The walls of veins are much thinner than the walls of arteries. Because the pressure in veins is low, veins contain one-way valves that help keep the blood flowing toward the heart. *Capillaries* are the smallest and most numerous of the blood vessels. They are very thin and connect arteries and veins. They move oxygen, nutrients, and waste products between blood and body cells through their walls.
- When the heart stops, the patient is said to be in *cardiac arrest.* The signs of cardiac arrest include sudden unresponsiveness, absent breathing, and no signs of circulation. Organ damage begins quickly after the heart stops. *Sudden cardiac death* is the unexpected loss of life occurring either immediately or within 1 hour of the onset of cardiac symptoms. Brain damage begins 4–6 minutes after the patient suffers a cardiac arrest. Brain damage becomes irreversible in 8–10 minutes.
- Chest compressions are used to circulate blood when the heart is not beating. Chest compressions are combined with rescue breathing to oxygenate the blood. The combination of rescue breathing and external chest compressions is called *cardiopulmonary resuscitation (CPR).*
- The *Chain of Survival* is the ideal series of events that should take place immediately after recognizing an injury or the onset of sudden illness. The chain consists of four steps:
  1. Early access
  2. Early CPR

3. Early defibrillation
4. Early advanced cardiac life support

- When a cardiac arrest occurs, CPR must be started as early as possible. However, even with the best CPR, CPR provides only about one third of the normal blood flow to the heart and brain. By itself, CPR is not enough to help someone survive a cardiac arrest. CPR can keep oxygen-rich blood flowing to the heart and brain until the arrival of an *automated external defibrillator (AED)* and advanced care. An AED is a machine that analyzes the patient's heart rhythm for any abnormalities. It administers an electric shock through the patient's chest to the heart.
- The steps of CPR include
  1. Checking the patient's level of responsiveness
     - Use the AVPU scale to quickly check the patient's level of responsiveness (mental status). For chest compressions to be effective, the patient must be positioned on a firm, level surface. If you find the patient in bed, move him or her to the floor. Place the patient's arms at his or her sides. Once the patient is lying face up, position yourself at the patient's side, so that you can provide rescue breathing and chest compressions if necessary.
  2. *A* = *Airway*
     - If the patient is unresponsive and you do not suspect trauma, open the airway using the head tilt–chin lift maneuver. If you suspect trauma, open the airway using the jaw thrust without head tilt.
  3. *B* = *Breathing*
     - After you have made sure that the patient's airway is open, assess his or her breathing. Look for the rise and fall of the chest. Listen and feel for air movement from the patient's nose or mouth. If the patient is not breathing, begin rescue breathing using a pocket mask or a mouth-to-barrier device.
  4. *C* = *Circulation*
     - Use the carotid artery to check the pulse of an unresponsive adult or child older than 1 year of age. Feel for a brachial pulse in an unresponsive infant. Feel for a pulse for about 10 seconds and look for other signs of circulation, such as coughing or movement in response to your rescue breaths. If there is no pulse or signs of circulation, you must begin chest compressions.
  5. *D* = *Defibrillation,* if necessary
     - You may need to use an AED during CPR.

► Tracking Your Progress

After reading this chapter, can you	Page Reference	Objective Met?
• List the reasons for the heart to stop beating?	208	☐
• Define the components of cardiopulmonary resuscitation?	209	☐
• Describe each link in the Chain of Survival and how it relates to the EMS system?	208–209	☐
• List the steps of one-rescuer adult CPR?	212–215	☐
• Describe the technique of external chest compressions on an adult patient?	212	☐
• Describe the technique of external chest compressions on an infant?	223	☐
• Describe the technique of external chest compressions on a child?	219–222	☐
• Explain when you, in your role as an Emergency Medical Responder, are able to stop CPR?	230	☐
• List the steps of two-rescuer adult CPR?	216–219	☐
• List the steps of infant CPR?	224–226	☐
• List the steps of child CPR?	220–222	☐
• Respond to the feelings that the family of a patient may be having during a cardiac event?	228	☐
• Demonstrate a caring attitude toward patients with cardiac events who request Emergency Medical Services?	230	☐
• Place the interests of the patient with a cardiac event as the foremost consideration when making any and all patient care decisions?	210	☐
• Communicate with empathy with family members and friends of the patient with a cardiac event?	230	☐

Chapter Quiz

Multiple Choice

In the space provided, identify the letter of the choice that best completes each statement or answers each question.

_____ **1.** When a patient experiences a cardiac arrest, brain damage becomes irreversible in

a. 30 seconds to 2 minutes.
b. 2 to 4 minutes.
c. 4 to 6 minutes.
d. 8 to 10 minutes.

_____ **2.** When a single rescuer is performing chest compressions on an infant, the rescuer should compress the chest

a. with the heel of one hand.
b. using two fingers.
c. using one finger.
d. using the heels of both hands.

_____ **3.** When checking an infant's pulse, you should feel the

a. aorta.
b. carotid artery.
c. brachial artery.
d. posterior tibial artery.

_____ **4.** When compressing the chest of an adult, press down

a. ½ to 1 inch.
b. 1 to 1½ inches.
c. 1 ½ to 2 inches.
d. 2 to 2½ inches.

_____ **5.** A 50-year-old man has collapsed at his desk. As you approach him, you see that he appears to be unresponsive. He does not appear to be breathing and his skin is pale. After ensuring that the scene is safe, your next action should be to

a. check for a femoral pulse.
b. check his level of responsiveness.
c. give 2 rescue breaths.
d. start chest compressions.

_____ **6.** The patient in question 5 has been moved to the floor. You have determined that he is not breathing. After giving 2 rescue breaths, what should your next action be?

a. Apply an AED.
b. Check for a carotid pulse.
c. Position the patient on his side in case he vomits.
d. Leave for a moment to phone for help.

_____ **7.** The patient in question 5 has no pulse. When performing chest compressions on this patient,

a. compress the chest at a rate of 80 compressions per minute.
b. give 5 compressions and 1 rescue breath.
c. use the heel of 1 hand.
d. give 30 compressions and 2 rescue breaths.

_____ **8.** In the patient in question 5, you should check for a pulse after how many cycles of rescue breaths and chest compressions?

a. 2
b. 5
c. 10
d. 15

True or False

Decide whether each statement is true or false. In the space provided, write T for true or F for false.

_____ **9.** During rescue breathing, you can minimize the amount of air that enters the patient's stomach by providing breaths with just enough force to see the chest rise.

_____ **10.** Infant and child CPR should be performed using 5 compressions and 1 ventilation.

Matching

Match the key terms in the left column with the definitions in the right column by placing the letter of each correct answer in the space provided.

_____ **11.** Veins

_____ **12.** Atria

_____ **13.** Pulmonary arteries

_____ **14.** Capillaries

_____ **15.** Aorta

_____ **16.** Arteries

_____ **17.** Pulse

_____ **18.** Dorsalis pedis artery

_____ **19.** Plasma

_____ **20.** Carotid artery

_____ **21.** Ventricles

_____ **22.** Cardiopulmonary resuscitation

_____ **23.** Posterior tibial artery

_____ **24.** Femoral artery

_____ **25.** Brachial artery

_____ **26.** Cardiac arrest

_____ **27.** Radial artery

_____ **28.** Sudden cardiac death

a. Two lower chambers of the heart
b. Major artery of the neck
c. Rhythmic contraction and expansion of the arteries with each heartbeat
d. Major artery of the thigh
e. Liquid portion of the blood
f. Artery of the lower leg
g. Vessels that return blood to the heart
h. Vessel that supplies the upper arm with blood
i. Two upper chambers of the heart
j. Smallest and most numerous of the blood vessels
k. Unexpected loss of life that occurs either immediately or within one hour of the onset of cardiac symptoms
l. Vessels that carry blood low in oxygen from the right ventricle to the lungs
m. Largest artery of the body
n. Major artery of the lower arm
o. Combination of rescue breathing and external chest compressions
p. Blood vessels that carry blood away from the heart to the rest of the body
q. Temporary or permanent cessation of the heartbeat
r. Artery in the foot

Module 4

Patient Assessment

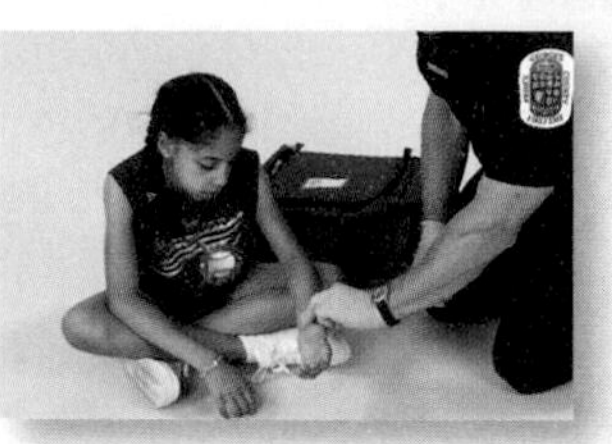

CHAPTER

8 Patient Assessment

By the end of this chapter, you should be able to

Knowledge Objectives ▶

1. Discuss the components of scene size-up.
2. Describe common hazards found at the scene of a trauma and a medical patient.
3. Determine if the scene is safe to enter.
4. Discuss common mechanisms of injury/nature of illness.
5. Discuss the reason for identifying the total number of patients at the scene.
6. Explain the reason for identifying the need for additional help or assistance.
7. Summarize the reasons for forming a general impression of the patient.
8. Discuss methods of assessing mental status.
9. Differentiate between assessing mental status in the adult, child, and infant patient.
10. Describe methods used for assessing if a patient is breathing.
11. Differentiate between a patient with adequate and inadequate breathing.
12. Describe the methods used to assess circulation.
13. Differentiate between obtaining a pulse in an adult, child, and infant patient.
14. Discuss the need for assessing the patient for external bleeding.
15. Explain the reason for prioritizing a patient for care and transport.
16. Discuss the components of the physical exam.
17. State the areas of the body that are evaluated during the physical exam.
18. Explain what additional questioning may be asked during the physical exam.
19. Explain the components of the SAMPLE history.
20. Discuss the components of the ongoing assessment.
21. Describe the information included in the Emergency Medical Responder hand-off report.

Attitude Objectives ▶

22. Explain the rationale for crew members to evaluate scene safety prior to entering.
23. Serve as a model for others by explaining how patient situations affect your evaluation of the mechanism of injury or illness.

24. Explain the importance of forming a general impression of the patient.
25. Explain the value of an initial assessment.
26. Explain the value of questioning the patient and family.
27. Explain the value of the physical exam.
28. Explain the value of an ongoing assessment.
29. Explain the rationale for the feelings that these patients might be experiencing.
30. Demonstrate a caring attitude when performing patient assessments.
31. Place the interests of the patient as the foremost consideration when making any and all patient care decisions during patient assessment.
32. Communicate with empathy during patient assessment to patients as well as with family members and friends of the patient.

Skill Objectives ▶

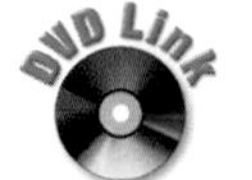

33. Demonstrate the ability to differentiate various scenarios and identify potential hazards.
34. Demonstrate the techniques for assessing mental status.
35. Demonstrate the techniques for assessing the airway.
36. Demonstrate the techniques for assessing if the patient is breathing.
37. Demonstrate the techniques for assessing if the patient has a pulse.
38. Demonstrate the techniques for assessing the patient for external bleeding.
39. Demonstrate the techniques for assessing the patient's skin color, temperature, condition, and capillary refill (infants and children < six years of age only).
40. Demonstrate questioning a patient to obtain a SAMPLE history.
41. Demonstrate the skills involved in performing the physical exam.
42. Demonstrate the ongoing assessment.

On The Scene

It is just after midnight when you are called to respond to a vehicle collision. You flick on your emergency response lights, radio your status, and proceed to the scene. En route, you realize that you will be the first Emergency Medical Responder on the scene. You can see the crash from the crest of a hill. A truck has crashed into a tree and shows major front-end damage. No fire or other danger is visible. You radio your report to the dispatcher. She repeats your size-up over the air so that all incoming units know what to expect. You grab your emergency kit, put on your protective gear, and head to the truck.

There is one person inside, moaning. Something doesn't look right. Despite major front-end damage to the vehicle, the driver's airbag has deployed. However, the passenger airbag has not. Another rescuer arrives. You warn him to stay clear of the passenger side—the undeployed bag could inflate suddenly, causing serious injury or death. You reach in and turn off the ignition.

The other rescuer firmly grasps the patient's head to maintain in-line stabilization. You say to the patient, "We're Emergency Medical Responders. We're here to help. Are you all right?" The patient's eyes open and he moans. You continue your exam. He is breathing, but the rate seems fast. You reach for his wrist and are glad to feel a fast, regular pulse. In the available light, it is hard to see his skin color, but it feels cool to the touch. There is a large bump forming on the side of his head. The patient also has a cut, which is bleeding. You hand gauze to your partner so that he can hold pressure on the wound while you continue your exam. ■

THINK ABOUT IT

As you read this chapter, think about the following questions:

- What personal protective gear is appropriate to wear on this call?
- Is this patient a high or low priority?
- What are your next priorities in the assessment and care of this patient?
- How quickly should you try to care for this patient on the scene prior to transport?

Introduction

The Importance of Patient Assessment

You will be taught many skills during your Emergency Medical Responder course. Of all the skills you will learn, the most important is patient assessment. Every decision you make about the care of your patient is based on what you find during your patient assessment. In this chapter, you will learn the steps needed to assess a patient properly. You will learn about sizing up the scene, forming a general impression, determining responsiveness, and assessing the patient's airway, breathing, and circulation. You will also learn how to determine the priorities of patient care.

Scene Size-Up

As an Emergency Medical Responder, you will be called to provide emergency care to patients in many different settings. Your patients will include infants, children, young adults, middle-aged adults, the elderly, and patients with special healthcare needs. These patients may experience an emergency due to trauma or a medical condition. These emergencies may occur in a person's home, on a busy highway, in a shopping mall, or in an office. In every situation, you must quickly look at the entire scene before approaching the patient (Figure 8-1). You must size up the scene

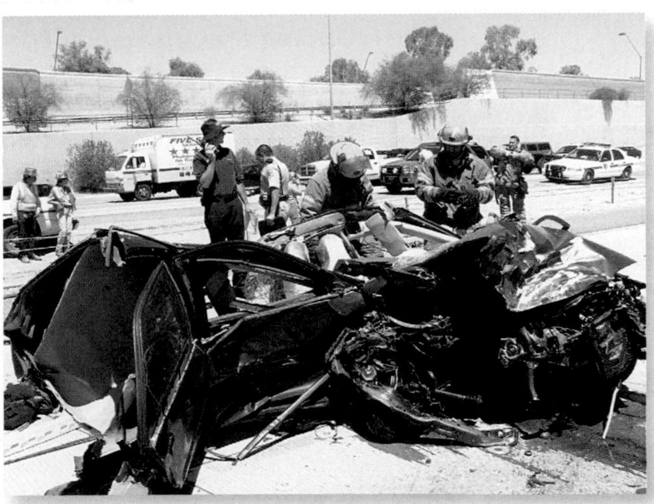

FIGURE 8-1 ▶ You must quickly survey the entire scene for safety on every emergency call. Courtesy of City of Tempe Fire Department, Tempe, Arizona

to find out if there are any threats that may cause injury to you, other rescuers, or bystanders or that may cause additional injury to the patient.

Objective 1 ▶

Scene size-up is the first phase of patient assessment and is made up of five parts:

1. Body substance isolation precautions
2. Evaluation of scene safety
3. Determining the mechanism of injury or the nature of the patient's illness
4. Determining the total number of patients
5. Determining the need for additional resources

The scene size-up begins with the information received about the emergency. The information the caller gives the EMS dispatcher may help you determine the following:

- The location of the emergency
- If the call is a trauma emergency (such as a motor vehicle crash) or a medical emergency (such as a seizure)
- The number of vehicles involved
- The number of patients involved
- The ages and genders of all patients
- When the emergency occurred
- If the call involves fire or other potential hazards such as leaking materials, downed power lines, broken gas lines, hazardous materials, a violent patient, or dangerous pets
- If law enforcement or fire department personnel are on the scene
- If Advanced Life Support personnel have been sent to the scene
- If special resources will be required, such as a hazardous materials team, a confined space rescue team, a water rescue team, extrication equipment, or air medical transport

Be prepared for the unexpected.

En route to the scene, try to create a mental picture of the call using the information the dispatcher has given you. What additional help might be needed on the scene? Law enforcement personnel? The fire department? A utility company? Advanced Life Support personnel? How will you gain access to the patient? What questions will you ask the patient or family?

Remember This!

The information the dispatcher gives you is often limited to that provided by the caller. You may arrive at the scene of an emergency to find the patient with injuries or a complaint that differs from that reported by the caller.

Body Substance Isolation (BSI) Review

You must take appropriate BSI precautions on *every* call. Consider the need for BSI precautions before you approach the patient. Put on appropriate personal protective equipment based on the information the dispatcher gives you and your initial survey of the scene (Figure 8-2). This equipment includes gloves, eye protection, mask, and gown, if necessary. Consider the following examples of real emergency situations:

- You are called to a fitness club for a woman with a rapid heart rate. The dispatcher tells you that the woman was using the treadmill when she felt weak, became dizzy, and felt her heart race. Because gloves should be worn before physical contact with *every* patient, put on gloves while en route to the scene.

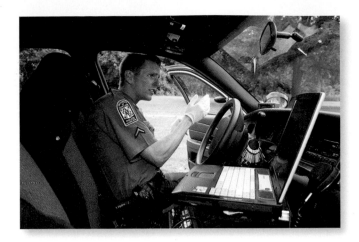

FIGURE 8-2 ► Based on the dispatch information you receive and your initial survey of the scene, put on appropriate personal protective equipment.

- You are called to respond to a single vehicle rollover. The bystander who called 9-1-1 said the vehicle rolled twice and is resting on its side. There is heavy damage to the vehicle. He believes there are three patients. En route to the scene, put on gloves because it is likely that blood will be present on the scene. Once on the scene, put on a chin-length face shield (or protective eyewear and mask) if you see serious bleeding that could spray or splash into your eyes, nose, or mouth. Put on a gown if there is a chance of splashing blood or other body fluids and your clothing is likely to be soiled. If you are trained in fire or rescue techniques, wear appropriate clothing to protect yourself from fire, glass, sharp edges and fragments, and other debris at the scene. Protective clothing includes turnout gear, puncture-proof gloves, a helmet, eye protection (safety glasses or goggles), and boots with steel toes.

You Should Know

Components of Scene Size-Up

- Body substance isolation precautions
- Evaluation of scene safety
- Determining the mechanism of injury or the nature of the patient's illness
- Determining the total number of patients
- Determining the need for additional resources

Scene Safety

Objective 3 ►

Objective 22 ►

Scene safety is an assessment of the entire scene and surroundings to ensure your well-being and that of other rescuers, the patient(s), and bystanders. Remember, you are of no help to the patient if you become a patient yourself.

Stop and Think!

Do not enter an unsafe scene. Scenes may be dangerous even if they seem safe. If the scene is unsafe, make it safe. If you cannot make it safe, do not enter. Call for appropriate personnel to handle the situation.

Personal and Other Rescuer Safety

Objective 2 ►

Study the scene before approaching the patient (Figure 8-3). Consider the following questions at a crash or rescue scene:

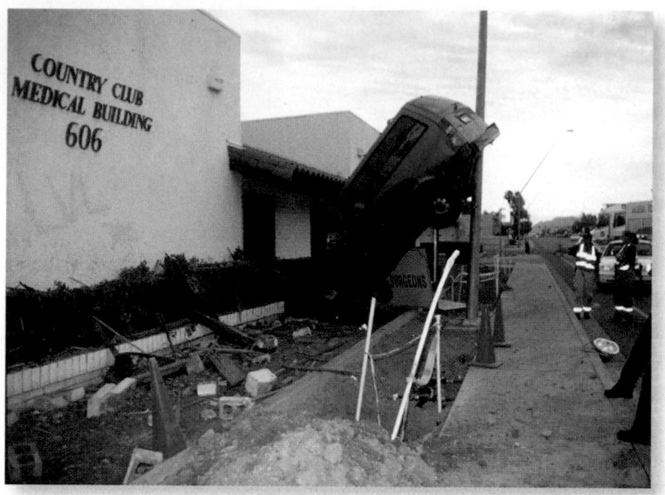

FIGURE 8-3 ► Before approaching the patient, study the scene. Look for possible hazards. Courtesy of City of Mesa Fire Department, Mesa, Arizona.

- Is the area marked by safety lights or flares?
- Is traffic controlled by law enforcement personnel?
- Does the vehicle, aircraft, or machinery appear stable?
- Do you see any leaking fluids?
- Are downed power lines present?
- Do you see fire, smoke, or potential fire hazards?
- Do you see entrapped victims?

At a scene involving toxic substances, obvious hazards may be present. At other scenes, the hazards may not be as obvious. Look for clues that suggest the presence of hazardous materials:

- Placards on railroad cars, storage facilities, or vehicles
- Vapor clouds or heavy smoke
- Unusual odors
- Spilled solids or liquids
- Leaking containers, bottles, or gas cylinders
- Chemical transport tanks or containers

When you arrive at a scene, park at a safe distance upwind or uphill from the incident. Contact your local hazardous materials response team immediately. Do not enter the area unless you are trained to handle hazardous materials and are fully protected with the proper equipment. Do not walk or drive an emergency vehicle through spilled liquids. Keep unnecessary people away from the area. Provide emergency care only after the scene is safe and the patient is decontaminated.

Emergencies that occur in a confined space, such as a mine, a well, a silo, or an unreinforced trench, may be low in oxygen (Figure 8-4). Rescues in these situations require specially trained personnel and equipment. Do not enter the area unless you have all the necessary equipment and have been trained in this type of rescue.

At a crime scene or hostile situation, assess the potential for violence. Clues include

- A knowledge of prior violence at a particular location
- Evidence of alcohol or other substance use
- Weapons visible or in use
- Loud voices, fighting, or the potential for fighting

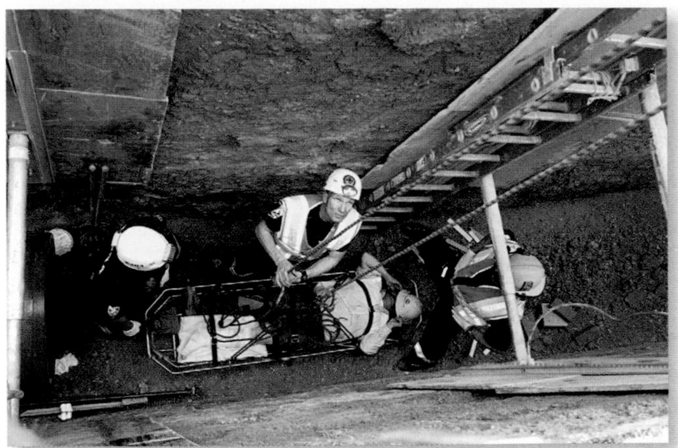

FIGURE 8-4 ▲ Confined space rescue requires specially trained personnel and equipment. Courtesy of City of Mesa Fire Department, Mesa, Arizona

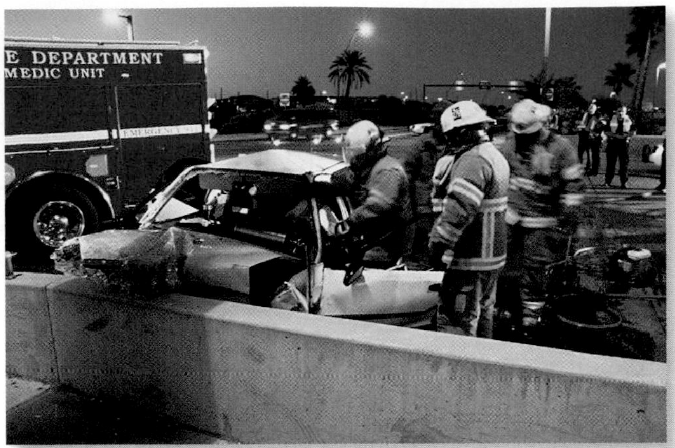

FIGURE 8-5 ▲ You are responsible for ensuring the patient's safety, including protecting the patient from glass and other debris during extrication procedures. Courtesy of City of Tempe Fire Department, Tempe, Arizona

Assess the crowd and look for hostile bystanders. *Never* enter a potential crime scene or a scene involving a family dispute, a fight, an attempted suicide, drugs, alcohol, or weapons until law enforcement personnel have secured the scene and declared it safe for you to enter and provide patient care.

Consider the environment before approaching the patient. If a surface or slope is unstable or if water, ice, fire, or downed power lines are present, call for specially trained personnel as needed. Do not enter a body of water unless you have been trained in water rescue. Do not enter fast-moving water or venture out onto ice unless you have been trained in this type of rescue. If the scene is safe but extremes of heat or cold are a concern, move the patient to an ambulance as quickly as possible.

Patient Safety

You are responsible for ensuring the patient's safety. This responsibility includes

- Protecting the patient from curious onlookers
- Assessing for traffic and other hazards
- Protecting the patient from glass and other debris during extrication procedures (Figure 8-5)
- Protecting the patient from environmental temperature extremes

Bystander Safety

At the scene of an emergency, bystanders may become so engrossed in the situation that they fail to watch out for themselves. Look for bystanders who may be in danger or who may endanger your safety or that of the patient. Help bystanders avoid becoming patients by preventing them from getting too close to the scene. If the scene is safe and you need assistance, ask bystanders to help you. Reassure your patient and bystanders by working confidently and efficiently.

The Mechanism of Injury or the Nature of the Illness

Objective 23 ▶

During the scene size-up, try to determine the nature of the patient's problem. A **trauma patient** is one who has experienced an injury from an external force. In trauma situations, look for the mechanism of injury. A **medical patient** is one whose condition is caused by an illness. In medical situations, try to determine the nature of the patient's illness.

Making a Difference

Trauma and medical emergencies can occur at the same time. For example, a patient with low blood sugar may be involved in a motor vehicle crash or a patient may have had a seizure before falling. A patient with a history of asthma may develop difficulty breathing after an airbag deploys in a motor vehicle crash. Don't get tunnel vision!

The Mechanism of Injury

Objective 26 ▶

The mechanism of injury (MOI) is the way in which an injury occurs, as well as the forces involved in producing the injury. **Kinetic energy** is the energy of motion. The amount of kinetic energy an object has depends on the object's mass (weight) and speed (velocity). **Kinematics** is the science of analyzing the mechanism of injury and predicting injury patterns. The amount of injury is determined by the following three elements:

If the patient is unresponsive, considering the mechanism of injury may be the only way you can determine what happened.

1. The type of energy applied
2. How quickly the energy is applied
3. To what part of the body the energy is applied

Survey the scene and talk to the patient, family, and bystanders to determine the mechanism of injury.

Making a Difference

When providing care for a seriously injured trauma patient, make every effort to limit your time on the scene to 10 minutes or less. These patients require definitive care at the hospital. The longer it takes to deliver a seriously injured patient to the hospital, the less likely patient survival becomes. As an Emergency Medical Responder, you are responsible for helping transport agencies assess the patient and prepare him or her for transport. Give only essential care at the scene. EMS transport personnel will provide further care en route to the hospital.

Objective 4 ▶

Trauma is generally divided into two categories: blunt and penetrating. **Blunt trauma** is any mechanism of injury that occurs without actual penetration of the body (Figure 8-6). Mechanisms of injury due to blunt trauma include motor vehicle crashes, falls, sports injuries, and assaults with a blunt object. Blunt trauma produces injury first to the body surface and then to the body's contents. This results in compression and/or stretching of the tissue beneath the skin.

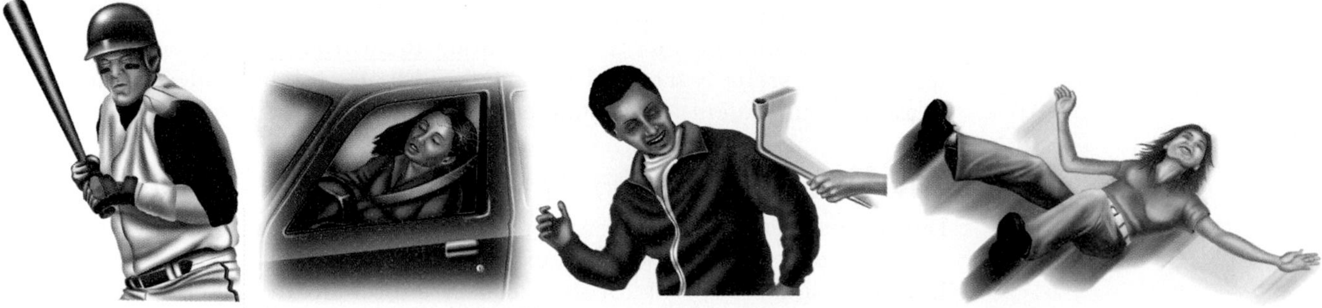

FIGURE 8-6 ▲ Blunt trauma is any mechanism of injury that occurs without actual penetration of the body.

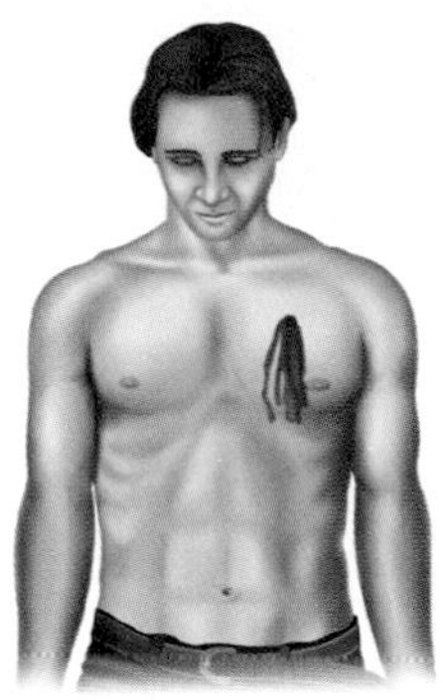
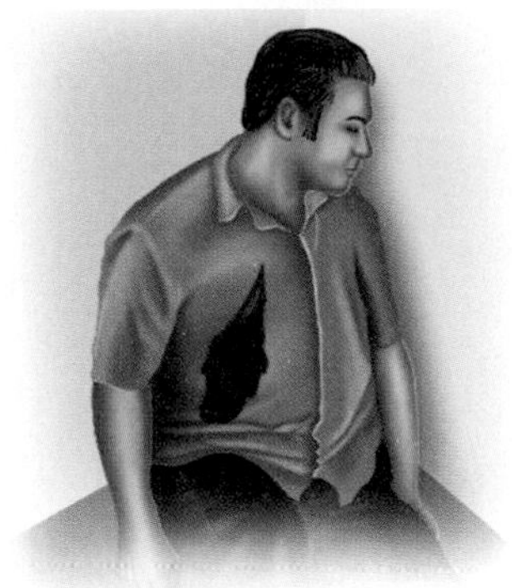
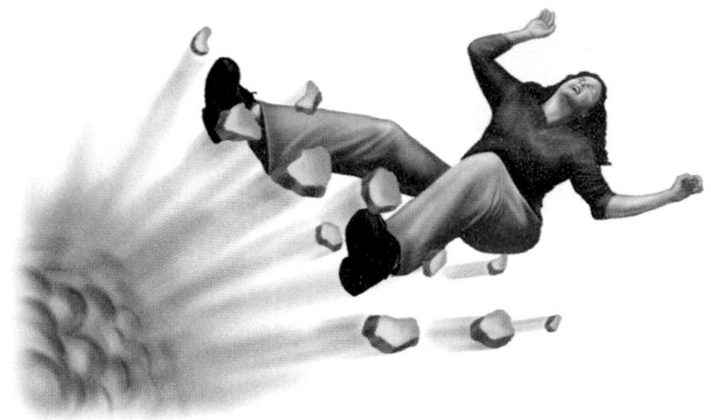

FIGURE 8-7 ▲ Penetrating trauma is any mechanism of injury that causes a cut in or piercing of the skin.

The amount of injury depends on how long the compression occurred, the force of the compression, and the area compressed.

Penetrating trauma is any mechanism of injury that causes a cut in or piercing of the skin (Figure 8-7). Mechanisms of injury due to penetrating trauma include gunshot wounds, stab wounds, and blast injuries. Penetrating trauma usually affects organs and tissues in the direct path of the wounding object.

Making a Difference

The extent and seriousness of a patient's injuries may not be obvious. When evaluating the mechanism of injury, try to picture the organs that may have been damaged. This technique will help you predict the patient's injuries.

Motor Vehicle Crashes

Most motor vehicle crashes (75%) occur within 25 miles of home. Most crashes also occur in areas where the speed limit is 40 mph or lower.

A motor vehicle crash (MVC) can involve automobiles, motorcycles, all-terrain vehicles (ATVs), and tractors. In an MVC, three separate impacts occur as kinetic energy is transferred (Figure 8-8):

1. The vehicle strikes an object.
2. The occupant collides with the interior of the vehicle. Interior elements include seat belts, airbags, and the dashboard.
3. Internal organs collide with other organs, muscle, bone, or other structures inside the body. The lungs, brain, liver, and spleen are particularly vulnerable to trauma. Note that a fourth impact may occur if loose objects in the vehicle become projectiles.

A motor vehicle crash is classified by the type of impact. The five types of impact are head-on (frontal), lateral (side), rear-end, rotational, and rollover (Figure 8-9). The injuries that result depend on the type of collision, the occupant's position inside the vehicle, and the use or nonuse of active or passive restraint systems.

Restraint systems are used to absorb the energy of the impact before the occupant hits something hard. They also limit the distance the body has to travel. As of October 2001, passenger airbags had killed 118 children in the United States. Twenty-two percent of those deaths had occurred among infants who had been placed in rear-facing child safety seats in front of the passenger seat airbag. Most of the children killed by airbags in motor vehicle crashes had been unrestrained or improperly restrained.

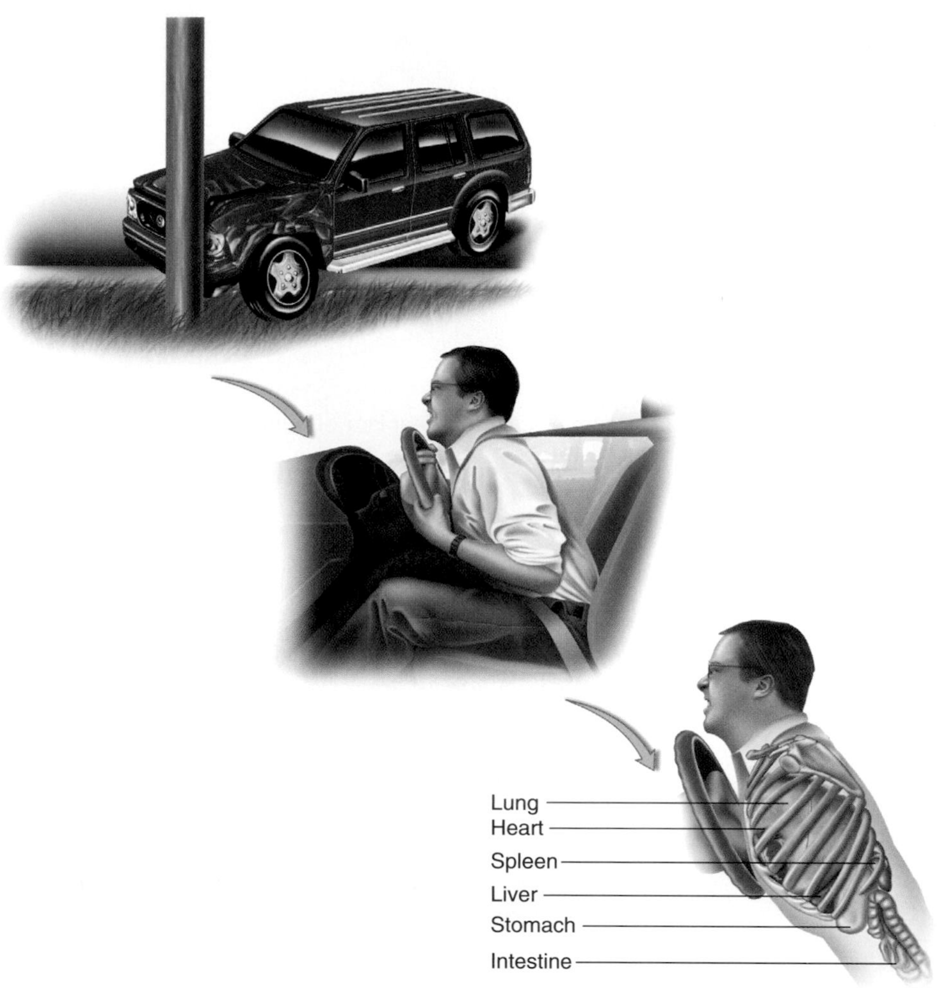

FIGURE 8-8 ▶ In an MVC, three separate impacts occur as kinetic energy is transferred: (1) The vehicle strikes an object, (2) the occupant collides with the interior of the vehicle, including the seat belt, airbag, or dashboard, (3) internal organs collide with other organs, muscle, bone, or other structures inside the body.

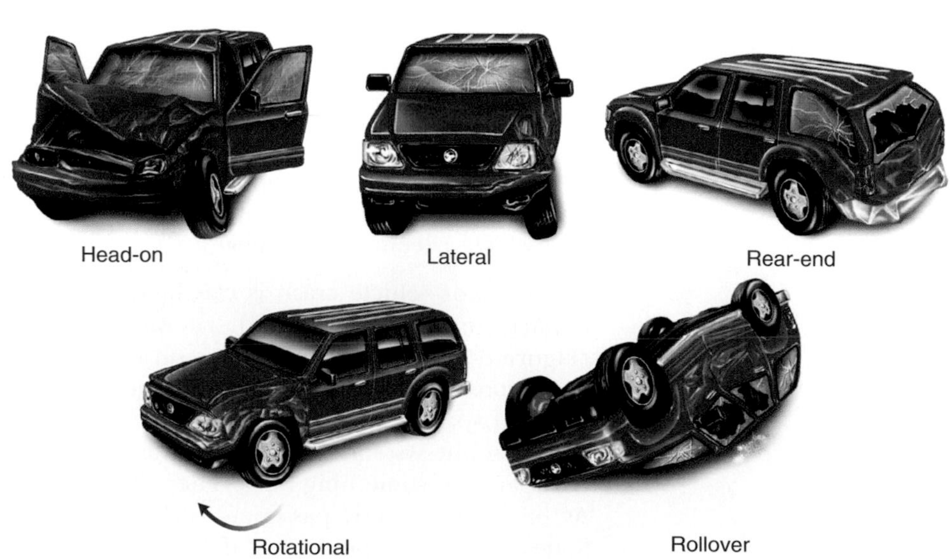

FIGURE 8-9 ▶ The five types of motor vehicle crashes are head-on (frontal), lateral (side), rear-end, rotational, and rollover.

You Should Know

Motor Vehicle Crash Statistics

- One out of four of all occupant deaths among children ages 0 to 14 years involve a drinking driver.
- Of children ages 0 to 14 years who were killed in motor vehicle crashes in the United States during 2002, 50% were unrestrained.
- Restraint use among young children often depends on the driver's restraint use. Almost 40% of children riding with unbelted drivers are themselves unrestrained.
- Physical frailty increases the injury risk of older adults in a crash. A crash that results in nonfatal injuries to a younger person may result in the death of an older adult driver or passenger.

Motor Vehicle–Pedestrian Crashes

Adult pedestrians will typically turn away if they are about to be struck by an oncoming vehicle. This action results in injuries to the side or back of the body. A child will usually face an oncoming vehicle, which results in injuries to the front of the body.

Among children five to nine years of age, pedestrian injuries are the most common cause of death from trauma. Children are susceptible to crashes due to the following factors:

- They have less accurate depth perception.
- They tend to dart into traffic.
- They cannot accurately judge the speed of a vehicle.

Children under the age of five years are at risk of being run over in the driveway. Most pedestrian injuries occur during the day, peaking in the period after school. About 30% of pedestrian injuries occur while the child is in a marked crosswalk.

Falls

Falls are a common mechanism of injury. The factors to consider in a fall are

- The height from which the patient fell
- The patient's weight
- The surface the patient landed on
- The part of the patient's body that struck first

Infants are more likely to fall from changing tables, countertops, and beds. Preschool children usually fall from windows. Older children fall more often from playground equipment. Adults who have jumped rather than fallen from a height tend to land on their feet and then fall onto their buttocks or outstretched hands. Of older adults who fall, 20–30% suffer moderate to severe injuries, such as hip fractures or head trauma.

You Should Know

Fall Statistics

- Falls are a leading cause of traumatic brain injuries.
- More than one third of adults 65 years or older fall each year.
- Among children, preschoolers are at greatest risk for falls.

Bicycle Crashes

Most severe and fatal bicycle injuries involve head trauma. Other injuries associated with bicycle crashes include trauma to the face, limbs, and abdomen (from striking the handlebars). The most common bicycle crashes include the following:

- Riding into a street without stopping
- Turning left or swerving into traffic that is coming from behind
- Running a stop sign
- Riding against the flow of traffic

Bicycle helmets protect against injuries to the mid- and upper face. They can also reduce the risk of head injury. A helmet absorbs some of the energy and disperses the blow over a larger area for a slightly longer time. It is estimated that helmets reduce the risk of head injury by 85% and brain injury by 88%.

The predictable injuries based on the common mechanisms of injury are listed in Table 8-1.

Making a Difference

Significant Mechanisms of Injury

If the patient has any of the following injuries, transport the patient to a trauma center:

- Penetrating injury to the head, neck, or torso (excluding superficial wounds in which the depth of the wound can be easily determined)
- Penetrating injury to the extremities above the elbow or knee
- Flail chest
- Combination trauma with burns
- Two or more proximal long-bone fractures
- Pelvic fractures
- Open or depressed skull fracture
- Paralysis
- Amputation above the wrist or ankle
- Major burns

Consider transport to a trauma center if the mechanism of injury is from any of the following causes:

- Ejection from a vehicle (including motorcycles, mopeds, all-terrain vehicles, the open beds of pickup trucks)
- Dead occupant in the same passenger compartment
- Falls of more than 15 feet (or three times the patient's height), falls greater than 10 feet if the patient is younger than 14 years or older than 55
- Vehicle rollover
- High-speed auto crash with an initial speed of more than 40 mph
- High-speed auto crash with major auto deformity of more than 20 inches
- High-speed auto crash with intrusion into the passenger compartment of more than 12 inches
- Injury from an auto-pedestrian or auto-bicycle crash with significant impact (more than 5 mph)

- Pedestrian thrown or run over
- Motorcycle crash at more than 20 mph or with separation of the rider from the bike

Also consider transport to a trauma center for significant mechanisms of injury for infants and children:

- Falls of more than 10 feet (or three times the child's height)
- Bicycle collision
- Vehicle collision at a medium speed
- Any vehicle collision in which the infant or child was unrestrained

TABLE 8-1 Predictable Injuries Based On Common Mechanisms of Injury

Mechanism of Injury		Predictable Injuries
Motor Vehicle Crashes	**Head-On Collision**	Below the steering wheel: • Lower-extremity fractures • Dislocated knees and hips At the level of and above the steering wheel: • Trauma to the head, brain, and face • Serious chest injuries
	Lateral (Side) Collision	• Head and cervical spine injuries • Injuries to the chest and pelvis • Internal injuries that may be present without outward signs of injury
	Rear-End Collision	• Head, brain, and cervical spine injuries • Possible chest, abdomen, long-bone, and soft-tissue injuries
	Rotational Collision	• Head and cervical spine injuries • Internal injuries that may be present without outward signs of injury
	Rollover	• Head and cervical spine injuries • Crushing injuries • Soft-tissue injuries, multiple broken bones
Motor Vehicle–Pedestrian Crashes	**Adult**	• Injuries to lower portions of both legs • Secondary injuries that may occur when the body strikes the hood of the car and then the ground
	Child	• Trauma to the lower extremities from the bumper • Chest and abdominal trauma from striking the hood • Injuries to the head and face from hitting the hood or windshield

TABLE 8-1 *(Continued)*

Mechanism of Injury		Predictable Injuries
Falls	**Adult**	• Compression injuries of the spine • Upper- or lower-extremity trauma
	Child	• Head, face, and neck trauma (young children tend to fall head first) • Upper- or lower-extremity trauma
Bicycle Crashes	**Without a Helmet**	• Injuries to the head, face, and spine; broken clavicles and ribs • Extremity fractures • Abdominal injuries (from striking the handlebars)
	With a Helmet	• Upper- or lower-extremity trauma • Abdominal injuries (from striking the handlebars)
Motorcycle Crashes	**Head-On Collision**	• At the level of and above the handlebars, lower-extremity fractures with serious soft-tissue injuries and blood loss • Head, face, and neck trauma likely on landing
	Lateral Collision	• Pelvic or lower-extremity injuries; crushing injuries
	Ejection	• The type and severity of injuries depend on how the victim lands and the nature of the object struck
	Laying Down of the Motorcycle	• Scrapes, burns, and possible fractures of the lower extremities
Penetrating Traumas	**Low-Velocity Weapons (e.g., Knife, Ice Picks)**	• Injury that is usually limited to the area penetrated • Blood loss
	Medium- and High-Velocity Weapons (e.g., Shotguns, High-Powered Rifles, and Assault Weapons)	• An injured area that is larger than the area penetrated • Fluid-filled organs (bladder, heart, great vessels, and bowel) that can burst because of the pressure waves generated • Liver, spleen, and brain, which are easily injured

The Nature of the Illness

The **nature of the illness (NOI)** is the medical condition that resulted in the patient's call to 9-1-1. Examples include fever, difficulty breathing, chest pain, headache, and vomiting. Try to find out the nature of the illness by talking to

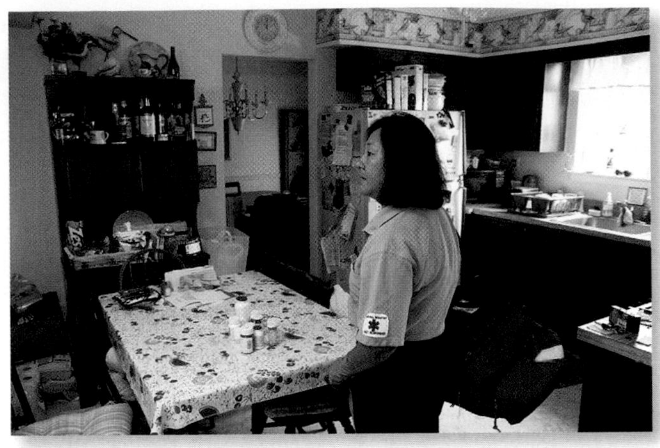

FIGURE 8-10 ▶ While in a patient's home, look around and note the orderliness, cleanliness, and safety of the home.

the patient, family, coworkers, and bystanders. If the patient is uncooperative or unresponsive, look to family members or others at the scene as sources of information. Look for clues to explain the patient's condition, such as pills, spilled medicine containers, and household or gardening chemicals.

While in a patient's home, look around you. Note the orderliness, cleanliness, and safety of the home (Figure 8-10). Look at the general appearance of the patient and other members of the family. Check if there are any medical devices the patient may use, such as home oxygen equipment or a breathing machine.

Sometimes homes are hazardous because of large collections of paper, trash, or animal waste.

The Number of Patients

Objective 4 ▶

Objective 5 ▶

At the scene, first you should take appropriate BSI precautions, evaluate scene safety, and determine the mechanism of injury or the nature of the patient's illness. After taking these steps, determine the total number of patients. Be alert for patients in addition to the first patient you observe at the scene. Look for clues that other patients may be present, including toys, diapers, bottles, schoolbooks, a purse, or a child safety seat.

It is important to quickly find out the number of patients on the scene in order to request additional resources if necessary. In most situations, one EMS professional is needed for each patient. If a patient is severely ill or injured, two or more EMS professionals may be needed to provide emergency care. If there are more patients than you can handle effectively, call for additional help.

Remember This!

Call for additional help *before* you make contact with the patient. Once you begin patient care, you will have fewer chances to make the call.

While waiting for the arrival of more resources, determine the patients who must be treated first. The process of sorting patients by the severity of their illness or injury is called **triage.** This information is covered in more detail in Chapter 14.

Additional Resources

Objective 6 ▶

Determine if more help is needed at the scene. The types of additional help that may be needed are shown in Table 8-2. Contact the dispatcher as soon you recognize the need for more resources.

TABLE 8-2 Scene Hazards and Possible Resources

Scene Hazards	Possible Resources
Traffic control, crime or violent scene	Law enforcement personnel
Complex extrication	Fire department, special rescue team
Hazardous materials	Fire department, hazardous materials team
Confined space	Fire department, special rescue team
Swift-water rescue	Fire department, special rescue team
High-angle rescue	Fire department, special rescue team
Trench rescue	Fire department, special rescue team
Downed power lines	Fire department, electric utility company
Natural gas leak	Fire department, gas utility company
Dangerous pets	Animal control
Mass casualty incident	Law enforcement, fire department, Advanced Life Support personnel, ground ambulances, air ambulances, municipal and public school bus services (if needed), Federal Emergency Management Agency (FEMA) (if needed), National Guard (if needed)

Remember This!

Scene size-up is an ongoing process. Alter your plan of action as necessary based on the information obtained at the scene, your patient assessment findings, and available resources.

Patient Assessment

An organized approach to patient assessment helps you make certain that no significant findings or problems are missed.

The ability to assess a patient properly is one of the most important skills you can master. You must learn to work quickly and efficiently in all types of situations. Some situations may include poor lighting conditions, temperature extremes, large numbers of people, and being in a moving ambulance. To work efficiently, you must approach patient assessment systematically. The emergency care you provide your patient will be based on your assessment findings.

Patient assessment consists of the following components (Table 8-3):

- Scene size-up
- Initial assessment
- Focused history and physical examination
- Detailed physical examination
- Ongoing assessment

TABLE 8-3 Components of Patient Assessment

Scene Hazards	Possible Resources
Scene Size-Up	• Take BSI precautions. • Evaluate scene safety. • Determine the mechanism of injury or the nature of the patient's illness. • Determine the total number of patients. • Determine the need for additional resources.
Initial Assessment	• Form a general (first) impression. • Assess the level of responsiveness and provide cervical spine protection if the mechanism of injury suggests a cervical spine injury. • Assess the airway. • Assess breathing. • Assess circulation. • Identify priority patients. • Provide an EMS report.
Focused History and Physical Examination	• Obtain a SAMPLE history and baseline vital signs. • Perform a focused physical examination.
Detailed Physical Examination	• Perform a head-to-toe physical examination.
Ongoing Assessment	• Repeat the initial assessment. • Reassess the patient's vital signs. • Repeat the focused assessment regarding the patient's complaint or injuries. • Reevaluate the emergency care.

The order in which the steps in a patient assessment is performed is generally the same. However, some specific parts of the assessment will vary, depending on the following:

- Whether the situation involves a medical condition or trauma
- Whether the patient is responsive or unresponsive

The patient assessment sequence for these situations is shown in Table 8-4.

Initial Assessment

Objective 25 ▶

You must perform an initial assessment on *every* patient. The initial assessment begins after the scene or situation has been found safe or made safe and you have gained access to the patient. The purpose of the initial assessment is to find and care for immediate life-threatening conditions. It usually requires less than 60 seconds to complete. However, it may take longer if you must provide emergency care to correct an identified problem. Remember to wear appropriate personal protective equipment (PPE) before approaching the patient.

TABLE 8-4 Patient Assessment Sequence

Medical Patient	Trauma Patient
Responsive patient: 1. Scene size-up 2. Initial assessment 3. SAMPLE history/vital signs 4. Focused physical exam 5. Ongoing assessment	With no significant mechanism of injury: 1. Scene size-up 2. Initial assessment 3. Focused physical exam 4. SAMPLE history/vital signs 5. Ongoing assessment
Unresponsive patient: 1. Scene size-up 2. Initial assessment 3. Detailed (head-to-toe) physical exam 4. SAMPLE history/vital signs 5. Ongoing assessment	With significant mechanism of injury: 1. Scene size-up 2. Initial assessment 3. Rapid trauma assessment (detailed or head-to-toe physical exam) 4. SAMPLE history/vital signs 5. Ongoing assessment

The initial assessment has several parts (Figure 8-11):

- General (first) impression
- Level of responsiveness and cervical spine protection
- Airway
- Breathing and ventilation
- Circulation with bleeding control
- Identification of priority patients
- Delivery of an EMS update

FIGURE 8-11 ▶ The initial assessment.

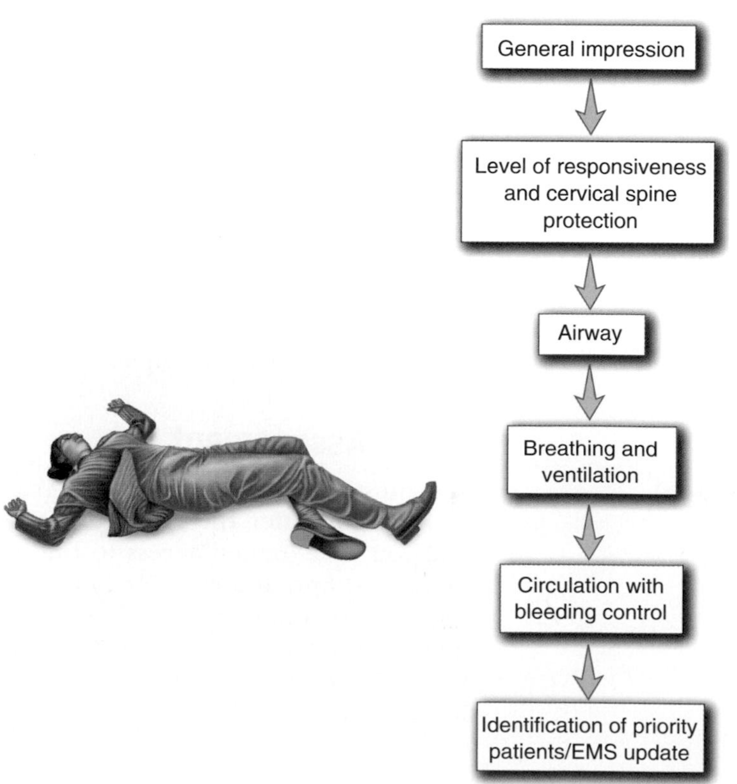

While performing an initial assessment, you will find out your patient's signs and symptoms. A **sign** is a medical or trauma condition that can be seen, heard, smelled, measured, or felt. Examples of signs are unusual chest movement, bleeding, swelling, pale skin, and a fast pulse. A **symptom** is a condition described by the patient. Shortness of breath, nausea, abdominal pain, chills, chest pain, and dizziness are examples of symptoms. You must provide emergency medical care based on the patient's signs and symptoms.

Patient assessment requires you to use your senses of sight (look), sound (listen), touch (feel), and smell:

- *Look.* You will use your sense of sight to assess parts of the patient's body and the patient's behavior. Does he or she look sick or poorly nourished? Do you see obvious problems, such as a rash, external bleeding, vomiting, seizures, an arm or a leg deformity, pale or flushed skin, or sweating?
- *Listen.* You will use your sense of hearing to find out why your patient called for assistance. You will also listen to find out if the patient is breathing normally, if the patient is having difficulty breathing, or if breathing is absent. You will use a stethoscope and blood pressure cuff if you are expected to take a blood pressure.
- *Feel.* You will use your sense of touch to find out important information about your patient. Using your hands, you can find out if the patient's skin is hot, warm, cool, or cold. You can also determine if a body part is hard, soft, or swollen. You will also determine if touching a part of the patient's body causes pain.
- *Smell.* You will use your sense of smell to identify smells associated with specific problems. For example, a sweetish (fruity) breath odor can indicate a diabetic problem. The smell of alcohol may explain why a patient is slow to answer your questions.

General Impression

Objective 7 ▶

Objective 24 ▶

Whenever you meet someone for the first time, you form a first impression—sometimes without realizing it. You will do the same thing with every patient. A general impression is an "across-the-room" assessment. You will form a general impression without the patient's telling you what the complaint is. You can complete it in 60 seconds or less. The purpose of forming a general impression is to decide if the patient looks "sick" or "not sick." If the patient looks sick, you must act quickly. As you gain experience, you will develop an instinct for recognizing quickly when a patient is sick and needing to act quickly.

Remember This!

Your patient's condition can change at any time. A patient that initially appears not sick may rapidly worsen and appear sick. Reassess your patient often.

A general impression is also called a first impression.

Before you speak to your patient and find out what is wrong, stop a short distance from the patient (Figure 8-12). Look and listen. What things stand out in your mind when you first see the patient?

- Does the patient look ill (medical patient) or injured (trauma patient)? If the patient looks ill, are there clues around you that suggest the nature of the illness? For example, the presence of an oxygen tank suggests that someone in the home has a chronic medical condition. If the patient is injured, what is the mechanism of injury?
- How old do you think the patient is? Is the patient male or female?
- Does the patient look sick? If so, the patient may have a life-threatening problem, which must be treated immediately. Life-threatening problems include unresponsiveness, a blocked airway, absent breathing (respiratory arrest), and severe bleeding. If you find a life-threatening condition, you must treat it before going on to the next step.

FIGURE 8-12 ▶ Form a general impression by pausing a short distance from the patient.

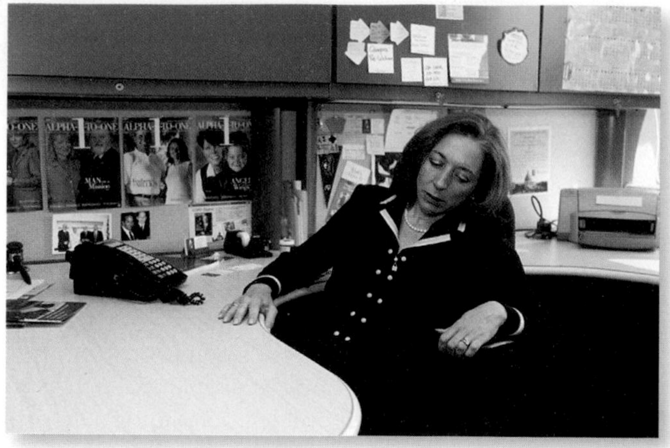

Making a Difference

Some say that intuition helps form a general impression of a patient. It is actually a combination of knowledge, careful observation, effective communication, and experience that forms your intuition.

You will base your general impression of a patient on three main factors: (1) appearance, (2) (work of) breathing, and (3) circulation:

Remember: Approach a patient only after making sure the scene is safe.

1. *Appearance.* Unless the patient is sleeping, her eyes should be open and should follow you as you move. If she looks agitated, limp, or appears to be asleep, approach her immediately and begin your focused assessment.
2. *(Work of) breathing.* With normal breathing, both sides of the chest rise and fall equally. Normal breathing is quiet, is painless, and occurs at a regular rate. Approach the patient immediately and begin your focused assessment if the patient
   - Looks as if she is struggling (laboring) to breathe
   - Has noisy breathing (gurgling, snoring, wheezing)
   - Is breathing faster or slower than normal
   - Looks as if her chest is not moving normally
3. *Circulation.* The patient's skin color should be normal for her ethnic group. Approach the patient immediately and begin your focused assessment if the patient's skin looks flushed (red), pale (whitish), gray, or blue (cyanotic).

If your general impression reveals an urgent problem, move quickly. Begin emergency care and arrange for immediate patient transport. If your general impression does not reveal an urgent problem, work at a reasonable pace and continue your patient assessment. Remember to explain to the patient and family what you are doing.

Level of Responsiveness and Cervical Spine Protection

Level of Responsiveness (Mental Status)

Objective 8 ▶

After forming a general impression, assess the patient's level of responsiveness. The best way to do this is to talk to the patient. If the patient appears to be awake, start by telling him your first name. Let him know you are an Emergency Medical Responder. Explain that you are there to help. Next, ask your patient a question, such as "Why did you call 9-1-1 today?" His answer will give you some important information. First, it will tell you his level of responsiveness. Level of responsiveness is also called *level of consciousness* or *mental status.* These terms refer to a patient's level of awareness. A patient's mental status is "graded" using a scale called the AVPU scale. Second, the patient's answer should be his **chief complaint.** A chief complaint is the reason EMS was called, usually in the patient's own words.

If the patient looks as if he is sleeping, gently rub his shoulder and ask, "Are you okay?" or "Can you hear me?" Unresponsiveness may indicate a life-threatening condition. Move the patient only if absolutely necessary. If the patient does not answer, family or bystanders may be able to supply information. You may ask, "Can you tell me what happened?"

Determine if the patient is awake and responds appropriately to questions. Evaluate the patient's orientation to the following:

- Person (the patient can tell you his name)
- Place (the patient can tell you where he is)
- Time (the patient can tell you the day, date, or time)
- Event (the patient can tell you what happened)

A patient who is speaking or crying is responsive (conscious), is breathing, and has a pulse.

A patient who is oriented to person, place, time, and event is said to be "alert and oriented × ('times') 4" or "A and O × 4." If your patient is awake but cannot answer these questions correctly, the patient is said to be confused or disoriented. For example, if your patient is awake and knows his name (alert and oriented to person) and where he is (alert and oriented to place) but does not know what day it is and cannot tell you what happened, he is said to be "alert and oriented times 2."

If the patient is not awake but responds appropriately when spoken to, he is said to "respond to verbal stimuli." For example, the patient will respond correctly to a request such as "squeeze my fingers." If the patient is not awake but responds to a painful stimulus, such as a pinch of the skin on the back of the hand or earlobe, he is said to "respond to painful stimuli" (Figure 8-13). The patient is unresponsive if he does not respond to a verbal or painful stimulus.

In a trauma patient, agitation and combativeness may be due to a decreased supply of oxygen.

As you continue your assessment, note any changes in the patient's mental status. The brain requires a constant supply of oxygen and sugar. Changes in the patient's level of responsiveness may result from a decreased supply of oxygen or sugar. These changes may also come from the use of alcohol or drugs, brain swelling due to injury, or other causes. Be sure to tell medical personnel about any changes in the patient's mental status. In your prehospital care report, document the patient's response to a specific stimulus and any changes in mental status—for example, "The patient opened her eyes on command," "The patient moaned in response to a pinch on the wrist," or "The patient knows his name but does not know the date, where he is, or what happened."

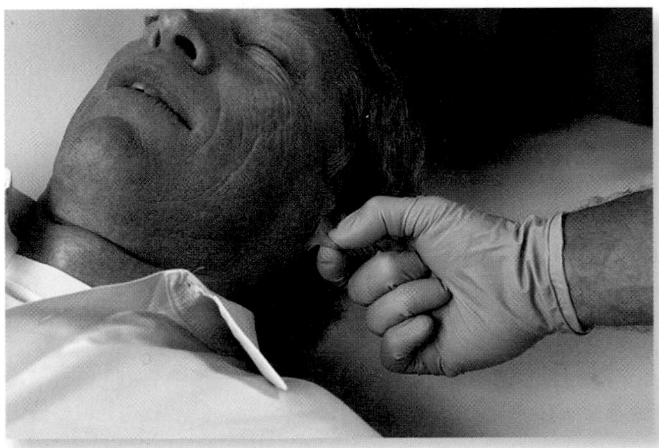

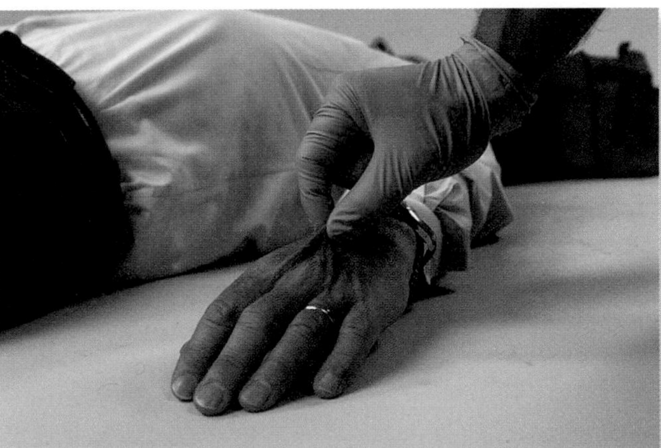

FIGURE 8-13 ▲ Determining the response to a painful stimulus.

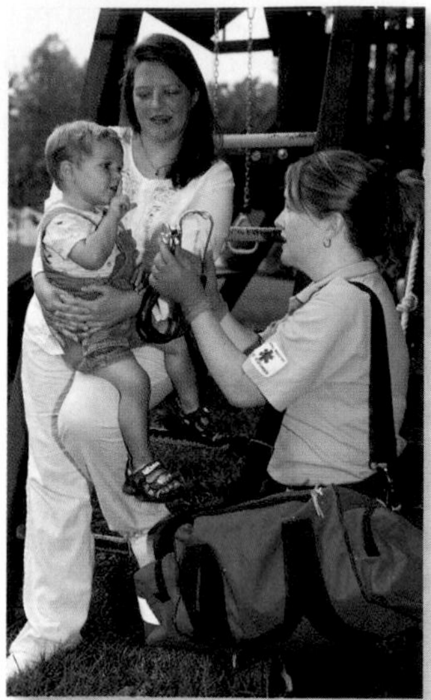

FIGURE 8-14 ▲ An alert infant or young child smiles, orients to sound, follows objects with his or her eyes, and interacts with others.

Remember This!

During the initial assessment, find the answers to these five questions:

1. Is the patient awake and alert?
2. Is the patient's airway open?
3. Is the patient breathing?
4. Does the patient have a pulse?
5. Does the patient have severe bleeding?

Infants and Children An alert infant or young child (younger than three years of age) smiles, orients to sound, follows objects with her eyes, and interacts with those around her (Figure 8-14). As the infant or young child's mental status decreases, the following changes may be seen (in order of decreasing mental status):

- The child may cry but can be comforted.
- The child may show inappropriate, persistent crying.
- The child may become irritable, agitated, and restless.
- The child may have no response (unresponsive).

Objective 9 ▶

Assessing the mental status of a child older than three years of age is the same as assessing that of an adult.

Making a Difference

Assessing a young child can be difficult. Toddlers distrust strangers and are likely to resist your attempts to examine them. They do not like having their clothing removed. They fear pain, separation from their caregiver, and separation from their favorite blanket or toy. When possible, assess the child in the arms or lap of the caregiver. Approach the child slowly and talk to him or her at eye level. Use simple words and phrases and a reassuring tone of voice. The child will understand your tone, even if he does not understand your words.

Cervical Spine Protection

For trauma patients and unresponsive patients with an unknown nature of illness, take **spinal precautions.** Spinal precautions are used to stabilize the head, neck, and back in a neutral position. This stabilization is done to minimize movement that could cause injury to the spinal cord. The technique used to minimize movement of the head and neck is called **in-line stabilization.** The term *in-line* refers to keeping the head and neck anatomically in line with the body. In-line stabilization is first performed using your hands. This is called manual stabilization.

The patient's head is not considered stabilized until it is secured to a long backboard.

If the patient is awake and you suspect trauma to the head, neck, or back, face the patient so that he does not have to turn his head to see you. Instruct him not to move his head or neck. Position your hands on both sides of the patient's head and spread your fingers apart (Figure 8-15). Place the patient's head in a neutral position (eyes facing forward and level) and in line with the body. If the patient complains of pain or you meet resistance when moving the head and neck to a neutral position, stop and maintain the head and neck in the position in which you found them. Once begun, manual stabilization of the patient's head and neck must be continued until additional EMS personnel have properly secured the patient to a backboard with the head and neck stabilized (Figure 8-16). The timing to begin manual stabilization is very important. If you are by yourself and begin manual stabilization too soon, you will be unable to complete the assessment.

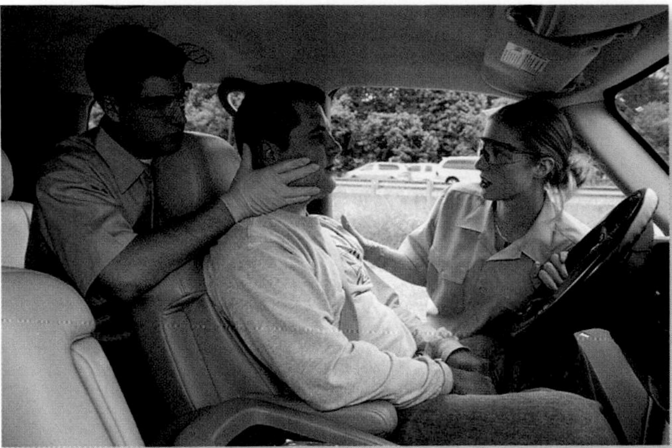

FIGURE 8-15 ▲ In-line stabilization requires keeping the head and neck anatomically in line with the body.

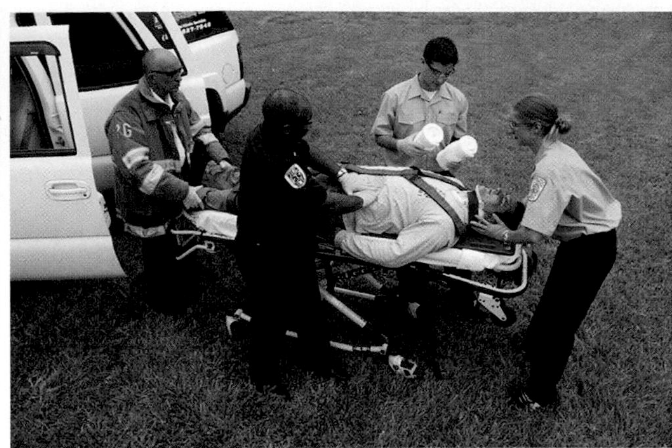

FIGURE 8-16 ▲ Manual stabilization of the patient's head and neck must be continued until additional EMS personnel have properly secured the patient to a backboard with the head and neck stabilized.

Airway

The airway is the pathway from the nose and mouth to the lungs.

The tongue is the most common cause of a blocked airway in an unresponsive patient.

The human body must have a continuous supply of oxygen to survive. Air containing oxygen enters the body through the nose and mouth. It travels down the throat (pharynx), through the windpipe (trachea), and into the lungs. In the lungs, oxygen is transferred to the blood. The oxygen-rich blood is circulated to every cell in the body. The cells of the body cannot live long without oxygen. Therefore, a life-threatening emergency can result if the flow of air is blocked (obstructed) or if oxygen-rich blood is not circulated throughout the body.

A patient who is alert and talking clearly or crying without difficulty has a **patent** (open) airway. If the patient is unable to speak, cry, cough, or make any other sound, the airway is completely obstructed. A patient who has noisy breathing, such as snoring or gurgling, has a partial airway obstruction.

If the patient is unresponsive and you do not suspect trauma, open the airway using the head tilt–chin lift maneuver (Figure 8-17). If the patient is unresponsive and you suspect trauma, open the airway using the jaw-thrust without head tilt (Figure 8-18). Both of these maneuvers lift the tongue away from the back of the

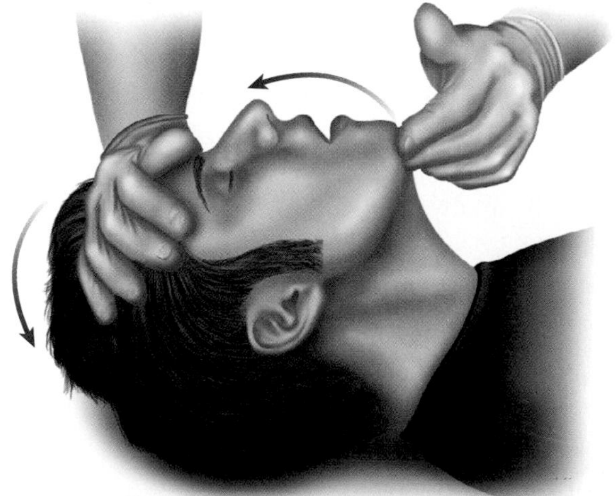

FIGURE 8-17 ▲ If you do not suspect trauma, use the head tilt–chin lift maneuver to open the airway of a patient who is unresponsive.

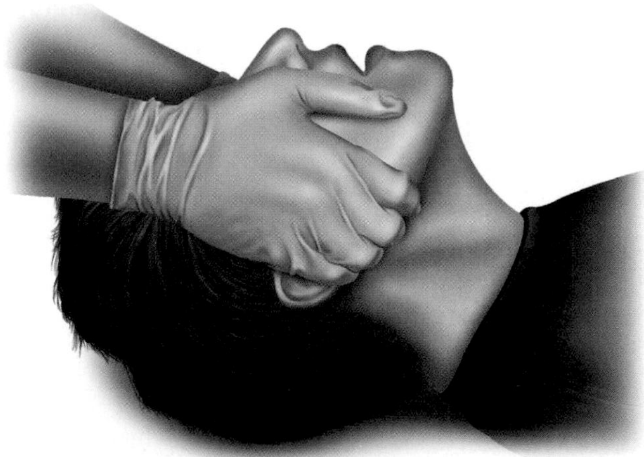

FIGURE 8-18 ▲ If you suspect trauma, use the jaw-thrust without head tilt to open the airway of a patient who is unresponsive.

FIGURE 8-19 ▶ If the patient is unresponsive, look, listen, and feel for breathing.

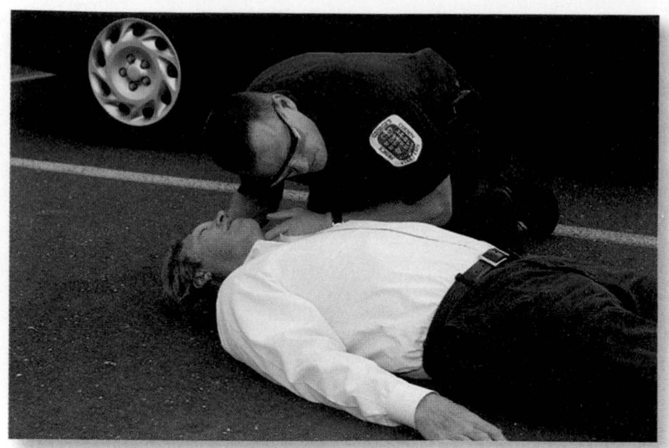

throat, allowing air to enter the lungs. If the patient is an unresponsive infant or child, do not hyperextend the neck when opening the airway.

Look for an actual or a potential airway obstruction, such as a foreign body, blood, vomitus, teeth, or the patient's tongue. If there is blood, vomitus, or other fluid in the patient's airway, clear it with suctioning.

Breathing

Objective 10 ▶

Objective 11 ▶

The priorities for assessing breathing and providing necessary treatment for infants and children are the same as for adults.

After you have made sure that the patient's airway is open, assess his breathing. If the patient is responsive, watch and listen to him as he breathes. Quickly determine if breathing is adequate or inadequate. Keep in mind that normal respiratory rates for infants and children are faster than those for adults. If the patient is unresponsive, look, listen, and feel for breathing (Figure 8-19). Look for a rise and fall of the chest. Because the diaphragm is the main muscle used for breathing in infants and young children, watch the abdomen when assessing breathing. Look at the chest to assess breathing in older children and adults. Listen for air movement. Determine if breathing is absent, quiet, or noisy. Feel for air movement from the patient's nose or mouth against your chin, face, or palm. If breathing is present, quickly determine if breathing is adequate or inadequate. Breathing that is too fast or too slow for the patient's age is a red flag that requires a search for the cause.

You Should Know

Characteristics of Adequate and Inadequate Breathing

Adequate Breathing

- The breathing effort (work of breathing) is quiet, relaxed, and effortless.
- The breathing rate is within normal limits for the patient's age.
- The breathing pattern is regular.
- Both sides of the chest rise and fall equally.
- The depth of breathing is adequate.
- Skin color is normal; skin is warm and dry to the touch.

Inadequate Breathing

- The patient's appearance is anxious; the patient concentrates on breathing.
- The patient is confused, restless.
- The breathing rate is too fast or slow for the patient's age.
- The breathing pattern is irregular.
- The depth of breathing is unusually deep or shallow.

- Breathing is noisy (snoring, gurgling, wheezing).
- The patient is sitting upright and leaning forward to breathe.
- The patient is unable to speak in complete sentences.
- The patient has pain with breathing.
- The patient's skin looks flushed, pale, gray, or blue and feels cold and sweaty.
- The chest rise and fall is unequal.
- The patient is using the muscles in the neck, above the collarbone, between the ribs, or below the rib cage to breathe.

If breathing is adequate and the patient is responsive, allow the patient to assume a comfortable position. If the patient is unresponsive and breathing is adequate, maintain an open airway. Use airway adjuncts, such as an oral airway, if needed. Place the patient in the recovery position if there are no contraindications. Provide oxygen by nonrebreather mask if it is available and you have been trained to use it. Watch the patient closely to make sure that adequate breathing continues.

If the patient is not breathing, the heart will stop beating unless you begin breathing for him or her.

If the patient is unresponsive and breathing is inadequate or if the patient is not breathing, begin rescue breathing using a pocket mask or mouth-to-barrier device. If the patient has dentures, leave them in place to help provide a good mask seal. If the dentures are loose, remove them so that they do not fall back into the throat and obstruct the airway. Watch the patient's chest while you breathe into the patient. If your breaths are going in, you should see the patient's chest rise gently with each breath. Continue breathing for the patient until he begins to breathe adequately on his own or another trained rescuer takes over.

Remember This!

When giving rescue breaths, give breaths with just enough force to see the patient's chest rise gently with each breath. If you breathe too fast or use too much force, you can blow air into the patient's stomach. Too much air in the stomach can cause vomiting.

If your breaths do not go in, gently reposition the patient's head and breathe for him again. If the breaths still do not go in, you must assume the airway is blocked. Attempt to clear the airway using the obstructed airway maneuvers discussed in Chapter 6. Use abdominal thrusts for children and adults. Use back blows and chest thrusts for infants.

Circulation

Objective 12 ▶

The assessment of circulation involves evaluating the following:

- Signs of obvious bleeding
- Central and peripheral pulses
- Skin color, temperature, and condition
- Capillary refill (in children younger than six years of age)

Obvious Bleeding

Objective 14 ▶

Look from head to toes for signs of significant external bleeding. Control major bleeding, if present. Apply direct pressure over the bleeding site. If the bleeding is from an extremity, elevate it unless doing so is contraindicated. If bleeding continues, apply pressure over arterial pressure points. Apply a pressure bandage if needed.

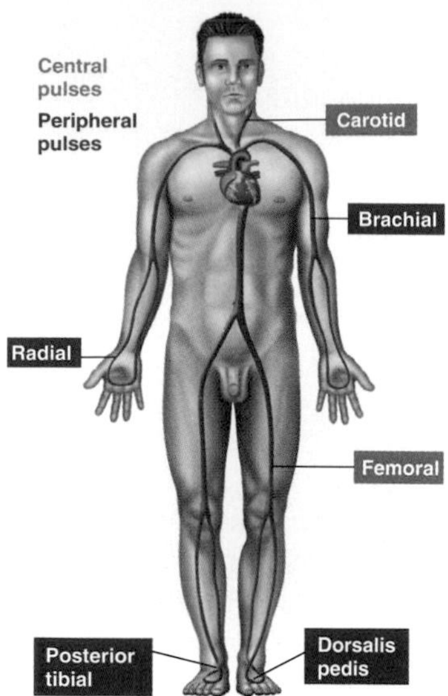

FIGURE 8-20 ▲ The location of the central (carotid and femoral) and peripheral pulses (radial, brachial, posterior tibial, and dorsalis pedis).

Stop and Think!

Dark clothing, waterproof clothing, and many layers of clothing may mask severe bleeding. Expose the injury site and look closely for bleeding in these situations.

Pulses

Arteries are large blood vessels that carry blood away from the heart to the rest of the body. Blood is forced into the arteries when the heart contracts. A **pulse** is the rhythmic contraction and expansion of the arteries with each beat of the heart. A pulse can be felt anywhere an artery passes near the skin surface and can be pressed against firm tissue, such as a bone.

A **central pulse** is a pulse found close to the trunk of the body (Figure 8-20). Examples of central pulses are the carotid pulse and femoral pulse. The carotid artery is the major artery of the neck. It supplies the head with blood. Pulsations can be found on either side of the neck (Figure 8-21). To find the carotid pulse, place your index and middle fingers in the soft, hollow area just to the side of the patient's windpipe. The femoral artery is located in the fold between the thigh and pelvis. In the field, a femoral pulse is not often used due to the presence of the patient's clothing. It may require more pressure than other sites to be felt adequately.

A peripheral pulse is located farther from the trunk of the body than a central pulse. A peripheral pulse can be felt at several locations:

- The radial pulse is located in the wrist at the base of the thumb (Figure 8-22). Check for a radial pulse first when assessing a responsive adult or a child one year of age or older.
- The brachial pulse is located on the inside of the upper arm, midway between the shoulder and the elbow (Figure 8-23). Always check for a brachial pulse in an infant.
- The posterior tibial pulse is located just behind the ankle bone.
- The dorsalis pedis pulse is located on the top surface of the foot.

Objective 13 ▶

Practice finding pulses on adults and children of various ages. Knowing how to find a normal pulse in a healthy patient will help you recognize what is abnormal.

When assessing a responsive adult or a child one year of age or older, first check the radial pulse in the wrist. Use the carotid artery in the neck to check the pulse of an unresponsive adult or a child older than one year of age. Feel for a brachial pulse in the upper arm in an infant. Feel for a pulse for about 10 seconds. A heart rate that is too fast or too slow for the patient's age is a red flag that requires a search for the cause. If there is no pulse, you must begin chest compressions.

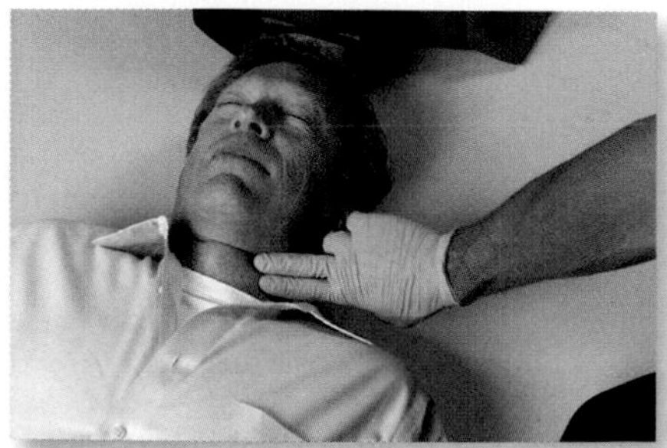

FIGURE 8-21 ▲ Use the carotid artery to check the pulse of an unresponsive adult or child older than one year of age.

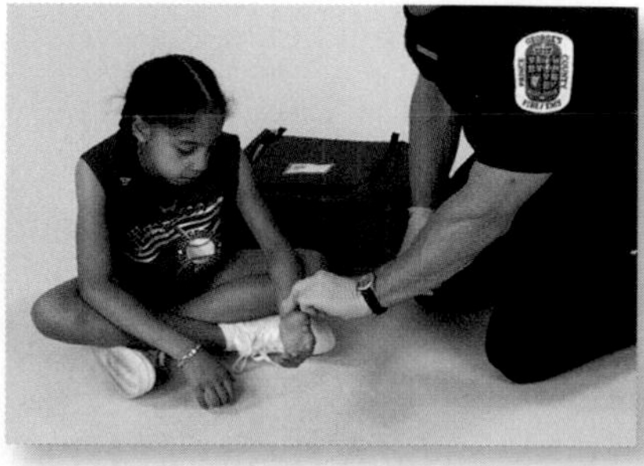

FIGURE 8-22 ▲ In a responsive adult or a child one year of age or older, check circulation by feeling for a radial pulse.

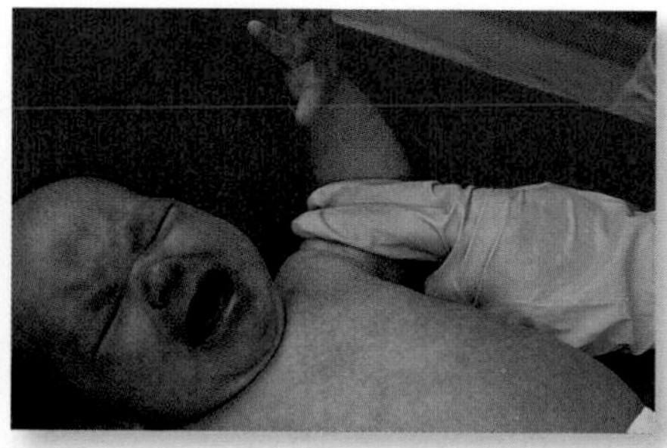

FIGURE 8-23 ▲ In infants, feel for a brachial pulse.

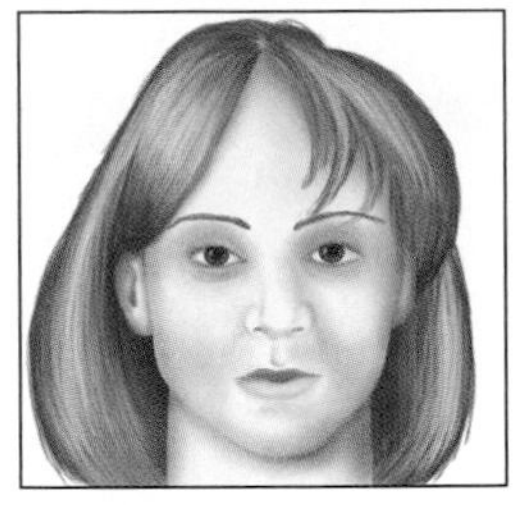
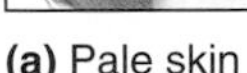

(a) Pale skin

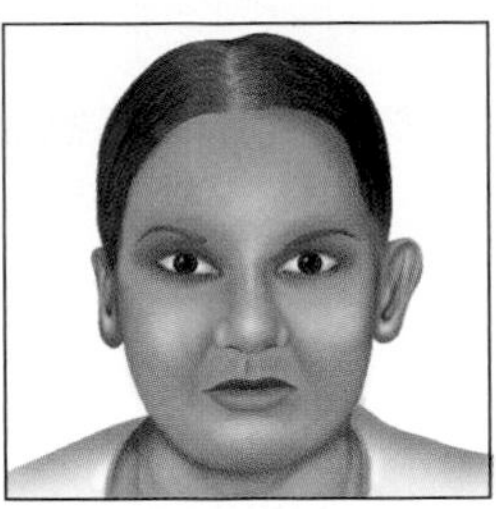

(b) Cyanosis

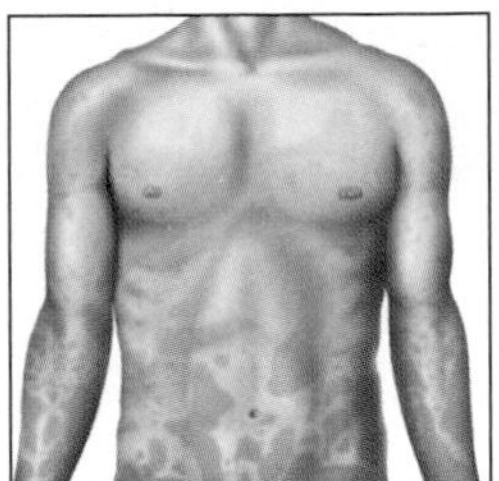

(c) Mottled skin

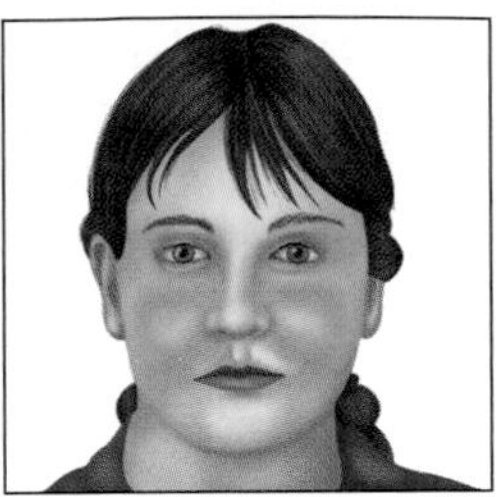

(d) Flushed skin

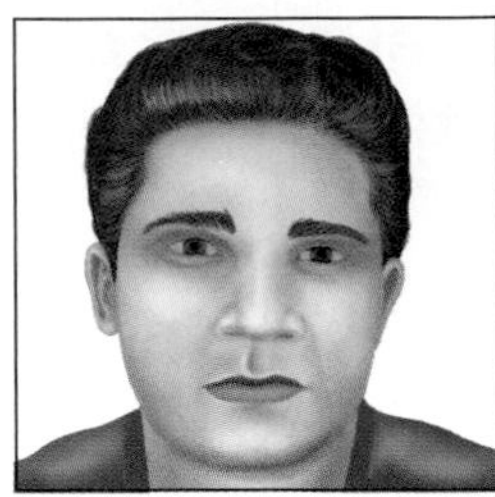

(e) Jaundice

FIGURE 8-24 ▲ Assess an adult patient's skin color in the nail beds, inside the mouth, and inside the eyelids. In infants and children, assess the palms of the hands and soles of the feet.

Skin Color, Temperature, and Condition

While assessing the patient's pulse, quickly check the patient's skin. Assessing the patient's skin condition can provide important information about the flow of blood through the body's tissues **(perfusion).** Perfusion is assessed by evaluating the following:

- Skin color
- Skin temperature
- Skin condition (moist, dry)
- Capillary refill (in infants and children younger than six years of age)

Assess the patient's skin color in the nail beds, inside the mouth, and inside the eyelids. In infants and children, assess the palms of the hands and soles of the feet. Pale (whitish) skin occurs when the blood vessels in the skin have severely narrowed (constricted); (Figure 8-24). This condition may be seen in shock, fright, anxiety, and other causes. **Cyanotic** (blue) skin suggests inadequate breathing or poor perfusion and often appears first in the fingertips or around the mouth. Cyanosis may be seen in

- Respiratory distress
- Airway obstruction
- Exposure to cold
- Blood vessel disease
- Shock
- Cardiac arrest

Mottling is an irregular or a patchy skin discoloration that is usually a mixture of blue and white. Mottled skin is usually seen in patients in shock, with hypothermia, or in cardiac arrest. Jaundiced (yellow) skin may be seen in patients with liver or gallbladder problems. Flushed (red) skin may be caused by the following:

- Heat exposure
- Late stages of carbon monoxide poisoning
- Allergic reaction
- Alcohol abuse
- High blood pressure

The back surfaces of the hands and fingers are used in assessing skin temperature. The skin in these areas is thin and sensitive to temperature changes.

Assess skin temperature by placing the back of your hand against the patient's face, neck, or abdomen (Figure 8-25). Normal skin temperature is warm. Hot skin may be caused by fever or heat exposure. Cool skin may be due to inadequate circulation or exposure to cold. Cold skin may be due to extreme exposure to cold or shock. Clammy (cool and moist) skin may be caused by shock, among many other conditions.

TABLE 8-5 Central and Peripheral Pulses

Central Pulses	
Carotid	• Major artery of the neck • Supplies the head with blood • Pulsations can be found on either side of the neck • Check this pulse first when assessing an unresponsive adult or child one year of age or older • Avoid excess pressure in elderly patients • Never assess the carotid pulse on both sides of the neck at the same time
Femoral	• Located in the fold between the thigh and pelvis • In the field, not often used due to the presence of patient clothing • May require more pressure than other sites to be felt adequately
Peripheral Pulses	
Radial	• Located in the wrist at the base of the thumb • Used to assess circulation in the upper extremities • Check this pulse first when assessing a responsive adult or a child one year of age or older
Brachial	• Located on the inside of the upper arm, midway between the shoulder and the elbow • Used to assess circulation in the upper extremities • Always check this pulse in an infant
Posterior tibial	• Located just behind the ankle bone • Used to assess circulation in the lower extremities
Dorsalis pedis	• Located on the top surface of the foot • Used to assess circulation in the lower extremities

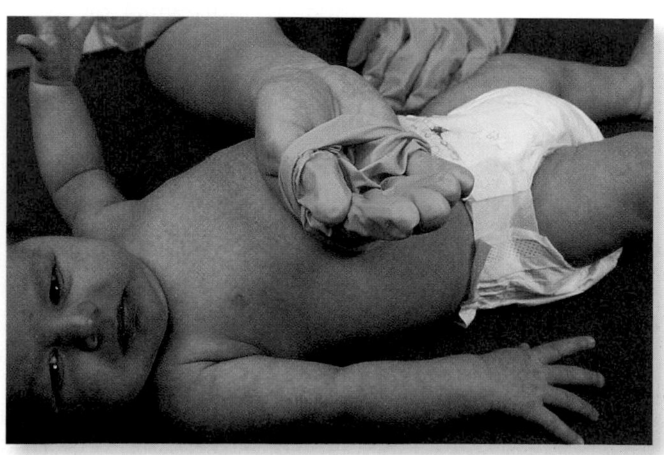

FIGURE 8-25 ▶ Assess your patient's skin temperature by placing the back of your hand against the patient's face, neck, or abdomen.

FIGURE 8-26 ► Assess capillary refill in infants and children less than six years of age.

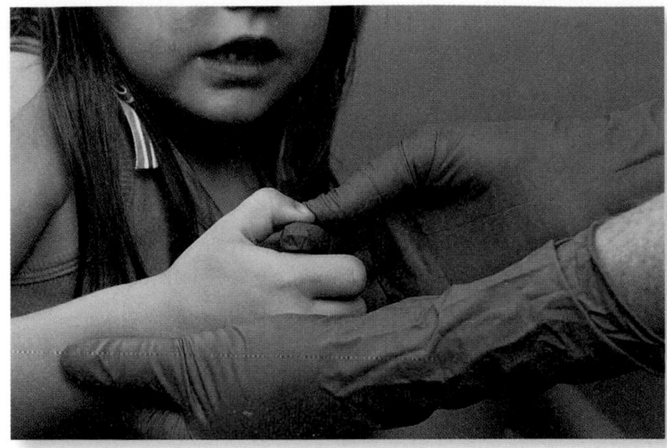

Assess the patient's skin condition (moisture). Normal skin is dry. Wet or moist skin may indicate shock, a heat-related illness, or a diabetic emergency. Excessively dry skin may indicate dehydration.

Capillary Refill

Assess capillary refill in infants and children younger than six years of age. To assess capillary refill, firmly press on the child's nail bed until it blanches (turns white) and then release (Figure 8-26). Observe the time it takes for the tissue to return to its original color. If the temperature of the environment is warm, color should return within two seconds. Other sites may be used to assess capillary refill, including the forehead, chest, abdomen, and fleshy part of the palm. A capillary refill time of three to five seconds is said to be *delayed.* This may indicate poor perfusion or exposure to cool temperatures. A capillary refill time of more than five seconds is said to be *markedly delayed* and suggests shock.

Identifying Priority Patients

Objective 15 ►

Determine if the patient requires on-scene stabilization or immediate transport with additional emergency care en route to a hospital. Patients who require immediate transport ("load and go") include the following:

- Patients who give a poor general impression
- Unresponsive patients
- Responsive patients who cannot follow commands
- Patients who have difficulty breathing
- Patients who are in shock
- Women who are undergoing a complicated childbirth
- Patients with chest pain and a systolic blood pressure less than 100 mm Hg
- Patients with uncontrolled bleeding
- Patients with severe pain anywhere

Providing an EMS Report

When you have completed your initial assessment, update the EMS unit responding to the scene with a brief report by phone or radio, if possible. Include the following patient information in your report:

- Number of patients
- Age and gender of the patient(s)
- Chief complaint
- Level of responsiveness
- Airway, breathing, and circulation status

Focused History and Physical Examination

After the initial assessment, you should obtain a SAMPLE history, complete a physical examination, and obtain baseline vital signs.

SAMPLE History

Objective 19 ▶

The **patient history** is the part of the patient assessment that provides pertinent facts about the patient's medical history. When possible, ask the patient questions. Try to avoid questions that the patient can answer with yes or no. Instead, ask questions that will give you as much information as possible. Then allow the patient time to answer. Do not anticipate what the patient is going to say and finish sentences for him. In some situations, the patient will not be able to answer your questions. For example, the patient may be unresponsive or too short of breath to provide detailed answers. If the patient is unresponsive, gather as much information as possible by looking at the scene. Also look for medical identification tags and question family members, coworkers, or others at the scene.

SAMPLE is a memory aid used to remind you of the information you should get from the patient. SAMPLE stands for

- *S*igns and symptoms
- *A*llergies
- *M*edications
- (Pertinent) *P*ast medical history
- *L*ast oral intake
- *E*vents leading to the injury or illness

With medical patients, take the patient's history before performing the physical exam. With trauma patients, perform the physical exam first.

Signs and Symptoms

A sign is any medical or trauma condition displayed by the patient that can be

- Seen, such as bleeding
- Heard, such as snoring or wheezing
- Smelled, such as an unusual breath odor
- Measured, such as a fast pulse or a fever
- Felt, such as cold skin

A symptom is any condition described by the patient. Examples of symptoms are nausea, shortness of breath, headache, and pain.

Allergies

Allergies are common and may be the reason you were called to the scene. Find out if the patient has an allergy to medications, food, environmental causes (such as pollen), and products (such as latex). Ask the patient (or bystanders if the patient is unresponsive),

- "Do you have any allergies to medications?"
- "Are you allergic to latex?"
- "Do you have any food allergies or allergies to pollen, dust, or grass?"

Check for a medical identification tag. The patient may be wearing a bracelet or necklace or carrying a wallet card that identifies a serious medical condition, allergies, or medications she is taking.

Medications

Find out if the patient is currently taking any medications. You will need to ask specific questions, because some patients do not consider some substances, such as vitamins and aspirin, to be medications. Questions to ask include

- Do you take any prescription medications? Is the medication prescribed for you? What is the medication for? When did you last take it? Are you taking birth control pills (if applicable)?
- Do you take any over-the-counter medications, such as aspirin, allergy medications, cough syrup, or vitamins? Do you take any herbs?
- Have you recently started taking any new medications? Have you recently stopped taking any medications?
- Do you use any recreational drugs (such as cocaine or marijuana)?

If the patient is taking medication, send the medication containers to the hospital with the patient. This action helps the hospital staff determine what his medical condition is, if he sees a doctor regularly, and if the patient has been taking the medication correctly.

Pertinent Past Medical History

Ask the patient about medical conditions he may have that would help you determine what the current problem is. If the patient is unresponsive, check for a medic alert tag. Questions to ask include the following:

- Are you seeing a doctor for any medical condition?
- Do you have a history of heart problems, respiratory problems, high blood pressure, diabetes, epilepsy, or another ongoing medical condition?
- Have you been in the hospital recently? Have you had any recent surgery?

Last Oral Intake

It is important to determine when the patient last ate or had anything to drink. This is especially important if the patient is a diabetic or may need immediate surgery. Determine what the patient last ate or drank, how much, and when.

Events Leading to the Injury or Illness

Ask the patient to tell you what happened. This information can provide important clues about the patient's current situation. For example, you arrive on the scene of a motor vehicle crash. After making sure there are no immediate life threats, you ask the patient what happened. She tells you she is a diabetic. She remembers taking her insulin this morning. She was running late for her doctor's appointment and did not have time to eat breakfast. She thinks she may have blacked out. The information provided by the patient tells you that although you must look for possible injuries due to the motor vehicle crash, some of the signs you will find during your physical exam may be caused by her medical condition.

If your patient is complaining of pain, OPQRST is a memory aid that may help identify the type and location of the patient's complaint:

- *O*nset: "What were you doing when the problem started?"
- *P*rovocation: "What makes the problem better or worse?"
- *Q*uality: "What does the pain feel like (dull, burning, sharp, stabbing, shooting, throbbing, pressure, or tearing)?"
- *R*egion/radiation: "Where is the pain?" "Is the pain in one area or does it move?" "Is the pain located in any other area?"
- *S*everity: "On a scale of 0 to 10, with 0 being the least and 10 being the worst, what number would you give your pain or discomfort?"
- *T*ime: "How long ago did the problem or discomfort begin?" "Have you ever had this pain before?" "When?" "How long did it last?"

Remember This!

SAMPLE History

*S*igns/symptoms
*A*llergies
*M*edications
*P*ertinent past medical history
*L*ast oral intake
*E*vents leading to the injury or illness

Detailed Physical Examination

Objective 16 ▶

Objective 27 ▶

The focused history and physical examination is also called the focused exam.

The term *physical examination* implies a head-to-toe assessment of the patient's entire body. A quick head-to-toe assessment of a trauma patient with a significant mechanism of injury is called a **rapid trauma assessment.** Seriously injured or unresponsive trauma patients require this type of physical exam in order to find out if they have life-threatening injuries.

Less seriously injured trauma patients do not require a head-to-toe physical exam. The term *focused physical examination* is used to describe an assessment of specific body areas that relate to the patient's illness or injury. For example, a physical examination of a patient with a cut finger would begin with an assessment of the injured body part. Other areas of the body would be examined as needed.

Making a Difference

Using the mechanism of injury, chief complaint, and initial assessment findings, you must be able to tell the difference between a seriously injured trauma patient who needs a rapid trauma assessment and a less seriously injured patient who needs a focused exam.

For an ill (medical) patient, perform a focused physical examination based on the patient's chief complaint as well as signs and symptoms.

The focused history and physical examination of a medical patient is guided by the patient's chief complaint and signs and symptoms. If your patient is responsive and ill, find out her medical history first. The information you receive will help guide where you look and what you are looking for in the focused physical exam. For example, if your patient is complaining of abdominal pain, your physical exam will be focused on that area. If your patient is unresponsive, perform a quick head-to-toe physical exam first. Doing so will help identify the patient's problem. Then proceed with getting the patient's vital signs. Try to get the patient's medical history from family, friends, and clues in the area. Some examples of clues are a "puffer" (inhaler), nitroglycerin tablets or other medications, and medical identification, such as a necklace or bracelet.

Remember This!

- If you find life-threatening injuries in the initial assessment, you may never get to perform the physical exam.
- If you find a serious injury, treat it when you find it.
- If the patient's condition worsens during the physical exam, go back and repeat the initial assessment. In such situations, you may never complete the physical exam.

Objective 29 ▶

Objective 30 ▶

Objective 31 ▶

Objective 32 ▶

Because it can cause pain, palpation should be performed last.

Be aware that your patient will be anxious about having his clothing removed and having an exam performed by a stranger. Ease your patient's fears by explaining what you are about to do and why it must be done. Remember to properly drape or shield an unclothed patient from the stares of others. Conduct the exam professionally and efficiently, and talk with the patient throughout the procedure. If your patient is a child, ask a parent or family member to help you. Doing so should lessen the child's anxiety.

When examining your patient, first look (inspect) and then feel (palpate) body areas to identify potential injuries. If you have a stethoscope, use it to listen to (auscultate) the movement of air into and out of the patient's lungs. If you have a stethoscope, perform the physical exam in the following order: inspect, auscultate, and feel.

DOTS is a helpful memory aid to remember what to look and feel for during a physical exam:

- *D*eformities
- *O*pen injuries
- *T*enderness
- *S*welling

Objective 17 ▶

A detailed (head-to-toe) physical examination is presented in Skill Drill 8-1. Remember that a focused physical exam may be more appropriate based on the patient's chief complaint, your initial assessment findings, and the mechanism of injury or the nature of the illness.

Begin the physical exam by checking the patient's head. Then examine the neck, chest, abdomen, pelvis, lower extremities, upper extremities, and back. Compare one side of the body with the other. For example, if an injury or a medical condition involves one side of the body, use the uninjured or uninvolved side as the normal finding for comparison.

Head

The head contains many blood vessels and wounds of the face or scalp may bleed heavily.

Before examining the head of a trauma patient, have someone stabilize the patient's head and neck to keep them from moving—if this has not already been done. Using your gloved hands, gently feel the patient's scalp for deformities, depressions, tenderness, and swelling (see Skill Drill 8-1, Step 1). Look for any open wounds or discolored areas. Run your fingers through the patient's hair and examine your gloves for the presence of blood. Gently slide your gloved hands behind the patient's head and feel for tenderness, swelling, or depressions that may indicate a skull fracture. If you feel a depression or an indentation in the skull, you may hear and feel crackling. This is called **crepitation** or **crepitus** and is caused by the grating of broken bone ends against each other. Control bleeding from a scalp wound by applying gentle, direct pressure with a dry, sterile dressing. If you suspect a skull fracture, do not apply direct pressure to the center of the wound. Doing so could force bone fragments down into the brain. Instead, apply gentle pressure around the edges of the wound and over a broad area.

Gently palpate the facial bones (see Skill Drill 8-1, Step 2). Look for bluish discoloration around the eyes (raccoon eyes). This sign suggests a possible skull fracture. Check that both sides of the face appear the same. In a patient who has had a stroke, one side of the face may appear to droop.

If you have one, use a penlight or flashlight to look in the ears, nose, and mouth and to examine the eyes.

Look for injury to the eyes, but do not touch the eyes to determine if an injury is present. Look at the color of the whites of the eyes (the sclerae). A yellow discoloration (jaundice) suggests liver disease. Check the size and shape of the pupils (see Skill Drill 8-1, Step 3). The pupils are normally equal and round, and they react briskly to light.

Look for blood or fluid leaking from the ears (see Skill Drill 8-1, Step 4). If fluid is observed in the ears, do not attempt to stop the flow. Cover the ear

Skill Drill 8-1

Performing a Detailed Physical Assessment

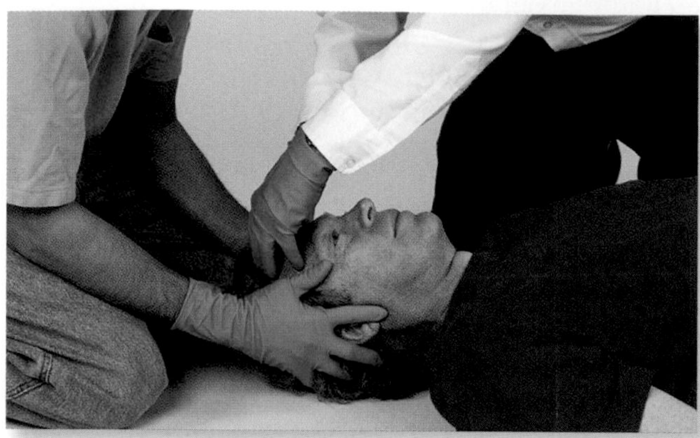

STEP 1 ▲ Using your gloved hands, gently feel the patient's scalp for deformities, depressions, tenderness, and swelling. Look for any open wounds or discoloration.

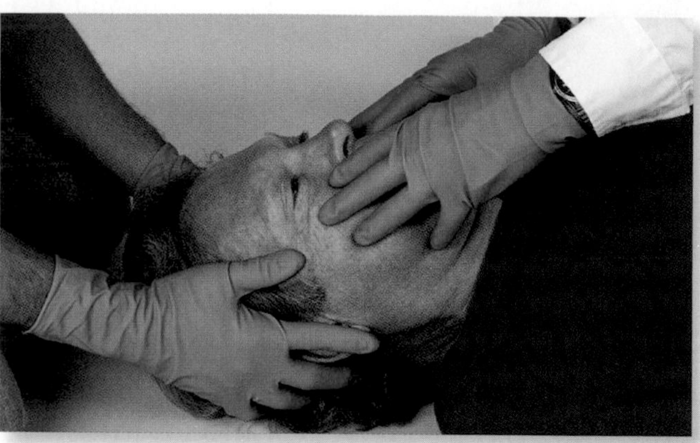

STEP 2 ▲ Gently palpate the facial bones.

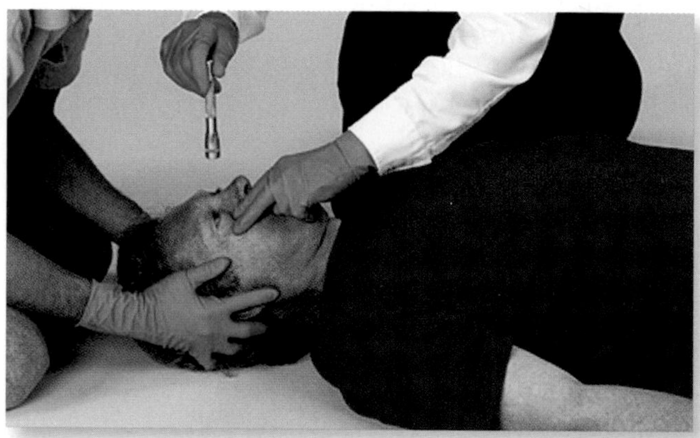

STEP 3 ▲ Look at the size and shape of the pupils and their response to light.

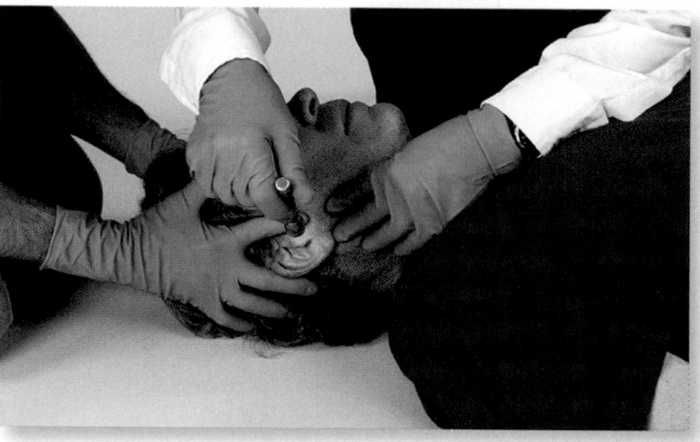

STEP 4 ▲ Look for blood or fluid leaking from the ears.

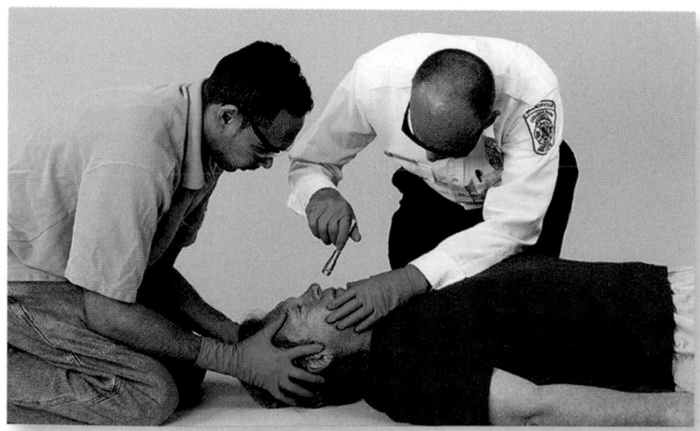

STEP 5 ▲ Look for blood or fluid from the nose and singed nasal hairs.

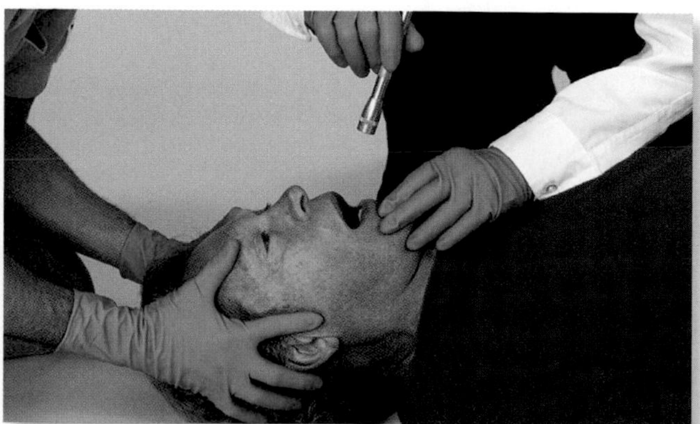

STEP 6 ▲ Look in the mouth for blood, vomitus, loose teeth, or foreign material.

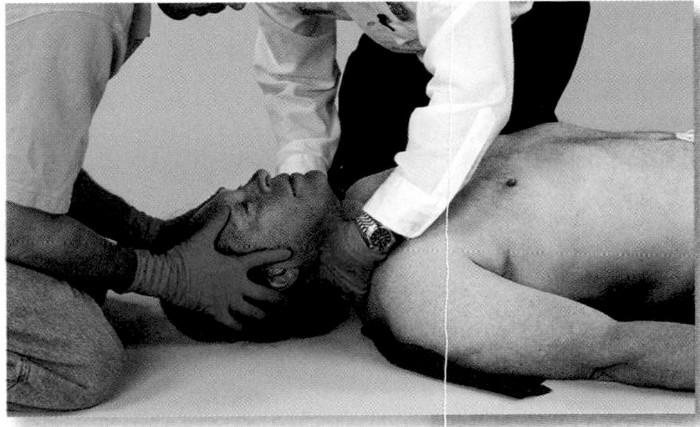

STEP 7 ▲ Gently feel the front and back of the neck to detect areas of tenderness or deformity.

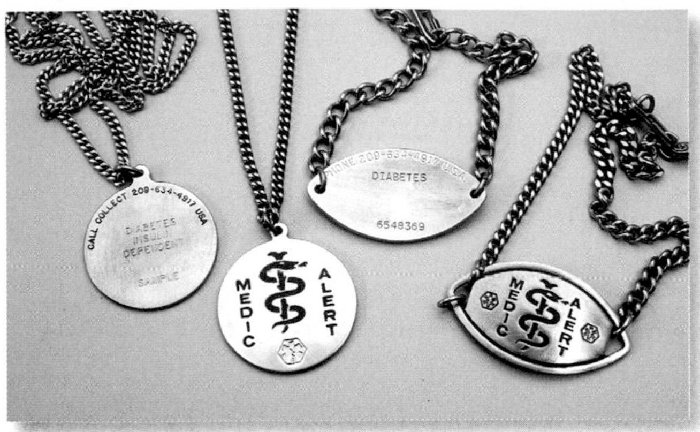

STEP 8 ▲ Medical alert tags may be worn on a necklace or bracelet. These ID tags contain important medical information, including the patient's medical condition, important prescription medications, and allergies.

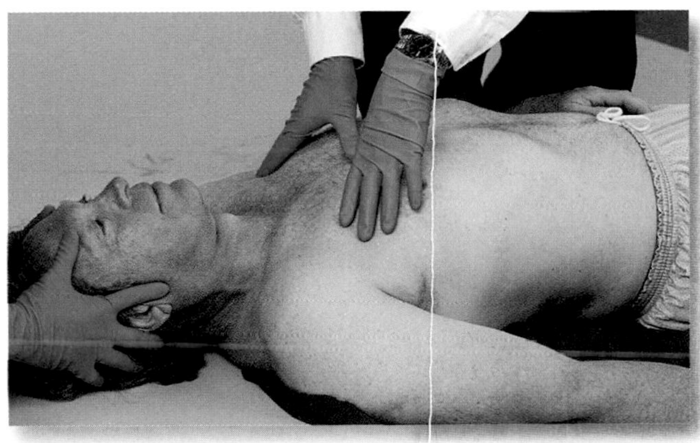

STEP 9 ▲ Feel the collarbones, shoulders, breastbone, and ribs for tenderness and deformity.

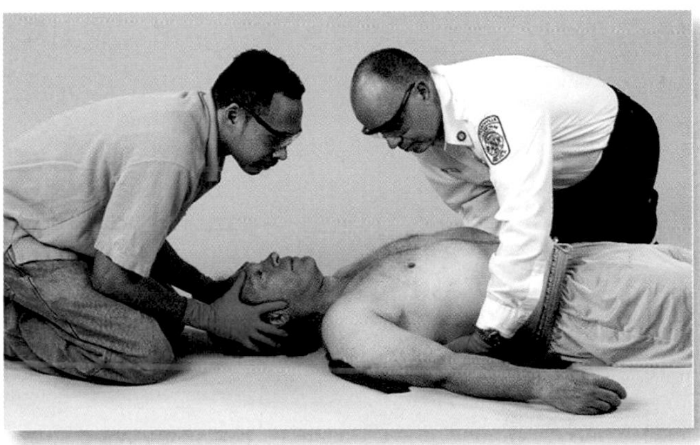

STEP 10 ▲ Gently reach under the patient to assess the back of the chest.

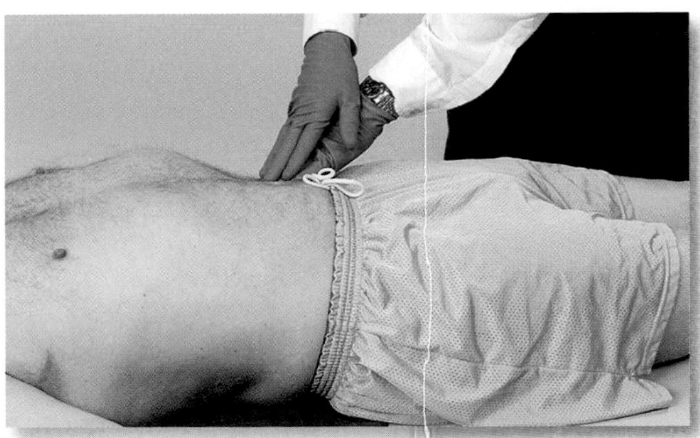

STEP 11 ▲ Using the pads of your fingers, gently feel the upper and lower areas of the abdomen for injuries or tenderness.

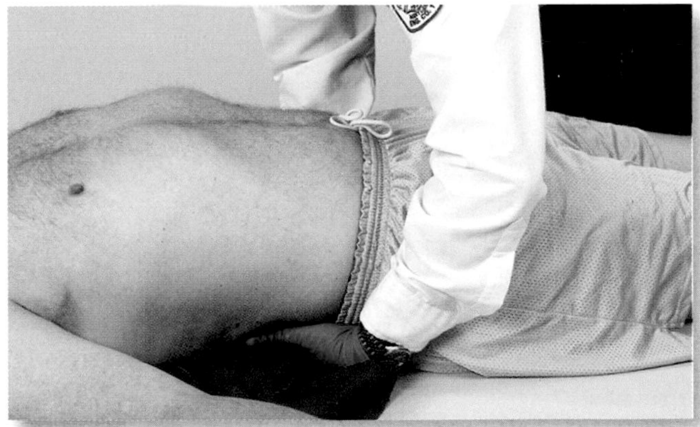

STEP 12 ▲ Gently reach under the patient to assess the lower back.

Continued on next page

Skill Drill 8-1

Performing a Detailed Physical Assessment *(continued)*

STEP 13 ▶ If the patient has not complained of pain and there are no obvious signs of pelvic injury, assess the pelvis by applying gentle, downward pressure on the pubic bone.

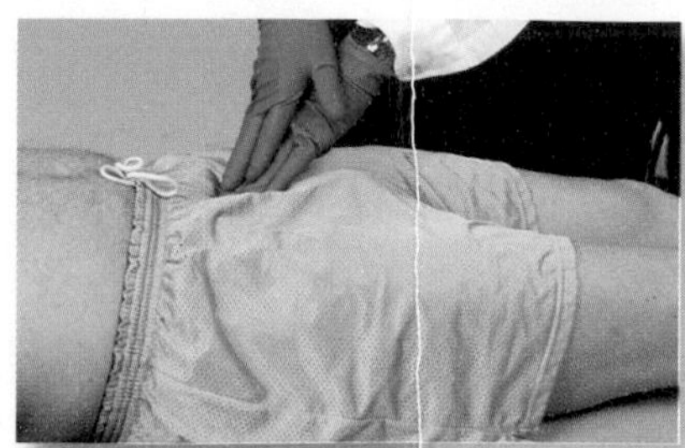

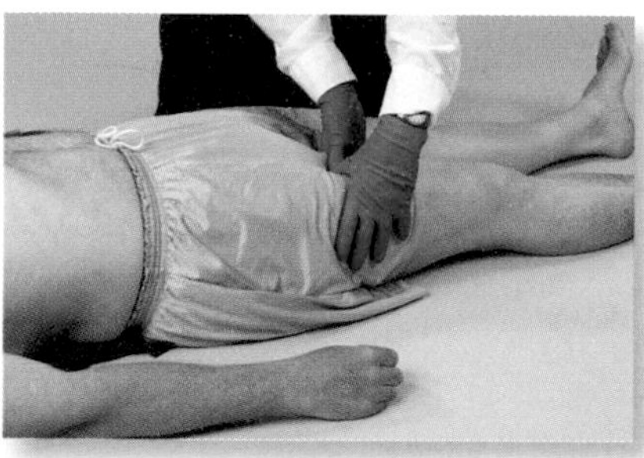

STEP 14 ▲ Examine the upper leg.

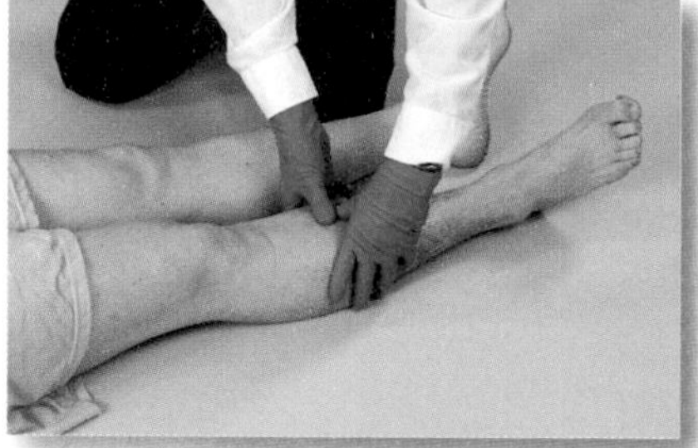

▲ Examine the lower leg.

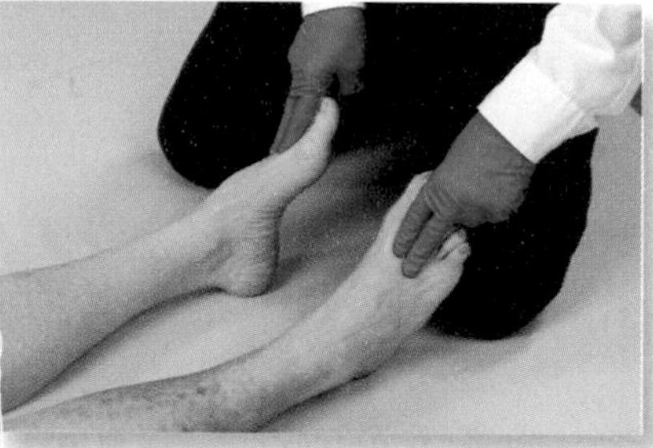

▲ Assess the dorsalis pedis pulse in each lower extremity. Remember to assess movement and sensation in each extremity.

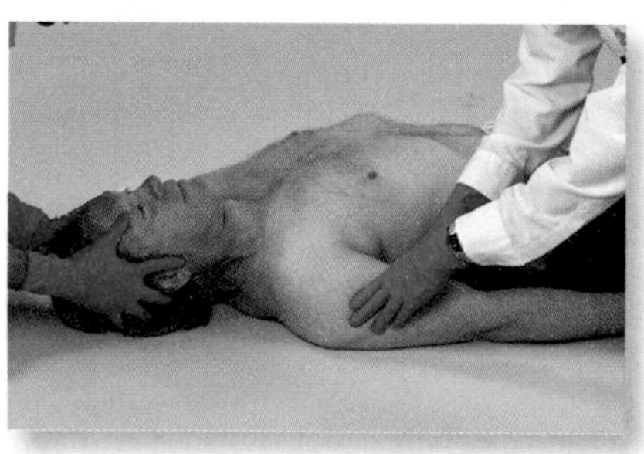

STEP 15 ▲ Examine the upper arm.

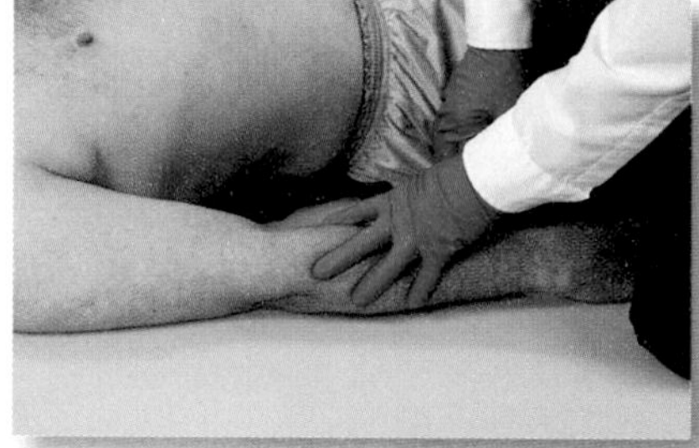

▲ Examine the lower arm.

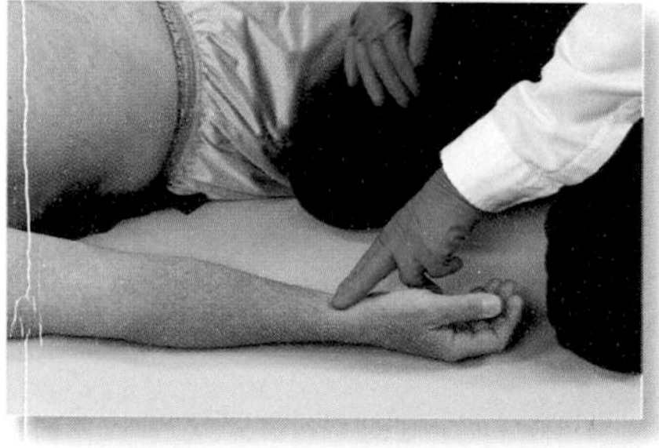

▲ Assess the radial pulse in each upper extremity.

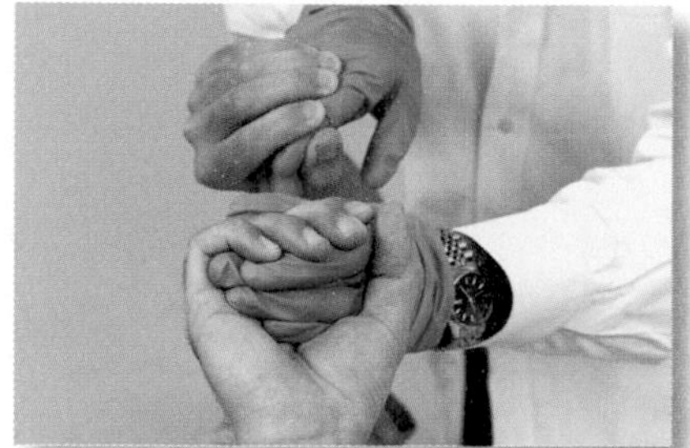

STEP 16 ▲

If the patient is awake, assess movement by asking the patient to squeeze your fingers.

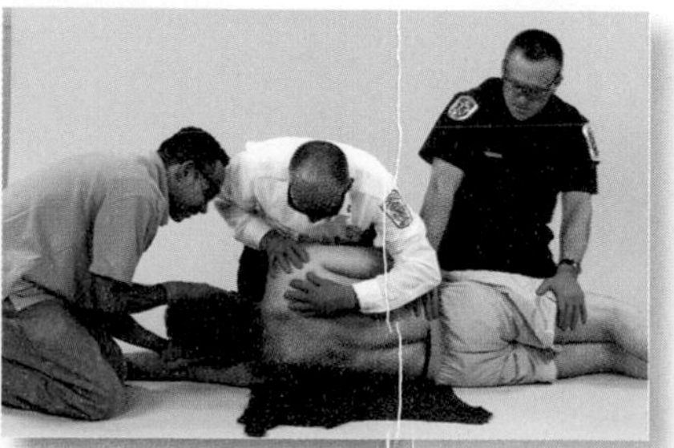

STEP 17 ▲

If there are enough personnel on the scene, log-roll the patient to assess the patient's back.

with a loose, sterile dressing. A bluish discoloration behind the ear (Battle's sign) is a sign of a possible skull fracture. Look for blood or fluid from the nose (see Skill Drill 8-1, Step 5). Also look for singed nasal hairs, which suggest a possible airway burn. Feel for stability of the bones of the nose. Look in the mouth for blood; vomitus; absent, broken, or loose teeth; and foreign material (see Skill Drill 8-1, Step 6). Look at the color of the inside of the mouth. Check if the tongue is injured or swollen. Make a note of any odors, such as alcohol. Suction the mouth to clear the airway if necessary.

Neck

Look at the neck for open wounds or the presence of a **stoma.** Gently feel the front and back of the neck to detect areas of tenderness or deformity (see Skill Drill 8-1, Step 7). Look for a medical ID (see Skill Drill 8-1, Step 8). Medical alert tags may be worn on a necklace or bracelet. These ID tags contain important medical information, such as the patient's medical condition, important prescription medications, and allergies.

If there is an open wound of the neck, cover the wound with an airtight (occlusive) dressing to prevent air from entering the wound. Examine the front and back of the neck of a trauma patient. Apply a cervical immobilization device if you have the equipment available, know how to apply it properly, and a spinal injury is suspected. Ask another responder to continue to maintain in-line spinal stabilization while you continue the assessment. Remember, once begun, manual stabilization must continue until additional help arrives and the patient has been completely immobilized on a long backboard.

Chest

It may be necessary to remove the patient's clothing to examine the patient's chest. Protect the patient's privacy and shield him or her from curious onlookers.

Assess the patient's work of breathing. Look for an equal rise and fall of the chest, bruises, open wounds, surgical scars, and obvious deformities. Look for uneven chest movement or evidence of difficulty breathing. If you see an open chest wound, immediately cover it with your gloved hand and then apply an airtight dressing. Tape the dressing to the chest on three sides. Leave the fourth side open to allow air to escape but not enter the wound. If the patient appears to worsen after covering the wound with the dressing (or your hand), remove it to let air escape. Then reapply your hand or the dressing to the wound. If you see an object impaled in the chest, such as a knife, do not try to remove it. Removing it can result in bleeding and the entry of air into the chest. Leave the object in place and stabilize it there with bulky dressings.

If you have been trained to use a stethoscope, listen to the movement of air into and out of the patient's lungs. Comparing from side to side, determine if breath sounds are present or absent, equal or unequal, clear or noisy. If you do not have a stethoscope and the patient is responsive, ask the patient to take a deep breath and then blow out the air. Watch and listen to see if the patient has any signs of difficulty breathing or pain with breathing.

Gently feel the collarbones, shoulders, breastbone, and ribs for tenderness and deformity (see Skill Drill 8-1, Step 9). Gently reach under the patient to assess the back of the chest (see Skill Drill 8-1, Step 10). Examine your gloves for the presence of blood.

Abdomen

Distention (swelling) can be caused by blood, fluid, or air. It is difficult to assess in obese patients.

When assessing the abdomen, look for the following:

- Surgical scars
- Bruising
- Open wounds

- Protruding abdominal organs
- An impaled object
- Signs of obvious pregnancy

Check if the abdomen appears distended (larger than normal). If exposed abdominal organs are present, do not attempt to reinsert them into the abdominal cavity. Cover them with a moist, sterile dressing. If you see an object impaled in the abdomen, leave the object in place and stabilize it there with bulky dressings.

During your examination, watch the patient's facial expression for signs of tenderness.

The abdomen is normally soft and is not painful or tender to touch. To examine the abdomen, place one hand on top of the other. Use the pads of the fingers of your lower hand and gently feel the upper and lower areas of the abdomen for injuries or tenderness (see Skill Drill 8-1, Step 11). If the patient is responsive, ask him to point to the area that hurts (point tenderness). Assess the area that hurts last. Determine if the abdomen feels soft or firm. Gently reach under the patient to assess the lower back (see Skill Drill 8-1, Step 12). Examine your gloves for the presence of blood.

Pelvis

Do not rock the pelvis.

The pelvic area contains large blood vessels. Therefore, an injury to the pelvic ring can result in life-threatening internal and external bleeding. If the patient complains of pain in the pelvic area or if obvious deformity is present, do *not* palpate or compress the pelvis. If the patient has not complained of pain and there are no obvious signs of pelvic injury, assess the pelvis by directing gentle downward pressure on the pubic bone using the heel of one hand (see Skill Drill 8-1, Step 13). If applying pressure results in tenderness, instability, or crepitation, suspect a pelvic fracture. When examining the pelvic area, check if the patient lost control of his bowels or bladder. This may occur in patients who experience a seizure, stroke, or cardiac arrest.

Remember This!

If the patient complains of pain in the pelvic area or if obvious deformity is present, do *not* palpate or compress the pelvis. Do not move the patient unless absolutely necessary until additional EMS personnel arrive.

Extremities

Check PMS in each extremity. PMS = pulse, movement, and sensation. Compare each extremity to the opposite extremity.

Look for open wounds, swelling, and abnormal positioning, such as unequal lengths. Look at the wrists and ankles for a medical ID tag. Gently examine the upper and lower portions of each extremity for bone or joint deformities and tissue swelling. Assess circulation in each extremity by feeling for pulses. Assess the dorsalis pedis pulse (on the top of the foot) in each lower extremity (see Skill Drill 8-1, Step 14). Assess the radial pulse in each upper extremity (see Skill Drill 8-1, Step 15).

Objective 18 ▶

Assess movement and sensation in each extremity. If the patient is awake, assess movement of the lower extremities by asking if the patient can push both feet into your hands at the same time. Assess movement of the upper extremities by asking the patient to squeeze your fingers, using both of the patient's hands at the same time (see Skill Drill 8-1, Step 16). Compare the strength of the patient's grips and note if they are equal or if one side appears weaker. If the patient is awake, assess sensation by touching the hands and toes of each extremity and asking the patient to tell you where you are touching. If the patient is unresponsive, assess movement and sensation by applying a pinch to each foot and hand. See if the patient responds to pain with facial or extremity movements.

Making a Difference

Assess the presence of pulses, movement, and sensation in each of your patient's extremities *before* and *after* immobilization. Make sure to document your findings.

Back

If there are enough personnel on the scene, log-roll the patient to assess the patient's back (see Skill Drill 8-1, Step 17). Make sure to maintain in-line spinal stabilization while rolling the patient. Look for obvious deformities, open wounds, and swelling. Feel for swelling, tenderness, instability, and crepitation. If there are any open wounds, cover them with an airtight dressing.

Vital Signs

Vital signs are assessments of breathing, pulse, temperature, pupils, and blood pressure. Measuring vital signs is an important part of patient assessment. Vital signs are measured to

- Detect changes in normal body function
- Recognize life-threatening situations
- Determine a patient's response to treatment

Baseline vital signs are an initial set of vital sign measurements. Later measurements are compared against baseline vital signs. When possible, take two or more sets of vital signs. Doing so will allow you to note changes (trends) in the patient's condition and response to treatment. For example, after obtaining the first set of vital signs (the baseline), you will be able to spot if the patient's heart rate is increasing, staying about the same, or decreasing when you take them the second or third time. Watching these trends in your patient's condition is very important. With this information and your patient assessment findings, you will be able to recognize life-threatening emergencies, such as shock.

To take a patient's vital signs, you will need

- A watch with a second hand or a digital watch that shows seconds. This will be used to count your patient's respirations and pulse as well as to note the time of events for your documentation.
- A penlight or flashlight. This will be used to look at your patient's pupils.
- A **stethoscope.** A stethoscope is an instrument used to hear sounds within the body, such as respirations. It is also used to measure blood pressure.
- A blood pressure cuff **(sphygmomanometer)** to take your patient's blood pressure
- A pen and paper to record your findings

Not all Emergency Medical Responders are expected to take a patient's blood pressure.

Pulse

To feel for a pulse,

- Use the pads of your index and middle fingers and apply gentle pressure to the artery (Figure 8-27). If you use too much pressure, you will cut off blood flow through the artery and will not be able to feel a pulse.
- Count the number of beats for 30 seconds. Then multiply the number by 2 to determine the number of beats per minute. If the pulse is irregular, count it for 1 full minute. Normal pulse rates for patients at rest are shown in Table 8-6.

The pads on the tips of the finger are used to detect a pulse, because they are the most sensitive areas. Do not use your thumb to assess a pulse—it has a pulse of its own and could be mistaken for the patient's pulse.

A patient's pulse rate varies with age and physical condition. When checking the pulse, note if the pulse rate feels very slow, very fast, or within the normal range

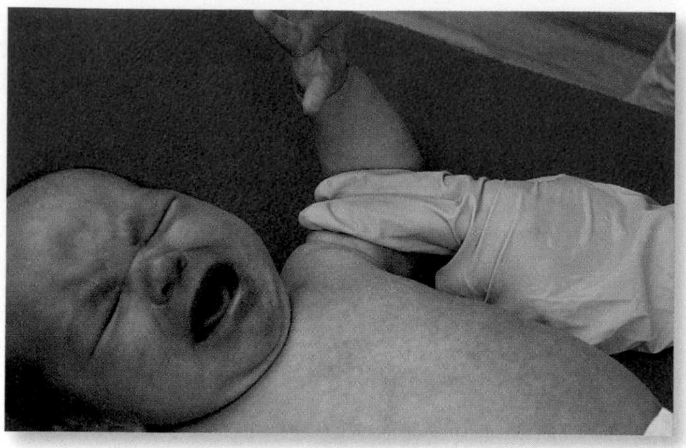

FIGURE 8-27 ▶ To feel for a pulse, use the pads of your index and third fingers and apply gentle pressure to the artery.

for the patient's age. Also note if the rhythm of the pulse is regular or irregular. A slow heart rate may be normal in well-conditioned athletes. However, a slow heart rate may occur because of a medical or trauma-related problem. A fast heart rate occurs as a normal response to the body's demand for more oxygen.

You Should Know

Possible Causes of a Slow Heart Rate

- Coughing
- Vomiting
- Straining to have a bowel movement
- Heart attack
- Head injury
- Very low body temperature (hypothermia)
- Sleep apnea
- Some medications

Possible Causes of a Rapid Heart Rate

- Fever
- Fear
- Pain
- Anxiety
- Infection
- Shock
- Exercise
- Heart failure
- Substances such as caffeine and nicotine
- Drugs such as cocaine, amphetamines, Ecstasy, and cannabis
- Some medications

Pulse quality refers to the strength of the heartbeat felt when taking a pulse.

A normal pulse is easily felt and the pressure is equal for each beat. This kind of pulse is said to be a strong pulse. A pulse is said to be weak if it is hard to feel. A pulse that is weak and fast is called a thready pulse. Pulses are normally of equal strength on both sides of the body.

TABLE 8-6 Normal Pulse Rates at Rest

	Age	Beats per Minute
Newborn	Birth to 1 month	120 to 160
Infant	1 to 12 months	80 to 140
Toddler	1 to 3 years	80 to 130
Preschooler	4 to 5 years	80 to 120
School-age child	6 to 12 years	70 to 110
Adolescent	13 to 18 years	60 to 100
Adult	18 years and older	60 to 100

Respirations

Respiration is the act of breathing air into the lungs (inhalation) and out of the lungs (exhalation). A single respiration consists of one inhalation and one exhalation. During inhalation, the chest rises and oxygen is taken into the lungs. During exhalation, the chest falls and carbon dioxide is moved out of the lungs.

To count a patient's respirations,

- Place the patient's arm across his chest or abdomen. Hold the patient's wrist as if you were assessing the radial pulse. Watch the rise and fall of the chest or abdomen. Begin counting when the chest or abdomen rises. Count each rise and fall of the chest or abdomen as one respiration (Figure 8-28). Watch to see if respirations are regular and if the chest rises equally.
- Count respirations for 30 seconds. Multiply the number by 2 to determine the rate for 1 minute. If the patient's respirations are irregular or slow, count the rate for 1 full minute.
- In infants and young children, it is often easier to observe the rise and fall of the abdomen to determine the respiratory rate. Count an infant's respirations for 1 full minute.

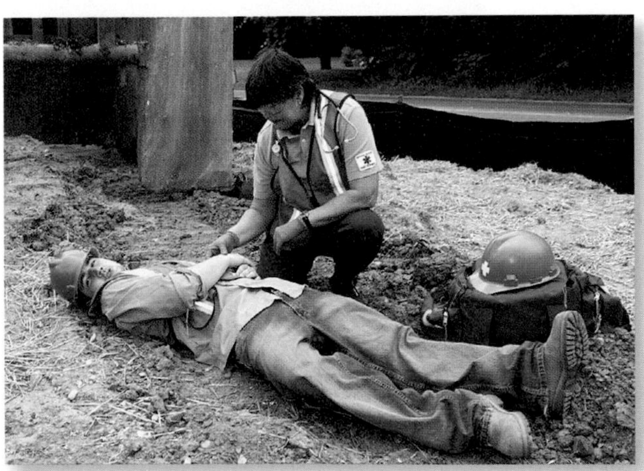

FIGURE 8-28 ► Counting a patient's respiratory rate.

Remember This!

- Do not tell the patient you are counting the respiratory rate. The patient may vary his or her breathing without realizing it if he or she knows it is being assessed.
- Make it a habit to count the patient's pulse first. When you have finished, keep your hands in place but shift your attention to the patient's chest and abdomen and count the respiratory rate.

The normal respiratory rates for an adult, a child, and an infant at rest are shown in Table 8-7. The number of respirations per minute can be influenced by many factors. For example, exercise, stress, anxiety, pain, fever, and the use of stimulants can increase the respiratory rate. The use of narcotics or sedatives decreases the respiratory rate.

Normal respirations are evenly spaced and of adequate depth. Infants and young children tend to breathe less regularly than adults do. Irregular respirations may be associated with conditions such as a diabetic emergency or a head injury. A patient is said to breathe *shallowly* if it is difficult to see movement of the chest or abdomen during breathing. Only a small volume of air is exchanged during shallow breathing.

Normal breathing is relaxed and effortless. *Labored* breathing is an increase in the work (effort) of breathing. If a patient is having difficulty breathing, he is usually irritable, anxious, or restless. You may see the following signs during labored breathing (Figure 8-29):

- Gasping for air
- Excessive widening of the nostrils with respiration (nasal flaring)
- The use of the neck muscles to assist with inhalation
- The use of the abdominal muscles and the muscles between the ribs to assist with exhalation
- A sinking in of the soft tissues between and around the ribs or above the collarbones (retractions)
- Skin color changes (blue, or cyanotic, skin)

Normal breathing is quiet. While counting the patient's respirations, listen for any abnormal respiratory sounds. Abnormal respiratory sounds include

TABLE 8-7 Normal Respiratory Rates at Rest

	Age	Breaths per Minute
Newborn	Birth to 1 month	30 to 50
Infant	1 to 12 months	20 to 40
Toddler	1 to 3 years	20 to 30
Preschooler	4 to 5 years	20 to 30
School-age child	6 to 12 years	16 to 30
Adolescent	13 to 18 years	12 to 20
Adult	18 years and older	12 to 20

FIGURE 8-29 ▶ Signs of respiratory distress.

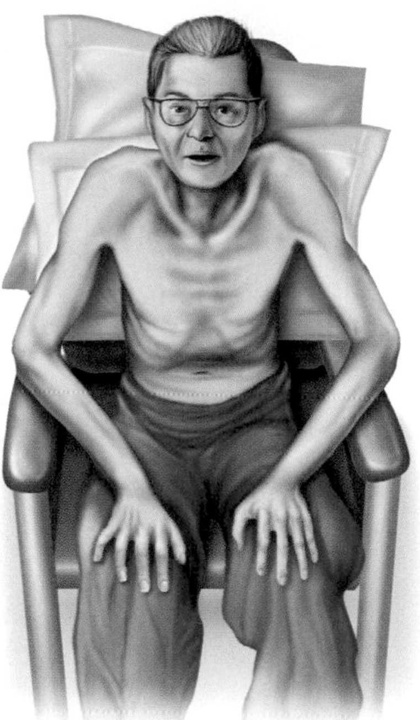

- **Stridor,** which is a harsh, high-pitched sound (like the bark of a seal). Stridor is associated with severe upper airway obstruction and is most often heard during inhalation.
- **Snoring,** which results from partial obstruction of the upper airway by the tongue
- **Wheezing,** which is a high-pitched whistling sound heard on inhalation or exhalation. This sound suggests a narrowed or partially obstructed airway.
- **Gurgling,** which is the sound heard as air passes through moist secretions in the airway
- **Crowing,** which is a long, high-pitched sound heard on inhalation

Pupils

Examine the patient's pupils. The pupils are normally equal in size, round, and equally reactive to light (Figure 8-30). Briefly shine a light into the patient's eyes and assess the size, equality, and reactivity of the patient's pupils.

- *Size.* Dilated (very big) pupils in the presence of bright light may be due to trauma, fright, poisoning, eye medications, or glaucoma. Constricted (small) pupils in a darkened area may be caused by narcotics, treatment with eye drops, or a nervous system problem.
- *Equality.* Unequal pupils are a normal finding in 2–4% of the population. In most patients, unequal pupils suggest a head injury, a stroke, the presence of an artificial eye, or cataract surgery on one eye.
- *Reactivity.* *Reactivity* refers to whether or not the pupils change in response to light. Normally, a light that is shined into the pupil of one eye will cause the pupils of both eyes to constrict. Nonreactive pupils do not change when exposed to light. This condition may occur due to medications or cardiac arrest. Unequally reactive pupils (one pupil reacts but the other does not) may occur because of a head injury or stroke.

Blood Pressure

Blood pressure is abbreviated *BP*.

Blood pressure is the force exerted by the blood on the walls of the arteries. Blood pressure is usually assessed using a blood pressure cuff and stethoscope.

FIGURE 8-30 ▶ Assess the size, equality, and reactivity of your patient's pupils.

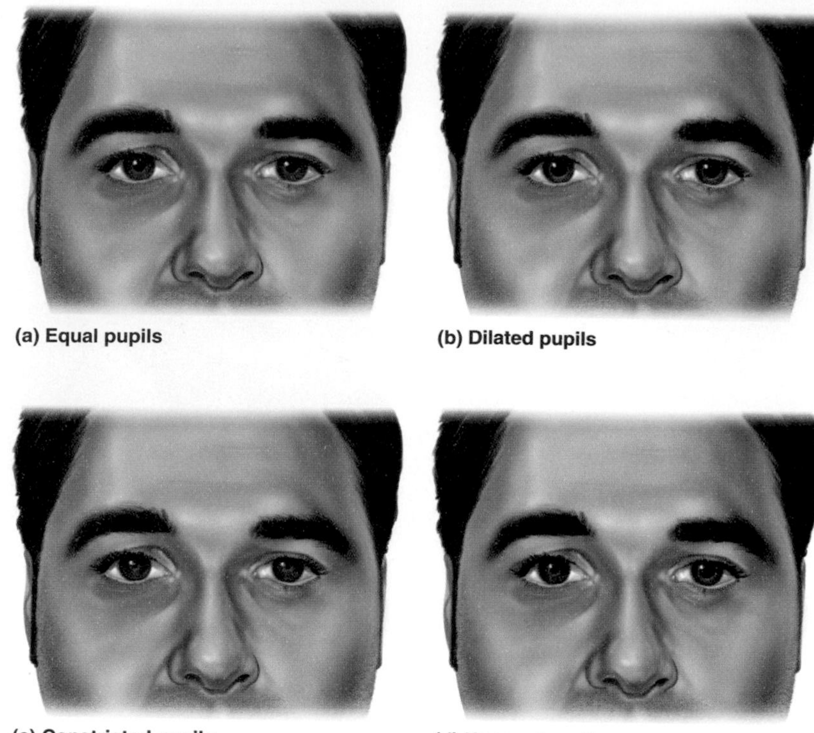

This method of taking a blood pressure is called *blood pressure by auscultation* because it involves the use of a stethoscope.

When a blood pressure cuff is applied to a patient's arm and inflated, blood flow in the artery under the cuff is momentarily cut off. If a stethoscope is applied over the artery, sounds can be heard that reflect the patient's blood pressure. As the cuff is slowly deflated, blood flow resumes through the partially compressed artery. The first sound heard is the systolic pressure. **Systolic pressure** is the pressure in an artery when the heart is pumping blood. As the pressure in the cuff continues to drop, a point is reached in which sounds are no longer heard because the artery is no longer compressed. The point at which the sound disappears is the diastolic pressure. **Diastolic pressure** is the pressure in an artery when the heart is at rest. A blood pressure measurement is made up of both the systolic and the diastolic pressure. It is written as a fraction (115/78), with the systolic number first. Skill Drill 8-2 explains how to assess a patient's blood pressure by auscultation.

Sometimes the presence of noise on the scene makes it impossible to hear sounds through a stethoscope. In such situations, assess the patient's blood pressure by palpation. Skill Drill 8-3 explains how to assess a patient's blood pressure using this method. When a blood pressure is obtained by palpation, the diastolic pressure cannot be measured. Document the patient's blood pressure as the systolic pressure over a capital *P*, such as 110/P.

Many factors can influence a patient's blood pressure. For example, anxiety, fear, fever, pain, emotional stress, and obesity increase blood pressure. Blood loss may decrease blood pressure. Table 8-8 shows normal blood pressures for patients of different ages.

When taking a blood pressure, it is important to use a blood pressure cuff of the correct size. The width of the cuff should not be more than two-thirds the length of the patient's upper arm. Blood pressure readings will be wrong if the cuff is the wrong size.

Measuring Blood Pressure by Auscultation

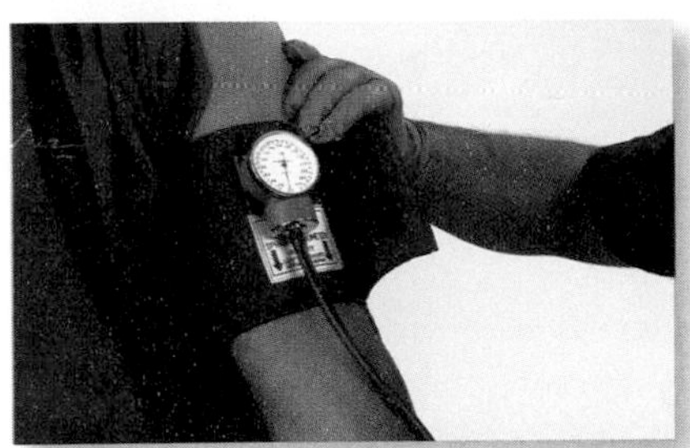

STEP 1 ▲

- Expose the patient's upper arm. Select the correct size of blood pressure cuff for the patient.
- Wrap the pressure cuff evenly around the patient's upper arm at least 1 inch above the elbow. Place the arrow on the cuff over the patient's brachial artery.

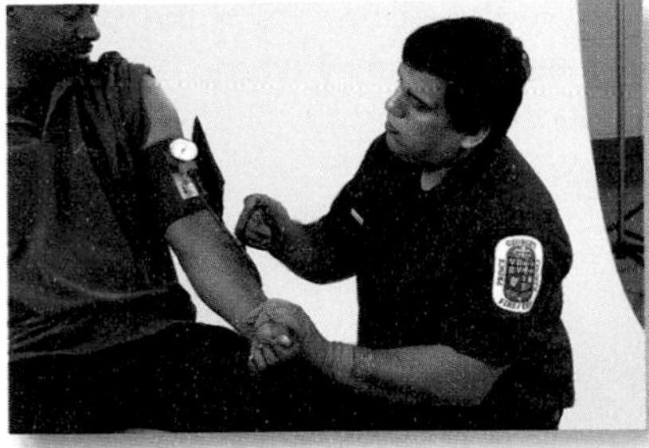

STEP 2 ▲

- Locate the patient's radial artery.
- Rapidly inflate the cuff until you can no longer feel the radial pulse. Inflate the cuff 30 mm Hg beyond the point at which you last felt the pulse.

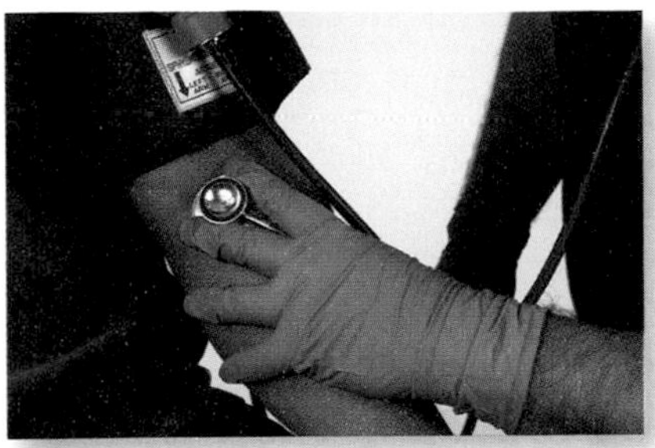

STEP 3 ▲

- Place the stethoscope in your ears.
- Place the diaphragm of the stethoscope over the brachial artery and hold it in place.

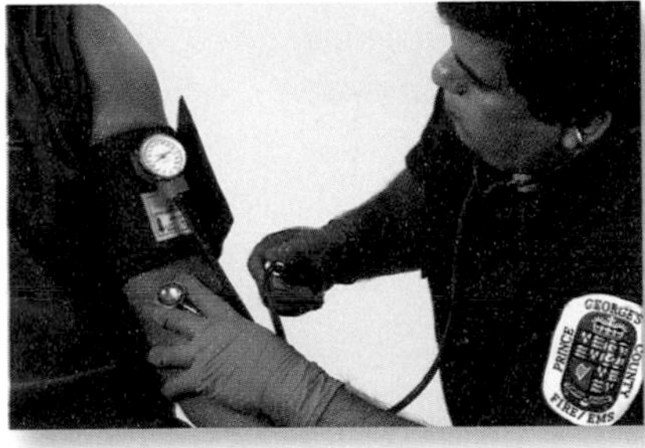

STEP 4 ▲

- While watching the gauge, deflate the cuff slowly and evenly at a rate of 2–3 mm Hg per second.
- Listen for sounds. The first sound is the systolic pressure and should be near the point at which the radial pulse disappeared.

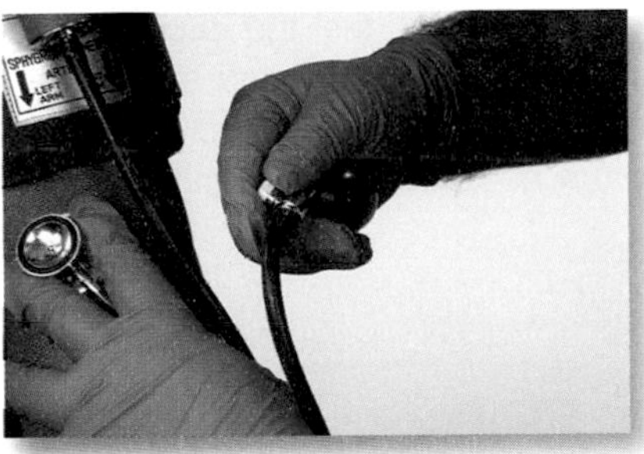

STEP 5 ▲

Continue to deflate the cuff, noting the point at which the sound disappears. This is the diastolic pressure.

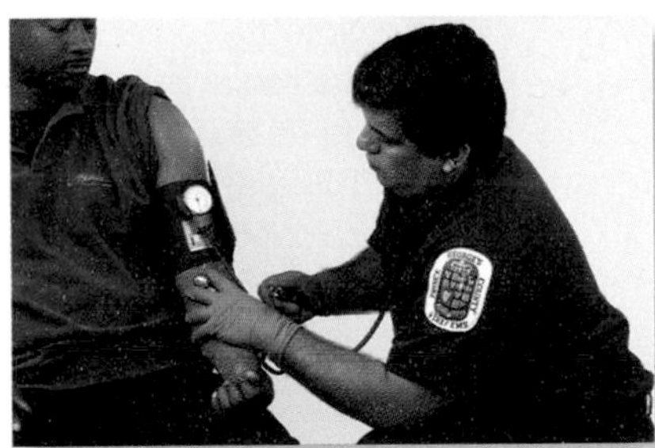

STEP 6 ▲

- Deflate the cuff completely.
- Record the blood pressure as systolic/diastolic pressure.

Skill Drill 8-3

Measuring Blood Pressure by Palpation

STEP 1 ▶
- Expose the patient's upper arm. Select the correct size of blood pressure cuff for the patient.
- Wrap the pressure cuff evenly around the patient's upper arm at least 1 inch above the elbow. Place the arrow on the cuff over the patient's brachial artery.

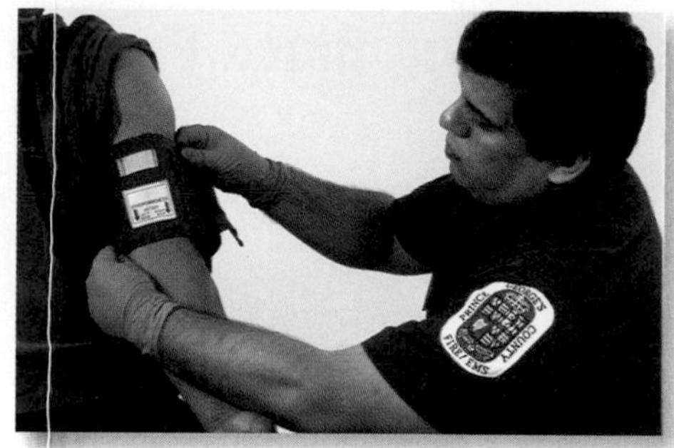

STEP 2 ▶
- Locate the patient's radial artery.
- Rapidly inflate the cuff until you can no longer feel the radial pulse. Inflate the cuff 30 mm Hg beyond the point at which you last felt the pulse.

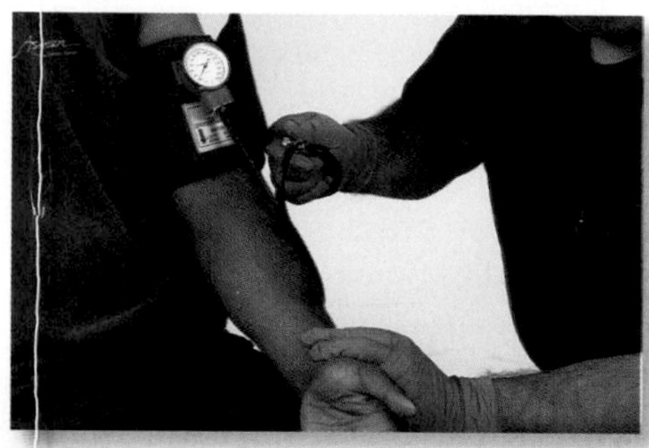

STEP 3 ▶
- While watching the gauge, deflate the cuff slowly and evenly at a rate of 2–3 mm Hg per second.
- Note the point on the gauge when you feel the return of the radial pulse. This is the systolic pressure and should be near the point at which the radial pulse disappeared. The diastolic pressure cannot be accurately measured by palpation.

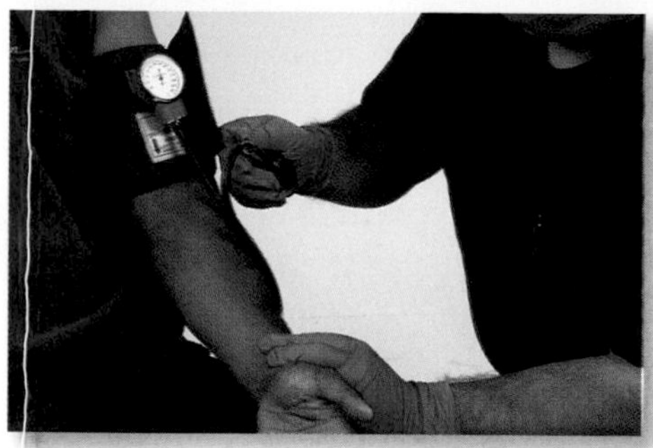

STEP 4 ▶
- Deflate the cuff completely.
- Record the blood pressure as systolic/P (for example, 148/P).

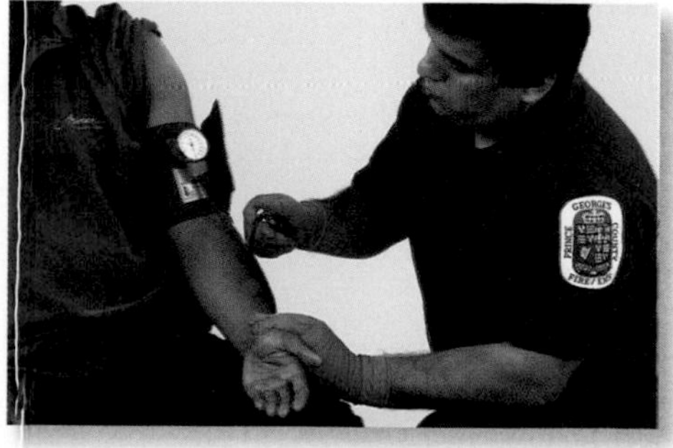

TABLE 8-8 Normal Blood Pressure Rates at Rest

	Age	Systolic Pressure	Diastolic Pressure
Newborn	Birth to 1 month	74 to 100	50 to 68
Infant	1 to 12 months	84 to 106	56 to 70
Toddler	1 to 3 years	98 to 106	50 to 70
Preschooler	4 to 5 years	98 to 112	64 to 70
School-age child	6 to 12 years	104 to 124	64 to 80
Adolescent	13 to 18 years	118 to 132	70 to 82
Adult	18 years and older	118 to 132	60 to 79

Remember This!

Common Errors in Blood Pressure Measurement

Errors That Produce a Falsely Low Reading

- The patient's arm is above the level of the heart.
- The cuff is too wide.

Errors That Produce a Falsely High Reading

- The cuff is deflated too slowly.
- The patient's arm is unsupported.
- The cuff is too narrow.
- The cuff is wrapped too loosely or unevenly.

Errors That Produce Either Falsely High or Low Readings

- Retaking a blood pressure too quickly may produce a falsely high systolic or low diastolic reading. Wait 2–3 minutes before reinflating the cuff.
- Deflating the cuff too quickly may produce a falsely low systolic and high diastolic reading. Deflate the cuff at a rate of 2–3 mm Hg per second.

For an unstable patient, vital signs should be assessed and recorded every 5 minutes. At a minimum, for a stable patient, vital signs should be assessed and recorded every 15 minutes. Remember, a stable patient can become unstable very quickly. Reassess frequently.

Remember This!

Learning to take accurate vital signs is very important. Because vital signs allow you to detect changes in your patient's condition, take them often.

Ongoing Assessment

Objective 20 ▶

While awaiting additional EMS resources, continue to assess the patient. Repeat the initial assessment every 15 minutes for a stable patient and every 5 minutes for an unstable patient. Reassess the patient's mental status and maintain an

Objective 28 ▶

open airway. Monitor the patient's breathing, pulse, skin color, temperature, and condition. Repeat the physical exam as needed. Check the treatments you provide to be sure that they are effective. Continue to calm and reassure the patient.

When EMS personnel arrive, provide a "hand-off" report. The information in your report should include the following patient information:

Objective 21 ▶

- Age and gender
- Chief complaint
- Level of responsiveness
- Airway and breathing status
- Circulation status
- Physical findings
- SAMPLE history
- Treatment provided
- Current condition

On The Scene

Wrap-Up

A quick head-to-toe exam is all you have time for before the ambulance arrives. You notice that the patient's tongue is cut and his pants are wet. He is wearing a medical necklace that says he has epilepsy. You help the ambulance crew remove the patient from the vehicle and secure him to a long backboard. As soon as the patient is loaded in the ambulance, the Paramedic places an oxygen mask on the patient. He asks you to cut off the patient's clothing, so that he can perform a more complete assessment. After the patient is exposed, you cover him with blankets and take his blood pressure. A second Paramedic carefully assesses the patient from head to toe to find any additional injuries. The patient has become progressively more alert since the Paramedics arrived. As they prepare to leave the scene, you hear the patient say he has not taken his seizure medicine for several days because he could not afford the prescription. ■

Sum It Up

- ▶ As an Emergency Medical Responder, you must look quickly at the entire scene before approaching the patient. You must size up the scene to find out if there are any threats that may cause injury to you, other rescuers, or bystanders or that may cause additional injury to the patient.
- ▶ *Scene size-up* is the first phase of patient assessment and is made up of five parts:
  1. Body substance isolation (BSI) precautions
  2. Evaluation of scene safety
  3. Determining the mechanism of injury or the nature of the patient's illness
  4. Determining the total number of patients
  5. Determining the need for additional resources
- ▶ You must take appropriate BSI precautions on *every* call. Consider the need for BSI precautions before you approach the patient. Put on appropriate personal protective equipment based on the information the dispatcher gives you and your initial survey of the scene. This equipment includes gloves, eye protection, mask, and gown, if necessary.

- ▶ *Scene safety* is an assessment of the entire scene and surroundings to ensure your well-being and that of other rescuers, the patient(s), and bystanders.
- ▶ During the scene size-up, try to determine the *mechanism of injury* or the *nature of the illness.*
  1. *The mechanism of injury (MOI)* is the way in which an injury occurs, as well as the forces involved in producing the injury. A trauma patient is one who has experienced an injury from an external force. In trauma situations, look for the mechanism of injury. Traumatic situations include motor vehicle crashes, motor vehicle–pedestrian crashes, falls, bicycle crashes, motorcycle crashes, and penetrating traumas.
  2. A medical patient is one whose condition is caused by an illness. The *nature of the illness (NOI)* describes the medical condition that resulted in the patient's call to 9-1-1. Examples are fever, difficulty breathing, chest pain, headache, and vomiting. You should try to find out the nature of the illness by talking to the patient, family, coworkers, and bystanders.
- ▶ The ability to assess a patient properly is one of the most important skills you can master. As an Emergency Medical Responder, you must learn to work quickly and efficiently in all types of situations. You must approach patient assessment systematically. Patient assessment consists of the following components:
  1. Scene size-up
  2. Initial assessment
     - You must provide emergency medical care based on the patient's signs and symptoms. A *sign* is a medical or trauma condition of the patient that can be seen, heard, smelled, measured, or felt. Examples are unusual chest movement, bleeding, swelling, pale skin, and a fast pulse. A *symptom* is a condition described by the patient. Shortness of breath, nausea, abdominal pain, chills, chest pain, and dizziness are examples of symptoms.
     - Using the *AVPU scale,* you must evaluate the patient's level of responsiveness (mental status):
       - *A* = *A*lert
       - *V* = Responds to *V*erbal stimuli
       - *P* = Responds to *P*ainful stimuli
       - *U*= *U*nresponsive
     - After assessing the patient's level of responsiveness, you should note the need for spinal precautions. You would then assess the patient's ABCs (airway, breathing, and circulation).
  3. Focused history and physical examination
     - After the initial assessment, you should obtain a SAMPLE history, complete a physical exam, and obtain baseline vital signs (an initial set of vital sign measurements against which later measurements are compared).
     - *SAMPLE* is an aid to remind you of the information you should get from the patient:
       - *S*igns and symptoms
       - *A*llergies
       - *M*edications
       - (Pertinent) *P*ast medical history
       - *L*ast oral intake
       - *E*vents leading to the injury or illness

- *DOTS* can help you remember what to look and feel for during physical exam:
  - *D*eformities
  - *O*pen injuries
  - *T*enderness
  - *S*welling
- Detailed physical examination
  - The term *physical exam* implies a head-to-toe assessment of the patient's entire body. A *focused physical examination* is an assessment of specific body areas that relate solely to the patient's illness or injury.
  - Before examining the head of a trauma patient, have someone stabilize the patient's head and neck to keep the patient from moving (if this has not already been done).
  - A quick head-to-toe assessment of a trauma patient with a significant mechanism of injury is called a *rapid trauma assessment.* Seriously injured or unresponsive trauma patients require this type of physical exam in order to find out if they have life-threatening injuries. Less seriously injured trauma patients do not require a head-to-toe physical exam.
  - Begin the physical exam by checking the patient's head. Then examine the neck, chest, abdomen, pelvis, lower extremities, upper extremities, and the back. Compare one side of the body with the other. If an injury or a medical condition involves one side of the body, use the uninjured or uninvolved side as the normal finding for comparison.
- *Vital signs* are assessments of breathing, pulse, temperature, pupils, and blood pressure. Measuring vital signs is an important part of patient assessment. Vital signs are measured to
  - Detect changes in normal body function
  - Recognize life-threatening situations
  - Determine a patient's response to treatment

4. Ongoing assessment

- While waiting for additional EMS resources, continue to assess the patient. Repeat the initial assessment every 15 minutes for a stable patient and every 5 minutes for an unstable patient. Reassess the patient's mental status and maintain an open airway. Monitor the patient's breathing, pulse, skin color, temperature, and condition. Repeat the physical exam as needed. Check the treatments you provide to be sure that they are effective. Continue to calm and reassure the patient.
- When EMS personnel arrive, provide a hand-off report. Your report should include the following patient information:
  - Age and gender
  - Chief complaint
  - Level of responsiveness
  - Airway and breathing status
  - Circulation status
  - Physical findings
  - SAMPLE history
  - Treatment provided
  - Current condition

▶ Tracking Your Progress

After reading this chapter, can you	Page Reference	Objective Met?
• Discuss the components of scene size-up?	240	☐
• Describe common hazards found at the scene of a trauma and a medical patient?	241–243	☐
• Determine if the scene is safe to enter?	241–243	☐
• Discuss common mechanisms of injury/nature of illness?	244–251	☐
• Discuss the reason for identifying the total number of patients at the scene?	251	☐
• Explain the reason for identifying the need for additional help or assistance?	251–252	☐
• Summarize the reasons for forming a general impression of the patient?	255	☐
• Discuss methods of assessing mental status?	256–258	☐
• Differentiate between assessing mental status in the adult, child, and infant patient?	256–258	☐
• Describe methods used for assessing if a patient is breathing?	260	☐
• Differentiate between a patient with adequate and inadequate breathing?	260–261	☐
• Describe the methods used to assess circulation?	261	☐
• Differentiate between obtaining a pulse in an adult, child, and infant patient?	262	☐
• Discuss the need for assessing the patient for external bleeding?	261	☐
• Explain the reason for prioritizing a patient for care and transport?	265	☐
• Discuss the components of the physical exam?	268	☐
• State the areas of the body that are evaluated during the physical exam?	268–272	☐
• Explain what additional questioning may be asked during the physical exam?	274	☐
• Explain the components of the SAMPLE history?	266–267	☐
• Discuss the components of the ongoing assessment?	283–284	☐
• Describe the information that you should include in the Emergency Medical Responder hand-off report?	284	☐
• Explain the rationale for crew members to evaluate scene safety prior to entering?	241	☐
• Serve as a model for others by explaining how patient situations affect your evaluation of the mechanism of injury or illness?	243	☐
• Explain the importance of forming a general impression of the patient?	255	☐
• Explain the value of an initial assessment?	253	☐
• Explain the value of questioning the patient and family?	244	☐

• Explain the value of the physical exam?	268	☐
• Explain the value of an ongoing assessment?	284	☐
• Explain the rationale for the feelings that these patients might be experiencing?	269	☐
• Demonstrate a caring attitude when performing patient assessments?	269	☐
• Place the interests of the patient as the foremost consideration when making any and all patient care decisions during patient assessment?	269	☐
• Communicate with empathy during patient assessment to patients as well as with family members and friends of the patient?	269	☐

Chapter Quiz

Multiple Choice

In the space provided, identify the letter of the choice that best completes each statement or answers each question.

_____ **1.** When arriving at the scene of an emergency, you should first

a. perform a scene size-up.
b. provide emergency care to the most seriously injured person.
c. find out why the patient called for help.
d. perform an initial assessment.

_____ **2.** You have been dispatched to a shopping mall for a possible shooting. The dispatcher said the caller indicated that there are three victims. The suspect is believed to still be in the area. Your best plan of action will be to

a. drive to the scene, enter the mall, and quickly remove all patients.
b. remain outside the entrance to the mall until law enforcement personnel tell you the scene is safe.
c. park a safe distance from the scene and wait for law enforcement personnel to tell you that the scene is safe.
d. enter the scene, quickly determine which patient is most seriously injured, and begin emergency care.

_____ **3.** What is the normal respiratory rate for an adult at rest?

a. 6 to 12 breaths per minute
b. 12 to 20 breaths per minute
c. 20 to 30 breaths per minute
d. 25 to 35 breaths per minute

_____ **4.** Which of the following represents a scale used to evaluate a patient's level of responsiveness?

a. AVPU
b. APGAR
c. OPQRST
d. SAMPLE

_____ **5.** The *P* in a SAMPLE history represents

a. pills.
b. painful stimulus.
c. pertinent past medical history.
d. posterior body.

_____ **6.** While forming a general impression of a patient, which of the following should be considered a life-threatening condition?

a. vomiting
b. major bleeding
c. abdominal pain
d. dizziness

_____ 7. After forming a general impression of a patient and evaluating mental status, you should next assess the patient's

a. circulation.
b. upper and lower extremities.
c. breathing.
d. airway.

_____ 8. What are vital signs?

a. the reason EMS was called, usually in the patient's own words
b. assessments of the entire scene and surroundings to ensure your well-being and that of other rescuers, the patient, and bystanders
c. assessments of breathing, pulse, skin, pupils, and blood pressure
d. the rhythmic contraction and expansion of the arteries with each heartbeat

True or False

Decide whether each statement is true or false. In the space provided, write T for true or F for false.

_____ 9. A trauma patient is a person whose condition is caused by an illness.

_____ 10. *Sphygmomanometer* is the medical term for a blood pressure cuff.

Matching

Match the key terms in the left column with the definitions in the right column by placing the letter of each correct answer in the space provided.

_____ 11. Nature of the illness
_____ 12. Chief complaint
_____ 13. Stethoscope
_____ 14. Cyanotic
_____ 15. Wheezing
_____ 16. Mechanism of injury
_____ 17. Mottling
_____ 18. Kinematics
_____ 19. Penetrating trauma
_____ 20. Jaundice
_____ 21. Diastolic pressure
_____ 22. Kinetic energy

a. Energy of motion
b. Any mechanism of injury that causes a cut in or piercing of the skin
c. Pressure in an artery when the heart is at rest
d. Instrument used to hear sounds within the body
e. Irregular or patchy discoloration of the skin; usually a mixture of blue and white
f. Medical condition that resulted in the patient's call to 9-1-1
g. Manner in which an injury occurs
h. Blue
i. High-pitched whistling sound heard on inhalation or exhalation that suggests a narrowed or partially obstructed airway
j. Science of analyzing the mechanism of injury and predicting injury patterns
k. Reason EMS is called, usually in the patient's own words
l. Yellow

Short Answer

Answer each question in the space provided.

23. List three common hazards found at the scene of a trauma patient.

1. _____________________
2. _____________________
3. _____________________

24. Why is it important to identify the total number of patients at an emergency scene?

____

____

____

25. List the four areas you should evaluate when assessing circulation in a five-year-old patient.

1. ____________________

2. ____________________

3. ____________________

4. ____________________

26. List four signs of adequate breathing.

1. ____________________

2. ____________________

3. ____________________

4. ____________________

27. DOTS is a memory aid used to remember what to look and feel for during a physical exam. What is the meaning of each of these letters?

D = ____________________

O = ____________________

T = ____________________

S = ____________________

28. Explain what is meant by the term *spinal precautions.*

____

____

____

Sentence Completion

In the blanks provided, write the words that best complete each sentence.

29. ______________ trauma is any mechanism of injury that occurs without actual penetration of the body.

30. A ______________ patient is a person who has experienced an injury from an external force.

Module 5

Illness and Injury

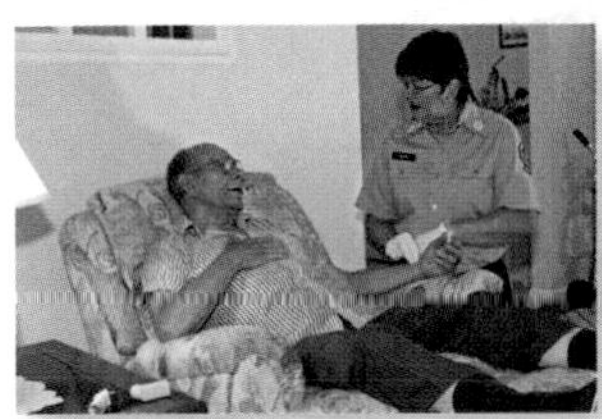

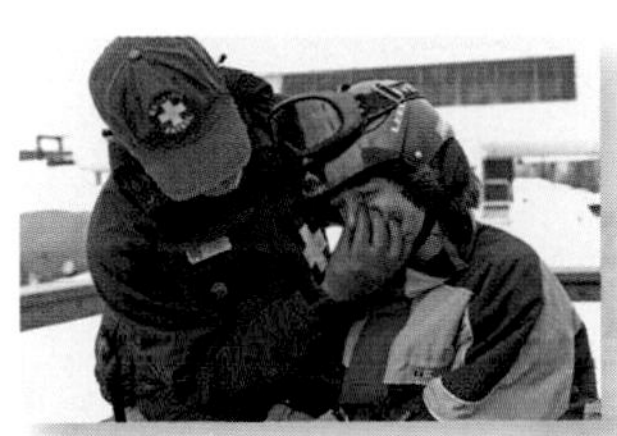

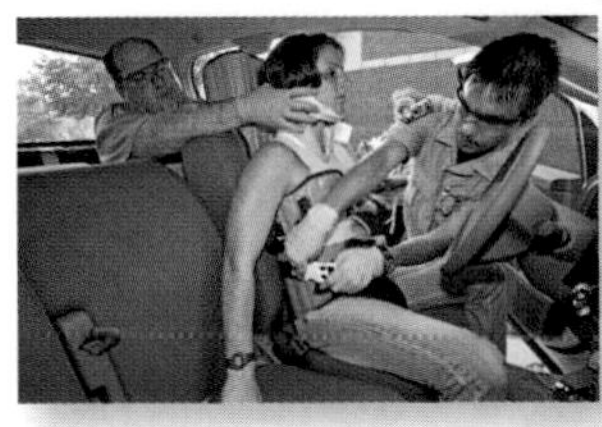

CHAPTER

9 Medical Emergencies

By the end of this chapter, you should be able to

Knowledge Objectives ▶

1. Identify the patient who presents with a general medical complaint.
2. Explain the steps in providing emergency medical care to a patient with a general medical complaint.
3. Identify the patient who presents with a specific medical complaint of altered mental status.
4. Explain the steps in providing emergency medical care to a patient with an altered mental status.
5. Identify the patient who presents with a specific medical complaint of seizures.
6. Explain the steps in providing emergency medical care to a patient with seizures.
7. Identify the patient who presents with a specific medical complaint of exposure to cold.
8. Explain the steps in providing emergency medical care to a patient with an exposure to cold.
9. Identify the patient who presents with a specific medical complaint of exposure to heat.
10. Explain the steps in providing emergency medical care to a patient with an exposure to heat.
11. Identify the patient who presents with a specific medical complaint of behavioral change.
12. Explain the steps in providing emergency medical care to a patient with a behavioral change.
13. Identify the patient who presents with a specific complaint of a psychological crisis.
14. Explain the steps in providing emergency medical care to a patient with a psychological crisis.

Attitude Objectives ▶

15. Attend to the feelings of the patient and/or family when dealing with the patient with a general medical complaint.
16. Attend to the feelings of the patient and/or family when dealing with the patient with a specific medical complaint.
17. Explain the rationale for modifying your behavior toward the patient with a behavioral emergency.

18. Demonstrate a caring attitude toward patients with a general medical complaint who request Emergency Medical Services.
19. Place the interests of the patient with a general medical complaint as the foremost consideration when making any and all patient care decisions.
20. Communicate with empathy to patients with a general medical complaint, as well as with family members and friends of the patient.
21. Demonstrate a caring attitude toward patients with a specific medical complaint who request Emergency Medical Services.
22. Place the interests of the patient with a specific medical complaint as the foremost consideration when making any and all patient care decisions.
23. Communicate with empathy to patients with a specific medical complaint, as well as with family members and friends of the patient.
24. Demonstrate a caring attitude toward patients with a behavioral problem who request Emergency Medical Services.
25. Place the interests of the patient with a behavioral problem as the foremost consideration when making any and all patient care decisions.
26. Communicate with empathy to patients with a behavioral problem, as well as with family members and friends of the patient.

Skill Objectives ▶

DVD Link

27. Demonstrate the steps in providing emergency medical care to a patient with a general medical complaint.
28. Demonstrate the steps in providing emergency medical care to a patient with an altered mental status.
29. Demonstrate the steps in providing emergency medical care to a patient with seizures.
30. Demonstrate the steps in providing emergency medical care to a patient with an exposure to cold.
31. Demonstrate the steps in providing emergency medical care to a patient with an exposure to heat.
32. Demonstrate the steps in providing emergency medical care to a patient with a behavioral change.
33. Demonstrate the steps in providing emergency medical care to a patient with a psychological crisis.

On The Scene

You are responding to a call to "Check welfare." A woman has called 9-1-1. She says she is worried. Her elderly neighbor has not been seen in two days and his newspapers are stacked up on the front walk. Approaching the house cautiously, you notice a person lying halfway on the living room floor, propped against a chair. You slide in through an open window and unlock the front door so that other rescuers can enter. You approach the elderly man and shake him gently as you say, "I'm an Emergency Medical Responder. Sir, are you all right?" There is no response. You place a hand on his forehead, lift his chin, and look, listen, and feel for breathing. He is breathing quietly, about 16 times per minute. When you reach to feel his radial pulse, you notice how cold and pale his skin is. His heart rate is 128 beats per minute. ■

THINK ABOUT IT

As you read this chapter, think about the following questions:

- What are some possible causes of this patient's altered level of consciousness?
- What additional assessment should you continue to perform?
- Is there more information that you should look for in his home?
- What treatment measures would be appropriate for this patient?

Introduction

Many patients are turning to EMS personnel for medical care that might otherwise be provided in a doctor's office.

Handling Medical Emergencies

As a healthcare professional, you will be called for a variety of emergencies. You will see some types of calls over and over again. Other types of calls will occur only once in your career. Just when you think you have "seen it all," something new will happen. This is especially true with patients who have a medical complaint. Emergency care professionals respond to calls involving medical complaints every day. A thorough patient assessment and careful history obtained from the patient, family, or others will often help you identify the underlying cause of the patient's complaint. Regardless of the cause, emergency care of the patient with a medical complaint focuses on the patient's airway, breathing, and circulation.

General Medical Complaints

Objective 1 ▸

When thinking about a medical call, what patient complaints might you encounter? General medical complaints can include the following:

- Tiredness, weakness
- Dizziness
- Nausea, vomiting
- Diarrhea
- Sore throat
- Headache
- Muscle cramps or spasms
- Stomach cramps
- Stuffy nose
- Cough

You should assess every patient and determine his chief complaint as well as his signs and symptoms. Give emergency medical care based on the patient's signs and symptoms. Keep in mind that some patient complaints may apply to more than one illness. For example, a patient who complains of difficulty breathing may have a problem with the respiratory system, such as pneumonia. Difficulty breathing may also result from a problem with the circulatory system. This can occur when the heart begins to fail and fluid backs up into the lungs. To determine the best care for your patient, you will need good interviewing skills and the ability to read between the lines.

Emergency Medical Responder Care

Scene Size-Up

Objective 2 ▶

When you are called for a medical emergency, consider the dispatch information you were given while en route to the call. Is the patient familiar to you because you have been frequently called to this address? If so, what do you remember from those calls? How might those experiences help you on this call?

Remember to wear appropriate PPE before approaching the patient.

When you arrive on the scene, make sure it is safe before entering. Survey the patient's environment for clues to the cause of the emergency. Quickly find out the nature of the patient's illness (Figure 9-1). You can usually get this information from the patient, family members, or bystanders as well as from your observations of the scene. Find out why you were called today. What is different today? What happened today that made the patient's condition worse than yesterday?

Determine the number of patients and the need for any additional resources. This is an excellent time to determine if Advanced Life Support personnel should be called to the scene. Although your patient may be experiencing a medical emergency, you should consider stabilizing the patient's spine if necessary. For example, suppose you are called to a person's home and find her unresponsive on the kitchen floor. The patient's daughter tells you she found the patient like this when she came home from school. Because no one saw the patient when she collapsed, you must consider the possibility that she hit her head on the floor. In situations like this, assume there is a head or neck injury and stabilize the patient's spine as necessary.

Initial Assessment

General Impression

You form a general impression without the patient telling you what his or her complaint is.

Begin your assessment of the patient from across the room. Form a general impression by looking at your patient's appearance, work of breathing, and skin color. What things stand out in your mind when you first see your patient? Does he look sick? Does he look as if he is having difficulty breathing? Does he look as if he must sit up to feel better? Does he look anxious, sad, or angry? Does his skin look pale?

Making a Difference

Forming a general impression is about trusting your instincts. If it looks bad, it probably is. Get assistance.

Objective 15 ▶

Objective 18 ▶

As you gain experience, you will develop an instinct for quickly recognizing when a patient is sick. You will also learn to recognize the need to act quickly. Learn to rely on your instincts and training. They will ultimately lead to the best outcome for your patients. Once your general impression is complete, perform a hands-on assessment. Show a caring attitude when performing your assessment and providing care. Be sure to comfort, calm, and reassure your patient while waiting for EMS help to arrive.

Level of Responsiveness and the Airway

A patient's mental status may dramatically improve—or worsen—during your care. Continuous reassessment is important to detect trends in the patient's condition.

After forming the general impression, you will next assess the patient's level of responsiveness and the patient's airway. The best way to do this is to ask your patient a question. If he can answer, you have just completed a couple of steps. First, you now know he has an open (patent) airway. Second, you know he is responsive to a verbal stimulus. When asking your patient questions,

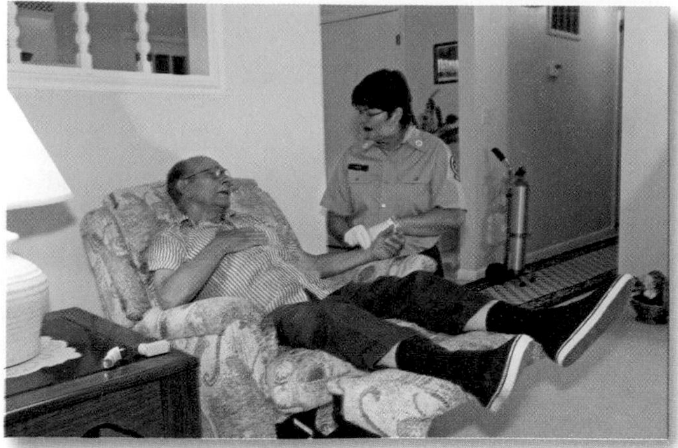

FIGURE 9-1 ▶ After making sure the scene is safe to enter, survey the patient's environment for clues to the cause of the emergency. Quickly find out the nature of the patient's illness.

pay attention to his answers. If his answers are appropriate, the patient is said to be alert and oriented to his surroundings.

Breathing

The next portion of the initial assessment is assessment of the patient's breathing. By simply looking at the patient, you can estimate his respiratory rate. Pay attention to the rate, depth, and regularity of his breathing. If any of these are unusual or if his breathing is noisy or labored, prompt emergency care is your best course of action. Provide initial care and find out what caused the patient's symptoms.

Circulation

Assessing circulation is the next step. Doing this properly will reveal several important facts about your patient. The first thing your assessment of circulation can tell you is the patient's heart rate. The second thing it can tell you is your patient's skin condition. You cannot accurately assess your patient's heart rate without touching him. While touching your patient, pay attention to his skin color, temperature, and condition (moisture). For example, if he is flushed, hot, and sweaty, there is an underlying problem. If he is pale, cool, and clammy, there is a different underlying problem.

Patient History

Objective 19 ▶

Objective 20 ▶

After the initial assessment, find out the patient's history. Show concern when speaking with the patient, his family members, and his friends. Perform a detailed or focused physical exam. You must determine which physical examination is appropriate based on your patient's chief complaint, your initial assessment findings, and the nature of the patient's illness. Provide appropriate emergency care based on your physical exam findings and the information gathered from the patient.

Specific Medical Complaints

Altered Mental Status

Objective 3 ▶

Altered mental status means a change in a patient's level of awareness. Altered mental status is also called an *altered level of consciousness (ALOC)*. The change in the patient's mental status may occur gradually or suddenly. A patient with an altered mental status may appear confused, agitated, combative, sleepy, difficult to awaken, or unresponsive. The length of the patient's altered mental status may be brief or prolonged. An altered mental status should be treated as a medical emergency.

A patient with an altered mental status can be challenging to care for because he usually cannot tell you what is wrong. You must obtain a careful history from the patient, the family, or others to find out the underlying cause of the patient's altered mental status.

You Should Know

Common Causes of Altered Mental Status

"A-E-I-O-U TIPPS = TIPPS over Vowels"

- *A*lcohol, abuse
- *E*pilepsy (seizures)
- *I*nsulin (diabetic emergency)
- *O*verdose, (lack of) oxygen (hypoxia)
- *U*remia (kidney failure)
- *T*rauma (head injury), temperature (fever, heat- or cold-related emergency)
- *I*nfection
- *P*sychiatric conditions
- *P*oisoning (including drugs and alcohol)
- *S*hock, stroke

Emergency Medical Responder Care of Patients with an Altered Mental Status

Objective 4 ►

Objective 16 ►

Regardless of the cause, emergency care of the patient with an altered mental status focuses on the airway, breathing, and circulation:

- Stabilize the patient's spine if trauma is suspected.
- Establish and maintain an open airway. If the patient cannot maintain his or her own airway, insert an oropharyngeal or a nasopharyngeal airway as needed. Suction as necessary.
- Provide oxygen if it is available and you have been trained to use it. If the patient's breathing is adequate, apply oxygen by mask at 15 liters per minute (LPM). If the patient's breathing is inadequate, assist his or her breathing with a bag-valve-mask (BVM) or mouth-to-mask device.
- Position the patient. If the patient is sitting or standing, help him or her to a position of comfort on a firm surface. If there is no possibility of trauma to the head or spine, place the patient in the recovery position.
- Remove or loosen tight clothing.
- Maintain body temperature.
- Comfort, calm, and reassure your patient and the family while waiting for help to arrive.

Remember This!

Many patients with serious medical conditions, such as diabetes, a drug allergy, or a heart condition, carry information with them about their condition. If your patient is unable to answer questions, look for a medical identification card or a medical ID necklace or bracelet, so that you can provide proper emergency care.

Making a Difference

The Cincinnati Prehospital Stroke Scale

A stroke is one possible cause of an altered mental status. If a person has an altered mental status, you can quickly assess three areas to find out if the patient might be having a stroke:

1. Ask the patient to smile. Both sides of the face should move equally. If one side droops, does not move at all, or does not move as well as the other side, request Advanced Life Support personnel right away.
2. Ask the patient to close his or her eyes and raise his or her arms out in front. Both arms should move the same or both arms should not move at all. If one arm does not move or one arm drifts down compared with the other, request Advanced Life Support personnel right away.
3. Ask the patient to repeat a simple sentence—for example, "You can't teach an old dog new tricks" or "The sky is blue in Cincinnati." The patient should be able to say the right words without slurring. Request Advanced Life Support personnel right away if the patient is unable to speak, slurs words, or uses the wrong words.

This technique is called the Cincinnati Prehospital Stroke Scale. You may be able to recognize key signs of a stroke using this simple test.

Reprinted from The Annals of Emergency Medicine, 33(4): Kothari RU, Pancioli A, Liu T, Broderick J, Cincinnati Prehospital Stroke Scale, pp. 373–378. © 1999, with permission from The American College of Emergency Physicians.

Seizures

Objective 5 ▶

A seizure is one possible cause of altered mental status.

A seizure is a temporary change in behavior or consciousness caused by abnormal electrical activity within one or more groups of brain cells. A seizure is a symptom (not a disease) of an underlying problem within the central nervous system.

The most common cause of adult seizures is the failure to take anti-seizure medication. The most common cause of seizures in infants and young children is a high fever. Epilepsy is a condition of recurring seizures in which the cause is usually irreversible.

You Should Know

Causes of Seizures

- Unknown cause
- Failure to take anti-seizure medication
- Rapid rise in body temperature (febrile seizure)
- Infection
- Low oxygen level (hypoxia)
- Head trauma
- Brain tumor
- Poisoning
- Low blood sugar level (hypoglycemia)
- Seizure disorder
- Previous brain damage
- Electrolyte disturbances
- Alcohol or drug withdrawal
- Eclampsia (seizures associated with pregnancy)
- Abnormal heart rhythm
- Genetic and hereditary factors
- Stroke

Types of Seizures

Tonic-clonic seizures were previously called grand mal seizures.

There are many types of seizures. When most people hear the word *seizure,* they think of the kind of seizure that involves stiffening and jerking of the patient's body. This type of seizure is called a tonic-clonic seizure. A tonic-clonic seizure usually has four phases:

1. Aura
2. Tonic phase
3. Clonic phase
4. Postictal phase

The jerking movements during the clonic phase are often called convulsions.

Do not try to place anything in the patient's mouth during a seizure.

Imagine the skeletal muscles of the body contracting at the same time. Even the most physically fit person would become tired afterward.

An aura is a peculiar sensation that comes before a seizure. Not all seizures are preceded by an aura. The aura is followed by a loss of consciousness. During the tonic phase, the body's muscles stiffen. The patient's breathing may be noisy and the patient may turn blue. This phase usually lasts 15–20 seconds. During the clonic phase, alternating jerking and relaxation of the body occurs. This is the longest phase of the seizure. It may last several minutes. The patient's heart rate and blood pressure are increased. The skin is usually warm, flushed, and moist. The patient may lose control of his bowels and bladder. Bleeding may occur if the patient bites his or her tongue or cheek.

The postictal phase is the period of recovery that follows a seizure. During this period, the patient often appears limp, has shallow breathing, and has an altered mental status. This altered mental status may appear as confusion, sleepiness, memory loss, unresponsiveness, or difficulty talking. During this phase, the patient slowly awakens. He or she may complain of a headache and muscle soreness. This phase may last minutes to hours.

You Should Know

Common Auras

- Unusual taste
- Dreamy feeling
- Feeling of fear
- Visual disturbance, such as a flashing or floating light
- Unpleasant odor
- Stomach pain
- Rising or sinking feeling in the stomach

Status epilepticus is

- A seizure that lasts longer than 30 minutes *or*
- A series of seizures occurring over a 30-minute period in which the patient remains unresponsive between seizures

Status epilepticus is a medical emergency. It can cause brain damage or death if it is not treated. The complications associated with status epilepticus include the following:

- Aspiration of vomitus and blood
- Long-bone and spine fractures
- Dehydration
- Brain damage due to a lack of oxygen or a depletion of glucose (sugar)

Assessment of a Patient with Seizures

Objective 21 ▶

Remember to put on appropriate PPE.

When you arrive on the scene, perform a scene size-up before starting emergency medical care. If the scene is safe, approach the patient and try to find out if the seizure is the result of trauma or an illness. Check for a medical ID. Look for evidence of burns or suspicious substances that might indicate poisoning or a toxic exposure. Are there signs of recent trauma? Perform an initial assessment and a physical exam. Demonstrate a caring attitude when performing your assessment and providing care.

Depending on its severity, injuries can occur during a seizure. Because the patient may bite her tongue or cheek during a seizure, be sure to look in her mouth for bleeding when the seizure is over. You may see scrapes on her head, face, or extremities because of the seizure. Fractures of the skull, arm, or leg can also occur.

Objective 23 ▶

When taking the patient's SAMPLE history, speak with kindness to her family members and friends. Show concern about the patient's condition and well-being. Find out if the patient has any allergies. Also find out if she is taking any medications (prescription and over-the-counter). Has there been any recent change in her medications (has she started taking a new medication, stopped taking a medication, or changed the dosage)? When finding out the patient's medical history, ask the following questions:

Obtaining a good history is very important when treating a seizure patient.

- Is this the patient's first seizure?
- If the patient has a history of seizures, is she on a seizure medication? Did the patient take her medications today?
- How often do the seizures usually happen? Does this seizure look like those the patient has had before?
- Does the patient have a history of stroke, diabetes (low blood sugar can cause seizures), or heart disease (an irregular heart rhythm can cause a low oxygen level and lead to seizures)?
- Does the patient use or abuse alcohol or drugs? (Alcohol or drug withdrawal can result in seizures.)

Your description of the seizure may be important in finding its cause.

When finding out the events that have led to a seizure, think about the following questions. If the seizure has stopped by the time you arrive, be sure to ask what the seizure looked like. If the seizure is in progress when you arrive, keep these questions in mind while watching the patient. You will need to describe what you saw (or what the family or bystanders described to you) to the EMS personnel who arrive on the scene.

- What was the patient doing at the time of the seizure? Did she hit her head or fall?
- Did the patient cry out or attract your attention in any way?
- What did the seizure look like? When did the seizure start? How long did it last?
- Did the seizure begin in one area of the body and progress to others?
- Did the patient lose bowel or bladder control?
- When the patient woke up, was there any change in her speech? Was she able to move her arms and legs normally?
- Did the patient exhibit any unusual behavior before, during, or after the seizure?

You Should Know

- Many cardiac arrests are called in to 9-1-1 as a seizure.
- More than 80 million people have had an unprovoked seizure.
- More than 30% of new patients with epilepsy will never know what causes their seizures.

Emergency Medical Responder Care of Patients with Seizures

Objective 6 ▶

Objective 22 ▶

Treating patients experiencing a seizure can be difficult. If the patients are postictal, they are sometimes combative or confused. They may not let you perform the skills that are necessary. As a result, frustration can set in on both sides. Keep in mind that you are on the scene for a purpose. That purpose is to provide the best emergency care possible. It may take you several attempts to get answers to questions, put oxygen on the patient, or get the patient loaded into the ambulance. Remember that as a patient becomes conscious in the postictal phase, confusion and combativeness are normal. No matter what caused the seizure, your emergency care must focus on the patient's airway, breathing, and circulation.

- Protect the patient's privacy. Ask bystanders (except the patient's family or caregiver) to leave the area.
- Position the patient. If the patient is sitting or standing, help her to the floor.
- If the patient is actively seizing, protect her from harm by moving furniture and other objects away from her (Figure 9-2). Protect the patient's head with a pillow or other soft material. Do not insert anything into the patient's mouth. This includes your fingers, an oropharyngeal airway, a padded tongue blade, or a bite block. Undo any tight clothing. Remove eyeglasses. Do not try to restrain body movements during the seizure.
- As soon as the seizure is over, make sure the patient's airway is open. Be sure to have suction available because the patient may vomit during or after the seizure. Gently suction the patient's mouth if secretions are present. Provide oxygen if it is available and you have been trained to use it. If the patient's breathing is adequate, apply oxygen by mask at 15 LPM. If the seizure is prolonged or if the patient's breathing is inadequate, assist her breathing with a bag-valve-mask or mouth-to-mask device. If the patient is confused or agitated, she may not tolerate an oxygen mask. In this case, blow-by oxygen is acceptable. When the patient is able to tolerate a mask, it should be applied. Place the patient in the recovery position if no trauma is suspected.
- Comfort, calm, and reassure the patient and the family while waiting for additional EMS personnel. Watch the patient very closely for repeat seizures.
- When EMS personnel arrive at the scene, pass on any patient information you have gathered. This should include how the scene looked and information from bystanders. You should also include what the patient looked like when you first arrived on the scene, the care you gave, and the patient's response to your care.
- Some patients are light sensitive (photophobic) after a seizure. Take care to reduce the patient's exposure to bright lights and loud noises. While rapid transport may be the best course of action, take care not to stimulate the patient more than necessary.

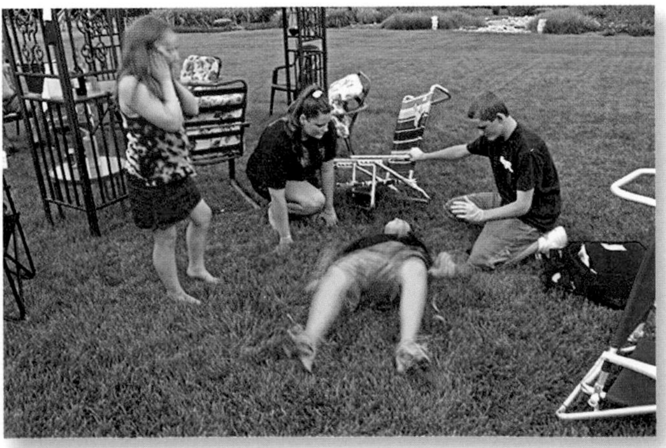

FIGURE 9-2 ▶ Protect a person who is having a seizure from harm by moving furniture and other objects away from him or her. If the patient is wearing eyeglasses, remove them. Undo any tight clothing.

Body temperature remains constant if the heat produced by the body equals the heat lost.

Exposure to Cold

Body Temperature

Body temperature is the balance between the heat produced by the body and the heat lost from the body. Body temperature is measured in heat units called degrees (°). The body is divided into two areas for temperature control: core temperature and peripheral (surface) temperature. The body core (the deep tissues of the body) includes the contents of the skull, vertebral column, thorax, abdomen, and pelvis. The body core is normally maintained at a fairly constant temperature, usually within 1°F (approximately 0.6°C) of normal, unless a person develops a fever.

You Should Know

When measured orally, the average normal temperature is between 98.0° and 98.6°F, which is approximately 37°C. The temperature measured in the armpit (the axillary temperature) or mouth (the oral temperature) is about 1°F (approximately 0.6°C) less than the rectal temperature.

When the body produces too much heat, the temperature can temporarily rise to as high as 101° to 104°F (38.3° to 40.0°C). This type of temporary rise in temperature can occur, for example, during strenuous exercise. When the body is exposed to cold, the temperature can often fall to below 96°F (35.6°C).

The peripheral area of the body includes the skin, subcutaneous tissue, and fat. The temperature of the body's extremities rises and falls in response to the environment. At room temperature, the temperature in the peripheral areas of the body is slightly below those of the body core.

Temperature Regulation

The skin plays a very important role in temperature regulation. Cold and warmth sensors (receptors) in the skin detect changes in temperature. These receptors relay the information to the hypothalamus. The hypothalamus (located in the brain) functions as the body's thermostat. It coordinates the body's response to temperature.

The cardiovascular system regulates blood flow to the skin. Blood vessels widen (dilate) and narrow (constrict) in response to messages from the hypothalamus. When high temperatures are sensed, blood vessels in the skin dilate. When low temperatures are sensed, blood vessels in the skin constrict (narrow). When these vessels narrow, sweating stops and the major body muscles shiver to increase heat.

Heat Production

Body heat is produced mainly by the conversion of food to energy (metabolism). Most of the heat produced in the body is made by the liver, brain, heart, and skeletal muscle during exercise. The heat made by skeletal muscle is important in temperature control. This is because muscle activity can be increased to produce heat when needed.

The body begins a series of actions when its cold sensors are stimulated. These actions are designed to conserve heat and increase heat production. One action is to produce more epinephrine and other hormones. The increased production of epinephrine and other hormones increases the rate at which the body converts food to energy, which increases heat production. Another action is to constrict peripheral blood vessels. This decreases blood flow and heat loss through the skin. It also keeps warm blood in the body's core. Muscle activity also increases. Muscle activity may be voluntary (such as walking, running, or moving about) or involuntary (such as shivering).

FIGURE 9-3 ► The body loses heat by radiation, convection, conduction, evaporation, and breathing.

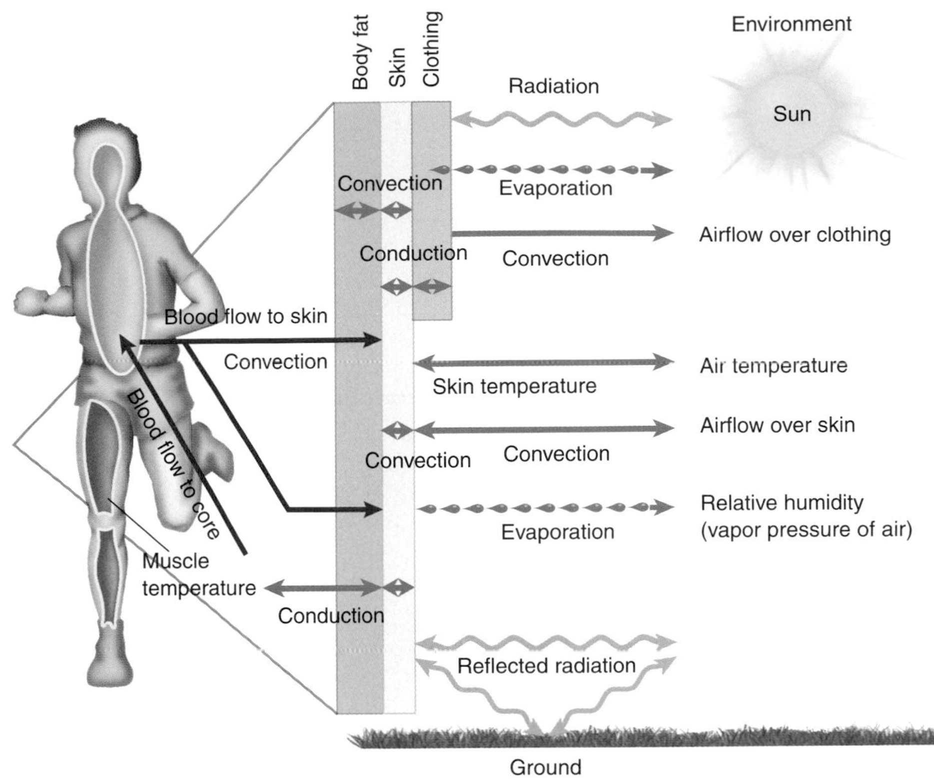

Heat Loss

You must know how the body loses heat when treating patients with a cold-related emergency. Knowing this information will allow you to prevent further heat loss.

The body loses heat to the environment in five ways (Figure 9-3):

1. Radiation
2. Convection
3. Conduction
4. Evaporation
5. Breathing

Most heat loss is transferred from the deeper body organs and tissues to the skin. From there it is lost to the air and other surroundings. Some heat loss occurs through the mucous membranes of the respiratory, digestive, and urinary systems.

More than half of the heat lost from the body occurs by radiation.

Radiation is the transfer of heat, as infrared heat rays, from the surface of one object to the surface of another without contact between the two objects. The heat from the sun is an example of radiation. When the temperature of the body is more than the temperature of the surroundings, the body will lose heat. Simple barriers (clothing) can reduce heat loss by radiation. **Convection** is the transfer of heat by the movement of air or water current. Wind speed affects heat loss by convection (wind-chill factor). **Conduction** is the transfer of heat between objects that are in direct contact. Heat flows from warmer areas to cooler ones. The amount of heat lost from the body by conduction depends on the following:

- The temperature difference between the body and the object
- The amount of time the objects are in contact
- The amount (surface area) of the body in contact with the object

Evaporation is a loss of heat by vaporization of moisture on the body surface. The body will lose heat by evaporation if the skin temperature is higher than the temperature of the surroundings. The body gains heat when the temperature of the surrounding air is higher than body temperature. As relative humidity rises, the effectiveness of body cooling by evaporation decreases.

The body also loses heat by breathing in cool air and exhaling the air that has become heated in the lungs. Additionally, the body continuously loses a relatively small amount of heat through the evaporation of moisture from within the lungs.

When the body's warmth sensors are stimulated, the body takes action to increase heat loss. Peripheral blood vessels dilate. Blood flow to the body surface increases. Heat escapes from the skin surface by radiation and conduction. When air currents pass across the skin, additional heat is lost by convection. This heat loss cools the body's core. The body's sweat gland secretion also increases. The sweat travels to the skin's surface. When air currents pass across the skin, heat is lost through evaporation.

Making a Difference

Consider a situation in which a patient is found lying on the ground or roadway after a motor vehicle crash. In cold climates, the patient may experience a cold-related emergency after lying on a cold surface. Taking a long time to assess the patient increases the amount of time he or she is exposed to the environment. In warm climates, patients have experienced severe burns from prolonged exposure to the hot ground or pavement. Even after being placed on a long backboard, patients have experienced burns on the back surfaces of their arms because they were left in contact with the pavement. Do not assume that a patient's complaints are related only to injuries from the crash. The complaints may also be related to the environment in which you have found him or her. Be sensitive to these types of situations.

Types of Cold Emergencies

Objective 7 ▶

There are two main types of cold emergencies: a generalized cold emergency (generalized hypothermia) and a local cold injury. A local cold injury is damage to a specific area of the body, such as fingers or toes. Local cold injury is discussed later in this chapter.

Hypothermia

Hypothermia is a core body temperature of less than 95°F (35°C). This condition results when the body loses more heat than it gains or produces. Hypothermia can be broken down into three stages: mild, moderate, and severe.

1. Mild hypothermia (core body temperature 93.2° to 96.8°F, or 34.0° to 37.0°C)
2. Moderate hypothermia (86.0° to 93.1°F, or 30.0° to 33.9°C)
3. Severe hypothermia (less than 86.0°F, or 30.0°C)

It is important to realize that the stages of hypothermia do not apply to everyone. Some patients may show signs and symptoms at different temperatures. It is also important to understand that these temperatures are core body temperatures. The usual methods for measuring temperature (oral and tympanic) may not accurately reflect core temperature. A rectal temperature gives the most accurate measure of core temperature. However, obtaining a rectal temperature in the field often raises issues of patient sensitivity and welfare, such as exposure to cold by removing clothing. In most cases, you will need to make judgments about hypothermia based on your patient's signs and symptoms.

Remember This!

Core body temperatures below 95°F (35°C) are significant because, at or below this temperature, the body typically does not generate enough heat to restore normal body temperature or maintain proper organ function.

Hypothermia can occur from exposure to conditions that result in excessive heat loss. Hypothermia can occur even in warm weather. For example, a person who remains in a cool environment, such as a swimming pool, can experience hypothermia. Hypothermia can also occur when the body loses its ability to maintain a normal body temperature. This can occur in patients who are in shock.

Some factors increase a person's risk of experiencing hypothermia. A person's age is one factor. For example, older adults are at risk for hypothermia due to the following:

- Lack of heat in the home
- Poor diet or appetite
- Loss of subcutaneous fat for body insulation
- Lack of activity
- Delayed circulation
- Decreased efficiency of temperature control mechanisms

Young children are at risk for hypothermia because they have less subcutaneous fat for body insulation. Their large surface area in relation to their overall size also results in a more rapid heat loss. Newborns are unable to shiver. Infants and very young children are unable to protect themselves from the cold. They cannot put on clothes and cannot move to warm surroundings without help.

Some illnesses and injuries increase a person's risk for hypothermia. These conditions include shock, head or spinal injuries, burns, generalized infection, and low blood sugar. The use of drugs or alcohol can affect a person's judgment, preventing him or her from taking proper safety measures. These safety measures might include wearing more clothing, increasing the room temperature, or coming in from the cold. Alcohol dilates the body's peripheral vessels and depresses the central nervous system. Heat loss may occur quickly due to dilated vessels. Sedation from alcohol can cause the sedation that comes from cold exposure to go unrecognized.

You Should Know

Factors That Contribute to Hypothermia

- Cold, windy weather conditions
- Prolonged exposure to a cool environment
- Immersion in water
- Improper, inadequate, or wet clothing
- Low body weight
- Poor physical condition
- Low blood sugar
- Recent trauma or burn injury
- Drug or alcohol intake
- Extremes in age (very young children, the elderly)
- Impaired judgment due to mental illness or Alzheimer's disease
- Preexisting medical conditions
- Previous cold exposure

A cold environment requires special safety considerations due to the presence of ice, snow, or wind.

Assessment of a Patient with a Cold-Related Injury

When you are called for a patient with a possible cold-related injury, carefully size up the scene on arrival. Look at the patient's environment for signs of cold exposure. The signs of exposure may be very obvious or very subtle. The signs of a subtle exposure include

- Alcohol ingestion
- Underlying illness
- Overdose or poisoning
- Major trauma
- Outdoor recreation
- Decreased room temperature (such as in the home of an older adult)

You may need to wait on the scene until the necessary equipment or rescue personnel arrive.

Removing the patient from the environment must be your main concern. Use trained rescuers for this purpose when necessary. While you assess the need for additional resources, think about what your department or agency can handle safely. For example, can your department handle safely removing a person who is trapped in freezing water? In all cases of cold-related emergencies, you should request Advanced Life Support personnel as soon as possible.

Stop and Think!

What equipment do you have in place right now to help you treat a cold-related emergency? Your answer to this question should be a reminder to check your seasonal equipment for use in an emergency setting.

As the patient's body temperature drops, there may be no clear difference between the stages of hypothermia.

After ensuring your safety, approach the patient and form a general impression. Notice the clothing the patient is wearing. Is it adequate for the climate you are in? What are the surroundings like? Perform an initial assessment, keeping in mind that you need to move the patient to a warm location as quickly and as safely as possible. Remove any cold or wet clothing. Protect the patient from the environment. This may include shielding the patient from the wind. Cover him to help preserve body heat. A lot of body heat is lost through the head. Covering the patient's head can help reduce heat loss. Stabilize his spine if needed.

Assess the patient's mental status, airway, breathing, and circulation. Keep in mind that mental status decreases as the patient's body temperature drops. The patient may show the following signs:

- Difficult (slow, slurred) speech
- Confusion
- Memory lapse (amnesia)
- Mood changes
- Combativeness
- Unresponsiveness
- Loss of motor skills and coordination
- Uncontrollable shivering and, later, a lack of shivering

Remember This!

A patient who has severe hypothermia may be alive but may have such a weak pulse or shallow breathing that you are unable to feel it. Do not assume a patient is dead until he or she is warm and has no pulse. Take longer than usual to assess the breathing and heart rate of a patient who has been exposed to cold before starting CPR. Assess breathing for 30–45 seconds. Also assess for a pulse for 30–45 seconds.

The patient's vital signs will also change as hypothermia worsens. The patient's breathing rate is initially increased, then slow and shallow, and finally absent. The heart rate is initially increased, then slow and irregular, and finally absent. Blood pressure may be normal at first and then low to absent. The pupils dilate and are slow to respond. The skin is initially red, then pale, then blue, and finally gray, hard, and cold to the touch. To assess the patient's general temperature, place the back of your hand between the patient's clothing and his abdomen. The patient experiencing a generalized cold emergency will have a cool or cold abdominal skin temperature.

Shivering stops below 86.0° to 89.6°F (30.0° to 32.0°C).

The patient's motor and sensory functions also change with the degree of hypothermia. The patient may initially complain of joint aches or muscle stiffness. He may show a lack of coordination and a staggering walk. Shivering is usually present initially. As hypothermia worsens, shivering gradually decreases until it is absent. The patient loses sensation and his muscles become rigid. Be certain to assess the patient for other injuries. Identify any life-threatening conditions and provide care based on your findings. The signs and symptoms of hypothermia are listed in Table 9-1.

If the patient is responsive, or if family members or bystanders are available, try to obtain a SAMPLE history. Keep in mind that some illnesses or injuries increase a person's risk for hypothermia. Find out if the patient has a history of alcohol abuse, thyroid disorder, diabetes, stroke, or trauma to the head, neck, or spine. When finding out what events have led to the patient's present situation, ask the following questions:

- How long has the patient been exposed to the cold?
- What was the source of the cold (for example, water or snow)? If the patient was exposed to water, what was the approximate water temperature?
- What was the patient doing when the symptoms began?

TABLE 9-1 Signs and Symptoms of Hypothermia

Mild	Moderate	Severe
• Increased heart rate • Increased respiratory rate • Cool skin (to preserve core temperature) • Shivering • Difficulty talking, slurred speech • Difficulty moving • Memory lapse (amnesia), mood changes, combative attitude • Joint aches, muscle stiffness • Altered mental status, confusion, poor judgment (patient may actually remove clothing)	• Shivering, which may gradually decrease and become absent; shivering becomes replaced with rigid muscles • Decreasing heart rate and respiratory rate • Irregular heart rate • Pale, blue (cyanotic), or mottled skin • Progressive loss of responsiveness • Dilated pupils • Blood pressure that is difficult to obtain	• Irrational attitude, which changes to unresponsiveness • Rigid muscles • Cold skin • Blue or mottled skin • Slow or absent breathing • Slowly responding pupils • Slow, irregular, or absent heart rate • A pulse that is hard to feel or absent • Low to absent blood pressure • Cardiopulmonary arrest

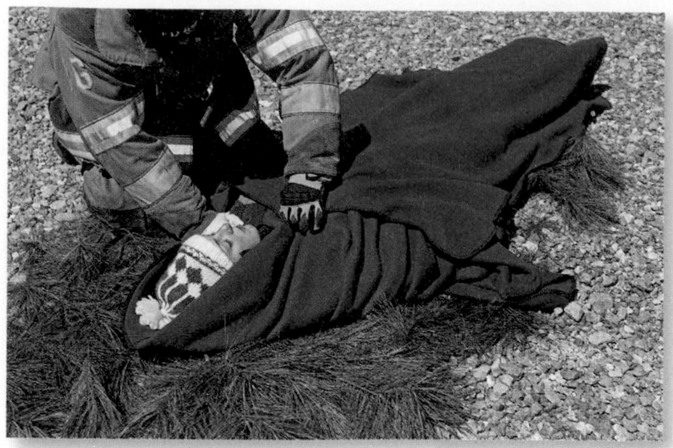

FIGURE 9-4 ► Protect the patient from the cold with available materials. Make sure to cover the patient's head, leaving the face exposed to watch the airway. Place insulating material between the patient and the surface on which he or she is lying.

Emergency Medical Responder Care of Patients with Hypothermia

Objective 8 ►

Remove the patient from the cold environment as quickly and as safely as possible to protect him from further heat loss. When moving the patient, keep in mind known or suspected injuries. Cut away cold or wet clothing rather than tugging and pulling at the patient's clothes. Protect the patient from the cold with available materials, such as blankets, a sleeping bag, newspapers, or plastic garbage bags (Figure 9-4). Make sure to cover the patient's head. However, leave his face exposed, so that you can watch his airway. Place insulating material between the patient and the surface on which he is lying. Protect the patient from drafts.

Handle the patient gently. Avoid rough handling. Do not allow the patient to walk or exert himself. Rough handling or exertion may force cold blood in the periphery to the body's core. Make sure the patient's airway is open and that suction is available. As the body cools, the cough reflex is depressed and respiratory secretions increase. Frequent suctioning may be necessary.

Provide oxygen if it is available and you have been trained to use it. If the patient's breathing is adequate, apply oxygen by mask at 15 LPM. If the patient's breathing is inadequate, assist his breathing with a BVM or mouth-to-mask device. Assess pulses for 30–45 seconds. If the patient has no pulse, begin CPR.

Stop and Think!

The decision to rewarm a hypothermic patient depends on your local protocol and the degree of hypothermia. Be sure to consult with medical direction before rewarming the patient.

There are two main types of rewarming: passive and active. Passive rewarming is the warming of a patient with minimal or no use of heat sources other than the patient's own heat production. Passive rewarming methods include placing the patient in a warm environment, applying warm clothing and blankets, and preventing drafts. Passive external rewarming is appropriate for all hypothermic patients.

Active rewarming involves adding heat directly to the surface of the patient's body. Active rewarming should not delay definitive care and may be used if the patient is alert and responding appropriately (follow local protocol):

- If the patient shows signs of mild hypothermia, apply warm blankets. Apply heat packs or hot water bottles to the groin, armpits, and back of the neck. To prevent burns, place a towel or dressings between the heat pack or hot water bottle and the patient's skin.

- If the patient shows signs of moderate hypothermia, apply warm blankets. Apply heat packs or hot water bottles to the torso only. Take care to avoid burning the underlying tissue.
- If the patient shows signs of severe hypothermia, apply warm blankets. Active rewarming will need to be done at the hospital.

Do not allow a patient to eat or drink stimulants (such as coffee, tea, or chocolate) or to drink alcohol. Do not rub or massage the patient's extremities. Doing so can cause cold blood to move from the extremities to the body core, causing a further decrease in temperature. During transport, turn up the heat in the patient area of the ambulance. If the patient is stable, perform ongoing assessments every 15 minutes. If the patient is unstable, perform ongoing assessments every 5 minutes.

Local Cold Injury

Hypothermia is often accompanied by frostbite.

When your body is exposed to cold, blood is forced away from your extremities to the body core. This puts your arms and legs at risk for local cold injury. Local cold injury (also called frostbite) involves tissue damage to a specific area of the body. It occurs when a body part, such as the nose, ears, cheeks, chin, hands, or feet, is exposed to prolonged or intense cold. Local tissue injury usually occurs when these areas are wet, poorly protected, or unprotected. Cold causes the blood vessels to narrow in the affected part. This narrowing decreases circulation to the involved area. Ice crystals form within the cells, which damages them.

Patients at risk for local cold injury include those with circulation problems, such as diabetics. Patients with a history of heart or blood vessel disease are also at risk. Alcohol, nicotine, and some medications decrease blood flow to the skin, increasing the risk for a local cold injury. Patients who have experienced a soft-tissue injury, such as a burn or a previous cold injury, are also at risk. Other factors that affect the risk for local cold injury include the following:

- Ambient temperature
- Wind-chill factor
- Length of exposure
- Type and number of clothing layers worn, including tight gloves and tight or tightly laced footwear
- Whether or not the patient was wet
- Whether or not the patient had direct contact with cold objects

A superficial cold injury involves the uppermost skin layers.

A local cold injury may be early (superficial frostbite) or late (deep frostbite). In a superficial cold injury, the skin of the exposed area first appears red and inflamed. With continued cooling, the area then becomes gray or white. When you press on the skin, normal color does not return (blanching). You may see a clear demarcation (a visible line of color change), although this sign may not present at the scene. The patient may complain of a loss of feeling in the injured area. The skin beneath the affected area remains soft. If the area is rewarmed, the patient experiences tingling or burning. This is followed by a "pins-and-needles" sensation as the area thaws and circulation improves.

A deep cold injury involves more tissue layers. This type of injury is more serious than superficial frostbite.

In a deep cold injury, the whitish skin color is followed by a waxy appearance. The affected area becomes frozen. It feels stiff and solid. The patient may complain of slight burning pain followed by a feeling of warmth and then numbness. Swelling may be present. Blisters may be present, usually appearing in one to seven days. If the affected area has thawed or partially thawed, the skin may appear flushed, with areas that are blue, purple, pale, or mottled.

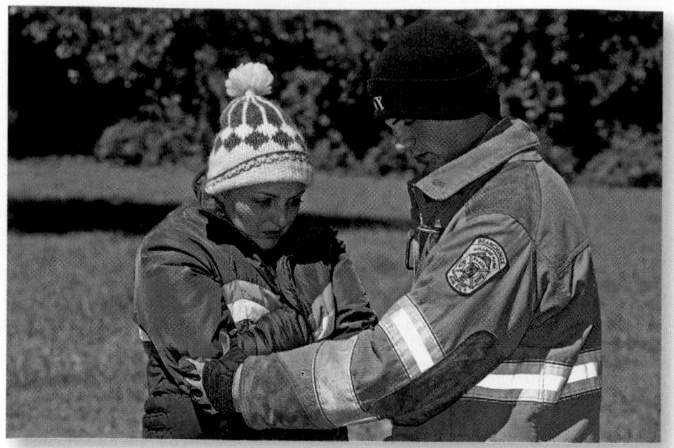

FIGURE 9-5 ▲ To care for an early (superficial) local cold injury, warm the affected part by placing it against a warm part of the body, such as the stomach or armpit.

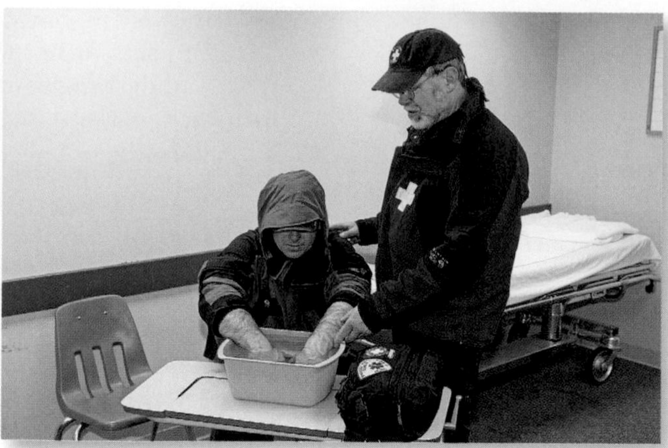

FIGURE 9-6 ▲ If you are instructed to do so, care for a late, or deep, local cold injury by placing the affected part in a warm (not hot) water bath.

Emergency Medical Responder Care of Patients with Local Cold Injury

Check your local protocol about care for local cold injuries.

Early (superficial) local cold injury is also called *frostnip.*

Complete a scene size-up before beginning emergency medical care. After making sure that the scene is safe, remove the patient from the cold environment. Protect the affected area from further injury. Provide oxygen if it is available and you have been trained to use it.

If the injury is early, or superficial, gently remove any jewelry or wet or restrictive clothing. If clothing is frozen to the skin, leave it in place. Rewarm the affected part by placing it against a warm part of the body, such as the stomach or armpit (Figure 9-5). Splint the affected extremity and apply soft padding. (Avoid pressure when applying the soft padding.) Loosely cover the affected area with dry sterile dressings or clothing. Do not rub or massage the affected area or reexpose the affected area to the cold. Doing so can cause damage to the skin and surrounding tissue.

If the injury is late, or deep, gently remove any jewelry or wet or restrictive clothing. If clothing is frozen to the skin, leave it in place. Loosely cover the affected area with dry, sterile dressings or clothing. Take care to avoid doing any of the following:

- Breaking blisters
- Rubbing or massaging the affected area
- Applying heat to or rewarming the affected area
- Allowing the patient to walk on an affected extremity

When an extremely long or delayed transport is certain, contact medical direction for instructions or follow your local protocol. Do not begin rewarming if there is a risk that the affected part will be exposed to the cold again. If you are instructed to begin active, rapid rewarming, be aware that the patient will complain of intense pain during thawing. Handle the affected area gently. Submerge the affected area in a warm water bath (100° to 105°F or 37.8° to 40.6°C; Figure 9-6.) Do *not* use hot water. If a thermometer is not available, test the water by pouring some of it over the inside of your arm. Check the temperature of the water often, adding more warm water as needed. Continuously stir the water around the affected part to keep the heat evenly distributed. Continue rewarming until the affected part is soft and color and sensation return. Gently dry the area after rewarming. Dress the area with dry, sterile dressings.

If the affected area is a hand or foot, place dry, sterile dressings between the fingers or toes. Elevate the affected extremity to decrease swelling. Protect against refreezing of the warmed part. Arrange for prompt patient transport.

Exposure to Heat

Heat cramps are the mildest form of heat-related emergencies. Heat stroke is the most severe.

Hyperthermia (a high core body temperature) results when the body gains or produces more heat than it loses. There are three main types of heat emergencies: heat cramps, heat exhaustion, and heat stroke.

Predisposing Factors

Cooling of the body through the evaporation of sweat becomes ineffective as humidity rises, particularly if the humidity is above 50%.

The climate can increase a person's risk for hyperthermia. High ambient temperature reduces the body's ability to lose heat by radiation. High relative humidity reduces the body's ability to lose heat by the evaporation of sweat. Exercise and strenuous activity can cause the loss of more than 1 liter (L) of sweat per hour.

Older adults are at higher risk for heat emergencies for many reasons, including the following:

- Medications
- Lack of mobility (the patient cannot escape the hot environment)
- Impaired ability to maintain a normal temperature
- Impaired ability to adapt to temperature changes
- Impaired sense of thirst

Newborns and infants are at a higher risk for heat-related emergencies. This higher risk is due to their impaired ability to maintain a normal temperature and their inability to remove their own clothing.

Some medications can increase the risk for hyperthermia. For example, amphetamines and cocaine increase muscle activity, which increases heat production. Alcohol impairs the body's ability to regulate heat. Tricyclic antidepressants and antihistamines weaken the body's ability to lose heat.

You Should Know

Conditions That Increase the Risk for a Heat-Related Emergency

- Heart disease
- Dehydration
- Obesity (due to increased insulation)
- Fever
- Fatigue
- Diabetes
- Thyroid disorder
- Parkinson's disease
- History of a heat-related emergency

Types of Heat-Related Emergencies

Objective 9 ▶

Heat cramps usually affect people who sweat a lot during strenuous activity in a warm environment. Water and electrolytes are lost from the body during sweating. This loss leads to dehydration. The loss of water and electrolytes causes painful muscle spasms, which usually occur in the arms, abdomen, and muscles at the back of the lower legs. The cramps usually improve with the patient's moving to a cool environment, drinking water, and resting.

Heat exhaustion is also a result of too much heat and dehydration. A patient who has heat exhaustion usually sweats heavily. Body temperature is usually normal or slightly elevated (up to 101 to 102°F, or 38.3 to 38.9°C). The patient's symptoms usually improve with moving him to a cool environment, the removal of excess clothing, and rest. The patient may drink water or a sports drink if awake, alert, and not nauseated. Severe heat exhaustion often requires intravenous (IV) fluids. Heat exhaustion may progress to heat stroke if it is not treated.

You Should Know

Signs and Symptoms of Heat Exhaustion

- Body temperature normal or slightly elevated (up to 101 to 102°F, or 38.3 to 38.9°C)
- Cool, pale, moist skin
- Muscle cramps
- Heavy sweating
- Fast heart rate
- Thirst
- Dizziness
- Tiredness
- Weakness
- Headache
- Nausea, vomiting
- Fainting

Heat stroke is severe hypovolemic shock. This form of heat-related illness is a medical emergency.

Prompt treatment may lower the death rate to between 15% and 20%.

Heat stroke is the most severe form of heat-related illness. It occurs when the body can no longer regulate its temperature. Most patients have hot, flushed skin and do not sweat. Athletes and firefighters who wear heavy uniforms and perform strenuous activity for long periods in a hot environment are at risk for heat stroke. Military recruits, athletes, construction workers, and foundry and laundry workers are also at risk.

A patient with heat stroke has a very high body temperature. She also has an altered mental status. She may have a seizure or become unresponsive. Of patients who experience heat stroke, 50–80% die. You must act quickly to lower the patient's body temperature and increase her chances of survival. Call for Advanced Life Support personnel as soon as possible. The patient will need IV fluids and further care at the hospital.

You Should Know

Signs and Symptoms of Heat Stroke

- Altered mental status
- Dry, hot, flushed skin
- A high body temperature (higher than 103°F, or 39.4°C, orally)
- A fast heart rate initially and then a slow heart rate
- Deep breathing followed by periods of shallow breathing
- Headache
- Dizziness
- Nausea
- Vision disturbances
- Muscle twitching, seizures
- Unresponsiveness

Emergency Medical Responder Care of Patients with Heat-Related Emergencies

Objective 10 ▶

The first step in the emergency care of a patient suffering from a heat-related illness is to remove the patient from the hot environment. Move the patient to a cool (air-conditioned) location.

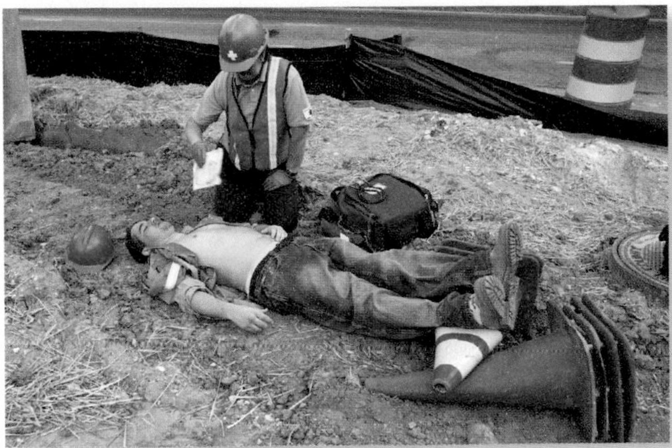

FIGURE 9-7 ▲ Remove as much of the patient's outer clothing as possible. Cool the patient by fanning. Elevate the patient's legs 8–12 inches (shock position).

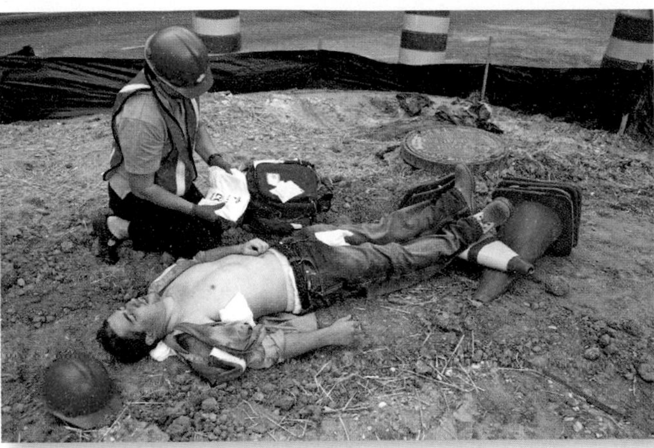

FIGURE 9-8 ▲ Remove as much of the patient's outer clothing as possible. Cool the patient by applying cool packs to the back of the neck, armpits, and groin. Wet the patient's skin and keep it wet by applying water with a sponge or wet towels.

Consult medical direction or follow local protocol.

Spray bottles filled with water are an excellent resource when trying to cool a patient who has been exposed to the heat.

Follow these guidelines if the patient has moist, pale skin that is normal to cool in temperature (Figure 9-7):

- Provide oxygen if it is available and you have been trained to use it. If the patient's breathing is adequate, apply oxygen by mask at 15 LPM. If the patient's breathing is inadequate, assist his breathing with a bag-valve-mask or mouth-to-mask device.
- Remove as much of the patient's outer clothing as possible. Loosen clothing that cannot be easily removed. Cool the patient by fanning. Do not cool the patient to the point of shivering, because shivering generates heat.
- Raise the patient's legs 8–12 inches (shock position). If the patient's mental status worsens and you do not suspect trauma, place him in the recovery position.
- If the patient is awake and alert and is not nauseated, have him slowly drink water or a sports drink. (Consult medical direction or follow local protocol.) If the patient has an altered mental status, is nauseated, or is vomiting, do *not* give fluids. Place the patient in the recovery position.
- Comfort, calm, and reassure the patient while waiting for help to arrive. If the patient is stable, perform ongoing assessments every 15 minutes. If the patient is unstable, perform ongoing assessments every five minutes.

Follow these guidelines if the patient has hot and dry or moist skin:

- Call for Advanced Life Support personnel as soon as possible. If ALS personnel are not available, arrange for patient transport to the closest appropriate facility.
- Provide oxygen if it is available and you have been trained to use it. If the patient's breathing is adequate, apply oxygen by mask at 15 LPM. If the patient's breathing is inadequate, assist his breathing with a bag-valve-mask or mouth-to-mask device.
- Start cooling the patient. Remove as much of the patient's outer clothing as possible. Apply cool packs to the back of the neck, armpits, and groin. Make sure to place a towel or dressings between the cool pack and the patient's skin to prevent local cold injury. Wet the patient's skin and keep it wet by applying water with a sponge or wet towels (Figure 9-8). Alternately, you can cover the patient with a sheet and keep the sheet wet. Fan the patient aggressively to promote evaporation and convective cooling. Note that fanning may not be effective if the humidity is high.
- Arrange for immediate patient transport. Comfort, calm, and reassure the patient while waiting for help to arrive. Perform ongoing assessments every five minutes.

Never try to cool a patient by placing him or her in an ice water bath.

Behavioral Emergencies

Behavior is the manner in which a person acts or performs. It includes any or all of a person's activities, including physical and mental activity. Abnormal behavior is a way of acting or conducting oneself that

- Is not consistent with society's norms and expectations
- Interferes with the individual's well-being and ability to function
- May be harmful to the individual or others

Objective 11 ▶

A **behavioral emergency** is a situation in which a patient displays abnormal behavior that is unacceptable to the patient, family members, or community. A behavioral emergency can be due to extremes of emotion that lead to violence or other inappropriate behavior. A behavioral emergency can also be due to a psychological or physical condition, such as mental illness, a lack of oxygen, or low blood sugar. Factors that may cause a change in a patient's behavior include alcohol or drugs, situational stressors, medical illnesses, and psychiatric illnesses or crises (Table 9-2). Psychological crises include panic, agitation, bizarre thinking and behavior, and destructive behavior. The patient who experiences a psychological crisis may be a danger to herself. She may show self-destructive behavior, such as suicide. She may also be a danger to others, acting in a threatening manner or even committing violence.

TABLE 9-2 Factors That May Cause Changes in Behavior

Mind-Altering Substances	• Alcohol, drugs	
Situational Stressors	• Rape • Loss of a job • Career change • Death of a loved one • Marital stress or divorce	• Physical or psychological abuse • Natural disasters (such as tornado, flood, earthquake, hurricane) • Human-made disasters (such as war, an explosion)
Medical Illnesses	• Poisoning • Central nervous system infection • Head trauma • Seizure disorder • Lack of oxygen (hypoxia)	• Low blood sugar • Inadequate blood flow to the brain • Extremes of temperature (excessive cold or heat)
Psychiatric Illnesses or Crises	• Panic • Agitation • Bizarre thinking and behavior	• Self-destructive behavior, suicide (danger to self) • Threatening behavior, violence (danger to others)

Remember This!

Do not assume that a patient has a psychiatric illness until you have ruled out possible physical causes for his or her behavior.

Psychological Crises

Anxiety and Panic

Objective 13 ▶

Anxiety is a state of worry and agitation that is usually triggered by a vague or an imagined situation. A person who is anxious is afraid of losing control or may feel that he will not be able to meet another's expectations. Some anxiety is good. To a point, it can increase awareness and performance. However, as one's level of anxiety increases, it drains energy, shortens one's attention span, and interferes with thinking and problem solving. Fear is usually triggered by a specific object or situation, such as a fear of losing a job or of being unable to pay the bills. Fear and anxiety are normal responses to a perceived threat. Fear and anxiety bring on various symptoms:

- Worry
- Confusion
- Apprehension
- Helplessness
- Negative thoughts

People show anxiety at different levels of intensity, ranging from uneasiness to a panic attack. Anxiety can be due to a medical cause.

You Should Know

Conditions Associated with Anxiety

- Asthma
- Diabetes
- Heart problems
- Thyroid disorder
- Seizure disorder
- Inner ear disturbances
- Premenstrual syndrome (PMS)
- Withdrawal from alcohol, sedatives, or tranquilizers
- Reactions to cocaine, amphetamines, caffeine, aspartame, or other stimulants

Anxiety disorders are the most common mental illness in the United States.

An **anxiety disorder** is more intense than normal anxiety. Anxiety normally goes away after the stressful situation that caused it is over. An anxiety disorder lasts for months and can lead to phobias. A patient with an anxiety disorder often has physical signs and symptoms that accompany the patient's intense worry. The common signs and symptoms are

- Tiredness
- Headaches
- Muscle tension
- Muscle aches
- Difficulty swallowing
- Trembling
- Twitching
- Irritability
- Sweating
- Hot flashes

Most panic attacks do not last longer than one-half hour.

A **panic attack** is an intense fear that occurs for no apparent reason. Panic attacks can build gradually over several minutes or hours or occur suddenly. The fear that accompanies a panic attack is very real to the patient. It is sometimes difficult for healthcare professionals to relate to that fear because there may be no obvious trigger. Do not minimize the patient's symptoms. Be supportive, calm, and reassuring.

You Should Know

Signs and Symptoms Common to Panic Attacks

- Numbness or tingling sensations (usually in the fingers, toes, or lips)
- Shortness of breath or a smothering sensation
- Heart palpitations (a rapid or irregular heartbeat)
- A fear of going crazy or being out of control
- Nausea or abdominal distress
- Choking
- Sweating
- Hot flashes or chills
- A feeling of detachment or being out of touch with oneself
- Trembling or shaking
- Dizziness or faintness
- Fear of becoming seriously ill or dying

Phobias

A phobia is a type of anxiety disorder.

A phobia is an irrational, constant fear of a specific activity, object, or situation. Some phobias are common and usually do not create a problem because the person simply avoids the activity, object, or situation. A phobic reaction resembles a panic attack. The signs and symptoms may include panic, sweating, difficulty breathing, and an increased heart rate.

You Should Know

Common Phobias

- Open spaces
- Driving, riding in vehicles
- Heights
- Darkness
- Enclosed spaces
- Flying
- Germs, bacteria
- Insects
- Public speaking
- Doctors, dentists
- Thunder, lightning
- Blood
- Animals
- Crossing bridges
- Water
- Being alone

Depression

More Americans suffer from depression than coronary heart disease, cancer, and AIDS combined.

Depression is a state of mind characterized by feelings of sadness, worthlessness, and discouragement. It often occurs in response to a loss. The loss may be the loss of a job, the death of a loved one, or the end of a relationship. The signs of depression vary with age. Depressed children may be sad, be irritable, or cry frequently. They may express anger by acting out toward parents, teachers, or other authority figures. Older children may have no appetite and may experience headaches or skin disorders. Depressed teens may behave unpredictably, run away, or change their physical and social activities. They may have no appetite, show no interest in their appearance, use alcohol or drugs excessively, or attempt suicide.

Depressed adults show a lack of interest in their job, home, or appearance. They focus on the negative aspects of life, past events, and failures. They may attempt suicide. Depression in older adults is often related to retirement. It may also be connected to the belief that they lack control over their lives, or it may result from a loss, such as the death of a spouse or another loved one. Older adults may feel useless or that they are a "burden." They may feel lonely as loved ones die or move away. Depressed older adults often withdraw, refuse to speak to anyone, and confine themselves to bed.

You Should Know

Signs and Symptoms of Depression

- Loss of appetite
- Diarrhea or constipation
- Tiredness
- Difficulty sleeping or sleeping too much
- Muscle aches
- Vague pains
- Constant feelings of sadness, irritability, or tension
- Significant weight loss or gain
- Loss of interest in usual activities or hobbies
- Crying spells
- Inability to make decisions or to concentrate
- Feelings of anger, helplessness, guilt, worthlessness, hopelessness, or loneliness
- Thoughts of suicide or death

Bipolar disorder is also known as manic-depressive illness.

Bipolar Disorder

Bipolar disorder is a brain disorder that causes unusual shifts in a person's mood, energy, and ability to function. A person with bipolar disorder has alternating episodes of mood elevation (mania) and depression. When manic, the person often appears restless. She may be extremely energetic and enthusiastic. Typically, a manic person is easily distracted, requires little sleep, and develops unrealistic plans. A person with bipolar disorder also usually experiences periods of depression in which she feels worthless. She may consider suicide. The person's mood is often normal between the periods of mania and depression.

Paranoia

Paranoia is a mental disorder characterized by excessive suspiciousness or delusions. **Delusions** are false beliefs that the patient believes are true, despite facts to the contrary. The common delusions of a paranoid patient include the following:

- Believing that people are following him, harassing him, plotting against him, reading his mind, or controlling his thoughts
- Believing that he possesses great power or special abilities
- Believing that he is a famous person

Hallucinations involve the senses. Delusions involve beliefs.

Paranoid patients may experience hallucinations. **Hallucinations** are false sensory perceptions. In other words, the patient sees, hears, or feels things others cannot. For example, a patient with visual hallucinations may think he sees worms or snakes crawling on the floor. An example of an auditory hallucination is hearing voices. An example of a tactile hallucination is feeling insects crawling on the skin.

Paranoid patients are suspicious, distrustful, and prone to argument. They often feel as if they are being mistreated and misjudged. These patients tend to carry grudges, recalling wrongs done to them years earlier. They are excitable and unpredictable, with outbursts of bizarre or aggressive behavior.

Schizophrenia

Schizophrenia is not the same as multiple personality disorder.

Schizophrenia is a group of mental disorders. Its symptoms include hallucinations, delusions, disordered thinking, rambling speech, and bizarre or disorganized behavior. Schizophrenic patients are often reserved, withdrawn, and indifferent to the feelings of others. They prefer to be alone and have few, if any, close friends. They can become combative and are at high risk for suicidal and homicidal behavior.

Suicide

Suicide is any willful act designed to end one's own life. Most people who commit suicide express their intentions beforehand. You should take every suicide threat or gesture seriously and arrange for patient transport for evaluation.

You Should Know

Risk Factors for Suicide

- Previous suicide attempt(s)
- History of mental disorders, particularly depression
- History of alcohol and drug abuse
- Family history of suicide
- Family history of child maltreatment
- Feelings of hopelessness
- Impulsive or aggressive tendencies
- Barriers to accessing mental health treatment
- Loss (relational, social, work, or financial)
- Physical illness
- Easy access to lethal methods
- Unwillingness to seek help because of the stigma attached to mental health and substance abuse disorders or suicidal thoughts
- Cultural and religious beliefs—for example, the belief that suicide is a noble resolution of a personal problem
- Local epidemics of suicide
- Isolation—a feeling of being cut off from other people

Depression is a factor that contributes to suicide. Arrest, imprisonment, or the loss of a job may be a source of depression. The risk for suicide is greatest in persons who have previously attempted suicide. The probability of successful suicide may increase with successive attempts, increasing the patient's risk. For example, a patient who ingested pills on her first attempt may slash her wrists on a second attempt.

Men commit suicide more frequently than women, although women *attempt* suicide more frequently than men.

The more well thought out the plan, the more serious the suicide risk. A patient who has chosen a lethal plan of action and has told others about it is at an increased risk. An unusual gathering of articles that could be used to commit suicide increases the risk (such as the purchase of a gun or a large volume of pills). If you've been told that the patient is suicidal, ask him about it. For example, ask the patient, "Your family says you've thought about killing yourself. Can you tell me about it?" If the

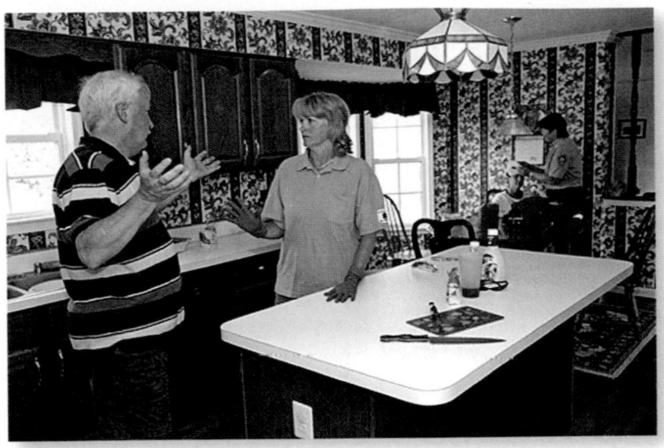

FIGURE 9-9 ► When you arrive on the scene of a possible behavioral emergency, carefully assess the scene for dangers, including the presence of weapons.

patient says he has had suicidal thoughts, ask if he has planned how he would carry it out. Then determine if he has a means to do it.

Assessment of Patients with Behavioral Emergencies

Calls to a scene involving a behavioral emergency cause healthcare professionals anxiety, because the scene is often unpredictable. Take steps to ensure your safety and that of other healthcare professionals responding to the scene. Start by considering the dispatch information you are given. Have you responded to this location in the past? If so, how many times? Were those calls violent? Find out from your dispatcher if law enforcement personnel are already on the scene. If they are not, ask that they respond to the scene. Remember, your safety comes first.

If you suspect a dangerous situation, do *not* enter the scene until law enforcement personnel are present and the safety of the scene is assured.

When you arrive on the scene, complete a scene size-up before beginning emergency medical care. Carefully assess the scene for possible dangers. Start by visually locating the patient. Visually scan the area for possible weapons (Figure 9-9). Look for signs of violence and evidence of substance abuse. Does the patient have a method or the means of committing suicide? Is this a domestic violence situation? Are there multiple patients? Also note the general condition of the environment. Look for signs of possible underlying medical problems, such as medications, home oxygen, or other medical equipment.

Never turn your back on a violent or potentially violent patient.

Check with the family and bystanders to see if the patient has threatened or has a history of violence, aggression, or combativeness. Patient postures that may indicate potential violence include

- Standing or sitting in a position that threatens the self or others
- Being unable to sit still, pacing nervously
- Clenching the fists or jaw
- Having an unsafe object in his or her hands

Throughout your assessment and care of the patient, maintain an alertness to danger.

Speech patterns may indicate potential violence. Examples include erratic speech, yelling, shouting, cursing, or threats of harm to the self or others. Watch the patient's movements closely. Movements that may indicate potential violence include

- Moving toward rescuers
- Carrying heavy or threatening objects
- Tensing the muscles
- Making quick, irregular movements

Other signs of potential violence include having a flushed face, being agitated, turning away when spoken to, and avoiding eye contact.

Objective 17 ▶

When you are called to the scene of a behavioral emergency, be prepared to spend time at the scene. Limit the number of people around the patient. Take time to calm the patient. Start by approaching the patient slowly and purposefully. Do *not* make any quick movements. If the patient is lying down, it is safest to approach her from the head.

Objective 12 ▶ Objective 14 ▶ Objective 25 ▶

Clearly identify yourself and try to build a connection with the patient. Explain who you are and what you are trying to do for her. As you talk with her, begin your assessment of the patient's mental status, airway, breathing, and circulation. Is she alert and oriented to person, place, time, and event? If the patient is confused, you will probably need to state more than once who you are and what you are doing. Respect the patient's personal space by limiting physical touch. Keep in mind that treating any life-threatening illness or injury that you find takes priority over the patient's behavioral problem.

Be aware of your position and posture when talking to your patient. Standing over her will immediately put her on the defensive. Face her and sit or stand at or below the patient's level while maintaining a comfortable distance from her. Maintain eye contact with the patient. Let her know what you expect and what she can expect from you. As you assess and provide care for your patient, keep her informed about what you are doing.

Do *not* place the patient between yourself and an exit.

Note the patient's appearance, speech, and mood. Is she speaking normally or is her speech garbled? Does she seem anxious, depressed, excited, agitated, angry, hostile, or fearful? If the patient appears disturbed or agitated, try to provide a safe, nonthreatening environment in which you can assess her. Pay attention to the patient's thought process. Does it appear disordered? Is the patient hearing or seeing things that are not there? Does she have unusual worries or fears?

Methods to Calm Patients with Behavioral Emergencies

Objective 24 ▶

Be polite and respectful when talking with a patient with a behavioral problem. Be careful not to talk down to him. Ask the patient open-ended questions using a calm, reassuring voice. Open-ended questions require more than a yes or no answer—for example, "Why were we called here today?" After asking a question, give the patient time to answer you. Allow him to tell you his story without being judgmental. Show you are listening by rephrasing or repeating part of what was said. Be aware of your own reactions to the situation and to what the patient is saying. For example, an anxious patient may make you anxious. A hostile patient may make you angry. Be careful not to allow your personal feelings to get in the way of your professional judgment. Do not threaten, challenge, or argue with disturbed patients.

Remember This!

- Do not assume you cannot talk with a patient until you have tried.
- Keeping your emotions in check when caring for a violent patient can be difficult. Monitor yourself. If your feelings and actions escalate, it is likely that the patient's feelings and actions will also escalate.

Objective 26 ▶

Give your patient honest reassurance. Answer his questions honestly—do not lie to him. However, do not make promises you cannot keep. If the patient is hearing or seeing things, do not "play along." In other words, do not tell the patient you are seeing or hearing the same things he is in an attempt to win his trust. Instead, let the patient know that you do not hear what he is hearing but are interested in knowing what he is hearing.

Stop and Think!

Never leave a patient who is experiencing a behavioral emergency alone.

If possible, involve trusted family members or friends in the patient's care. However, if family members or bystanders are disruptive as you attempt to assess the patient, or if they interfere with your care of the patient, ask law enforcement personnel to remove them from the area.

Restraining Patients with Behavioral Emergencies

Be aware that, after a period of combativeness and aggression, some apparently calm patients may cause unexpected and sudden injury to you, themselves, or others.

Avoid restraining a patient unless the patient is a danger to you, herself, or others. When using restraints, have police present, if possible, and get approval from medical direction. If you must use restraints, apply them with the help of law enforcement and other EMS personnel.

Avoid the use of unreasonable force. Reasonable force depends on what force is necessary to keep the patient from injuring you, herself, or others. You can determine what is reasonable by looking at all the circumstances involved. These circumstances include the following:

- The patient's size and strength
- The type of abnormal behavior
- The patient's gender and mental state
- The method of restraint

Avoid acts or physical force that may cause injury to the patient.

When applying restraints, make certain you have enough assistance. You will need at least four healthcare or law enforcement personnel (one for each extremity). Have a plan. Decide who will do what before attempting to restrain the patient. Be sure to take BSI precautions for protection against body fluids.

Use only the force necessary for restraint.

Estimate the range of motion of the patient's arms and legs. Stay beyond that range until you are ready to restrain the patient. Once the decision has been made to restrain, act quickly. One EMS professional should talk to the patient throughout the procedure. Tell the patient you are restraining her for her safety and for the safety of those around her. At least four people should approach the patient. Each one should be assigned to each of the patient's extremities ("limb assignments"; Figure 9-10). Restrain on cue to gain rapid control of the patient.

Secure the patient's extremities with restraints approved by medical direction, such as soft leather or cloth. Secure the patient on her back to the stretcher with chest, waist, and thigh straps (Figure 9-11). If the patient is spitting, cover her face with a disposable surgical mask. Reassess the patient's airway, breathing, and circulation frequently. Suction as necessary. Chest straps should not hinder the patient's breathing. Reassess distal pulses in each extremity to make sure circulation is not impaired by the restraints. When using restraints, be careful to avoid doing any of the following:

- Inflicting unnecessary pain
- Using unreasonable force
- Leaving a restrained patient unattended
- Removing the restraints once they have been applied

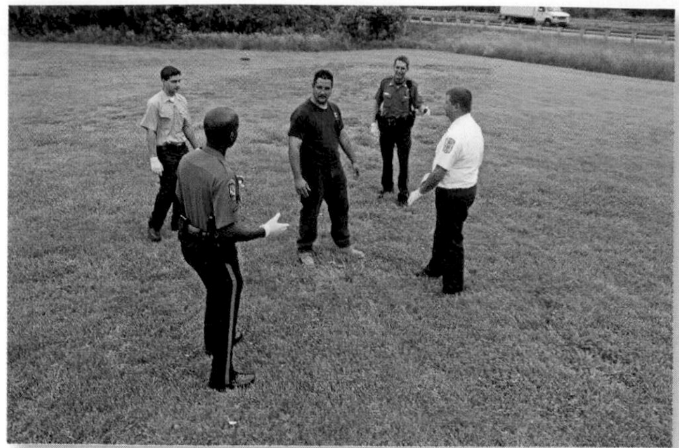

FIGURE 9-10 ▲ Once the decision has been made to restrain a patient, act quickly. One EMS professional should talk to the patient throughout the procedure. At least four persons should approach the patient, one assigned to each of the patient's extremities. Restrain on cue to gain rapid control of the patient.

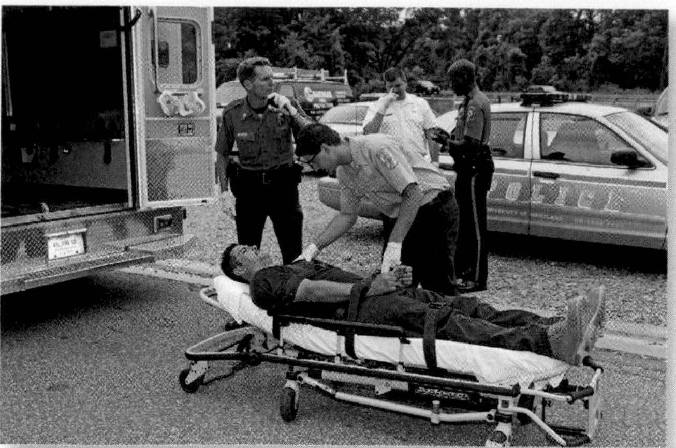

FIGURE 9-11 ▲ Secure the patient on his or her back to the stretcher with chest, waist, and thigh straps. Reassess the patient's airway, breathing, and circulation frequently.

You Should Know

Acceptable Restraints

- Soft leather straps
- Padded cloth straps
- Nylon restraints
- Velcro straps

Stop and Think!

A restrained patient must *never* be left alone. You must constantly monitor the status of the patient's airway, breathing, and circulation while the patient is in your care.

Some states may require an involuntary petition to be completed before a person is forcibly transported against his or her will. Check your state regulations and local protocol.

It is important to document the use of restraints. Make sure to document your findings each time you reassess the patient while she is in restraints and in your care.

Remember This!

Documenting the Use of Restraints

When caring for a patient in restraints, document the following information:

- The reason for the restraints
- The number of personnel used to restrain the patient
- The type of restraint used
- The time the restraints were placed on the patient
- The status of the patient's ABCs and distal pulses before and after the restraints were applied
- The reassessment of the patient's ABCs and distal pulses

Medical and Legal Considerations

Emotionally disturbed patients may falsely accuse EMS and law enforcement personnel of unprofessional conduct, including sexual misconduct. To protect yourself against false accusations, it is very important that you document the patient's abnormal behavior. If possible, have witnesses present when you provide patient care. This is especially important during transport. When possible, use attendants of the same gender as the patient and involve third-party witnesses.

Emotionally disturbed patients will often resist treatment. To provide care against the patient's will, you must have a reasonable belief that the patient would harm you, himself, or others. If the patient is a threat to you, himself, or others, the patient may be transported without consent after you have contacted medical direction and have received approval to do so. Law enforcement personnel are usually required.

On The Scene

Wrap-Up

By the time the ambulance arrives, you have obtained the patient's blood pressure. It is 96/54. You did not find any other abnormal findings in your examination. You give a report and the Paramedics apply oxygen by mask at 15 LPM. They start an IV and check the patient's blood sugar, which is normal. They recheck his vital signs and notice that his breathing is now more labored, so they insert an oral airway. You begin to assist his breathing with a BVM until they insert the breathing (endotracheal) tube.

A police officer performs a quick search of his home and finds his prescribed medicines, but nothing else that is unusual. The ambulance leaves the scene with lights and sirens on to hasten their arrival to the hospital.

You wonder what caused this patient's condition. Later, Paramedics tell you that he had a stroke with bleeding in his brain. Apparently, the stroke happened a day or two ago. His body temperature was low from lying immobile on the floor for so long. Unfortunately, his condition rapidly worsened at the hospital and he died an hour after arrival. ■

Sum It Up

- As an Emergency Medical Responder, you should assess every patient and determine the chief complaint, as well as the signs and symptoms. Give emergency medical care based on the patient's signs and symptoms. Keep in mind that some patient complaints apply to more than one illness.
- Your initial assessment of the patient begins from across the room. Form a general impression by looking at your patient's appearance, work of breathing, and skin color. Once your general impression is complete, perform a hands-on assessment and gather the patient's history. Show a caring attitude when performing your assessment and providing care.
- An *altered mental status* is a change in a patient's level of awareness. It is also called an *altered level of consciousness (ALOC)*. A change in the patient's mental status may occur gradually or suddenly. It may last briefly or be prolonged. A patient with an altered mental status may appear confused, agitated, combative, sleepy, difficult to awaken, or unresponsive. An altered mental status should be treated as a medical emergency. Regardless of the cause of the altered mental status, emergency care focuses on airway, breathing, and circulation.

- A *seizure* is a temporary change in behavior or consciousness caused by abnormal electrical activity within one or more groups of brain cells. A seizure is a symptom of an underlying problem within the central nervous system. The most common cause of adult seizures is the failure to take anti-seizure medication. The most common cause of seizures in infants and young children is a high fever. Epilepsy is a condition of recurring seizures; the cause is usually irreversible.
  - The type of seizure that involves stiffening and jerking of the patient's body is called a *tonic-clonic seizure* (formerly called a *grand mal seizure*). This type of seizure typically has four phases:
    1. Aura—a peculiar sensation that comes before a seizure
    2. Tonic phase—the body's muscles stiffen, the patient's breathing may be noisy, and the patient may turn blue
    3. Clonic phase—alternating jerking and relaxation of the body occurs
    4. Postictal phase—the period of recovery that follows a seizure; the patient often appears limp, has shallow breathing, and has an altered mental status
  - *Status epilepticus* is a seizure that lasts longer than 30 minutes *or* a series of seizures occurring over a 30-minute period in which the patient remains unresponsive between seizures. Status epilepticus is a medical emergency. It can cause brain damage or death if it is not treated.
    - No matter what caused the seizure, your emergency care must focus on the patient's airway, breathing, and circulation. In addition, remember the following:
      1. Protect the patient's privacy.
      2. If the patient is actively seizing, protect the patient from harm by moving furniture and other objects away from the patient.
      3. Do not insert anything into the patient's mouth. Remove eyeglasses. Do not try to restrain body movements during the seizure.
      4. As soon as the seizure is over, make sure the patient's airway is open.
      5. Some patients are light sensitive (photophobic) after a seizure. Take care to reduce the patient's exposure to bright lights and loud noises.
- The skin plays a very important role in temperature regulation. Cold and warmth sensors (receptors) in the skin detect changes in temperature. These receptors relay the information to the hypothalamus. The hypothalamus (located in the brain) functions as the body's thermostat. It coordinates the body's response to temperature.
- The body loses heat to the environment in five ways:
  1. Radiation
     - *Radiation* is the transfer of heat from the surface of one object to the surface of another without contact between the two objects. When the temperature of the body is more than the temperature of the surroundings, the body will lose heat.
  2. Convection
     - *Convection* is the transfer of heat by the movement of air current. Wind speed affects heat loss by convection (wind-chill factor).
  3. Conduction
     - *Conduction* is the transfer of heat between objects that are in direct contact. Heat flows from warmer areas to cooler ones.
  4. Evaporation
     - *Evaporation* is a loss of heat by the vaporization of moisture on the body surface. The body will lose heat by evaporation if the skin temperature is higher than the temperature of the surroundings.

5. Breathing
    - The body loses heat through breathing. With normal breathing, the body continuously loses a relatively small amount of heat through the evaporation of moisture.

- *Hypothermia* is a core body temperature of less than 95°F (35°C). This condition results when the body loses more heat than it gains or produces.
    - A rectal temperature gives the most accurate measure of core temperature. However, obtaining a rectal temperature in the field often raises issues of patient sensitivity and welfare, such as exposure to cold by removing clothing.
    - Your main concern in providing care should be to remove the patient from the environment. Use trained rescuers for this purpose when necessary. Perform an initial assessment, keeping in mind that you need to move the patient to a warm location as quickly and as safely as possible. Remove any cold or wet clothing. Protect the patient from the environment. Assess the patient's mental status, airway, breathing, and circulation. Keep in mind that mental status decreases as the patient's body temperature drops.
    - You may need to rewarm the patient. The two main types of rewarming are passive and active.
        - *Passive rewarming* is the warming of a patient with minimal or no use of heat sources other than the patient's own heat production. Passive rewarming methods include placing the patient in a warm environment, applying warm clothing and blankets, and preventing drafts.
        - *Active rewarming* should be used only if sustained warmth can be ensured. Active rewarming involves adding heat directly to the surface of the patient's body. Warm blankets, heat packs, and/or hot water bottles may be used, depending on how severe the hypothermia is.
- Local cold injury *(frostbite)* involves tissue damage to a specific area of the body. It occurs when a body part, such as the nose, ears, cheeks, chin, hands, or feet, is exposed to prolonged or intense cold. When the body is exposed to cold, blood is forced away from the extremities to the body's core. A local cold injury may be early (superficial frostbite) or late (deep frostbite).
- When the body gains or produces more heat than it loses, *hyperthermia* (a high core body temperature) results. The three main types of heat emergencies are heat cramps, heat exhaustion, and heat stroke.
    1. *Heat cramps* usually affect people who sweat a lot during strenuous activity in a warm environment. Water and electrolytes are lost from the body during sweating. This loss leads to dehydration and causes painful muscle spasms.
    2. *Heat exhaustion* is also a result of too much heat and dehydration. A patient with heat exhaustion usually sweats heavily. His or her body temperature is usually normal or slightly elevated. Severe heat exhaustion often requires intravenous (IV) fluids. Heat exhaustion may progress to heat stroke if it is not treated.
    3. *Heat stroke* is the most severe form of heat-related illness. It occurs when the body can no longer regulate its temperature. Most patients have hot, flushed skin and do not sweat. Individuals who wear heavy uniforms and perform strenuous activity for long periods in a hot environment are at risk for heat stroke.
- The first step in the emergency care of a patient suffering from a heat-related illness is to remove the patient from the hot environment. Move the patient to a cool (air-conditioned) location and follow treatment guidelines based on the patient's degree of heat-related illness.

- As an Emergency Medical Responder, you will likely encounter various *behavioral emergencies.* A behavioral emergency is a situation in which a patient displays abnormal behavior that is unacceptable to the patient, family members, or community. A behavioral emergency can be due to extremes of emotion or to psychological or physical conditions. A number of factors can result in these emergencies, including mental illness, a lack of oxygen, low blood sugar, alcohol or drugs, situational stressors, medical illnesses, and psychiatric illnesses or crises.
  - *Anxiety* is a state of worry and agitation that is usually triggered by a vague or an imagined situation.
  - An *anxiety disorder* is more intense than normal anxiety. Anxiety normally goes away after the stressful situation that caused it is over. An anxiety disorder lasts for months and can lead to phobias.
  - A *panic attack* is an intense fear that occurs for no apparent reason. Panic attacks can build gradually over several minutes or hours or can occur suddenly. The fear that accompanies a panic attack is very real to the patient. It is sometimes difficult for healthcare professionals to relate to that fear because there may be no obvious trigger.
  - A *phobia* is an irrational, constant fear of a specific activity, object, or situation. Some phobias are common and usually do not create a problem because the person simply avoids the activity, object, or situation. A phobic reaction resembles a panic attack. The signs and symptoms include panic, sweating, difficulty breathing, and an increased heart rate.
  - *Depression* is a state of mind characterized by feelings of sadness, worthlessness, and discouragement. It often occurs in response to a loss. The loss may be of a job, a loved one, or a relationship. The signs of depression vary with age.
  - *Bipolar disorder* is a brain disorder that causes unusual shifts in a person's mood, energy, and ability to function. A person with bipolar disorder has alternating episodes of mood elevation (mania) and depression. When manic, the person often appears restless. He or she may be extremely energetic and enthusiastic. A person with bipolar disorder also usually experiences periods of depression, in which he or she feels worthless. The person may consider suicide. The person's mood is often normal between the periods of mania and depression.
  - *Paranoia* is a mental disorder characterized by excessive suspiciousness or delusions. Paranoid patients are suspicious, distrustful, and prone to argument. They often feel as if they are being mistreated and misjudged. These patients tend to carry grudges, recalling wrongs done to them years before. They are excitable and unpredictable, with outbursts of bizarre or aggressive behavior.
  - *Delusions* are false beliefs that the patient believes are true, despite facts to the contrary.
  - *Hallucinations* are false sensory perceptions. The patient sees, hears, or feels things that others cannot.
  - *Schizophrenia* is a group of mental disorders. Its symptoms include hallucinations, delusions, disordered thinking, rambling speech, and bizarre or disorganized behavior. Schizophrenic patients are often reserved, withdrawn, and indifferent to the feelings of others. They prefer to be alone and have few, if any, close friends. They can become combative and are at high risk for suicidal and homicidal behavior.
  - *Suicide* is any willful act designed to end one's own life. Most people who commit suicide express their intentions beforehand. You should take every suicide threat or gesture seriously and arrange for patient transport for evaluation.
- When called to a scene that involves a behavioral emergency, remember that the scene may be unpredictable. Take steps to ensure your safety and that of other

healthcare professionals responding to the scene. Complete a scene size-up before beginning emergency medical care. Carefully assess the scene for possible dangers. Start by visually locating the patient. Visually scan the area for possible weapons. Be prepared to spend time at the scene. Limit the number of people around the patient. Take time to calm the patient.

- Avoid restraining a patient unless the patient is a danger to you, him- or herself, or others. When using restraints, have police present, if possible, and get approval from your medical director. If you must use restraints, apply them with the help of law enforcement and other EMS personnel.
- When caring for a patient in restraints, document the following information:
    - The reason for the restraints
    - The number of personnel used to restrain the patient
    - The type of restraint used
    - The time the restraints were placed on the patient
    - The status of the patient's ABCs and distal pulses before and after the restraints were applied
    - The reassessment of the patient's ABCs and distal pulses

▶ Tracking Your Progress

After reading this chapter, can you	Page Reference	Objective Met?
• Identify the patient who presents with a general medical complaint?	294	☐
• Explain the steps in providing emergency medical care to a patient with a general medical complaint?	295–296	☐
• Identify the patient who presents with a specific medical complaint of altered mental status?	296–297	☐
• Explain the steps in providing emergency medical care to a patient with an altered mental status?	297	☐
• Identify the patient who presents with a specific medical complaint of seizures?	298–301	☐
• Explain the steps in providing emergency medical care to a patient with seizures?	301	☐
• Identify the patient who presents with a specific medical complaint of exposure to cold?	304	☐
• Explain the steps in providing emergency medical care to a patient with an exposure to cold?	308–311	☐
• Identify the patient who presents with a specific medical complaint of exposure to heat?	311–312	☐
• Explain the steps in providing emergency medical care to a patient with an exposure to heat?	312–313	☐
• Identify the patient who presents with a specific medical complaint of behavioral change?	314	☐
• Explain the steps in providing emergency medical care to a patient with a behavioral change?	319–321	☐
• Identify the patient who presents with a specific complaint of a psychological crisis?	315–319	☐

• Explain the steps in providing emergency medical care to a patient with a psychological crisis?	320–321	☐
• Attend to the feelings of the patient and/or family when dealing with the patient with a general medical complaint?	295	☐
• Attend to the feelings of the patient and/or family when dealing with the patient with a specific medical complaint?	297	☐
• Explain the rationale for modifying your behavior toward the patient with a behavioral emergency?	320	☐
• Demonstrate a caring attitude toward patients with a general medical complaint who request Emergency Medical Services?	295	☐
• Place the interests of the patient with a general medical complaint as the foremost consideration when making any and all patient care decisions?	296	☐
• Communicate with empathy to patients with a general medical complaint, as well as with family members and friends of the patient?	296	☐
• Demonstrate a caring attitude toward patients with a specific medical complaint who request Emergency Medical Services?	300	☐
• Place the interests of the patient with a specific medical complaint as the foremost consideration when making any and all patient care decisions?	301	☐
• Communicate with empathy to patients with a specific medical complaint, as well as with family members and friends of the patient?	300	☐
• Demonstrate a caring attitude toward patients with a behavioral problem who request Emergency Medical Services?	320–321	☐
• Place the interests of the patient with a behavioral problem as the foremost consideration when making any and all patient care decisions?	320	☐
• Communicate with empathy to patients with a behavioral problem, as well as with family members and friends of the patient?	320–321	☐

Chapter Quiz

Multiple Choice

In the space provided, identify the letter of the choice that best completes each statement or answers each question.

_____ **1.** Most heat is lost from the body by the process of

a. breathing.
b. radiation.
c. conduction.
d. convection.

_____ **2.** You are called to care for an elderly man found unresponsive in an alley. It is a cold January night. You see no obvious signs of life as you approach the patient. You should check the patient's breathing and pulse for

a. no more than 10 seconds.
b. 30–45 seconds.
c. 45–60 seconds.
d. 1–2 minutes.

_____ **3.** The signs and symptoms of mild hypothermia include

a. rigid muscles.
b. a progressive loss of responsiveness.
c. an increased heart rate and respiratory rate.
d. cardiopulmonary arrest.

_____ **4.** What is the most commonly used method of suicide in the United States?

a. hanging
b. pills
c. firearms
d. alcohol

_____ **5.** You are called to the home of a 21-year-old man who has called 9-1-1. He had threatened to kill himself with an overdose of sleeping pills. You arrive to find your patient sitting quietly in his bedroom. After sizing up the scene, your next step should be to

a. contact medical direction for instructions.
b. quickly look around the room for items the patient might use to kill himself.
c. prepare to restrain the patient.
d. perform a head-to-toe physical examination.

True or False

Decide whether each statement is true or false. In the space provided, write T for true or F for false.

_____ **6.** An altered mental status is often a medical emergency.

_____ **7.** A person does not have to be exposed to cold environmental temperatures in order for hypothermia to occur.

Short Answer

Answer each question in the space provided.

8. List five causes of an altered mental status.

1. _____________________
2. _____________________
3. _____________________
4. _____________________
5. _____________________

9. List the two types of a local cold injury.

1. _____________________
2. _____________________

10. Why are infants and young children at an increased risk for hypothermia?

____

____

____

11. You are called for an unresponsive patient who is a victim of cold exposure. Describe how you should assess this patient's general temperature.

____

____

____

12. Name four body parts that are prone to a local cold injury.

1. ______________

2. ______________

3. ______________

4. ______________

13. List the three main types of heat emergencies.

1. ______________

2. ______________

3. ______________

14. A patient experiencing a behavioral emergency required physical restraint. The procedure was accomplished successfully. You recall that it is very important to document the use of restraints. List the areas that must be covered in your documentation of this procedure.

____

____

____

CHAPTER

10 Bleeding and Soft-Tissue Injuries

By the end of this chapter, you should be able to

Knowledge Objectives ▶

1. Differentiate between arterial, venous, and capillary bleeding.
2. State the emergency medical care for external bleeding.
3. Establish the relationship between body substance isolation precautions and bleeding.
4. List the signs of internal bleeding.
5. List the steps in the emergency medical care of the patient with signs and symptoms of internal bleeding.
6. Establish the relationship between body substance isolation precautions and soft-tissue injuries.
7. State the types of open soft-tissue injuries.
8. Describe the emergency medical care of the patient with a soft-tissue injury.
9. Discuss the emergency medical care considerations for a patient with a penetrating chest injury.
10. State the emergency medical care considerations for a patient with an open wound to the abdomen.
11. Describe the emergency medical care for an impaled object.
12. State the emergency medical care for an amputation.
13. Describe the emergency medical care for burns.
14. List the functions of dressing and bandaging.

Attitude Objectives ▶

15. Explain the rationale for body substance isolation precautions when dealing with bleeding and soft-tissue injuries.
16. Attend to the feelings of the patient with a soft-tissue injury or bleeding.
17. Demonstrate a caring attitude toward patients with a soft-tissue injury or bleeding who request Emergency Medical Services.
18. Place the interests of the patient with a soft-tissue injury or bleeding as the foremost consideration when making any and all patient care decisions.
19. Communicate with empathy to patients with a soft-tissue injury or bleeding, as well as with family members and friends of the patient.

Skill Objectives ▶

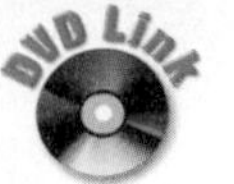

20. Demonstrate direct pressure as a method of emergency medical care for external bleeding.
21. Demonstrate the use of diffuse pressure as a method of emergency medical care for external bleeding.
22. Demonstrate the use of pressure points as a method of emergency medical care for external bleeding.
23. Demonstrate the care of the patient exhibiting signs and symptoms of internal bleeding.
24. Demonstrate the steps in the emergency medical care of open soft-tissue injuries.
25. Demonstrate the steps in the emergency medical care of a patient with an open chest wound.
26. Demonstrate the steps in the emergency medical care of a patient with open abdominal wounds.
27. Demonstrate the steps in the emergency medical care of a patient with an impaled object.
28. Demonstrate the steps in the emergency medical care of a patient with an amputation.
29. Demonstrate the steps in the emergency medical care of an amputated part.

On The Scene

The call went out: "House fire, people trapped." You can see the dark smoke curling up over the hill before you even arrive on the scene. You are on the third unit arriving at the fire—the nearest ambulance will be another 20 minutes. A firefighter crawls out through the gray smoke belching out of the front door, pulling an elderly man behind him. The Incident Commander tells you to take the patient. His clothes are smoldering slightly, so you roll him on the ground and then quickly remove them. The patient moans as you douse his obvious burns with a bottle of water from your truck. "Call for a helicopter," you order, knowing that he will need to be taken to a burn center. As you apply oxygen, you assess him and can see blistered burns over his face and that his eyebrows are singed. The front of his chest and abdomen are covered with burns. Some burns are yellow, others are waxy white, and scattered charred areas are present. His right arm is burned completely around. ■

THINK ABOUT IT

As you read this chapter, think about the following questions:

- What depth of burns does this patient have?
- How can you calculate the percentage of his body that has been burned?
- Is there any evidence that he has an inhalation injury?
- Why will he need the specialized resources of a burn center?
- What additional assessment and care will you need to perform?

Introduction

Managing Bleeding and Treating Soft-Tissue Injuries

Soft tissues are the layers of the skin and the fat and muscle beneath them.

Traumatic injuries and bleeding are some of the most dramatic situations you will encounter. Your first steps will be to perform the scene size-up and make sure the scene is safe. After assessing and managing the patient's airway and breathing, you must control any bleeding from an artery or vein, if it is present. **Soft-tissue** injuries range from bruises, cuts, and scrapes to amputations and full-thickness burns. Although soft-tissue injuries are common and impressive to look at, they are rarely life-threatening. You must be able to recognize the different types of soft-tissue injuries and give appropriate emergency care. This care includes controlling bleeding, preventing further injury, and reducing contamination.

Perfusion

Perfusion is the circulation of blood through an organ or a part of the body. In order to have adequate perfusion, the heart, vessels, and blood flow must function properly. When the body's tissues are adequately perfused, oxygen and other nutrients are carried to the cells of all the organ systems and waste products are removed. **Shock** is the inadequate circulation of blood through an organ or a part of the body. Uncontrolled bleeding that leads to depleted blood volume is one cause of shock.

Bleeding

A **wound** is an injury to the soft tissues. A **closed wound** occurs when the soft tissues under the skin are damaged but the surface of the skin is not broken. A bruise is an example of a closed wound. When the skin surface is broken, it is called an **open wound**. Cuts and scrapes are open wounds.

Hemorrhage may be internal or external.

If a blood vessel is torn or cut, bleeding occurs. Bleeding can occur from capillaries, veins, or arteries. The larger the blood vessel, the more blood that flows through it. Therefore, the larger the blood vessel, the greater the bleeding and blood loss if the vessel is injured. **Hemorrhage** (also called **major bleeding**) is an extreme loss of blood from a blood vessel. It is a life-threatening condition that requires *immediate* attention. If it is not controlled, hemorrhage can lead to shock and, possibly, to death.

When a blood vessel is cut or torn, the body's normal response is an immediate contraction (spasm) of the wall of the blood vessel. This action slows the flow of blood from the injured vessel by reducing the size of the hole. Next, platelets rush to the area to plug the torn vessel. Layers upon layers of platelets stick to each other like glue to fill the hole. Usually within seconds of the injury, a clot begins to form at the site of the torn vessel. This process is activated by substances from the wall of the injured vessel and from the platelets at the injury site. Clotting is usually complete within 6–10 minutes.

Some conditions affect blood clotting. For example, **hemophilia** is a disorder in which the blood does not clot normally. A person with hemophilia may have major bleeding from minor injuries and may bleed for no apparent reason. Some medications, such as aspirin and Coumadin (a blood thinner), can interfere with blood clotting. A serious injury may also prevent effective clotting.

Types of Bleeding

Objective 1 ►

The three types of bleeding are arterial, venous, and capillary. The characteristics of these types of bleeding are noted in Table 10-1.

TABLE 10-1 Types of Bleeding

	Arterial	Venous	Capillary
Color	Bright red	Dark red, maroon	Dark red
Blood Flow	Spurts with each heartbeat	Flows steadily	Oozes slowly
Bleeding Control	Difficult to control	Usually easier to control than arterial bleeding; bleeding from deep veins may be hard to control	Often clots and stops by itself within a few minutes

Arterial Bleeding

Arterial bleeding is life-threatening.

Arterial bleeding is the most serious type of bleeding. The blood from an artery is bright red, oxygen-rich blood. When an artery bleeds, blood spurts from the wound because the arteries are under high pressure (Figure 10-1). Each spurt represents a heartbeat. A bleeding artery can quickly lead to the loss of a large amount of blood. Arterial bleeding can be difficult to control due to high pressure within the artery.

Venous Bleeding

Bleeding from a vein is more serious than capillary bleeding.

Bleeding occurs more often from veins than arteries because veins are closer to the skin's surface. Blood lost from a vein flows as a steady stream and is dark red or maroon, because it is oxygen-poor blood. Venous bleeding is usually easier to control than arterial bleeding, because it is under less pressure. Bleeding from deep veins (such as those in the thigh) can cause major bleeding that is hard to control.

Capillary Bleeding

Capillary bleeding is usually not serious.

Capillary bleeding is common because the walls of the capillaries are fragile and many are close to the skin's surface. When a capillary is torn, blood oozes slowly from the site of the injury because the pressure within the capillaries is low. Bleeding from capillaries is usually dark red. Capillary bleeding often clots and stops by itself within a few minutes.

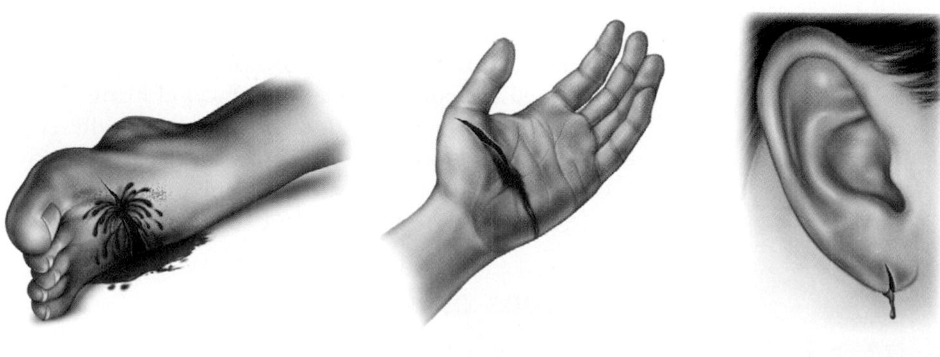

FIGURE 10-1 ▶ Arterial bleeding, venous bleeding, and capillary bleeding.

External Bleeding

Capillary bleeding is the most common type of external bleeding.

External bleeding is bleeding that you can see. You can see this type of bleeding because the blood flows through an open wound, such as a cut, scrape, or puncture. Clotting normally occurs within minutes. However, external bleeding must be controlled with your gloved hands and dressings until a clot is formed and the bleeding has stopped.

Remember This!

External bleeding may be hidden by clothing.

Emergency Medical Responder Care of External Bleeding

Objective 2 ▶

Objective 3 ▶

Objective 15 ▶

When you arrive at the scene of an emergency, first consider your personal safety. During the scene size-up, evaluate the mechanism of injury or the nature of the illness before approaching the patient. Personal protective equipment (PPE) *must* be worn when an exposure to blood or other potentially infectious material can be reasonably anticipated. HIV and the hepatitis virus are examples of diseases to which you may be exposed that can be transmitted by exposure to blood. Remember to put on disposable gloves before physical contact with the patient. Additional PPE, such as eye protection, mask, and gown, should be worn if there is a large amount of blood. PPE should also be worn when the splashing of blood or body fluids into your face or eyes is likely.

Stop and Think!

- *Never* touch blood or body fluids with your bare hands.
- *Always* wear PPE during *every* patient contact.
- Wash your hands immediately after exposure to blood and/or body fluids and after removing disposable gloves.
- If you were not wearing gloves and had contact with blood or body fluids, wash your hands with soap and water for at least two minutes.
- Remember to throw away contaminated gloves and other PPE in clearly labeled biohazard bags or containers.
- Report all exposures to your supervisor or Risk Management Department immediately.

After the scene size-up, form a general impression of the patient and then perform an initial assessment. Bleeding may be obvious when you approach the patient. However, remember that making sure the patient has an open airway and adequate breathing takes priority over other care. Stabilize the cervical spine if needed. During your assessment of the patient's circulation, look for the presence of major (severe) bleeding. If it is present, you will need to control it during the initial assessment.

Objective 16 ▶

Objective 17 ▶

If the patient is bleeding, keep in mind that the sight of blood is frightening for most patients. Conduct your examination professionally and efficiently. Remember to talk with your patient while you are providing care. Because clothing can hide and absorb large amounts of blood, cut or remove your patient's clothing as needed to see where the bleeding is coming from. Remember that your patient will often be anxious about having clothing removed and having an exam performed by a stranger. Ease your patient's fears by explaining what you are doing and why it must be done.

TABLE 10-2 Measures of Severe Blood Loss

Patient Type	Normal Blood Volume	Severe Blood Loss
Adult	5,000–6,000 mL	Loss of 1,000 mL or more
Child	2,000 mL	Loss of 500 mL or more
Infant	800 mL	Loss of 100–200 mL or more

As you remove the patient's clothing, remember to drape or shield him or her properly from the view of others not providing care.

When you donate blood, you are giving about 500 mL of blood. If a child lost that much blood, he or she would develop shock.

An average adult man has a normal blood volume of about 5–6 liters (5,000–6,000 mL). In a previously healthy patient, a sudden episode of blood loss will usually not produce vital sign changes until the patient has lost 15–30% of his blood volume (Table 10-2). Therefore, estimate the severity of blood loss based on the patient's signs and symptoms. If the patient shows signs and symptoms of shock, consider the bleeding severe.

Control bleeding by using direct pressure, elevation, pressure points, splints, or, as a last resort, a tourniquet. If bleeding is severe, give oxygen if it is available and you have been trained to use it. If signs of shock are present, treat the patient for shock. These techniques are described in the section "Controlling External Bleeding".

After completing the initial assessment, decide if the patient needs on-scene stabilization or immediate transport with additional emergency care en route to a hospital. When you have completed your initial assessment, update the EMS unit responding to the scene with a brief report by phone or radio, if possible.

Making a Difference

Although covering a bleeding wound is important for any patient, it is especially important if your patient is a young child. A young child may fear that "all of my blood will leak out" if the wound is not covered quickly.

Controlling External Bleeding

Most bleeding can be controlled with direct pressure.

Six methods may be used to control external bleeding:

1. Applying direct pressure to the wound
2. Elevating the affected extremity
3. Applying pressure to an arterial pressure point
4. Applying a splint to immobilize the extremity
5. Applying a pressure splint (air splint)
6. Applying a tourniquet (*only* as a last resort)

Direct Pressure

To control external bleeding, begin by applying **direct pressure** to the bleeding site. Applying direct pressure slows blood flow and allows clotting to take place. Place a sterile **dressing** (such as a gauze pad) or a clean cloth (such as a towel or washcloth) over the wound. If you do not have a dressing or clean cloth available, use your gloved hand to apply firm pressure to the bleeding site until a dressing can be applied (Figure 10-2). Use your gloved fingertips if the bleeding site is small. If the patient has a large, open wound, you may need to apply direct pressure to the site with the palm of your gloved hand. Hold continuous, firm

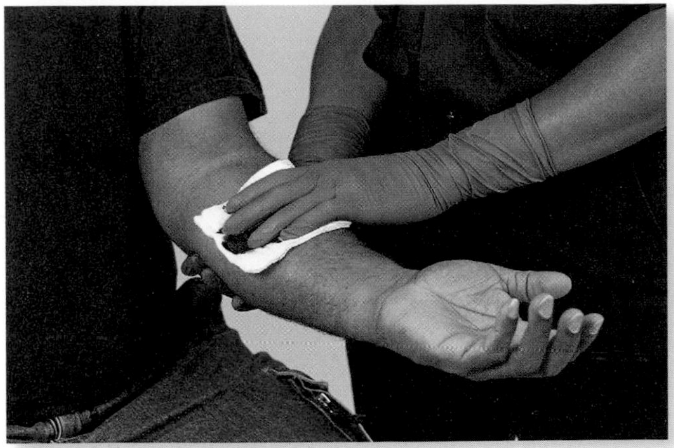

FIGURE 10-2 ▲ Apply direct pressure to a bleeding wound.

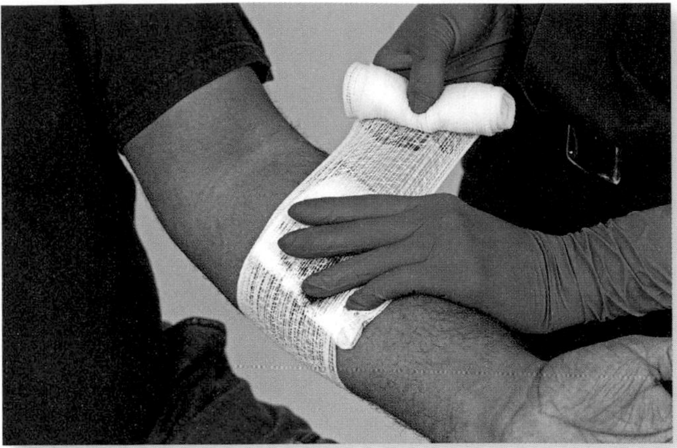

FIGURE 10-3 ▲ Continue direct pressure by applying a pressure bandage.

pressure to the bleeding site while the body works to plug the wound with a clot. If the bleeding does not stop within 10 minutes, press more firmly over a wider area.

A pressure bandage that is wrapped too loosely will not be effective in controlling bleeding. A bandage that is applied too tightly can cause tissue damage.

If the bleeding site is on an extremity, continue direct pressure by applying a **pressure bandage.** Wrap roller gauze snugly over the dressings to hold them in place on the wound (Figure 10-3). Apply the pressure bandage snugly enough to control the blood loss. Make sure that it is not so tight that there is no blood flow past the dressing. For example, if you have applied a pressure bandage to a wound on a patient's lower arm, you should be able to feel a pulse at the wrist if the bandage has been applied properly.

If blood soaks through the dressings, do not remove them. Removing the original dressings could disturb any blood clots that may be forming and cause more bleeding. Add another dressing on top of the first and continue to apply direct pressure.

Stop and Think!

If PPE is not available and you must provide care for a bleeding patient, use whatever materials are readily available to help protect yourself against disease. For example, use a plastic bag, plastic wrap, or other waterproof material to apply direct pressure to the wound. If the patient is able to help you, ask him or her to apply direct pressure to the wound with his or her own hand. When you have finished providing care, be sure to wash your hands with soap and water for at least two minutes.

Elevation

Direct pressure and elevation are used together to control bleeding from an arm or a leg.

If bleeding continues from an arm or a leg, elevation may help control the bleeding (Figure 10-4). If possible, elevate the extremity above the level of the heart while continuing to apply direct pressure. Raising the extremity above the heart reduces pressure at the wound site by reducing blood flow to it. This action allows blood to pool and clot. Do not elevate the extremity if pain, swelling, or deformity is present.

FIGURE 10-4 ► Elevation can be used with direct pressure to control bleeding.

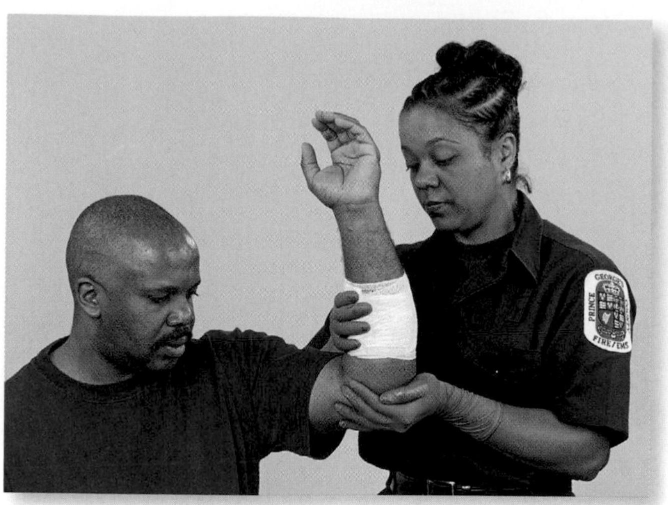

Remember This!

Methods to Control External Bleeding

- Direct pressure
- Elevation
- Pressure points
- Splint
- Pressure (air) splint
- Tourniquet

Pressure Points

Using a pressure point to control bleeding is useless if you do not know where to find the pressure points.

If bleeding continues from an arm or a leg, pressure points (also called pulse points) may be used to slow severe bleeding. When applying pressure at a pressure point, continue to apply direct pressure to the bleeding site. To slow bleeding in the lower arm, locate the brachial artery in the upper arm. Use your first three fingers and press the brachial artery firmly against the upper-arm bone (the humerus). To slow bleeding in the leg, use your fingers to locate the femoral artery in the groin. Press the femoral artery firmly against the pelvic bone using the palm of your hand (Figure 10-5).

Splint

A broken bone that penetrates the skin is called an **open**, or **compound, fracture.**

The sharp ends of broken bones can pierce the skin and cause major bleeding. Unless a broken bone is immobilized, the movement of bone ends or bone fragments can damage soft tissues and blood vessels, which results in more bleeding. Dress and bandage the wound and then apply a splint. A **splint** is a device used to limit the movement of an injured arm or leg to reduce pain and further injury. After applying the splint, be sure to check the patient's fingers (or toes) often for color, warmth, and feeling.

Pressure (Air) Splint

Dress and bandage the wound before applying an air splint.

A pressure splint (also called an air or a pneumatic splint) can help control the bleeding associated with soft-tissue injuries or broken bones. It also helps stabilize a broken bone. An air splint acts as a pressure bandage, applying even pressure to the entire arm or leg (Figure 10-6). After applying any splint, be sure to check the patient's fingers (or toes) often for color, warmth, and feeling. Direct

FIGURE 10-5 ► Pressure points may be used to slow severe bleeding from an arm or a leg. To slow bleeding in the lower arm, press the brachial artery firmly against the humerus. To slow bleeding in the leg, press the femoral artery firmly against the pelvic bone using the palm of your hand.

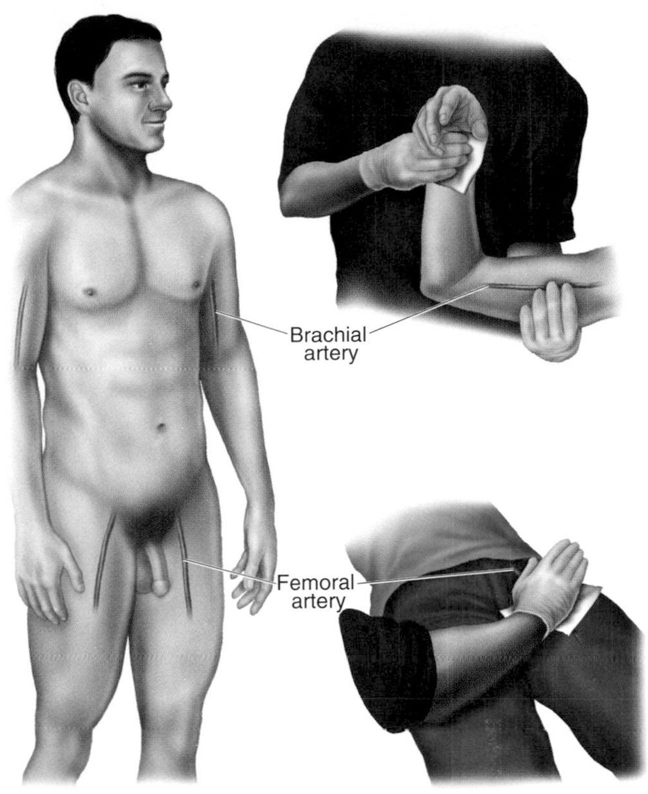

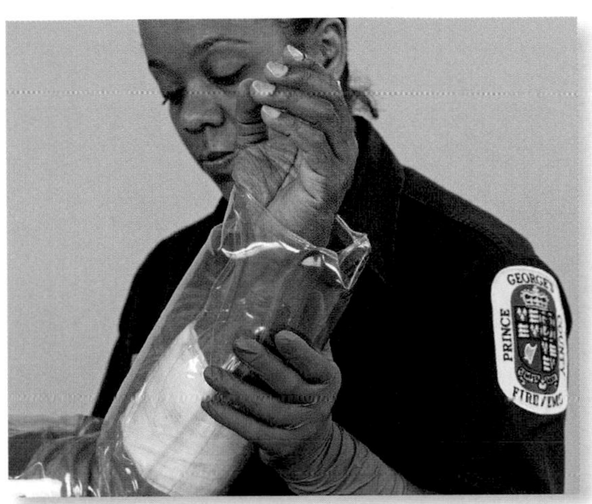

FIGURE 10-6 ▲ An air splint acts as a pressure bandage, applying even pressure to the entire arm or leg.

pressure can be applied with an air splint in place. This may be necessary to control arterial bleeding from an arm or a leg.

In most EMS systems, an Emergency Medical Responder can help apply a PASG under direct supervision.

The pneumatic antishock garment (PASG) is used in some EMS systems. This garment is also called the Military Antishock Trousers (MAST). This device can be used as an effective pressure splint to help control severe bleeding from the legs or pelvis (Figure 10-7). The PASG has three separate compartments that can be inflated: the abdomen, left leg, and right leg. If there is an injury to one leg, that leg compartment is inflated. If both legs are injured, both leg compartments are inflated. All three compartments are inflated if there is an injury to the pelvis. The abdominal compartment is *never* used without inflating both leg compartments. When the PASG is positioned on the patient, the top edge of the garment must be below the patient's lowest ribs. If the garment is positioned higher on the patient, the pressure caused by inflating the abdominal compartment could hamper the patient's breathing.

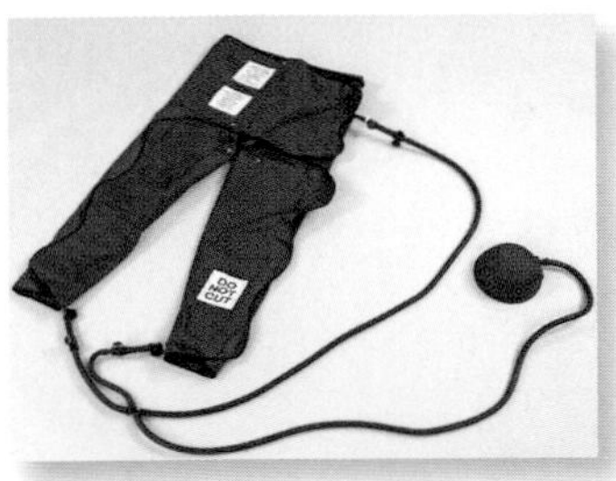

FIGURE 10-7 ▲ The pneumatic antishock garment (PASG) is used in some EMS systems to stabilize a pelvic fracture. It is also used to control bleeding from the lower extremities and pelvis.

Tourniquet

A **tourniquet** is a tight bandage that surrounds an arm or a leg. It is used to stop the flow of blood in an extremity. A tourniquet is rarely needed to control bleeding. It should be used *only* as a last resort to control life-threatening bleeding in an arm or a leg when you absolutely cannot control the bleeding by any other means. A tourniquet can cause permanent damage to nerves, muscles, and blood vessels, resulting in the loss of the affected extremity.

Stop and Think!

A tourniquet is used *only* when all other methods of bleeding control have failed. When you apply a tourniquet, you stop arterial and venous blood flow to the affected extremity. Remember that arteries carry oxygenated blood to the body's tissues. Without oxygenated blood, all the tissues of the extremity, both injured and uninjured, will die. The use of a tourniquet may result in surgical amputation of the lower portion of the extremity. Be absolutely sure that you have exhausted all other methods of bleeding control before considering the use of a tourniquet.

Note the exact time the tourniquet is applied.

To apply a tourniquet, use the following steps:

1. Use a bandage at least 4 inches wide and 6–8 layers deep.
2. Wrap the bandage around the extremity twice. Choose an area above the bleeding but as close to the wound as possible (Figure 10-8a).
3. Tie a single knot in the bandage and place a stick or rod on top of the knot (Figure 10-8b).
4. Tie the ends of the bandage over the stick in a square knot. Twist the stick until the bleeding stops (Figure 10-8c).
5. After the bleeding has stopped, secure the stick or rod in place.
6. Write the initials *TK*, for *tourniquet*, on a piece of adhesive tape and the time the tourniquet was applied. Place the adhesive tape on the patient's forehead. The information must be clearly visible to all who provide care to the patient (Figure 10-8d).
7. Notify the EMS personnel who take over patient care that you have applied a tourniquet.

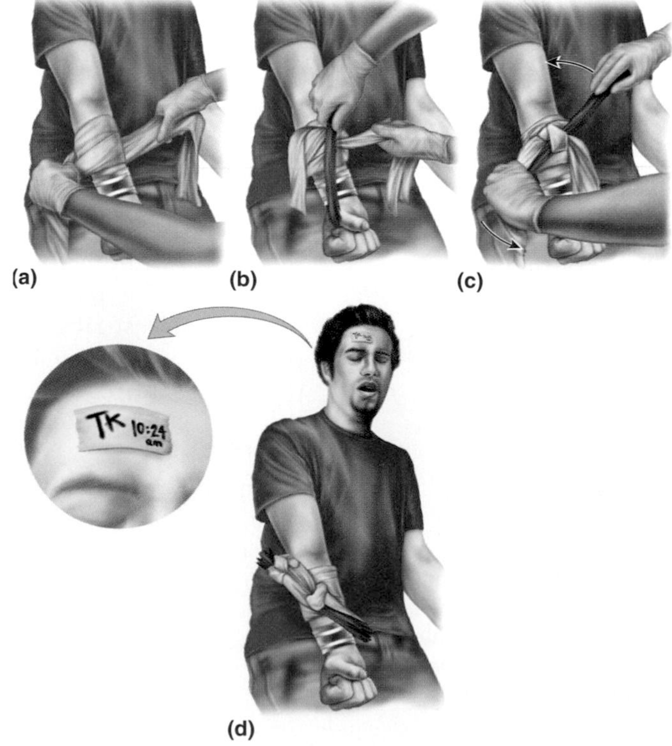

FIGURE 10-8 ► (a) To apply a tourniquet, use a bandage at least 4 inches wide and 6–8 layers deep. Wrap the bandage around the extremity twice. Choose an area above the bleeding but as close to the wound as possible. (b) Tie a single knot in the bandage and place a stick or rod on top of the knot. (c) Tie the ends of the bandage over the stick in a square knot. Twist the stick until the bleeding stops. Note the exact time the tourniquet is applied. (d) Write *TK* on a piece of adhesive tape and the time the tourniquet was applied. Place the adhesive tape on the patient's forehead.

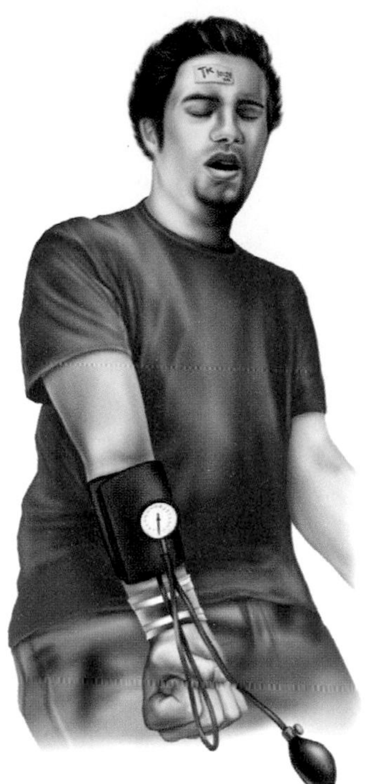

FIGURE 10-9 ▲ A blood pressure cuff may be used as a tourniquet. Place the cuff above the bleeding area. Inflate the cuff just enough to stop the bleeding.

Remember This!

A blood pressure cuff may be used as a tourniquet. Place the cuff above the bleeding area. Inflate the cuff just enough to stop the bleeding (Figure 10-9). Check the gauge on the cuff often to make sure there is no drop in pressure in the cuff.

You Should Know

Precautions for Tourniquet Use

Whenever you apply a tourniquet, make sure to take the following precautions:

- Always use a wide bandage. Never use wire, rope, a belt, or any other material that may cut into the skin and underlying tissue.
- Do not remove or loosen the tourniquet once it is applied unless you are directed to do so by a physician.
- Leave the tourniquet in open view so that it is readily seen by others. Do not cover the tourniquet with a bandage, a sheet, or the patient's clothing.
- Never apply a tourniquet directly over a joint. Place the tourniquet as close to the injury as possible.

Internal Bleeding

Internal bleeding can result in blood loss severe enough to cause shock and death.

The body contains hollow and solid organs. The hollow abdominal organs include the stomach, intestines, gallbladder, and urinary bladder. When hollow abdominal organs rupture, they empty their contents into the abdominal cavity. This rupture irritates the abdominal lining and causes pain. The solid abdominal organs include the liver, spleen, and kidneys. Solid organs are protected by bony structures and do not move around much. Solid organs bleed when injured and can result in a large amount of blood loss. **Internal bleeding** is bleeding that occurs inside body tissues and cavities. A **bruise** is a collection of blood under the skin due to bleeding capillaries. A bruise is an example of internal bleeding that is not life-threatening.

Internal bleeding may result from blunt or penetrating trauma. It can also be due to medical conditions, such as an ulcer. The two most common causes of internal bleeding are (1) injured or damaged internal organs and (2) fractures, especially fractures of the femur and pelvis. Internal bleeding may occur in any body cavity. However, major bleeding is most likely to occur in the abdominal cavity, chest cavity, digestive tract, or tissues surrounding broken bones. An injury to the liver or spleen can result in a loss of massive amounts of blood into the abdominal cavity in a short time. A fracture of a long bone can result in a loss of 500–1,000 mL of blood into the surrounding tissues. A femur fracture can produce a blood loss of up to 1,000 mL. The only signs of internal bleeding may be localized swelling and bruising.

Internal bleeding can cause blood to pool in a body cavity. This buildup of blood can cause pressure on vital organs. For example, a stab wound to the chest may hit a chamber of the heart. If bleeding escapes from the heart's chamber into the sac around the heart (the pericardial sac), the heart's ability to pump decreases. As blood fills the sac, the pressure in the sac increases and does not allow the heart muscle to expand during relaxation. If a blood vessel in the chest is torn, as much as 1,500 mL of blood can build up in the pleural cavity of each

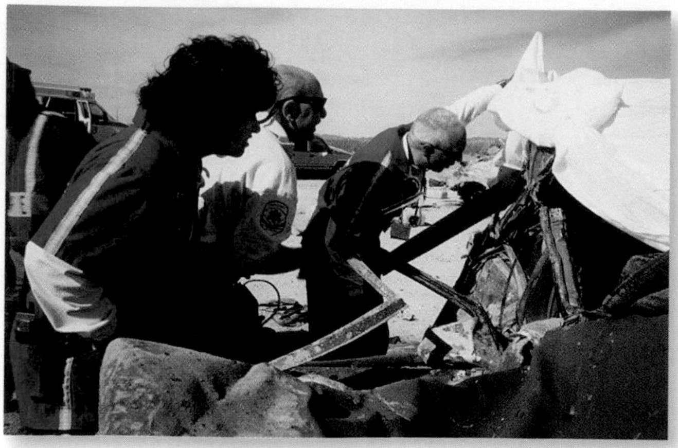

FIGURE 10-10 ▶ When the mechanism of injury suggests that the patient's body has been affected by severe force, suspect internal bleeding. © The McGraw-Hill Companies, Inc./Carin Marter, photographer

lung. Breathing may be compromised as the blood builds up, crushing the air-filled lung.

Emergency Medical Responder Care of Internal Bleeding

Internal bleeding is difficult to assess, because you cannot see it. Therefore, you should suspect it based on the mechanism of injury or the nature of the illness, as well as your patient's signs and symptoms. Suspect internal bleeding when the mechanism of injury suggests that the patient's body has been affected by severe force (Figure 10-10). Examples include penetrating trauma and blunt trauma, such as falls, motorcycle crashes, pedestrian impacts, automobile collisions, and blast injuries.

Trauma is a common cause of internal bleeding. It may also occur in patients with medical emergencies. For example, internal bleeding may occur because of a problem in the digestive tract, such as an ulcer. A patient with bleeding in the digestive tract may vomit blood or have bloody diarrhea. A patient with bleeding in the urinary tract may have blood in the urine.

Depending on the amount of bleeding, the signs and symptoms of internal bleeding may develop quickly or may take hours or days to develop. The signs and symptoms of internal bleeding include the following:

Objective 4 ▶

- Pain, tenderness, swelling, or discoloration of the skin (bruising) in the injured area
- A weak, rapid pulse
- Pale, cool, moist skin
- Broken ribs or bruising on the chest
- Vomiting or coughing up of bright red blood or dark, "coffee-ground" blood
- A tender, rigid, and/or swollen abdomen
- Bleeding from the mouth, rectum, vagina, or another body opening
- Black (tarry) stools or stools with bright red blood

Objective 5 ▶

To provide emergency care to a patient with the signs and symptoms of internal bleeding, use the following steps:

1. Conduct a scene size-up and ensure your safety. Evaluate the mechanism of injury or the nature of the illness before approaching the patient. Put on appropriate PPE.
2. Form a general impression and determine the urgency of further assessment and care.

3. Perform an initial assessment to identify and treat any life-threatening conditions. Manage the patient's airway and breathing. Stabilize the cervical spine if needed. After completing the initial assessment, update the EMS unit responding to the scene with a brief report by phone or radio, if possible.
4. Perform a physical examination. Identify the signs and symptoms of internal bleeding. Take the patient's vital signs, gather the patient's medical history, and document the information.
5. If you suspect internal bleeding, give oxygen if it is available and you have been trained to use it. A patient with internal bleeding may vomit. Watch the patient closely to make sure the airway remains clear. If he vomits and has no injury to his head or spine, place him on his left side in the recovery position.
6. A patient with internal bleeding is a priority patient and needs rapid transport to the closest appropriate hospital. The best you can do at the scene is to make the patient as comfortable as possible, provide reassurance, and keep him warm. Perform ongoing assessments every five minutes. If signs of shock develop, treat the patient for shock, as explained in the section "Shock (Hypoperfusion)."

Stop and Think!

Never give a patient who may have internal bleeding or who may be in shock anything to eat or drink. The patient may need surgery and should not have anything in his or her stomach.

Shock (Hypoperfusion)

Shock is a life-threatening condition. It requires *immediate* emergency care.

Shock is the inadequate flow of blood through an organ or a part of the body. Shock can be caused by failure of the body's pump (heart), fluid (blood), or container (blood vessels).

Cardiogenic shock is a pump problem.

- *Pump failure.* The amount of blood the heart pumps throughout the body depends on how many times the heart beats and the force of the contractions. **Cardiogenic shock** can result if the heart beats too quickly or too slowly or if the heart muscle does not have enough force to pump blood effectively to all parts of the body. This type of shock can occur because of a heart attack, a heart rhythm that is too fast or too slow, an injury to the heart, or other conditions that affect the heart's ability to pump.

Hypovolemic shock is the most common type of shock. Hypovolemic shock is a volume problem.

- *Fluid loss.* Shock can result if there is not enough blood for the heart to pump through the cardiovascular system. Shock caused by severe bleeding is called **hemorrhagic shock.** The bleeding may be internal, external, or both. However, blood is not the only type of fluid that may be lost from the body. For example, you may lose body fluid because of vomiting or diarrhea. You may lose plasma due to a burn. You can also lose fluid due to excessive sweating or urination. Shock caused by a loss of blood, plasma, or another body fluid is called **hypovolemic shock**.

Container failure is a pipe problem.

- *Container failure.* Normally, blood vessels work with the nervous system to increase or decrease the amount of blood sent to different areas of the body. When an area needs more blood, the vessels expand to provide it with more blood and constrict in areas that do not need it. When shock due to container failure occurs, the blood vessels lose their ability to adjust the flow of blood. Instead of expanding and constricting as needed, the blood vessels remain enlarged. The amount of fluid in the body remains constant (there is no actual loss of fluid), but blood pools in the outer areas of the body. As a result, there is an inadequate amount of blood to fill the enlarged vessels and the vital organs are not perfused. The four major causes of this type of shock are

- Injury to the spinal cord (neurogenic shock)
- Severe infection (septic shock)
- Severe allergic reaction (anaphylactic shock)
- Severe drug reaction

Regardless of the type of shock, cells are starved for enough oxygen-rich blood. When the body's cells and organs are not supplied with oxygen and nutrients, they begin to break down and waste products build up. Unless adequate perfusion is quickly restored, death may soon follow. It is not important that you be able to determine the cause of the patient's shock. What is important is that you can promptly recognize the signs and symptoms of shock. Promptly recognizing and treating shock are critical to your patient's survival.

You Should Know

Without an adequate supply of oxygen-rich blood,

- The brain, heart, and lungs will suffer damage after 4–6 minutes.
- The kidneys and liver will suffer damage after 45–90 minutes.
- The skin and muscles will suffer damage after 4–6 hours.

The Stages of Shock

Shock occurs in stages: early (compensated), late (decompensated), and irreversible (terminal).

Early Shock

Early shock is sometimes called "shock with a normal blood pressure."

In early shock, the body's defense mechanisms attempt to protect the vital organs—the brain, heart, and lungs (Figure 10-11). You can recognize signs of early shock by assessing the patient for the following:

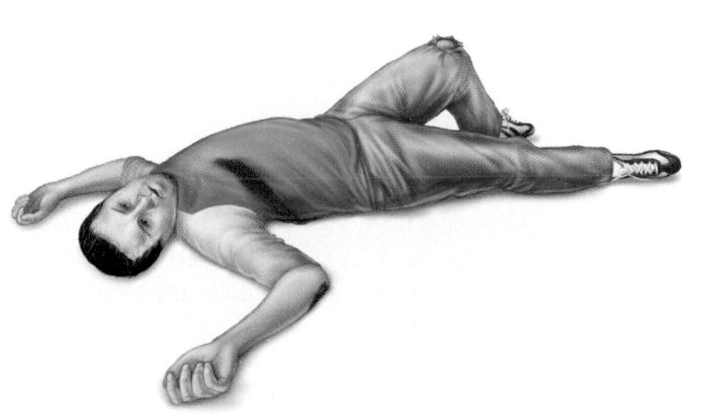

FIGURE 10-11 ▶ The signs and symptoms of early (compensated) hypovolemic shock.

- *Mental status.* Some of the earliest signs of shock can be seen as changes in the patient's mental status. A patient in early shock will appear anxious and restless. Some patients are combative. These changes occur because the brain is not receiving an adequate supply of oxygenated blood.
- *Breathing.* As the body attempts to draw in more oxygen, the bronchioles expand to draw in more air and the patient's breathing rate increases.
- *Skin color, temperature, and condition (moisture).* As blood is shunted from the skin and muscles to the patient's vital organs, the patient's skin will look pale and feel cool and moist. You may notice that the patient's face appears pale, especially around the mouth and nose. You may see beads of sweat on the patient's skin. Sweating is usually first visible on the upper lip and around the hairline.
- *Heart rate.* The patient's pulse will feel slightly faster than normal because the heart picks up its pace to pump oxygenated blood throughout the body.
- *Strength of the peripheral pulses.* Pulses in the arms and legs often feel weak because blood is being shunted away from them to protect the body's vital organs.
- *Capillary refill (in children younger than six years of age).* Delayed capillary refill (three to five seconds) may indicate poor perfusion or exposure to cool temperatures. A capillary refill time longer than five seconds is markedly delayed and suggests shock.

Remember This!

It may be difficult to determine pale skin color in a dark-skinned person. Look at the patient's nail beds, the mucous membranes of the eyes, or inside the mouth. If these areas are pale, consider possible shock.

During shock, the body will divert blood to the areas that are most dependent on a continuous, rich supply of oxygen. The patient's skin appears pale because the body diverts blood from the skin first.

Early shock is often difficult to recognize. Remember to look for it and to consider the patient's mechanism of injury or the nature of the illness when assessing your patient. For example, an increased heart rate can be caused by many things. Fever, fear, pain, anxiety, stress, and exercise can all increase a person's heart rate. However, an increased heart rate accompanied by pale, cool skin and anxiety in a victim of a motorcycle crash should make you think immediately of shock. The sooner shock is recognized and appropriate treatment is begun, the better your patient's chance for survival. Early shock is usually reversible if it is recognized and the patient receives emergency care to correct the cause of the shock. If early shock is not recognized or corrected, it will progress to the next stage.

You Should Know

Signs and Symptoms of Early Shock

- Anxiety, restlessness
- Thirst
- Nausea, vomiting
- Increased respiratory rate
- Slight increase in the heart rate
- Pale, cool, moist skin
- Delayed capillary refill (more than two to three seconds) in an infant or a young child
- Blood pressure in the normal range

FIGURE 10-12 ► The signs and symptoms of late (decompensated) hypovolemic shock.

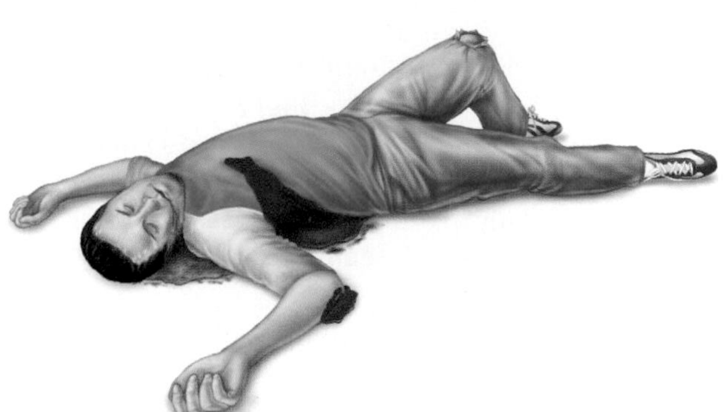

The presence of low blood pressure is the main difference between early (compensated) shock and late (decompensated) shock.

Late Shock

When an adult patient's systolic blood pressure drops to less than 90 mm Hg, late (decompensated) shock is present. In late shock, the body's defense mechanisms lose their ability to make up for the lack of oxygenated blood. A patient in late shock looks very sick (Figure 10-12). He is usually slow to respond, confused, or he may even be unresponsive. His breathing is shallow, labored, and irregular. The patient's skin is cool and moist, and it may be pale, blue, or mottled. His pulse is fast and hard to feel (thready) or may be absent in his arms and legs. The signs of late shock are more obvious than those of early shock, but late shock is more difficult to treat. It is still reversible if the cause of the problem is quickly corrected.

You Should Know

Signs and Symptoms of Late Shock

- Slowness to respond or being confused or unresponsive
- Extreme thirst (if the patient is awake)
- Nausea, vomiting
- Shallow, labored, irregular breathing
- Rapid heart rate
- Cool, moist skin that is pale, blue, or mottled
- Delayed capillary refill (more than two to three seconds) in an infant or a young child
- Low blood pressure

You will not know the point at which a patient moves from late to irreversible shock. Your goal should be to treat the patient as early as possible for shock to prevent the development of this lethal stage.

Irreversible Shock

Irreversible shock is also called terminal shock. At this stage, the body's defense mechanisms have failed. You will feel an irregular pulse as the patient's heart becomes irritable and begins to beat irregularly. As shock continues, the patient's

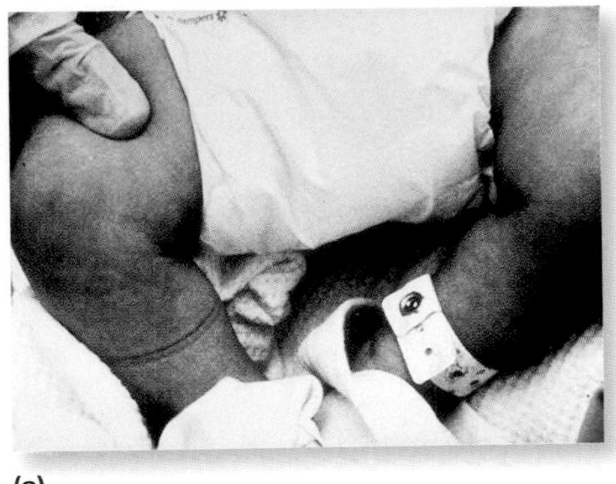

(a)

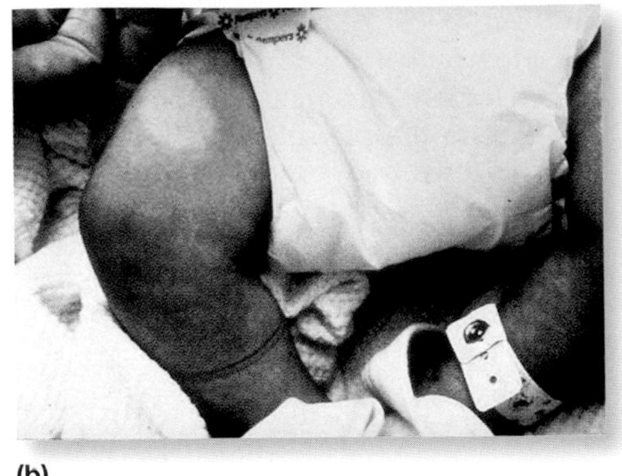

(b)

FIGURE 10-13 ▲ (a) Assess capillary refill in children younger than six years of age. (b) Delayed capillary refill in an infant. EMSC Slide Set (CD-ROM). 1996. Courtesy of the Emergency Medical Services for Children Program, administered by the U.S. Department of Health and Human Service's Health Resources and Services Administration, Maternal and Child Health Bureau.

heart rhythm becomes more chaotic and it can no longer pump blood effectively. Permanent damage occurs to the vital organs because the cells and organs have been without oxygenated blood for too long. Eventually, the heart stops, breathing stops, and death results.

Infants and Children

Suspect shock in an infant or a child who is very listless and whose muscle tone appears floppy.

Infants and children can maintain a normal blood pressure until more than half their blood volume is gone. By the time their blood pressure drops, they are close to death. Although children in shock tend to compensate longer, they also get worse faster when their compensatory mechanisms fail. To spot the signs of shock in a child, pay particular attention to the child's mental status and capillary refill (Figure 10-13). Also pay special attention to the child's skin temperature, color, and moisture (Figure 10-14), as well as to the strength of the child's pulses.

Emergency Medical Responder Care of Shock

To treat a patient in shock, use the following steps:

1. Conduct a scene size-up and ensure your safety. Evaluate the mechanism of injury or the nature of the illness before approaching the patient. Put on appropriate PPE.

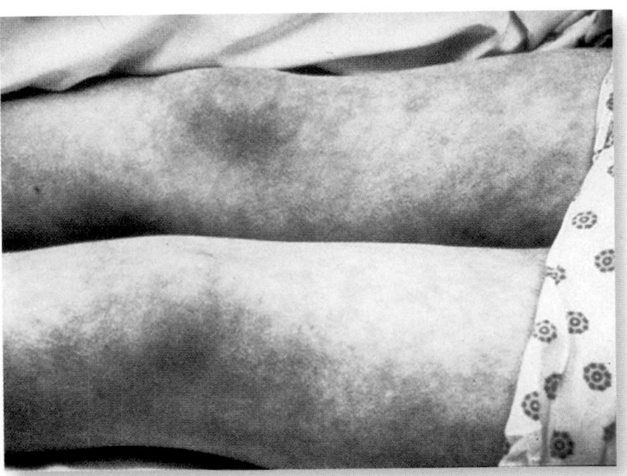

FIGURE 10-14 ▶ Mottled skin in a child. EMSC Slide Set (CD-ROM). 1996. Courtesy of the Emergency Medical Services for Children Program, administered by the U.S. Department of Health and Human Service's Health Resources and Services Administration, Maternal and Child Health Bureau.

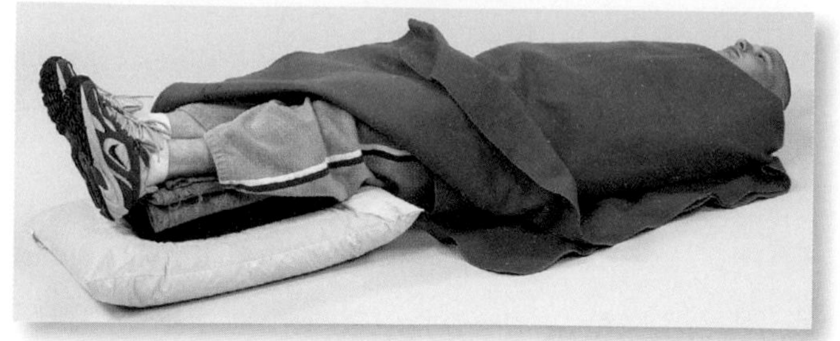

FIGURE 10-15 ► If you suspect shock, have the patient lie down and elevate his or her legs approximately 8–12 inches. Do not elevate the patient's legs if there is an injury to the head, spine, chest, abdomen, pelvis, or legs.

2. Form a general impression and determine the urgency of further assessment and care.
3. Perform an initial assessment to identify and treat any life-threatening conditions. Manage the patient's airway and breathing. Stabilize the cervical spine if needed.
4. The heart can pump only the blood it receives. Therefore, there must be an adequate volume of blood in the system and a steady volume of blood returning to the right side of the heart. One way to increase the amount of blood returning to the right side of the heart is to raise the patient's legs. If you suspect shock, place the patient on his back and raise his legs approximately 8–12 inches (shock position). Only elevate the patient's legs if he has no injuries to his head, spine, chest, abdomen, pelvis, or legs (Figure 10-15). A woman in late pregnancy should be positioned on her left side instead of on her back. When a woman in late pregnancy is placed on her back, the weight of the fetus compresses major blood vessels, such as the inferior vena cava and aorta. This compression decreases the amount of blood returning to the mother's heart and lowers her blood pressure. Positioning the patient on her left side shifts the weight of her uterus off the abdominal vessels.

Do not elevate the patient's legs if there is an injury to the head, spine, chest, abdomen, pelvis, or legs.

5. Give oxygen if it is available and you have been trained to use it. Prevent heat loss by placing blankets under and over the patient. A patient in shock often has an altered mental status. Many patients are also nauseated and may vomit. Watch the patient closely to make sure his airway remains clear. If he vomits or is bleeding from the mouth and has no injury to his head or spine, place him on his left side in the recovery position.
6. Control all obvious external bleeding. If possible, update the EMS unit responding to the scene with a brief report by phone or radio, if possible.
7. Perform a physical exam. Take the patient's vital signs and gather the patient's medical history. Splint any bone or joint injuries.
8. A patient in shock is a priority patient and needs rapid transport to the closest appropriate hospital. Comfort, calm, and reassure the patient while waiting for EMS personnel. Perform an ongoing assessment every five minutes.

Soft-Tissue Injuries

Soft-tissue injuries damage the layers of the skin and the fat and muscle beneath them. The skin can be damaged by sharp or blunt objects, falls, or impacts with motionless objects. Chemicals, radiation, electricity, and extreme hot or cold temperatures can also cause injury to the skin.

Soft-tissue injuries may be open or closed. A soft-tissue injury that is associated with a break in the skin surface is an open wound. A closed wound is one in which the skin surface remains intact. The signs of a soft-tissue injury are usually obvious. Do not allow the appearance of a soft-tissue injury to distract you from performing an initial assessment and treating any life-threatening injuries. These injuries may be impressive to look at. However, you must remember that soft-tissue injuries are usually not the patient's most serious injuries—unless they compromise the airway or are associated with severe bleeding. Because of the risk of exposure to blood and body fluids, PPE must always be worn when dealing with soft-tissue injuries.

Objective 6 ▶

Closed Wounds

Because there is no break in the skin, there is no external bleeding.

A **closed soft-tissue injury** occurs when the body is struck by a blunt object. There is no break in the skin, but the tissues and vessels beneath the skin surface are crushed or ruptured.

Knowing the "age" of bruises can be important if you suspect abuse. Does the age of the bruises match the story about the person's injuries? If not, make sure to pass along that information to the appropriate authorities.

A **contusion** (bruise) is the most common type of closed wound (Figure 10-16). A contusion results when an area of the body experiences a blunt force, such as a kick, fall, or blow. The outer skin layer, the epidermis, remains intact. However, the tissue layers and small blood vessels beneath it are damaged. The blunt force causes a small amount of internal bleeding in the area that was struck. Swelling, pain, and discoloration of the skin occur as blood leaks from the torn vessels into the surrounding tissue. At first, a contusion usually appears as a red area or as tiny red dots or splotches on the skin. The color changes to purple or blue in 2–5 days. After 5–10 days, the color changes to green and then yellow. It becomes brownish-yellow 10–14 days after the injury and then gradually disappears. Most contusions heal and disappear within 2–3 weeks.

The patient may lose 1 or more liters of blood under the skin.

If large blood vessels are torn beneath a bruised (contused) area, a **hematoma** forms (see Figure 10-16). A hematoma is a localized collection of blood beneath the skin due to a tear in a blood vessel. Hematomas often occur with trauma of enough force to break bones. Although similar to a contusion, a hematoma involves a larger amount of tissue damage.

Crush injuries may be open or closed injuries.

Crush injuries are caused by a crushing force applied to the body from blunt trauma (see Figure 10-16). An example of a minor crush injury is a hammer striking a thumb. Localized swelling and bruising are often present. In a severe crush injury, such as a car running over the chest and abdomen of a toddler, the extent of the injury may be hidden. You may see only minimal bruising, yet the force of the injury may cause internal organ rupture. Internal bleeding may be severe and lead to shock.

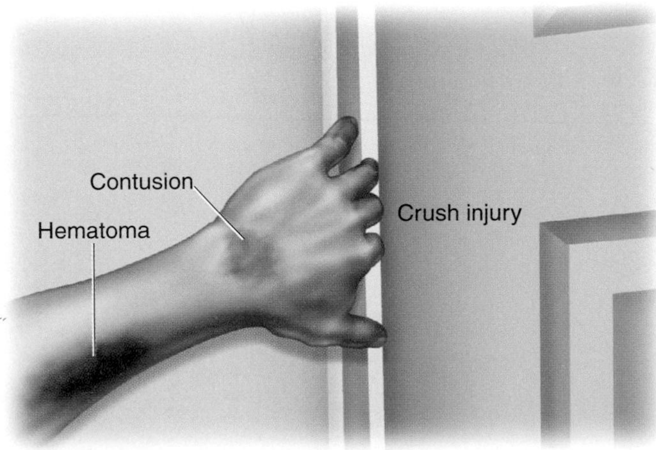

FIGURE 10-16 ▶ A contusion, a hematoma, and a crush injury without a break in the skin are closed wounds.

When assessing a closed wound, look carefully at the surface damage on the patient's skin and consider the mechanism of injury. With your knowledge of anatomy and how the injury occurred, try to visualize the possible damage to the organs and blood vessels beneath the area that was struck. For example, injuries to the upper abdomen can injure the liver, spleen, or pancreas. An injury to the lower abdomen can injure the bladder. An injury to the middle of the back can damage the kidneys. An injury to the neck can damage large blood vessels, the windpipe (trachea), and the spinal cord.

Emergency Medical Responder Care of Closed Wounds

Remember to consider carefully the mechanism of injury and the patient's signs and symptoms when making treatment decisions about a closed wound.

To treat a patient with a closed wound, use the following steps:

1. Conduct a scene size-up and ensure your safety. Evaluate the mechanism of injury before approaching the patient. Put on appropriate PPE.
2. Form a general impression and determine the urgency of further assessment and care.
3. Perform an initial assessment to identify and treat any life-threatening conditions. Stabilize the cervical spine if needed. If signs of shock are present or if internal bleeding is suspected, treat for shock.
4. Perform a physical exam. Take the patient's vital signs and gather the patient's medical history.
5. Splint any bone or joint injuries.
6. If an extremity is injured, raise it above the level of the heart unless there are signs or symptoms of a possible fracture, such as pain, swelling, or deformity. Apply an ice bag or a cold pack. Place a cloth or bandage between the patient's skin and the cold source. Applying cold to the wound helps reduce pain, constrict injured blood vessels (thereby reducing bleeding), and reduce swelling.
7. Comfort, calm, and reassure the patient while waiting for EMS personnel. Perform ongoing assessments every 5 minutes for a patient in shock and every 15 minutes if the patient is stable.

Never apply ice, an ice bag, or a cold pack directly to the skin. Doing so can cause tissue damage by freezing the tissue. Always use an insulating material, such as a towel, between the cold source and the skin.

Open Wounds

Objective 7 ▶

In an **open soft-tissue injury,** a break occurs in the skin. Because of the break in the skin, open wounds are at risk of external bleeding and infection. Properly dressing the wound helps protect against infection and helps control bleeding.

An **abrasion** occurs when the outermost layer of skin (epidermis) is damaged by rubbing or scraping (Figure 10-17). Little or no oozing of blood (capillary bleeding)

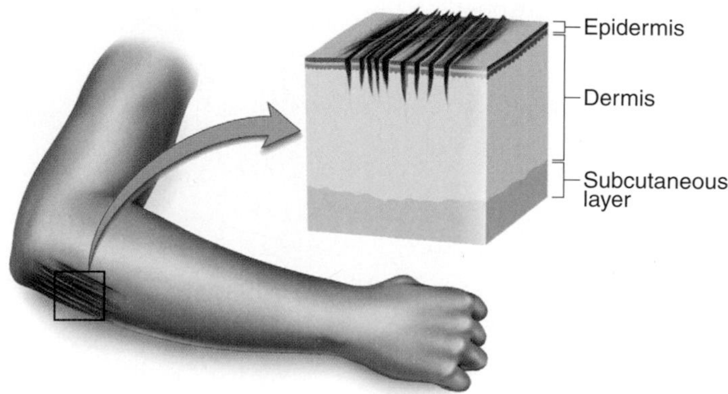

FIGURE 10-17 ▶ An abrasion results when the outermost layer of skin (epidermis) is damaged by rubbing or scraping.

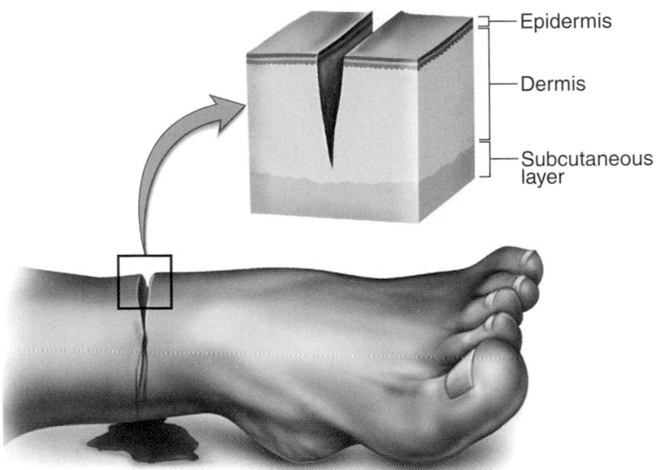

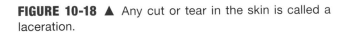

FIGURE 10-18 ▲ Any cut or tear in the skin is called a laceration.

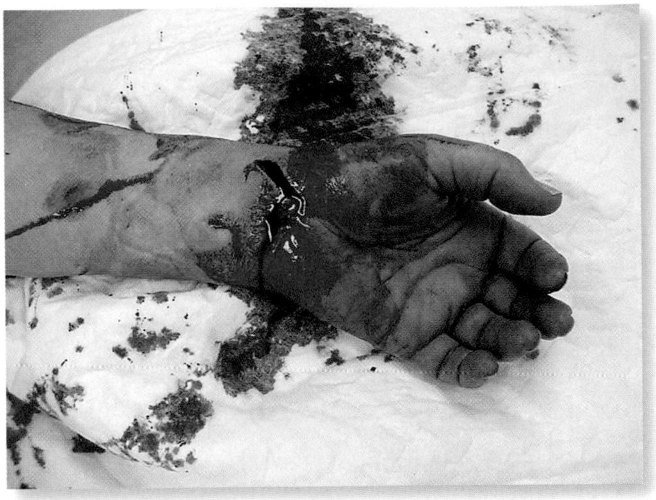

FIGURE 10-19 ▲ Laceration of the radial artery.
Trauma.org Image

An abrasion is a scrape. It is the most common type of open wound.

occurs. Although an abrasion is superficial, it can be very painful. Because the pain associated with the injury is like that of a second-degree burn, an abrasion is often called road rash, a rug burn, or a friction burn. Dirt and other foreign material can become ground into the skin with this type of injury. This greatly increases possible infection in a wound that is not properly cleansed with warm, soapy water or a fluid such as normal saline.

A laceration may occur by itself or with other types of soft-tissue injury.

A **laceration** is a cut or tear in the skin of any length, shape, and depth (Figure 10-18). A laceration can be made by a blunt object tearing the skin. It can also be made by a sharp instrument cutting through the skin, such as a knife, a razor blade, or broken glass. This type of laceration is said to be linear, or regular. A stellate laceration is irregularly shaped and is usually caused by forceful impact with a blunt object. Bleeding may be severe if a laceration is in an area of the body where large arteries lie close to the skin surface, such as in the wrists (Figure 10-19). You must control bleeding from a laceration and cover the wound to reduce the risk of infection.

Some animal bites, such as those from cats, typically leave a deep puncture wound.

A **penetration** or **puncture wound** results when the skin is pierced with a sharp, pointed object (Figure 10-20). Common objects that cause puncture wounds include nails, needles, pencils, splinters, darts, ice picks, pieces of glass, bullets, and knives. An object that remains embedded in an open wound is called

FIGURE 10-20 ► A penetration or puncture wound results when the skin is pierced with a sharp, pointed object.

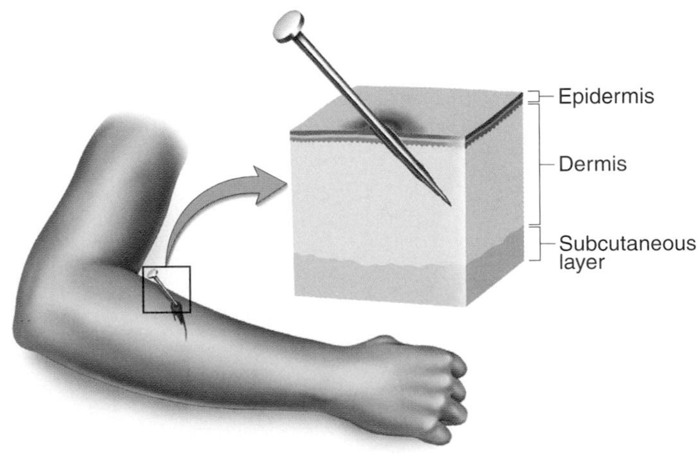

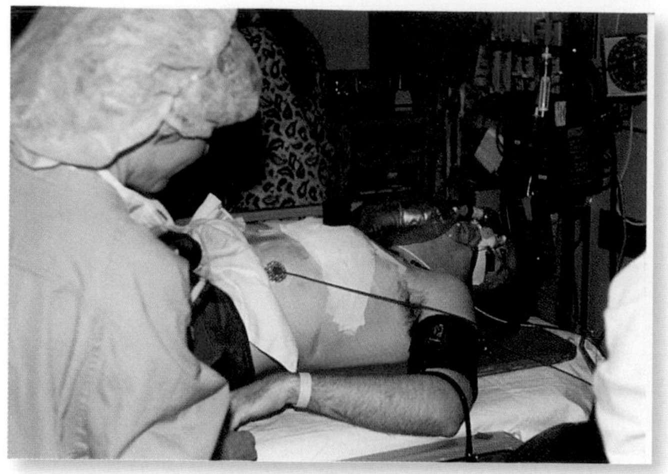

FIGURE 10-21 ► An object that remains embedded in an open wound is called an impaled object.

an **impaled object** (Figure 10-21). The severity of a puncture wound depends on where the injury is located. It also depends on how deep the wound is, the size of the penetrating object, and the forces involved in creating the injury. There is an increased risk of infection with this type of injury because the penetrating object may carry dirt and germs deep into the tissues. There may be little or no external bleeding with a puncture wound. However, internal bleeding may be severe. Assess the patient closely for signs and symptoms of shock if the puncture wound is in the chest or abdomen.

Assume that any penetrating injury to the chest has involved the abdomen. Assume that a penetrating abdominal wound has involved the chest.

Gunshot and stab wounds are types of puncture wounds that can go completely through the body or body part. This creates both an entrance and an exit wound. An entrance wound from a bullet usually looks like a puncture wound. A bullet's exit wound is typically larger and more irregular than the entrance wound. If a bullet breaks apart, it may create several exit wounds or none at all. Carefully examine your patient to find all wounds.

Stop and Think!

A bullet that enters the body can travel in many directions. Suspect a possible spinal injury in every patient who has suffered a gunshot wound to the head, neck, chest, or abdomen.

Remember This!

At a crime scene, disturb the patient and his or her clothing as little as possible while performing your assessment and during treatment. Cut around rather than through the areas penetrated by the weapon.

Care for completely avulsed tissue like an amputated part.

An **avulsion** is an injury in which a piece of skin or tissue is torn loose or pulled completely off. If the tissue is not totally torn from the body, it often hangs loose, like a flap (Figure 10-22). The amount of bleeding varies with the extent and depth of the injury. A common avulsion injury is an avulsion of the forehead. This type of injury can occur when an unrestrained motor vehicle occupant is thrown through the windshield. In a degloving avulsion injury, the skin and fatty tissue are stripped away from an extremity, like a glove.

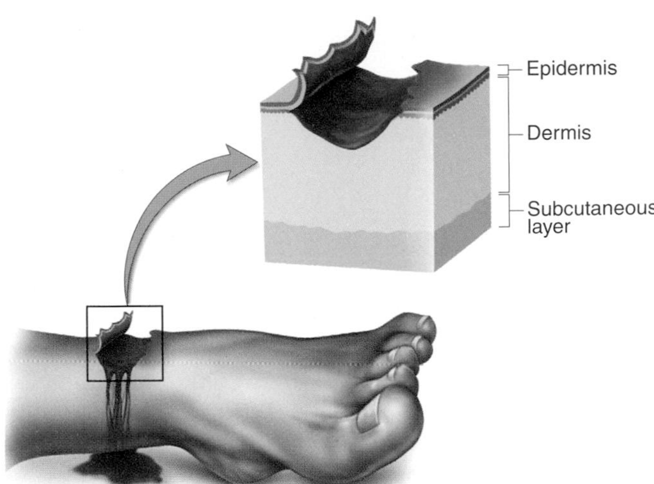

FIGURE 10-22 ▲ In an avulsion, a flap of skin or tissue is torn loose or pulled completely off. If the tissue is not totally torn from the body, it often hangs loose, like a flap.

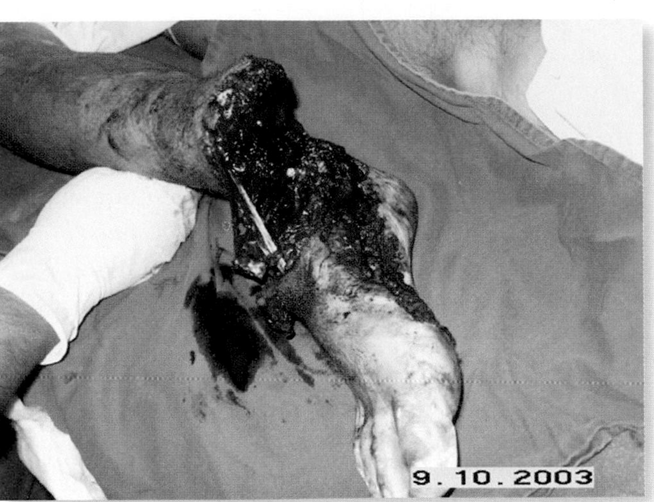

FIGURE 10-23 ▲ A 22-year-old with a traumatic amputation caused by a gear. Trauma.org Image

Be sure to send the severed body part to the hospital with the patient.

An **amputation** is the separation of a body part from the rest of the body. If the body part is forcefully separated from the body, the edges of the wound are usually ragged (Figure 10-23). The remaining tissue may look shredded, with bones or tendons exposed. Massive bleeding may be present. Alternately, bleeding may be limited because blood vessels normally constrict and pull in at the point of injury when damaged. Bleeding can usually be controlled with direct pressure applied to the stump.

A crush injury occurs when a part of the body is caught between two compressing surfaces. In an open crush injury, broken bone ends may stick out through the skin (Figure 10-24). Internal bleeding may be present and can be severe enough to cause shock.

FIGURE 10-24 ► In an open crush injury, fractured bone ends may stick out through the skin.

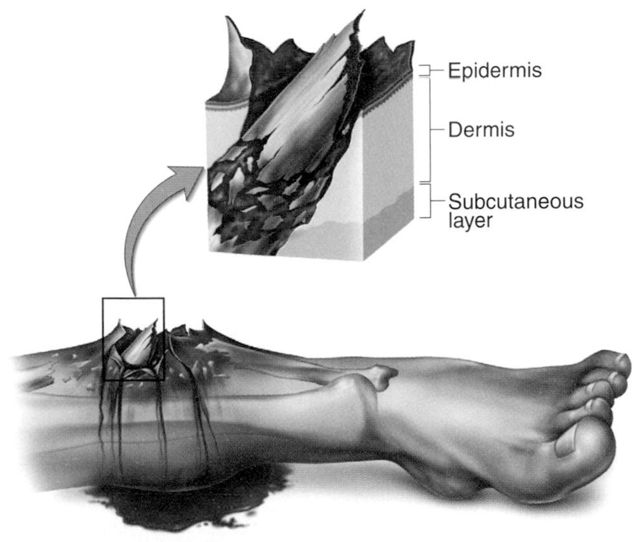

You Should Know

Types of Open Wounds

- Abrasion
- Laceration
- Penetration, puncture wound
- Avulsion
- Amputation
- Open crush injury

Objective 8 ▶

Emergency Medical Responder Care of Open Wounds

To treat a patient with an open wound, use the following steps:

1. Conduct a scene size-up and ensure your safety. Evaluate the mechanism of injury before approaching the patient. Put on appropriate PPE.
2. Form a general impression and determine the urgency of further assessment and care.
3. Perform an initial assessment to identify and treat any life-threatening conditions. Stabilize the cervical spine if needed. If major bleeding is present from an open wound, expose the wound to assess the injury. You may need to remove and cut away clothing. Control bleeding. If signs of shock are present or major external bleeding is present, treat for shock.
4. Once major bleeding is controlled, apply a sterile dressing to prevent further contamination of the wound. Bandage the dressing securely in place.
5. Perform a physical exam. Take the patient's vital signs and gather the patient's medical history.
6. Splint any bone or joint injuries.
7. Comfort, calm, and reassure the patient while waiting for EMS personnel. Perform ongoing assessments every 5 minutes for a patient in shock and every 15 minutes if the patient is stable.

Special Considerations

The following soft-tissue injuries require special consideration:

- Penetrating chest injuries
- Eviscerations
- Impaled objects
- Amputations
- Neck injuries
- Eye injuries
- Mouth injuries
- Ear injuries
- Nosebleeds

Penetrating Chest Injuries

A penetrating (open) chest injury is a break in the skin over the chest wall. This type of injury results from penetrating trauma, such as gunshot wounds, stabbings, blast injuries, or an impaled object. The severity of an open chest injury depends on the size of the wound. If the chest wound is more than two-thirds the diameter of the patient's windpipe, air will enter the chest wound rather than move through the trachea with each breath. You may hear a sucking or gurgling sound escaping from the

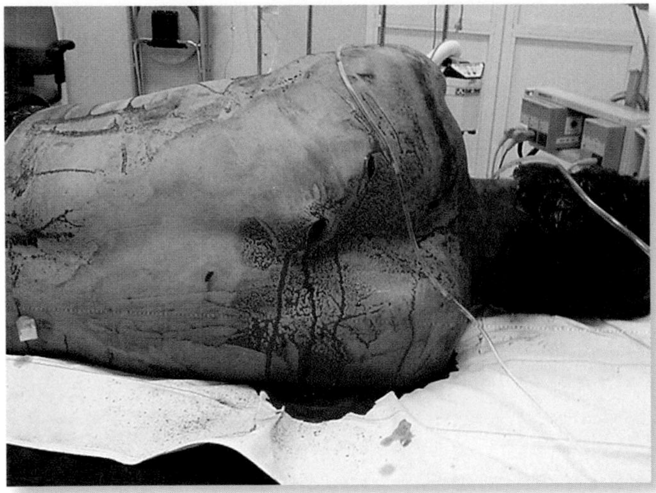

FIGURE 10-25 ▲ The front of this patient's chest showed visible bleeding but no obvious injury. When the patient's back was assessed, multiple wounds were found. Remember, the back is part of the chest. *Always* remember to check the back. Trauma.org Image

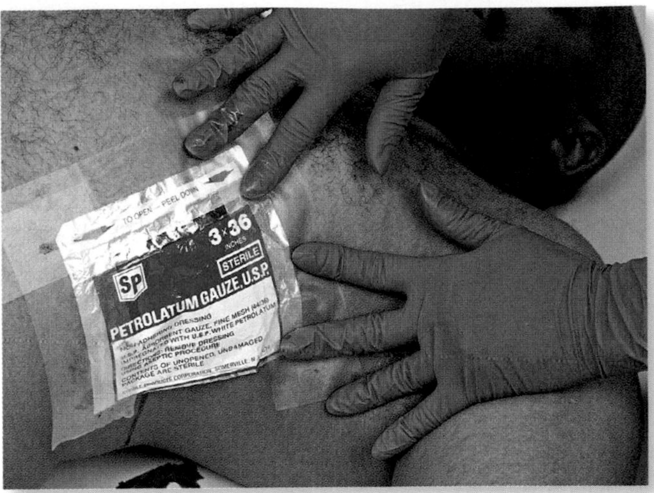

FIGURE 10-26 ▲ Cover an open chest wound with an airtight dressing taped on three sides.

wound when the patient breathes in. This sound occurs as air moves into the pleural cavity through the open chest wound. This type of injury is called a sucking chest wound. It is a life-threatening injury because the open wound can cause the lung on the injured side to collapse, affecting the patient's breathing (Figure 10-25).

Objective 9 ▸

You should consider *any* open chest wound a sucking chest wound. If an open chest wound is present, apply an occlusive (airtight) dressing to the wound. Examples of occlusive dressings include petroleum gauze, aluminum foil, and a piece of plastic wrap. Tape the dressing on three sides (Figure 10-26). The dressing will be sucked over the wound as the patient breathes in, preventing air from entering the chest. The open end of the dressing allows air that is trapped in the chest to escape as the patient breathes out. After covering the wound, provide oxygen if it is available and you have been trained to use it. Place the patient in a position of comfort if no spinal injury is suspected. If spinal injury is suspected, the patient should be placed on a long backboard.

Eviscerations

Objective 10 ▸

Never cover exposed organs with a dressing that will stick to them. Do *not* use aluminum foil. Exposure to the sun may literally bake the organs.

An **evisceration** occurs when an organ sticks out through an open wound. In an abdominal evisceration, abdominal organs stick out through an open wound in the wall of the abdomen. Do not touch or try to place the exposed organ back into the body. Carefully remove clothing from around the wound. Lightly cover the exposed organs and wound with a thick, moist dressing. Secure the dressing in place with a large bandage to keep moisture in and prevent heat loss (Figure 10-27). Place the patient in a position of comfort if no spinal injury is suspected. Keep the patient warm. Assess for signs of shock and treat if present.

Impaled Objects

Objective 11 ▸

An impaled object is also called an embedded object.

An **impaled object** is an object that remains embedded in an open wound. Do not remove an impaled object unless it interferes with CPR or is impaled through the cheek and interferes with care of the patient's airway. After removing an object from the cheek, apply direct pressure to the bleeding by reaching inside the patient's mouth with gloved fingers.

Leave the object in the wound and manually secure it to prevent movement. Shorten the object only if necessary. Any movement of the object can cause further damage to nerves, blood vessels, and other surrounding tissues. Expose the wound

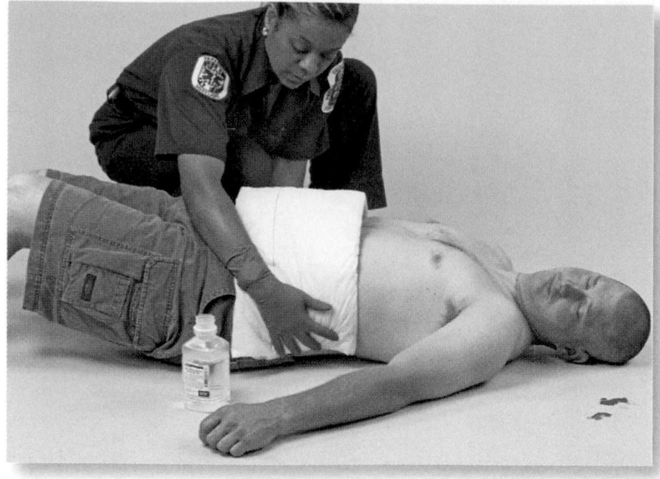

FIGURE 10-27 ▶ Cover the exposed organs and wound by applying a thick, moist dressing lightly over the organs and wound. Secure the dressing in place with a large bandage to retain moisture and prevent heat loss.

area and control bleeding. Stabilize the object with bulky dressings and bandage them in place. Assess the patient for signs of shock and treat if present.

Amputations

Objective 12 ▶

In the case of an amputated body part, control bleeding at the stump. In most cases, direct pressure will be enough to control the bleeding. While providing care for the patient, ask an assistant to find the amputated part. The amputated part may be able to be reattached at the hospital. Because reattaching an amputated part is attempted only in very limited situations, do not suggest to the patient that it will be done.

Put the amputated part in a dry plastic bag or waterproof container. Seal the bag or container and place it in water that contains a few ice cubes (Figure 10-28). Immobilize the injured area to prevent further injury. Treat the patient for shock and keep him or her warm. Comfort, calm, and reassure the patient while waiting for EMS personnel. Perform ongoing assessments every five minutes. Transport the amputated part with the patient to an appropriate facility.

FIGURE 10-28 ▶ Place an amputated part in a dry plastic bag or waterproof container. Seal the bag or container and place it in water that contains a few ice cubes.

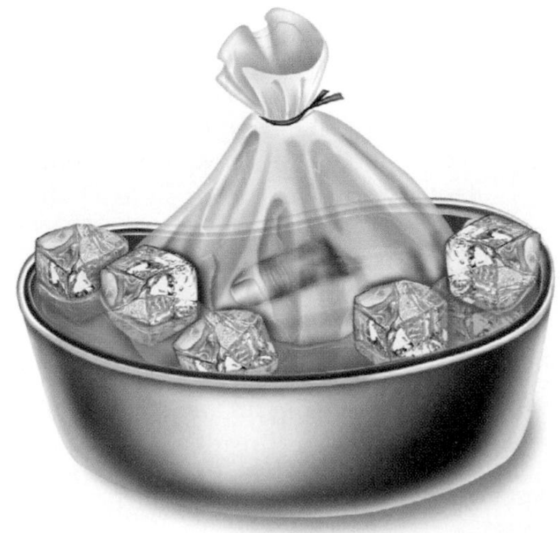

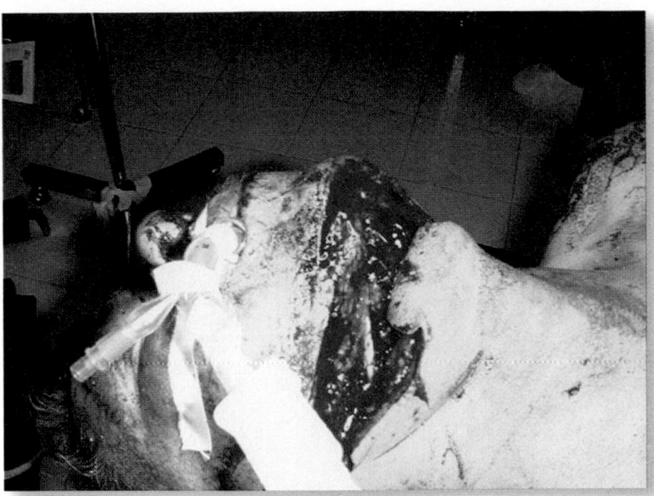

FIGURE 10-29 ▶ This patient is a 33-year-old man involved in a motor vehicle crash. He wore no seat belt and hit the windshield of the car he was driving. Despite the appearance of the injury, there were no injuries to the major blood vessels, trachea, or esophagus. The patient underwent surgery and was sent home 72 hours later. Trauma.org Image

Remember This!

When faced with a situation involving an amputated part, remember the following:

- Never use dry ice to keep an amputated part cool.
- Do not allow an amputated part to freeze.
- Never place an amputated part directly on ice or in water.

Neck Injuries

Consider an injury to the neck an injury to the spine. Immobilize the patient accordingly.

The possible causes of a neck injury include the following:

- A hanging
- Impact with a steering wheel
- "Clothesline" injuries in which a person runs into a stretched wire or cord and strikes his or her throat
- Knife or gunshot wounds

The neck contains many important blood vessels and airway structures. Swelling can cause an airway obstruction. A penetrating injury to the neck can result in severe bleeding (Figure 10-29). The signs and symptoms of a neck injury include shortness of breath, difficulty breathing, and a hoarse voice.

If a blood vessel is torn and exposed to the air, air can be sucked into the vessel and travel to the heart, lungs, brain, or other organs. This condition is called an **air embolism.** The air displaces blood and prevents tissue perfusion. Sometimes if a neck injury has damaged the airway, air will leak into the tissues. If this happens, there may be obvious swelling. When you palpate the skin, you will feel a "popping," as if there were crisped rice cereal trapped beneath it. This is a very important finding to report to other healthcare professionals.

To care for an open neck wound,

- Immediately place a gloved hand over the wound to control bleeding.
- Cover the wound with an airtight (occlusive) dressing.
- Apply a bulky dressing over the occlusive dressing. To control bleeding, apply pressure over the dressing with a gloved hand. Compress the carotid artery only if absolutely necessary to control bleeding. When applying pressure, make sure

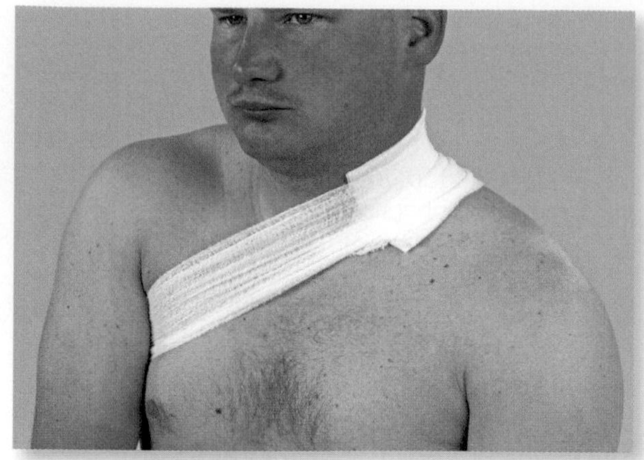

FIGURE 10-30 ► To care for an open neck wound, control bleeding and cover the wound with an airtight dressing. Apply a pressure bandage. Wrap it across the injured side of the neck and under the opposite armpit.

not to press on the trachea or you may cause an airway obstruction. Do not press on both carotid arteries at the same time. Doing so can slow blood flow to the brain. It can also slow the patient's heart rate.

- Apply a pressure bandage. Wrap it across the injured side of the neck and under the opposite armpit (Figure 10-30). *Never apply a circular bandage around a patient's neck.* Strangulation can occur.
- Treat the patient for shock.

Eye Injuries

Eye injuries are common and often occur due to blunt and penetrating trauma. Swelling, bleeding, and the presence of a foreign object in the eye are common signs of an eye injury and are easily seen. A foreign body, such as dirt, sand, and metal or wood slivers, may enter the eye and cause severe pain. Blurred vision, a loss of vision, and excessive tearing are also signs and symptoms of an eye injury.

You Should Know

Causes of Eye Injuries

- Motor vehicle crashes
- Sports and recreational activities
- Violence
- Chemical exposure from household and industrial accidents
- Foreign bodies
- Animal bites and scratches

Do not exert any pressure on the eye.

If a foreign body is in the eye, try flushing it out. Hold the patient's eyelid open and gently flush the eye with warm water. Flush from the nose side of the affected eye toward the ear, away from the unaffected eye. It is important to flush *away* from the uninjured eye so that foreign bodies or chemicals are not transferred to the uninjured eye. Make sure to use a gentle flow of water when flushing the eye. A bulb or irrigation syringe, nasal cannula, or bottle can be used for this purpose (Figure 10-31). If none of these devices is available, try placing the patient's head under a gently running faucet and rinse the eye. Flush the eye for at least five minutes. If you are unable to remove the foreign body, cover both eyes and arrange for patient transport to the nearest appropriate medical facility.

Do not attempt to remove the object.

If a foreign body is protruding from the eye, stabilize the object and arrange for patient transport as quickly as possible. If the object is long, stabilize it with bulky gauze. Then cover the eye with a paper or Styrofoam cup secured with tape to keep the object from moving (Figure 10-32). If the object is short, make

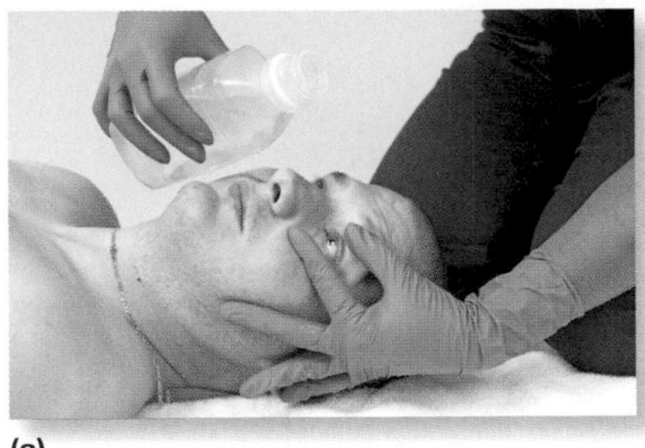

(a)

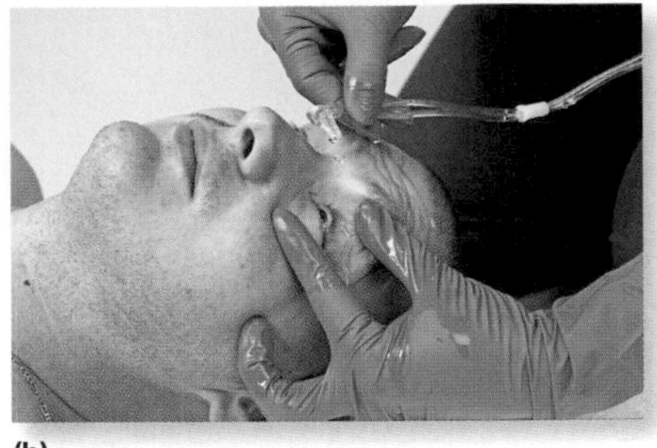

(b)

FIGURE 10-31 ▲ (a) To flush a foreign body from the eye, hold the patient's eyelid open and gently flush the eye with warm water. (b) Flush from the nose side of the affected eye toward the ear, away from the unaffected eye.

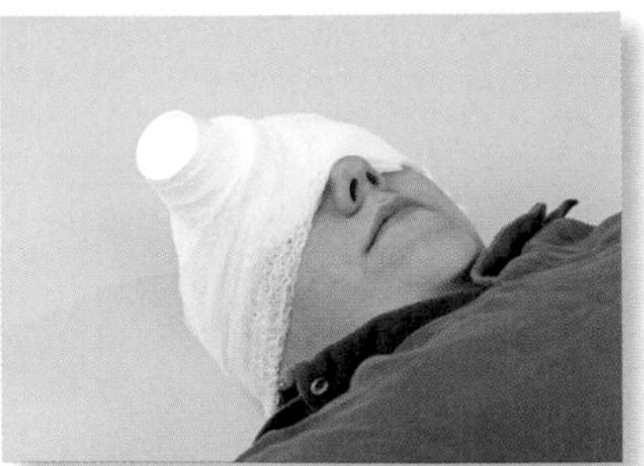

FIGURE 10-32 ▲ If a foreign body is protruding from the eye, stabilize it with bulky gauze. Then cover the eye with a paper or Styrofoam cup secured with tape to keep the object from moving. Cover the unaffected eye to limit movement of the affected eye.

a doughnut-shaped base from roller gauze or a triangular bandage and place it around the eye. Be careful not to bump the object. Because both eyes normally move together, you will also need to cover the unaffected eye with a dressing.

Chemical burns cause 7–10% of all eye injuries.

A chemical burn is the most urgent eye injury. The damage to the eye depends on the type and concentration of the chemical. The length of exposure and the elapsed time until treatment also affect the extent of damage. The early signs and symptoms of a chemical burn include

- Pain
- Redness
- Irritation
- Tearing
- An inability to keep the eye open
- A sensation of something in the eye
- Swelling of the eyelids
- Blurred vision, usually due to pain or tearing of the eye

Alkali burns are more dangerous than acid burns because they penetrate more deeply and rapidly. Common household substances that contain alkalis include lye, cement, lime, and ammonia. Sulfuric acid is found in automobile batteries and is one of the most common chemicals associated with acid burns of the eye. These exposures usually occur because of an automobile battery explosion.

Ask the patient if he is wearing contact lenses. If he is, have the patient remove them as soon as possible. If the lenses are left in, the irrigating solution will not be able to reach parts of the eye. If the patient is not wearing contact lenses or if the lenses have been removed, immediately flush the eye with water or normal saline. Continue flushing the eye for at least 20 minutes. Flush away from the unaffected eye (as previously described). Arrange for immediate patient transport. Irrigation should be continued throughout transport.

You Should Know

Pepper spray is an irritant that causes significant pain when sprayed into the eyes. Vision is not usually affected and it rarely causes eye damage. Flushing the affected eye for five minutes with warm water will generally stop further irritation.

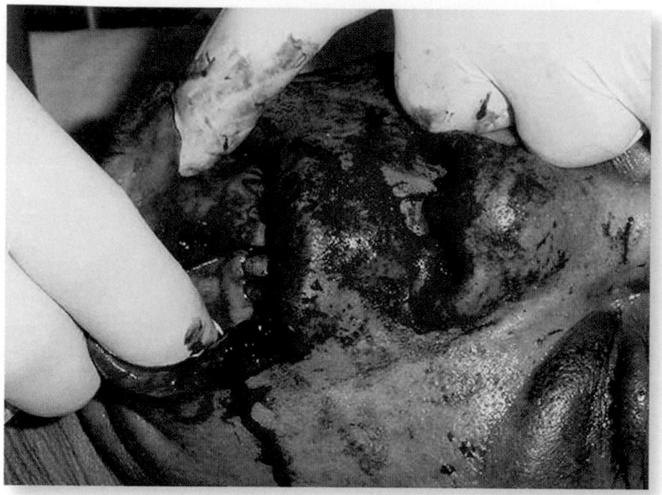

FIGURE 10-33 ▶ Jaw fracture due to direct frontal trauma. Trauma.org Image

If you cover both eyes, be sure to tell the patient everything that you are doing. The patient may be frightened when he or she cannot anticipate movements and other procedures.

A nonchemical burn to the eye can be caused by heat, radiation, lasers, infrared rays, and ultraviolet light (such as sunlight, arc welding, and bright snow). The patient will complain of severe pain in the eyes one to six hours after the exposure. Emergency care for a nonchemical burn to the eye includes covering both eyes with moist pads. Darken the room to protect the patient from further exposure to light. Arrange for patient transport for further evaluation and treatment.

Mouth Injuries

If the patient is unable to open his or her mouth or move his or her lower jaw side to side without pain, suspect a fracture.

An injury to the mouth can result in an airway obstruction due to severe swelling or bleeding. Because the tongue is attached to the lower jaw (mandible), a lower-jaw fracture may allow the tongue to fall against the back of the throat, blocking the airway. The signs and symptoms depend on the area of the jaw affected. Tenderness, bruising, and swelling are common (Figure 10-33).

The upper jawbone (maxilla) is often fractured in high-speed crashes. The patient's face is thrown forward into the windshield, steering wheel, and dashboard. A fracture of the maxilla is often accompanied by a black eye. The patient's face may appear unusually long. Swelling and pain are usually present.

A patient with a jaw fracture should receive spinal immobilization because of the mechanism of injury. Carefully look in the patient's mouth for teeth, blood, vomitus, and other potential obstructions. Suction as necessary. Look in the mouth for broken or missing teeth. If dentures or missing teeth are found, they should be transported with the patient. If a knocked-out tooth is found, handle only the top (crown) of the tooth. Rinse the tooth with water, place it in milk, and transport it with the patient. Control bleeding and treat for shock if indicated.

Ear Injuries

Never put anything into the ear to control bleeding.

A blow to the ear can result in bruising of the outer (external) portion of the ear. A severe blow can result in damage to the eardrum with pain, bleeding, or both. Suspect a possible skull fracture if you see blood or fluid draining from a patient's ear. Place a sterile dressing loosely over the ear to absorb the drainage and bandage it in place. If the ear is avulsed, collect the avulsed part and care for it as you would an amputated part. Make sure that the avulsed part is transported with the patient to the hospital. An ear laceration is treated like any other soft-tissue injury (Figure 10-34).

Nosebleeds

Swallowed blood can make people feel sick to their stomachs, increasing the chance of vomiting.

Most nosebleeds come from a bleeding blood vessel in the front of the nose. This type of nosebleed is called an anterior nosebleed. It is usually easy to control. Tell the patient with a nosebleed not to blow her nose or sniffle. Doing

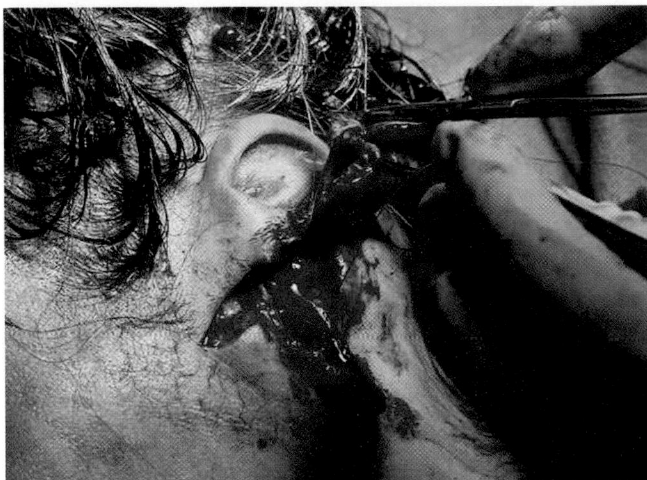

FIGURE 10-34 ▲ Ear laceration. Trauma.org Image

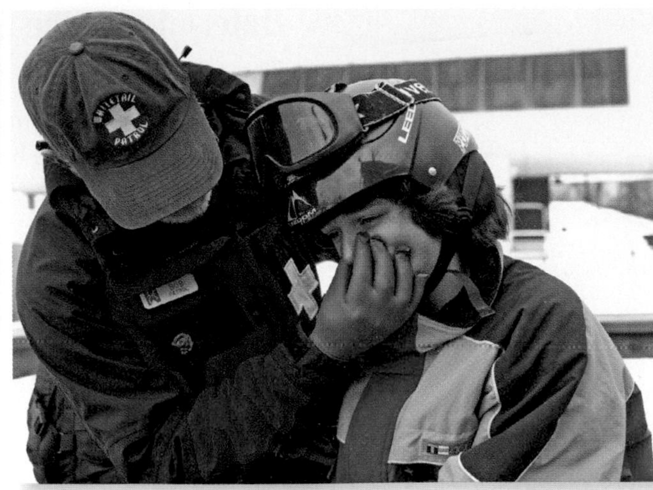

FIGURE 10-35 ▲ To stop a nosebleed, have the patient sit up, with the patient's head tilted forward. Pinch the fleshy part of the patient's nostrils together with your thumb and two fingers for 15 minutes.

so can prevent clots from forming or can break clots that have already developed. Do not put anything in the nose to try to control bleeding. If the patient can help you, have her sit up and lean her head forward. This position helps keep blood from draining into the back of the patient's throat. If the patient cannot sit up, have her lie down with her head raised. Tell the patient to breathe through her mouth. Pinch the fleshy part of the patient's nostrils together with your thumb and two fingers for 15 minutes (Figure 10-35).

A posterior nosebleed occurs most often in older adults.

Some nosebleeds come from a bleeding blood vessel in the back of the nose. This type of nosebleed is called a posterior nosebleed. A posterior nosebleed is difficult to control and the patient can develop shock. A patient with this type of nosebleed needs rapid transport to the hospital. Treat for shock if present.

Burns

Objective 13 ▶

Burns occur because of exposure to heat (thermal burn), chemicals, electricity, or radiation. Most burns are thermal burns that result from flames, scalds, or contact with hot substances. Chemical burns are caused by substances that produce chemical changes in the skin, resulting in tissue damage on contact. Acids and alkalis are substances that are commonly associated with a chemical burn. An electrical burn occurs when a person comes into contact with a source of electricity, including lightning. Body organs may be injured from the heat generated as the electrical current enters the body and travels through the tissues. Burns may also result from a high level of radiation exposure. Radiation burns are the least common type of burn.

The skin is the body's largest organ.

Remember that the skin

- Helps regulate body temperature
- Senses heat, cold, touch, pressure, and pain
- Helps maintain fluid balance
- Protects underlying tissues from injury

When the skin is disrupted because of a burn, many of these functions are affected. The body loses fluid, and the skin becomes less effective in helping maintain body temperature. Because the skin surface is no longer intact, the body is at an increased risk of infection.

Determining the Severity of a Burn

The severity of a burn is determined by a number of factors:

- The depth of the burn (how deeply the burn penetrates the skin)
- The extent of the burn (how much of the body surface is burned)
- The location of the burn
- The patient's age
- The medical or surgical conditions present before the burn
- Associated factors (such as the mechanism of injury)

Depth of the Burn

A burn wound continues to change up to 24 hours after the injury.

Burns are classified by how deeply the body's skin layers are affected. There are three categories of burns:

- Superficial (first-degree) burn
- Partial-thickness (second-degree) burn
- Full-thickness (third-degree) burn

Superficial Burns

Blistering does not occur with a superficial burn.

A superficial (first-degree) burn affects only the epidermis. It results in only minor tissue damage (Figure 10-36). A sunburn is a superficial burn. The skin is red, tender, and very painful (Figure 10-37). This type of burn does not usually require medical care and heals in two to five days with no scarring.

Partial-Thickness Burns

Not all partial-thickness burns blister. However, if blistering is present, it is a partial-thickness burn.

A partial-thickness (second-degree) burn involves the epidermis and dermis. The hair follicles and sweat glands are spared in this degree of burn (Figure 10-38). These burns commonly result from contact with hot liquids or flash burns from gasoline flames. A partial-thickness burn produces intense pain and some swelling. Blistering may be present (Figure 10-39). The skin appears pink, red, or mottled and is sensitive to air current and pressure. This type of burn usually

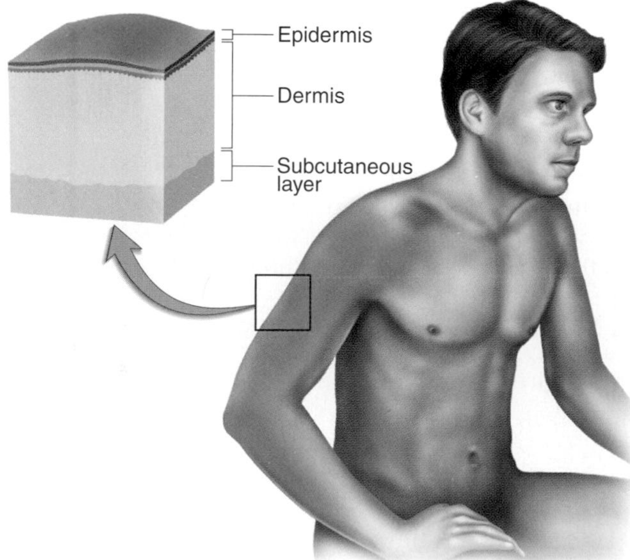

FIGURE 10-36 ▲ A superficial (first-degree) burn affects only the epidermis.

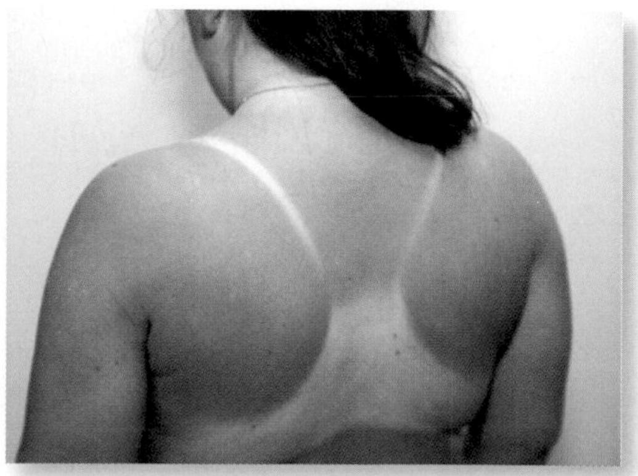

FIGURE 10-37 ▲ Superficial (first-degree) burn.

heals within 5–35 days. Scarring may or may not occur, depending on the depth of the burn.

Full-Thickness Burns

A full-thickness (third-degree) burn destroys both the epidermis and dermis and may include subcutaneous tissue, muscle, and bone (Figure 10-40). The color of the patient's skin varies from yellow or pale to black. The skin has a dry, waxy, or leathery appearance (Figure 10-41). A full-thickness burn is numb because the burn destroys nerve endings in the skin. However, many

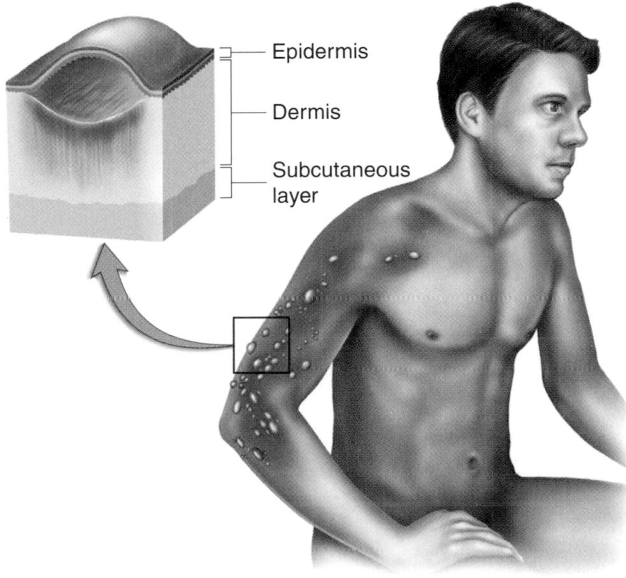

FIGURE 10-38 ▲ A partial-thickness (second-degree) burn affects the epidermis and dermis.

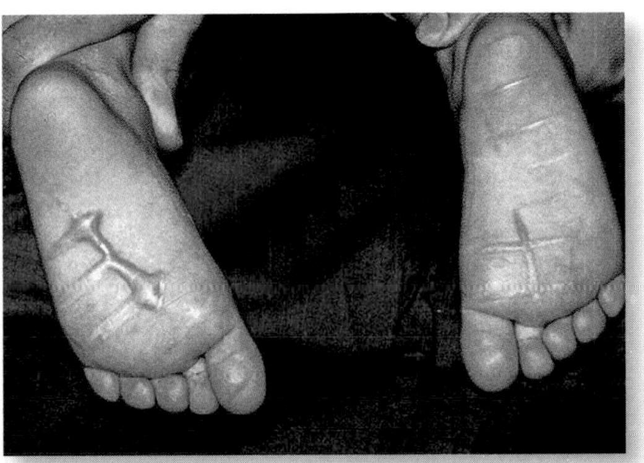

FIGURE 10-39 ▲ Partial-thickness (second-degree) burn. EMSC Slide Set (CD-ROM). 1996. Courtesy of the Emergency Medical Services for Children Program, administered by the U.S. Department of Health and Human Service's Health Resources and Services Administration, Maternal and Child Health Bureau.

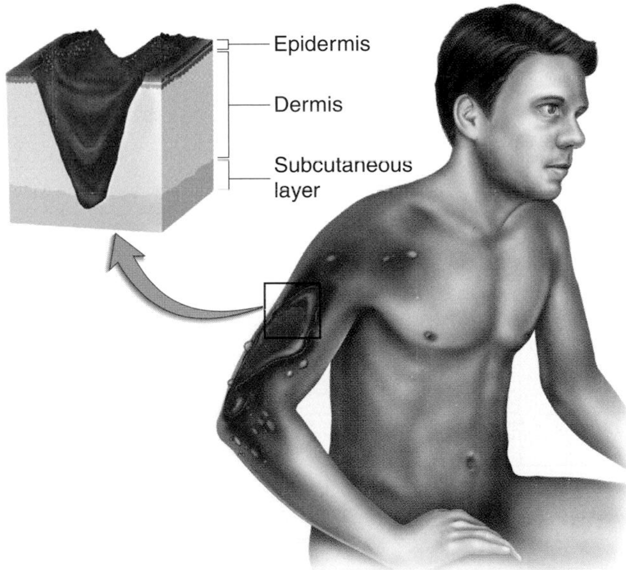

FIGURE 10-40 ▲ A full-thickness (third-degree) burn causes damage to all layers of the epidermis and dermis and may include subcutaneous tissue, muscle, and bone.

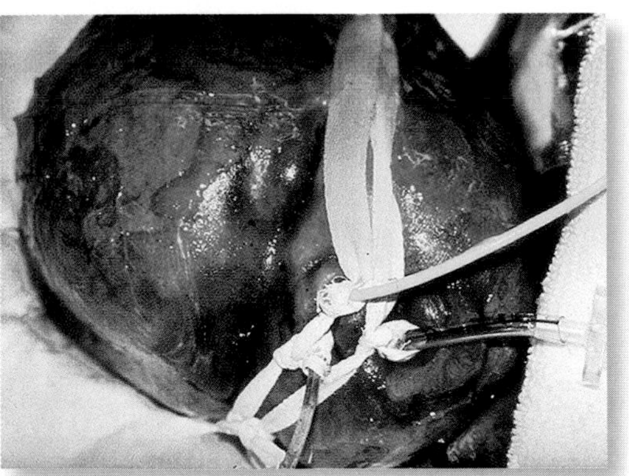

FIGURE 10-41 ▲ Full-thickness (third-degree) burn. EMSC Slide Set (CD-ROM). 1996. Courtesy of the Emergency Medical Services for Children Program, administered by the U.S. Department of Health and Human Service's Health Resources and Services Administration, Maternal and Child Health Bureau.

FIGURE 10-42 ▶ The rule of nines for an infant, a child, and an adult.

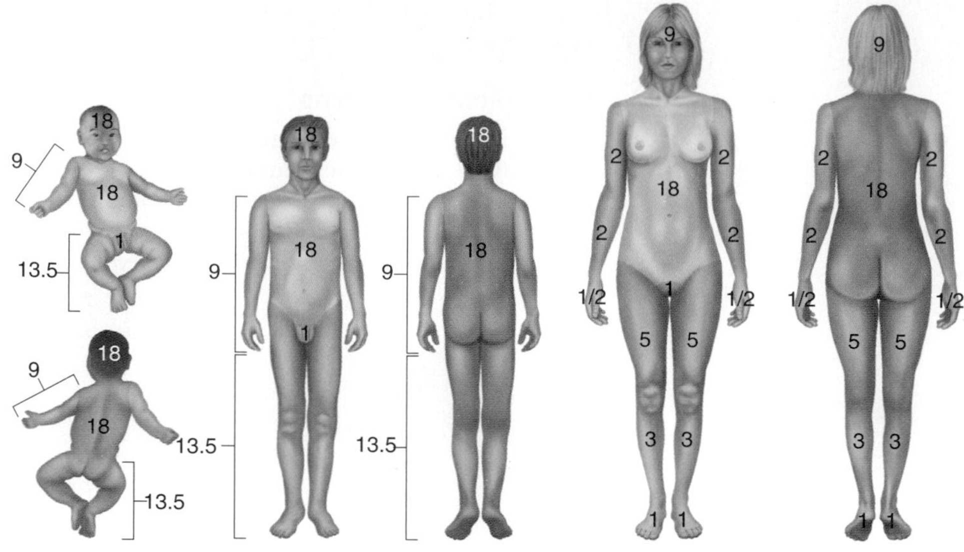

full-thickness burns are surrounded by areas of superficial and partial-thickness burns, which are painful. A large full-thickness burn requires skin grafting. Small areas may heal from the edges of the burn after weeks. Because the skin is so severely damaged in this type of burn, it cannot perform its usual protective functions. Rapid fluid loss often occurs. Be ready to treat the patient for shock.

Extent of the Burn

Only partial-thickness and full-thickness burns are included when calculating the extent of a burn.

When determining the seriousness of a burn, the extent of the burned area is more important than the depth of the burn. The "rule of nines" is a guide used to estimate the affected body surface area (BSA). The rule of nines divides the adult body into sections that are 9% or are multiples of 9% (Figure 10-42). The rule of nines has been modified for children and infants. To estimate the extent of a burn using the rule of nines, add the percentages of the areas burned. For example, if an adult is burned in the front of the trunk (18%), the front and back of one arm (9%), and the front and back of one leg (18%), 45% of his or her BSA is burned (Table 10-3).

TABLE 10-3 The Rule of Nines

Body Area	Adult	Child	Infant
Head and neck	9%	18%	18%
Front of trunk	18%	18%	18%
Back of trunk	18%	18%	18%
Each arm (shoulder to fingertips)	9%	9%	9%
Each leg (groin to toe)	18%	13.5%	13.5%
Genitals	1%	1%	1%

Remember This!

The "rule of palms" can be used for small or irregularly shaped burns or burns that are scattered over the patient's body. The palm of the *patient's* hand equals 1% of the patient's BSA. If the patient's palm would fit over the burned area eight times, the extent of the burn is 8% of the BSA.

Other Factors Related to Burn Severity

The Location of the Burn

The location of a burn is an important factor when determining burn severity. Burns to the face can cause breathing difficulty. Burns of the face and neck can interfere with the ability to eat or drink. Burns of the hands and feet can interfere with the patient's ability to walk, work, feed him- or herself, and perform other daily activities. Burns of the genitalia are prone to infection.

Preexisting Medical Conditions

A preexisting medical problem may increase a patient's risk of death or complications following a burn injury. A burn is considered severe if the patient is younger than 5 years or older than 55. The skin of infants, young children, and elderly people is thin. Burns in these patients may be more severe than they initially appear.

Remember This!

Burn Considerations for Infants and Children

- Children have a larger surface area in relation to total body size. This larger surface area results in greater fluid and heat loss.
- Children who are burned are more likely than adults to develop shock or airway problems.
- Consider the possibility of child abuse when treating a burned child. A common burn associated with child abuse is caused by dipping the child in scalding water. "Stocking-like" burns with no associated splash marks are often present on the buttocks, genitalia, or extremities (Figure 10-43). Report all suspected cases of abuse to law enforcement or emergency department personnel.

Burn Considerations for Older Adults

- Many older adults have thin skin and poor circulation. These factors affect the depth of a burn and slow the healing process.
- In older adults, the mechanisms and severity of burn injury are related to living alone. Older adults also tend to wear loose-fitting clothing while cooking and fall asleep while smoking. In addition, these patients tend to have declining vision, hearing, and sense of smell. Older adults may have a slowed reaction time and problems with balance and/or memory.
- Burns in older adults most often occur in the home. Scalds and flame burns are the most common type of burns in this age group.
- Older adults are more likely to have a preexisting medical condition, which increases their risk of complications after a burn. In some cases, the preexisting condition may be the cause of the burn. For example, an older adult may collapse because of a stroke while smoking or cooking.

FIGURE 10-43 ▶ "Stocking-like" burns with no associated splash marks are caused by dipping a child in scalding water. This type of injury is usually seen in children younger than two years. The child's caregiver punishes the child, for example, for an "accident" when he or she is being potty trained. EMSC Slide Set (CD-ROM). 1996. Courtesy of the Emergency Medical Services for Children Program, administered by the U.S. Department of Health and Human Service's Health Resources and Services Administration, Maternal and Child Health Bureau.

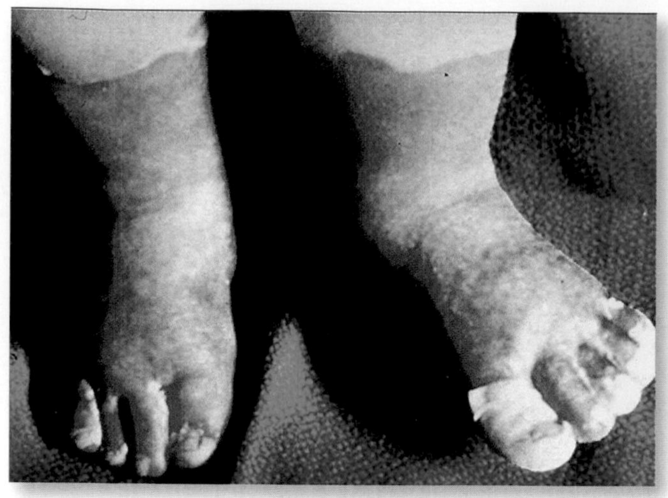

Burns Best Treated in a Burn Center

Although most burns are minor, some types of burns are best treated in a burn center. A burn center offers specialized care—including services, equipment, and staff trained to treat serious burn injuries. A patient with any of the following types of burns should be transported to a burn center:

- Partial-thickness (second-degree) burns involving more than 10% of the total body surface area (TBSA) in adults or 5% of the TBSA in children
- Chemical burns
- All burns involving the hands, face, eyes, ears, feet, genitalia, or circumferential burns of the torso or extremities
- Any full-thickness (third-degree) burn in a child
- All inhalation injuries
- Electrical burns, including lightning injuries
- All burns complicated by fractures or other trauma
- All burns in high-risk patients, including older adults, the very young, and those with preexisting conditions, such as diabetes, asthma, and epilepsy

Emergency Medical Responder Care of Thermal Burns

To treat a patient with a thermal burn, use the following steps:

1. Conduct a scene size-up and ensure your safety. Evaluate the mechanism of injury before approaching the patient. Put on appropriate PPE.
   - If the patient is still in the area of the heat source, remove the patient from the area. If the patient's clothing is in flames, "stop, drop, and roll." Place the patient on the floor or ground. Roll him or her in a blanket to smother the flames.
   - Remove smoldering clothing and jewelry. If the patient's clothing is stuck to the burned area, do not attempt to remove it. Instead, cut around the clothing, leaving the burn untouched.
2. Form a general impression and determine the urgency of further assessment and care.
3. Perform an initial assessment to identify and treat any life-threatening conditions. Manage the patient's airway and breathing. Stabilize the cervical spine if needed.
4. If the patient was in a confined space and was exposed to smoke, flames, or steam, be alert for potential airway problems. Patients who have signs of an

Examples of confined spaces include a room, vehicle, silo, pit, vessel, or vault.

inhalation injury likely have inhaled poisonous gases, such as carbon monoxide or cyanide. These gases are produced as a byproduct of substances that burn. High-flow oxygen is always indicated in these situations.

- Check the pulses in all extremities. Burn swelling that encircles an extremity (a circumferential burn) can act as a tourniquet.

5. After completing the initial assessment, update the EMS unit responding to the scene with a brief report by phone or radio, if possible.

After all immediate life threats have been managed, care for the burn itself.

6. Perform a physical exam. Quickly determine the severity of the burn. Take the patient's vital signs and gather the patient's medical history.
   - Consider the following questions about the burn:
     - How long ago did the burn occur?
     - How did it occur?
     - What was done to treat the burn before you arrived?
   - Keep in mind that even after being removed from the heat source, burned tissue will continue to burn. Cool the burn with cold water as soon as possible. Continue until pain is relieved. Do not use ice or ice water for longer than 10 minutes to cool a thermal burn, especially if the burn is large (>20% BSA).
   - Cover the burned area with a dry dressing or sheet. Cover the patient with clean, dry sheets and blankets to keep him or her warm. The sheet does not have to be sterile.
   - Remove all jewelry as soon as possible. Swelling of the hands and fingers may occur soon after a burn.
   - Look for other injuries and signs of shock. Treat and immobilize possible fractures. Treat any soft-tissue injuries. Treat shock if present.
   - Keep burned extremities elevated above the level of the heart.
   - Arrange for transport to the nearest appropriate hospital. Comfort, calm, and reassure the patient while waiting for EMS personnel. Perform an ongoing assessment every 5 minutes if the patient is unstable and every 15 minutes if the patient is stable.

Because burned tissue loses its ability to regulate temperature, cover the patient even when the outside temperature is warm.

You Should Know

Signs and Symptoms of Possible Inhalation Injury

- Facial burns
- Soot in the nose or mouth
- Singed facial or nasal hair
- Swelling of the lips or the inside of the mouth
- Coughing
- An inability to swallow secretions
- A hoarse voice

Remember This!

- Do not apply ice, butter, oils, sprays, lotions, or ointments to a burn.
- If a blister has formed, do not break it.
- Do not place ice or wet sheets on a burn.
- Do not transport a burn patient on wet sheets, wet towels, or wet clothing.

Chemical Burns

In some cases, the damage caused by chemicals is not limited to the skin. Some chemicals, such as hydrofluoric acid, can be absorbed into the body and cause damage to internal organs.

It has been estimated that more than 25,000 chemicals are currently in use that are capable of burning the skin or mucous membranes. Chemical burns can result from contact with wet or dry chemicals. The degree of injury in a chemical burn is based on the following:

- The chemical's mechanism of action
- The chemical's strength
- The chemical's concentration and amount
- How long the patient was in contact with the chemical
- The body part in contact with the chemical
- The extent of tissue penetration

Emergency Medical Responder Care of Chemical Burns

To treat a patient with a chemical burn, use the following steps:

Your personal safety must be your primary concern.

1. Conduct a scene size-up and ensure your safety. Evaluate the mechanism of injury before approaching the patient. Take the necessary scene safety precautions to protect yourself from exposure to hazardous materials. Wear gloves, eye protection, and other PPE as necessary. Additional resources, such as law enforcement, the fire service, the state or local hazardous materials team, and special rescue personnel, may be needed to secure the scene before you can safely enter the area.
2. Form a general impression and determine the urgency of further assessment and care.
3. Perform an initial assessment to identify and treat any life-threatening conditions.
   - Manage the patient's airway and breathing. Stabilize the cervical spine if needed.
   - Remove the patient's jewelry and clothing, including shoes and socks, which can trap concentrated chemicals. Place the items in plastic bags to limit others' exposure to the chemical.
4. After completing the initial assessment, update the EMS unit responding to the scene with a brief report by phone or radio, if possible.
5. Perform a physical exam. Take the patient's vital signs and gather the patient's medical history.
   - Stop the burning process by removing the chemical.
     - Brush off dry chemicals from the patient's skin using towels, sheets, or your gloved hands. Brush the chemical *away* from the patient.
     - Flush the burn with large amounts of room temperature water at low pressure. If the burn covers a large area, put the patient in the shower or use a garden hose, if available. Chemical burns should be flushed for at least 20 minutes.
   - Treat any other injuries.

Wet chemicals can be flushed with water. Brush away dry chemicals before flushing.

6. The patient should be decontaminated before transport to the hospital. If the patient is not fully decontaminated before transport, the receiving hospital should be notified as soon as possible. This notification will allow the hospital time to prepare to decontaminate the patient when he or she arrives at the facility.
7. Comfort, calm, and reassure the patient while waiting for EMS personnel. Perform an ongoing assessment every 5 minutes.

Stop and Think!

The severity of a chemical burn can be misleading. The skin may not appear to be significantly damaged, yet a severe injury may be present. You may be contaminated by the chemical if you do not use appropriate precautions.

Electrical Burns

The severity of an electrical injury is related to the following:

- The amperage (the flow of the current)
- The voltage (the current's force)
- The type of current (alternating current or direct current)
- The current's pathway through the body
- The resistance of tissues to the current
- The duration of contact with the current

Normally, the skin is a resistor to the flow of electric current into the body. When electricity enters the body, it is converted to heat. Inside the body, the current follows the paths of blood vessels, nerves, and muscles. This results in major damage to the body's internal organs. The skin may show no signs or only minimal signs of injury, despite massive internal damage.

Emergency Medical Responder Care of Electrical Burns

To treat a patient with an electrical burn, use the following steps:

Law enforcement, fire service, and utility company personnel may be needed to secure the scene before you can safely enter the area

1. Conduct a scene size-up and make sure the scene is safe before entering. Evaluate the mechanism of injury before approaching the patient. Take the necessary scene safety precautions to protect yourself from exposure to electrical hazards. Wear gloves, eye protection, and other PPE as necessary. If the patient is still in contact with the electrical source, you may need to contact the appropriate resources before approaching the patient. These resources may include law enforcement, fire service, and utility company personnel (Figure 10-44). Do not attempt to remove the patient from the electrical source unless you have been trained to do so. If the patient is still in contact with the electrical source or you are unsure, do not touch the patient.
2. Form a general impression and determine the urgency of further assessment and care (Figure 10-45).

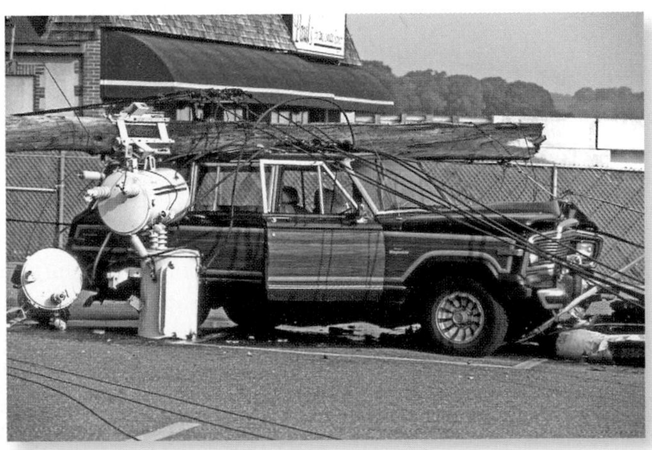

FIGURE 10-44 ► In situations involving electricity, additional resources, such as law enforcement, fire service, and utility company personnel, may be needed to secure the scene before you can safely enter the area.

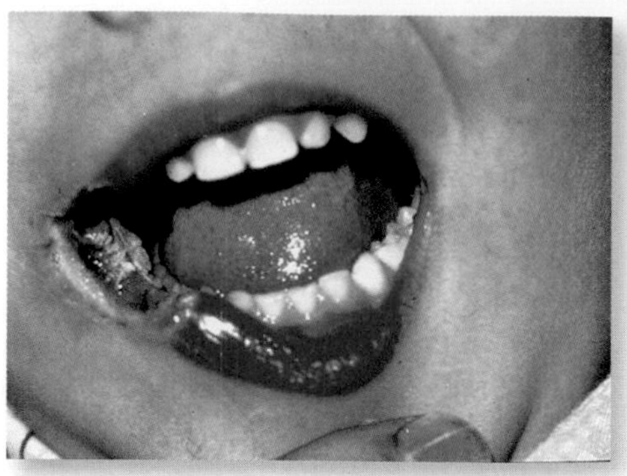

FIGURE 10-45 ▲ Electrical burn. EMSC Slide Set (CD-ROM). 1996. Courtesy of the Emergency Medical Services for Children Program, administered by the U.S. Department of Health and Human Service's Health Resources and Services Administration, Maternal and Child Health Bureau.

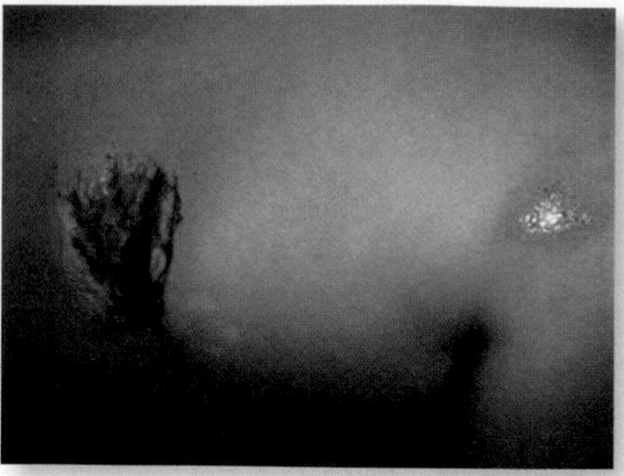

FIGURE 10-46 ▲ Electrical burn showing typical entrance and exit wounds. Trauma.org Image

Cardiac arrest due to an electrical injury usually responds to treatment if defibrillation is performed quickly.

3. Perform an initial assessment to identify and treat any life-threatening conditions. Manage the patient's airway and breathing. Stabilize the cervical spine if needed. Monitor the patient closely for respiratory and cardiac arrest. Make sure an automated external defibrillator is immediately available to you. After completing the initial assessment, update the EMS unit responding to the scene with a brief report by phone or radio, if possible.
4. Perform a physical exam. Take the patient's vital signs and gather the patient's medical history. Provide oxygen if it is available and you have been trained to use it.
5. Look for and treat any other injuries. The patient may have fallen or been thrown from the electrical source. Treat the soft-tissue injuries associated with the burn.
6. Look for both an entrance and an exit wound. The entrance wound may look dry and leathery. The exit wound is usually much larger (Figure 10-46).
7. *All* electrical burns should be evaluated by a physician. Arrange for patient transport to the hospital.
8. Comfort, calm, and reassure the patient while waiting for EMS personnel. Perform an ongoing assessment every five minutes.

Remember This!

Because electrical burns do more damage on the inside of the body than they do on the outside, it will be impossible for you to tell how bad an electrical burn really is. *All* electrical burns need to be evaluated at a hospital.

Emotional Support

Objective 18 ▶

Bleeding and soft-tissue injuries are dramatic injuries. The emergency care that you provide for bleeding and soft-tissue injuries is very important. It is also important to consider the psychological impact of these injuries. The patient and/or family members may experience many emotions because of the injury. Remember that, although grief is most often associated with death, *any* change of circumstance can cause a person to experience grief. A patient who has suffered a massive soft-tissue injury or

Objective 19 ►

major burn often goes through the stages of the grief process. You may see the emotions of fear, anger, guilt, and depression. Provide emotional support for the patient and family.

Always place the interests of the patient first when making patient care decisions.

Some of the injuries you will care for will be the result of a suicide attempt. After an unsuccessful suicide attempt, the patient may want to talk with you about it or may deny the attempt. Other injuries you will care for may be the result of child, elder, or spousal abuse. If you suspect abuse, share your concerns privately with the arriving EMS personnel. You should also report all suspected cases of abuse to law enforcement or emergency department personnel. Although these situations may be difficult, you must not be confrontational with the patient, family members, or others at the scene.

When providing care for bleeding and soft-tissue injuries, you may experience anger, anxiety, frustration, fear, grief, and feelings of helplessness, especially if you are unable to relieve a patient's suffering or if a patient dies despite your care. You may feel sick at the sight of these injuries. These emotions are common and expected. You should not feel embarrassed or ashamed when these situations affect you. Seek the help of a peer counselor, mental health professional, social worker, or member of the clergy when you need help coping with these situations.

Making a Difference

The physical care you provide for a patient's illness or injury is very important. Good emergency care involves attending to the patient's physical *and* emotional needs in a professional, caring, concerned, and sensitive way.

Dressings and Bandages

Objective 14 ►

A **dressing** is an absorbent material placed directly over a wound. A **bandage** is used to secure a dressing in place. The functions of dressing and bandaging wounds include

- Helping to stop bleeding
- Absorbing blood and other drainage from the wound
- Protecting the wound from further injury
- Reducing contamination and the risk of infection

Dressings

When choosing a dressing, select one that is lint-free and large enough to cover the wound. A dressing of the right size should extend beyond the edges of the wound. If available, use a sterile dressing whenever possible because the dressing will be in direct contact with the open wound. When applying the dressing to the wound, wear gloves and hold the dressing by a corner. Place the dressing right over the wound—do not slide it in place.

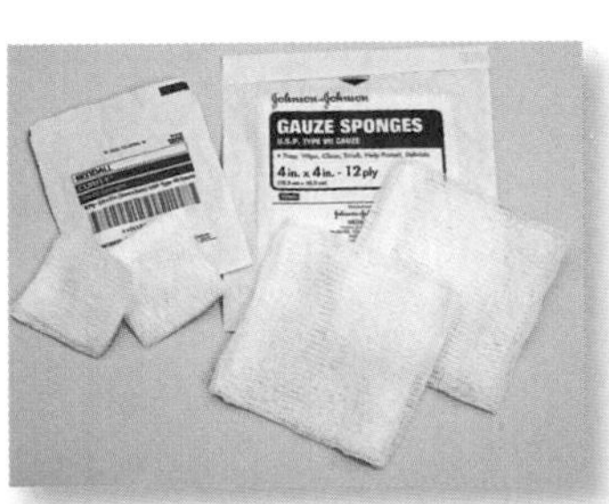

FIGURE 10-47 ▲ Sterile gauze pads come in different shapes and sizes.

Types of Dressings

The types of dressings commonly used in emergency care are sterile gauze pads, trauma dressings, occlusive dressings, and non-adherent pads.

Sterile Gauze Pads

Sterile gauze pads are the most commonly used dressings (Figure 10-47). They come in different shapes and sizes and are made of loosely woven material. This woven

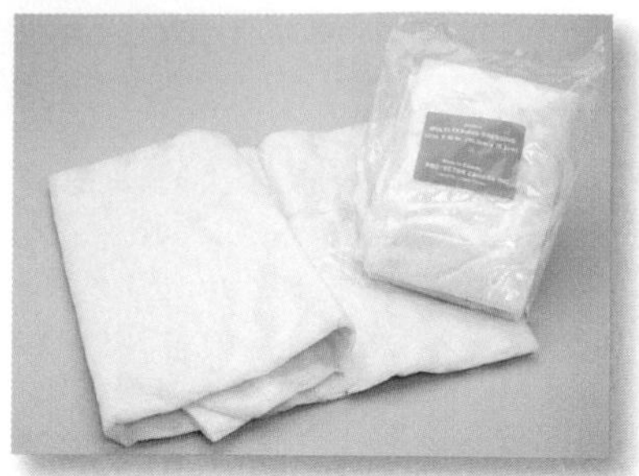

FIGURE 10-48 ▲ Trauma dressings are thick dressings that are used for large wounds. They are available in different sizes.

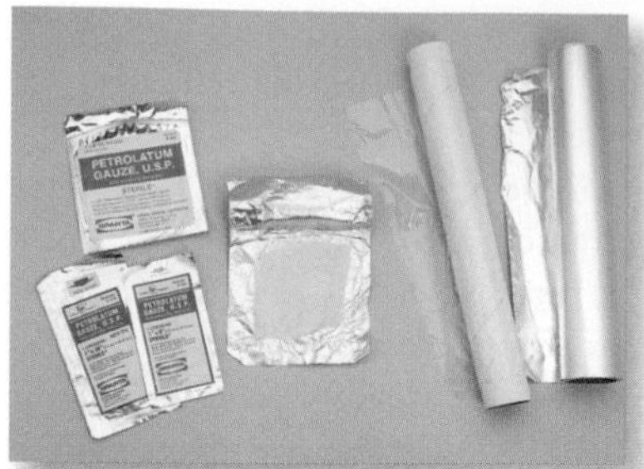

FIGURE 10-49 ▲ An occlusive dressing is used to cover an open wound and create an airtight seal. This type of dressing is made of nonporous material. Although commercially made occlusive dressings are available, plastic wrap or aluminum foil may also be used.

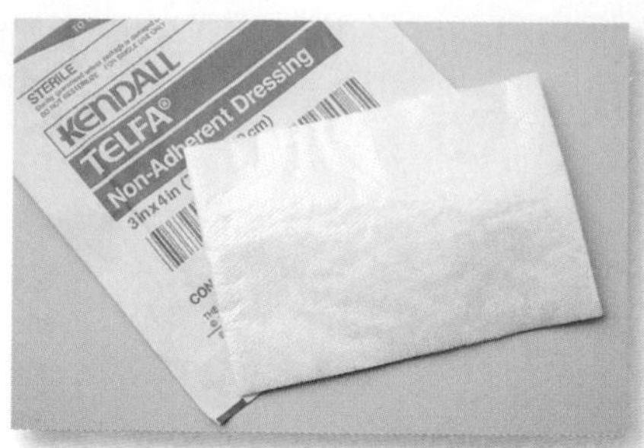

FIGURE 10-50 ▲ Non-adherent pads are used to cover an open wound, but they do not stick to it.

Do not place a gauze pad directly on an open wound that is leaking fluid because it will stick.

If blood soaks through a dressing, do not remove it. Apply more dressings and another bandage.

material allows blood and fluids to pass through the material and be absorbed. Small gauze pads are classified by their size in inches. For example, a 2 by 2 is a small dressing that is 2 inches long and 2 inches wide.

Trauma Dressings

Trauma dressings are thick dressings available in various sizes (Figure 10-48). They are made of two layers of gauze with absorbent cotton in the center. A trauma dressing is used for large wounds. It can also be used to pad an injured arm or leg inside a splint.

Occlusive Dressings

An occlusive dressing is a dressing made of nonporous material. This type of dressing is used to cover an open wound of the chest or neck, creating an airtight seal. Although commercially made occlusive dressings are available, plastic wrap or aluminum foil may also be used (Figure 10-49).

Non-Adherent Pads

Non-adherent pads are gauze pads that have a special coating. They are used to cover an open wound, such as a scrape or burn, that is leaking fluid, but they do not stick to the wound (Figure 10-50). Eye pads are used to cover the eyes after a minor eye injury (Figure 10-51). They may also be used to cover a small wound, such as a puncture. Adhesive strips, such as Band-Aids™, are a combination of a sterile dressing and a bandage.

Bandages

A bandage is applied to keep a dressing in place. Because a dressing separates the wound and the bandage, the bandage does not have to be sterile. Before applying a bandage on an extremity, remove the patient's jewelry and check the pulse distal to the wound. Tape is used to secure most dressings in place. Most of the tape used in first aid and EMS kits is made of silk, paper, or plastic because some patients are allergic to adhesive tape.

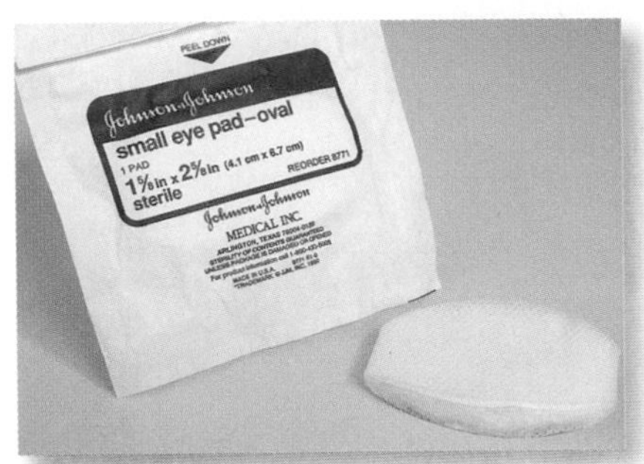

FIGURE 10-51 ▲ Eye pads are used to cover the eyes after a minor eye injury.

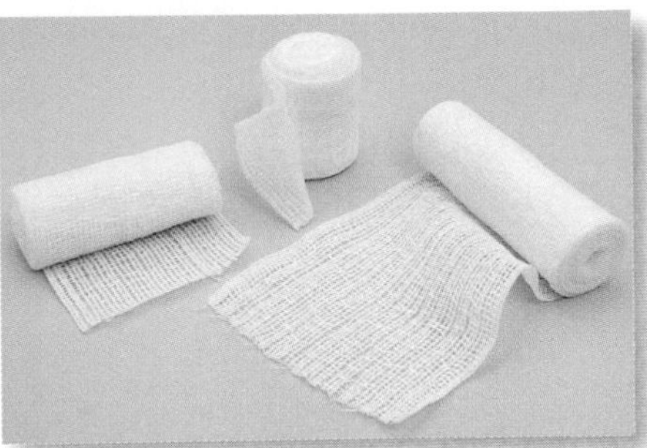

FIGURE 10-52 ▲ Roller gauze.

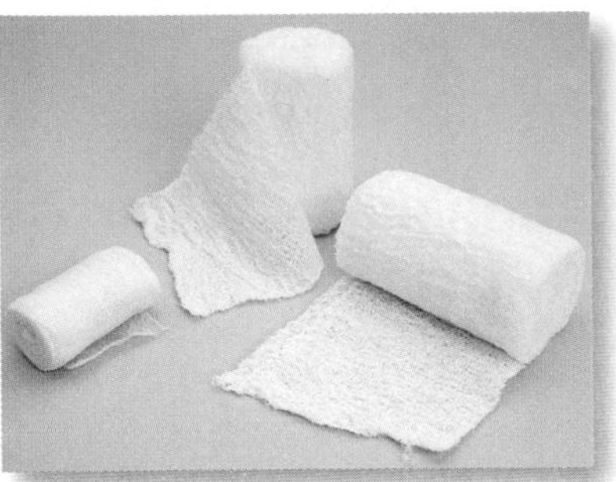

FIGURE 10-53 ▲ Roller bandage.

Types of Bandages

Fingertip and knuckle bandages are adhesive strips that are sterile dressing and bandage combinations. A knuckle bandage is made of cloth shaped like an H. This type of bandage is useful for covering minor cuts or abrasions on a knuckle, an elbow, a heel, or the chin.

Roller gauze (often called by the brand name Kling™) is wrapped around and around a dressing to secure it in place. This type of bandage comes in different widths and lengths (Figure 10-52). Pick a roller bandage width that is appropriate for the body part to be bandaged. A 1-inch roll is used to bandage fingers, and a 2-inch roll is used for wrists, hands, and feet. A 3-inch roll can be used for elbows and upper arms. A 4- to 6-inch roll is used for ankles, knees, and legs.

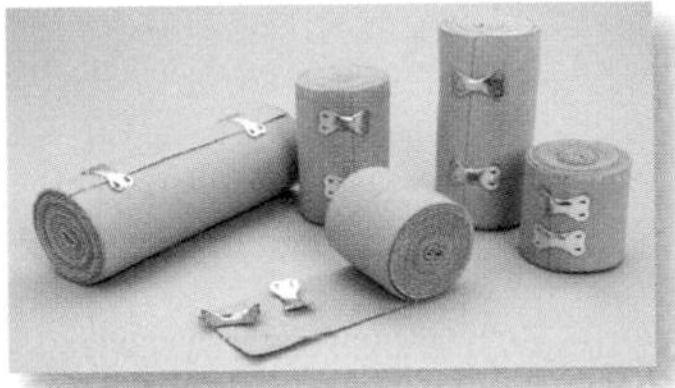

FIGURE 10-54 ▲ Elastic bandage.

A roller bandage (often called by the brand name Kerlix™) is made of soft, slightly elastic material and is available in various widths (Figure 10-53). Elastic bandages (such as an Ace™ bandage or elastic wrap) should not be used to secure a dressing in place (Figure 10-54). If the injured area swells, the elastic bandage may act as a tourniquet. A triangular bandage is a large piece of muslin that can be folded and used as a bandage or sling (Figure 10-55). A triangular bandage that has been folded is called a cravat.

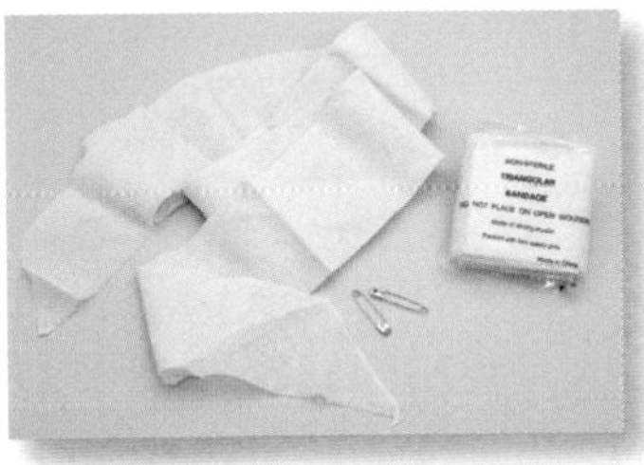

FIGURE 10-55 ▲ Triangular bandage.

Coban™ and Kimberly-Clark® Self-Adherent Wrap are elastic wraps coated with a self-adhering material that functions as tape (Figure 10-56). No pins or clips are required to hold the bandage in place. This type of bandage is often used as a pressure bandage.

A pressure bandage is a bandage with which enough pressure is applied over a wound site to control bleeding. To apply a pressure bandage,

- Cover the wound with several sterile gauze dressings or a bulky dressing.
- Apply direct pressure to the wound until bleeding is controlled.
- Secure the dressing firmly in place with a bandage. Assess the patient's pulse distal to the bandage.
- If possible, do not cover fingers or toes so that you can determine if the bandage is too tight. A bandage may be too tight if the fingers or toes become cold to the touch, the fingers or toes begin to turn pale or blue, or the patient complains of numbness in the extremity.

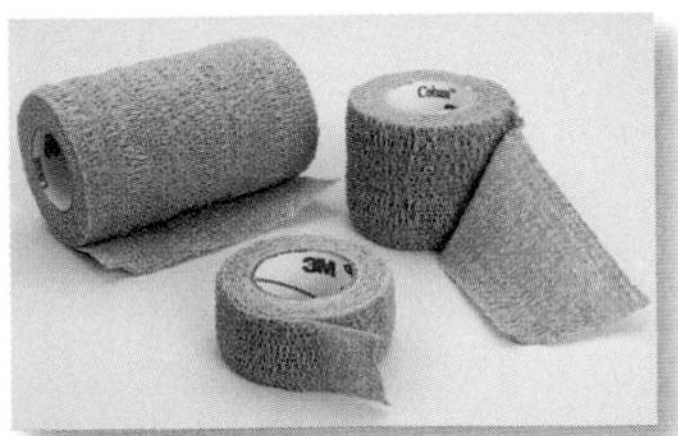

FIGURE 10-56 ▲ Coban™ is a self-adherent elastic wrap.

Skill Drill 10-1 shows the steps used to apply a roller bandage. Figures 10-57 through 10-62 show the bandaging techniques for different soft-tissue injuries.

Skill Drill 10-1

Applying a Roller Bandage

STEP 1 ▶ Start below the wound and work upward, applying the bandage directly over the sterile dressing on the wound.

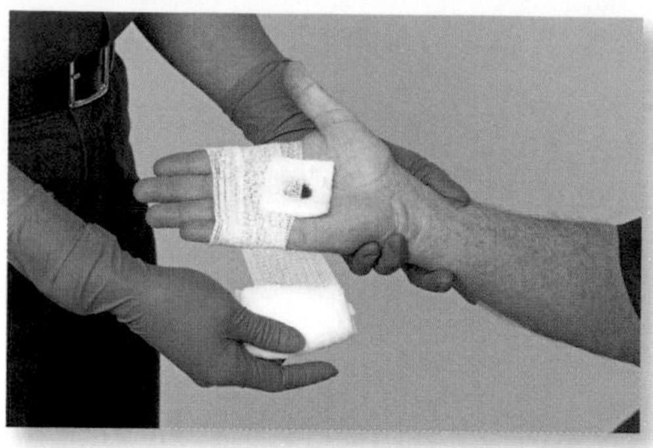

STEP 2 ▶ Using overlapping turns, cover the dressing completely. Unless the fingers are injured, leave them exposed to assess circulation.

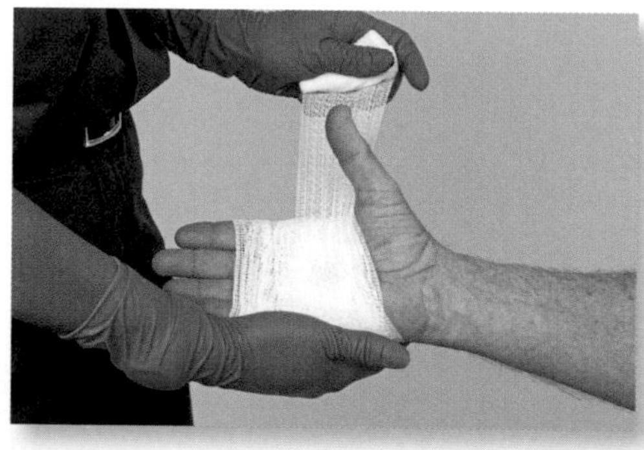

STEP 3 ▶ Tape or tie the bandage in place.

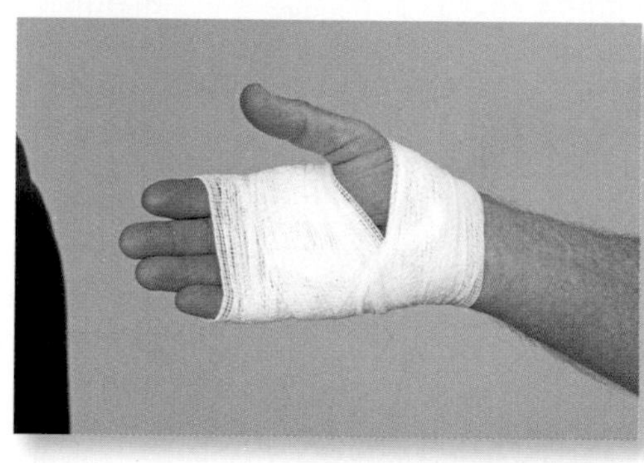

STEP 4 ▶ To make sure the bandage is not too tight, check a pulse distal to the wound site, the color of the fingers, and the temperature of the skin.

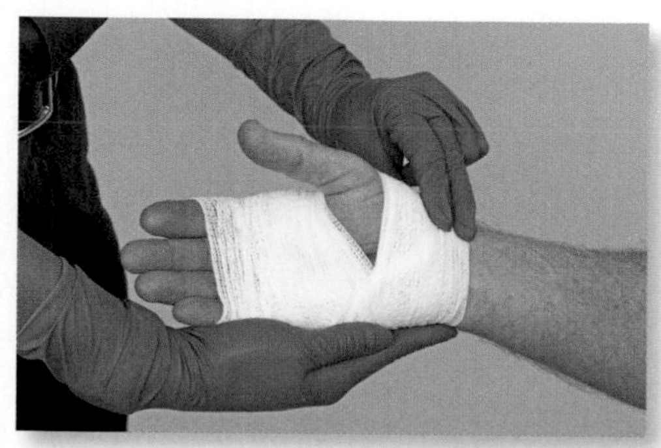

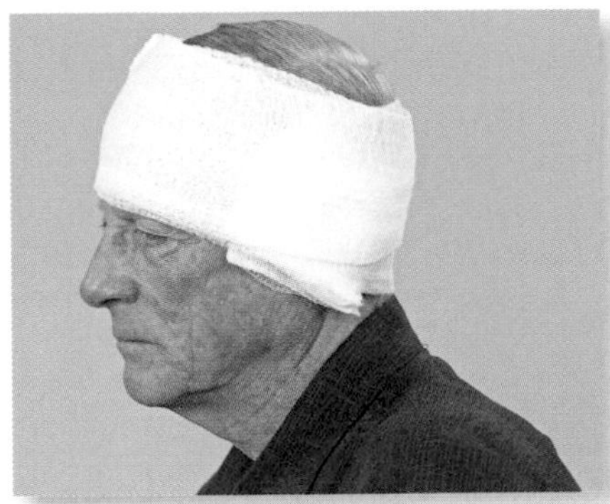

FIGURE 10-57 ▲ Head or ear bandage.

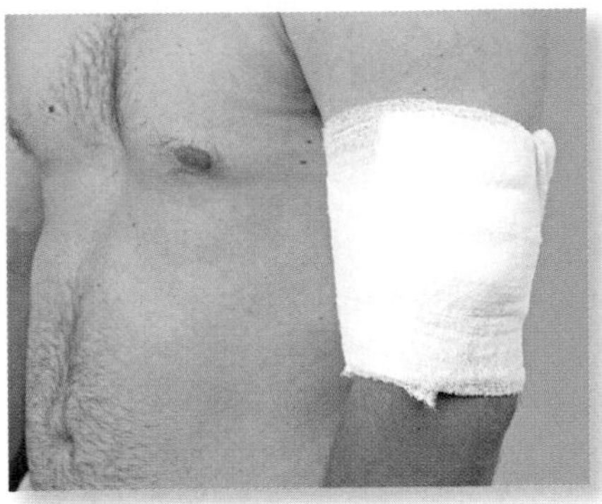

FIGURE 10-58 ▲ Upper arm bandage.

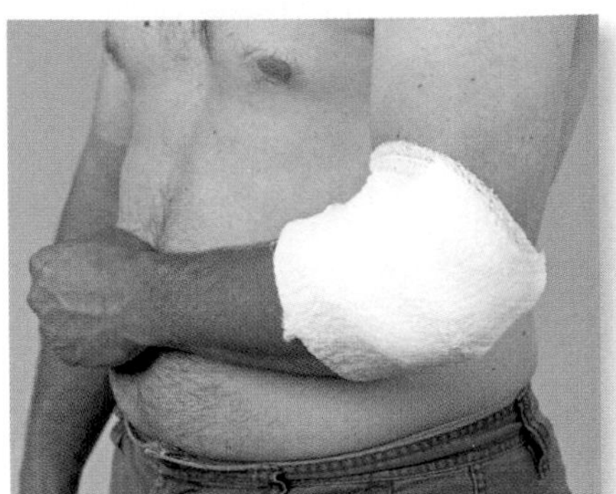

FIGURE 10-59 ▲ Elbow bandage.

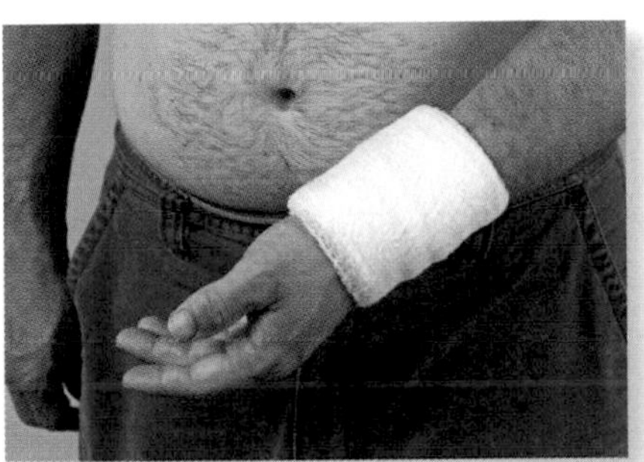

FIGURE 10-60 ▲ Wrist or forearm bandage.

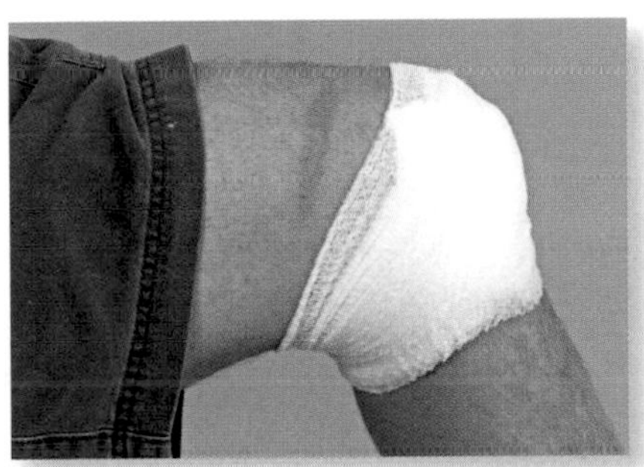

FIGURE 10-61 ▲ Knee bandage.

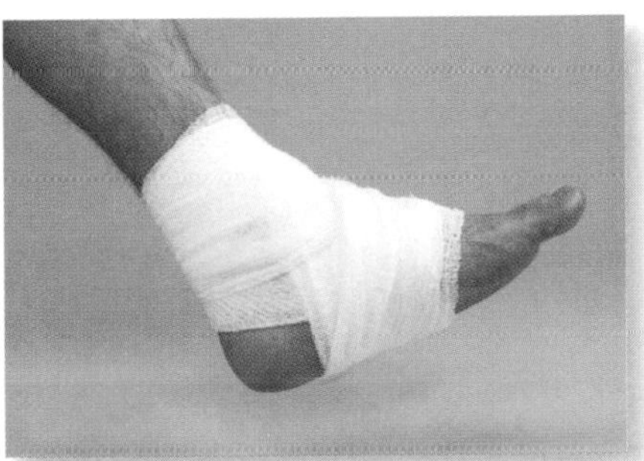

FIGURE 10-62 ▲ Foot or ankle bandage.

On The Scene

Wrap-Up

The helicopter has another 5-minute ETA. You cover the patient with a clean sheet and then a warm blanket. He is responsive to painful stimulus only. His vital signs are BP 104/70 mm Hg, pulse 128/min., respirations 24/min. As you continue your assessment, you can hear some wheezing noises in his lungs. You are worried about his right arm because his fingers are pale and cold and you cannot feel a radial pulse in that arm. As the aircraft lands, the patient's breathing rate increases. He is using neck muscles to breathe and is making a high-pitched noise with each inhalation. The flight crew springs into action. They start an IV, give him some drugs, and place a breathing tube before they move him to the helicopter. As they lift off, your partner shakes his head, commenting, "When will people learn that they can't smoke in bed?" ■

Sum It Up

- *Perfusion* is the circulation of blood through an organ or a part of the body. *Shock* is the inadequate circulation of blood through an organ or a part of the body. Uncontrolled bleeding that leads to depleted blood volume is one cause of shock.
- A *wound* is an injury to soft tissues. A *closed wound* occurs when the soft tissues under the skin are damaged but the surface of the skin is not broken (for example, a bruise). An *open wound* results when the skin surface is broken (for example, a cut or scrape).
- *Hemorrhage* (also called *major bleeding*) is an extreme loss of blood from a blood vessel. It is a life-threatening condition that requires *immediate* attention. If it is not controlled, hemorrhage can lead to shock and potentially to death.
- *Hemophilia* is a disorder in which the blood does not clot normally. A person with hemophilia may have major bleeding from minor injuries and may bleed for no apparent reason. Some medications or a serious injury may also prevent effective clotting.
- *Arterial bleeding* is the most serious type of bleeding. The blood from an artery is bright red, oxygen-rich blood. When an artery bleeds, blood spurts from the wound because the arteries are under high pressure. A bleeding artery can quickly lead to the loss of a large amount of blood. Arterial bleeding can be difficult to control due to high pressure within the artery.
- Bleeding occurs more often from veins than arteries because veins are closer to the skin's surface. *Venous bleeding* is usually easier to control than arterial bleeding because it is under less pressure. Blood lost from a vein flows as a steady stream and is dark red or maroon because it is oxygen-poor blood.
- *Capillary bleeding* is common because the walls of the capillaries are fragile and many are close to the skin's surface. Bleeding from capillaries is usually dark red. When a capillary is torn, blood oozes slowly from the site of the injury because the pressure within the capillaries is low. Capillary bleeding often clots and stops by itself within a few minutes.
- *External bleeding* is bleeding that you can see. The blood flows through an open wound, such as a cut, scrape, or puncture. Clotting normally occurs within minutes. However, external bleeding must be controlled with your gloved hands and dressings until a clot is formed and the bleeding has stopped.
- As an Emergency Medical Responder, you *must* wear personal protective equipment (PPE) when you anticipate exposure to blood or other potentially infectious material. HIV and the hepatitis virus are examples of diseases to which you may be exposed that can be transmitted by exposure to blood. Remember to put on disposable gloves before physical contact with the patient. Eye protection, a mask, and gown should be worn if there is a large amount of blood. PPE should also be worn when the splashing of blood or body fluids into your face or eyes is likely.
- Six methods may be used to control external bleeding:
  1. Applying direct pressure to the wound
     - Applying direct pressure slows blood flow and allows clotting to take place.
  2. Elevating the affected extremity
     - If an arm or a leg is bleeding, elevation may help control the bleeding. If possible, elevate the extremity above the level of the heart while continuing to apply direct pressure. Raising the extremity above the heart reduces pressure at the wound site by reducing blood flow to it. This action allows blood to pool and clot. Do not elevate the extremity if pain, swelling, or deformity is present.

3. Applying pressure to an arterial pressure point
   - If bleeding continues from an arm or a leg, pressure points (also called pulse points) may be used to slow severe bleeding.
4. Applying a splint to immobilize the extremity
   - A *splint* is a device used to limit the movement of an injured arm or leg and reduce bleeding. After applying the splint, make sure to check the patient's fingers (or toes) often for color, warmth, and feeling.
5. Applying a pressure splint (air splint)
   - A *pressure splint* (also called an *air* or *pneumatic splint*) can help control bleeding from soft-tissue injuries or broken bones. It can also help stabilize a broken bone. An air splint acts as a pressure bandage, applying even pressure to the entire arm or leg. After applying any splint, be sure to check the patient's fingers (or toes) often for color, warmth, and feeling.
   - The *pneumatic antishock garment (PASG)* is used in some EMS systems. (This garment is also called the *Military Antishock Trousers [MAST]*.) This device can be used as an effective pressure splint to help control severe bleeding from the legs or pelvis.
6. Applying a tourniquet (*only* as a last resort)
   - A *tourniquet* is a tight bandage that surrounds an arm or a leg. It is used to stop the flow of blood in an extremity. A tourniquet is rarely needed to control bleeding. It should be used *only* as a last resort to control life-threatening bleeding in an arm or a leg when you absolutely cannot control the bleeding in any other way. A tourniquet can cause permanent damage to nerves, muscles, and blood vessels, resulting in the loss of the affected extremity.

▶ *Internal bleeding* is bleeding that occurs inside body tissues and cavities. A *bruise* is a collection of blood under the skin due to bleeding capillaries. A bruise is an example of internal bleeding that is not life-threatening.

- Internal bleeding is difficult to assess because you cannot see it. You should suspect it based on the mechanism of injury or the nature of the illness as well as your patient's signs and symptoms. Suspect internal bleeding when the mechanism of injury suggests that the patient's body has been affected by severe force. Examples include penetrating trauma and blunt trauma, such as falls, motorcycle crashes, pedestrian impacts, automobile collisions, and blast injuries.

▶ *Shock* is the inadequate flow of blood through an organ or a part of the body. Shock can be caused by failure of the body's pump (heart), fluid (blood), or container (blood vessels).

- *Cardiogenic shock* can result if the heart beats too quickly or too slowly or if the heart muscle does not have enough force to pump blood effectively to all parts of the body. This type of shock can occur as a result of a heart attack, a heart rhythm that is too fast or too slow, an injury to the heart, or other conditions that affect the heart's ability to pump.
- Shock can result if there is not enough blood for the heart to pump through the cardiovascular system. Shock caused by severe bleeding is called *hemorrhagic shock*. The bleeding may be internal, external, or both.
- Blood is not the only type of fluid that can be lost from the body. For example, you can lose body fluid because of vomiting or diarrhea. You can lose plasma due to a burn. You can also lose fluid due to excessive sweating or urination. Shock caused by a loss of blood, plasma, or another body fluid is called *hypovolemic shock*.

▶ *Early shock* is often difficult to recognize. Remember to look for it and to consider the patient's mechanism of injury or the nature of the illness when assessing your patient. The sooner shock is recognized and appropriate treatment is begun, the better your patient's chance for survival. Early shock is usually reversible if it is recognized and the patient receives emergency care to correct the cause of the shock.

- *Late (decompensated) shock* results when the patient's systolic blood pressure drops to less than 90 mm Hg. In this phase of shock, the body's defense mechanisms lose their ability to make up for the lack of oxygenated blood. A patient in late shock looks very sick. The signs of late shock are more obvious than those of early shock, but late shock is more difficult to treat. It is still reversible if the cause of the problem is quickly corrected.
- *Irreversible shock* is also called *terminal shock.* You will feel an irregular pulse as the patient's heart becomes irritable and begins to beat irregularly. As shock continues, the patient's heart rhythm becomes more chaotic and can no longer effectively pump blood. Permanent damage occurs to the vital organs because the cells and organs have been without oxygenated blood for too long. Eventually, the heart stops, breathing stops, and death results.
- An *evisceration* occurs when an organ sticks out through an open wound. In providing care, do not touch or try to place the exposed organ back into the body. Carefully remove clothing from around the wound. Lightly cover the exposed organs and wound with a thick, moist dressing. Secure the dressing in place with a large bandage to keep moisture in and prevent heat loss.
- An *impaled object* is an object that remains embedded in an open wound. Do not remove an impaled object unless it interferes with CPR or is impaled through the cheek and interferes with care of the patient's airway. Control bleeding and stabilize the object with bulky dressings, bandaging them in place. Assess the patient for signs of shock and treat if present.
- In the case of an amputated body part, control bleeding at the stump. In most cases, direct pressure will be enough to control the bleeding. Ask an assistant to find the amputated part as it may be able to be reattached at the hospital. Put the amputated part in a dry plastic bag or waterproof container. Seal the bag or container and place it in water that contains a few ice cubes.
- There are three categories of burns:
  - A *superficial (first-degree) burn* affects only the epidermis. It results in only minor tissue damage (such as sunburn). The skin is red, tender, and very painful. This type of burn does not usually require medical care and heals in 2–5 days with no scarring.
  - A *partial-thickness (second-degree) burn* involves the epidermis and dermis. The hair follicles and sweat glands are spared in this degree of burn. A partial-thickness burn produces intense pain and some swelling. Blistering may be present. The skin appears pink, red, or mottled and is sensitive to air current and pressure. This type of burn usually heals within 5–35 days. Scarring may or may not occur, depending on the depth of the burn.
  - A *full-thickness (third-degree) burn* destroys both the epidermis and dermis and may include subcutaneous tissue, muscle, and bone. The color of the patient's skin varies from yellow or pale to black. The skin has a dry, waxy, or leathery appearance. Because the skin is so severely damaged in this type of burn, it cannot perform its usual protective functions. Rapid fluid loss often occurs. Be ready to treat the patient for shock.
- The rule of nines is a guide used to estimate the affected body surface area. The rule of nines divides the adult body into sections that are 9% or are multiples of 9%. This guideline has been modified for children and infants. To estimate the extent of a burn using the rule of nines, add the percentages of the areas burned.

- ▶ A *dressing* is an absorbent material placed directly over a wound. A *bandage* is used to secure a dressing in place. A *pressure bandage* is a bandage applied with enough pressure over a wound site to control bleeding. Dressings and bandages serve the following functions:
  - Help stop bleeding
  - Absorb blood and other drainage from the wound
  - Protect the wound from further injury
  - Reduce contamination and the risk of infection

▶ Tracking Your Progress

After reading this chapter, can you	Page Reference	Objective Met?
• Differentiate between arterial, venous, and capillary bleeding?	333–334	☐
• State the emergency medical care for external bleeding?	335–336	☐
• Establish the relationship between body substance isolation precautions and bleeding?	335	☐
• List the signs of internal bleeding?	342	☐
• List the steps in the emergency medical care of the patient with signs and symptoms of internal bleeding?	342–343	☐
• Establish the relationship between body substance isolation precautions and soft-tissue injuries?	349	☐
• State the types of open soft-tissue injuries?	350–353	☐
• Describe the emergency medical care of the patient with a soft-tissue injury?	354–361	☐
• Discuss the emergency medical care considerations for a patient with a penetrating chest injury?	355	☐
• State the emergency medical care considerations for a patient with an open wound to the abdomen?	355	☐
• Describe the emergency medical care for an impaled object?	355–356	☐
• State the emergency medical care for an amputation?	356	☐
• Describe the emergency medical care for burns?	361–364	☐
• List the functions of dressing and bandaging?	371	☐
• Explain the rationale for body substance isolation precautions when dealing with bleeding and soft-tissue injuries?	335	☐
• Attend to the feelings of the patient with a soft-tissue injury or bleeding?	335	☐
• Demonstrate a caring attitude toward patients with a soft-tissue injury or bleeding who request Emergency Medical Services?	335	☐
• Place the interests of the patient with a soft-tissue injury or bleeding as the foremost consideration when making any and all patient care decisions?	370	☐
• Communicate with empathy to patients with a soft-tissue injury or bleeding, as well as with family members and friends of the patient?	371	☐

Chapter Quiz

Multiple Choice

In the space provided, identify the letter of the choice that best completes each statement or answers each question.

_____ **1.** An average adult man has a normal blood volume of about

a. 3 to 4 liters. **b.** 4 to 5 liters. **c.** 5 to 6 liters. **d.** 6 to 7 liters.

_____ **2.** A 23-year-old man has been stabbed multiple times in his chest and abdomen. As you approach him and form your general impression, you see he is having difficulty breathing. There is a large pool of blood around him and his shirt is soaked with blood. In this situation, you should first

a. cover all wounds with a dressing.
b. assess and manage the patient's airway and breathing.
c. apply direct pressure to the most severe wounds.
d. assess for signs of internal bleeding.

_____ **3.** The head and neck of an infant is equal to about _____ of his or her total body surface area.

a. 9% **b.** 18% **c.** 27% **d.** 36%

_____ **4.** A 22-year-old woman has attempted suicide by slashing her left wrist. After taking body substance isolation precautions, you find that the immediate life threat that is present is the bright red blood spurting from her left wrist. There is a large amount of blood on the floor around her. You have applied a dressing with direct pressure to the wound and have elevated the extremity, but the wound is still bleeding. You should now

a. apply an air splint.
b. apply a tourniquet.
c. apply pressure at the brachial artery.
d. place the patient on her back with her lower legs elevated 12–18 inches.

True or False

Decide whether each statement is true or false. In the space provided, write T for true or F for false.

_____ **5.** Only partial-thickness and full-thickness burns are included when calculating the extent of a burn using the rule of nines.

_____ **6.** You should stop the burning process by applying cold water to a burn for at least 15 minutes.

_____ **7.** A triangular bandage may be used as a bandage or splint.

_____ **8.** You should use sterile dressings whenever possible.

Matching

Match the key terms in the left column with the definitions in the right column by placing the letter of each correct answer in the space provided.

_____ **9.** Shock
_____ **10.** Contusion
_____ **11.** Hemorrhage
_____ **12.** Perfusion
_____ **13.** Puncture
_____ **14.** Blood volume
_____ **15.** Laceration
_____ **16.** Circumferential wound
_____ **17.** Closed wound
_____ **18.** Rule of nines

a. Excessive loss of blood from a blood vessel
b. Circulation of blood through an organ or a part of the body
c. Bruise
d. Injury that encircles an extremity
e. Inadequate circulation of blood through an organ or a part of the body
f. Guide used to estimate the body surface area burned
g. Total amount of blood circulating within the body
h. Injury in which damage occurs to the soft tissues under the skin but the surface of the skin is not broken
i. Injury that results when the skin is pierced with a sharp, pointed object
j. Cut or tear in the skin of any length, shape, and depth

Short Answer

Answer each question in the space provided.

19. List six methods that may be used to control bleeding.

1. ____________________

2. ____________________

3. ____________________

4. ____________________

5. ____________________

6. ____________________

20. List four signs or symptoms of early shock.

1. ____________________

2. ____________________

3. ____________________

4. ____________________

21. How often should you perform ongoing assessments for a patient in shock?

____

____

____

22. What are the two most common causes of internal bleeding?

____

____

____

23. List four types of open wounds.

1. ____________________

2. ____________________

3. ____________________

4. ____________________

24. A 25-year-old man has been stabbed in the abdomen. Your assessment reveals that abdominal organs are protruding from the wound.

a. What is the name of this type of injury?

____

b. Describe how to care for the injury.

____

____

____

25. What is the most urgent type of injury to the eye?

____

____

____

26. A 33-year-old man has been found unresponsive in an apartment fire. The patient is breathing and has a pulse. List four signs or symptoms that should alert you to possible airway problems in this patient.

1. ______________________________
2. ______________________________
3. ______________________________
4. ______________________________

27. The mother of a 12-year-old boy is anxious because her son's nose will not stop bleeding. She says her son has a history of allergies but is otherwise healthy. The nosebleed started about 15 minutes ago. You find the boy standing in the bathroom of his home, holding a bloody towel to his face. After taking body substance isolation precautions, you perform an initial assessment. No life-threatening injuries are present. How will you care for the patient's nosebleed?

____

____

____

Sentence Completion

In the blanks provided, write the words that best complete each sentence.

28. A(n) ______________ is the most common type of closed wound.

29. A(n) ______________ burn affects only the epidermis and results in only minor tissue damage.

30. An occlusive dressing prevents ______________ from entering a wound.

CHAPTER

11 Injuries to Muscles and Bones

By the end of this chapter, you should be able to

Knowledge Objectives

1. Describe the function of the musculoskeletal system.
2. Differentiate between an open and a closed painful, swollen, deformed extremity.
3. List the emergency medical care for a patient with a painful, swollen, deformed extremity.
4. Relate mechanism of injury to potential injuries of the head and spine.
5. State the signs and symptoms of a potential spine injury.
6. Describe the method of determining if a responsive patient may have a spine injury.
7. List the signs and symptoms of an injury to the head.
8. Describe the emergency medical care for injuries to the head.

Attitude Objectives

9. Explain the rationale for the feeling patients who have need for immobilization of the painful, swollen, deformed extremity.
10. Demonstrate a caring attitude toward patients with a musculoskeletal injury who request Emergency Medical Services.
11. Place the interests of the patient with a musculoskeletal injury as the foremost consideration when making any and all patient care decisions.
12. Communicate with empathy to patients with a musculoskeletal injury, as well as with family members and friends of the patient.

Skill Objectives

13. Demonstrate the emergency medical care of a patient with a painful, swollen, deformed extremity.
14. Demonstrate opening the airway in a patient with suspected spinal cord injury.
15. Demonstrate evaluating a responsive patient with a suspected spinal cord injury.

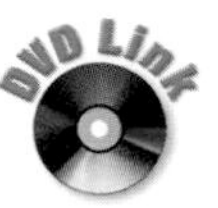

16. Demonstrate stabilizing of the cervical spine.

On The Scene

It must be the tenth time you have glanced at your watch, hoping your relief will arrive when the alarm tones sound. The dispatch speaker crackles, "Respond to 22 St. Louis Lane. Person has fallen." When you get there, your 80-year-old patient is lying in a crumpled heap at the bottom of 10 steps. Her husband says she was carrying a load of laundry, lost her footing, and fell from the top step. She is alert but is moaning. She says she has pain in her arms and leg. Your partner holds in-line immobilization of her head as you continue your exam. Her skin is pink and warm, but she is grimacing and there are beads of sweat on her forehead. Her vital signs are BP 168/100, P 116/min., and R 20/min. When you touch the back of her neck, she says that it hurts. She has no pain or obvious injury in her chest, abdomen, or pelvis. Her left leg has obvious swelling between the knee and hip. The same leg seems to be rotated slightly. Her left upper arm is very tender and swollen between her shoulder and her elbow. Her right wrist is angled strangely and she groans loudly when you touch the area. "We're going do a few things to help your pain, Mrs. Brown," you tell your patient as your partner heads back to your rescue truck for supplies.

THINK ABOUT IT

As you read this chapter, think about the following questions:

- Why did you hold in-line immobilization before you knew that the patient had neck pain?
- What bones are likely to be injured based on the information that you have now?
- How will you splint her injuries?
- What additional assessments should you perform?
- Which injuries could cause the patient to develop shock?

Introduction

Treating Musculoskeletal Injuries

Injuries to the musculoskeletal system are some of the most common traumatic injuries you will encounter. Most of these injuries are not life-threatening but they may be very dramatic. Although an injury may not be life-threatening, it may have a sudden impact on a patient physically as well as emotionally and socially. You must be able to recognize a musculoskeletal injury and provide appropriate emergency care. This care includes preventing further injury, reducing pain, and decreasing the likelihood of permanent damage.

The Musculoskeletal System

Objective 1 ▸

The musculoskeletal system

- Gives the body its shape
- Provides a rigid framework that supports and protects internal organs
- Provides for body movement
- Maintains posture

- Helps stabilize joints
- Produces body heat

The human skeleton provides the support for the body, much like the internal framework of a house. The skeleton provides a frame for other parts of the musculoskeletal system to attach to, including ligaments, tendons, and muscles. All parts of the musculoskeletal system work together to enable movement.

The Skeletal System

The skeletal system

- Gives the body shape, support, and form
- Works with muscles to provide for body movement
- Stores minerals, such as calcium and phosphorus
- Produces red blood cells
- Protects vital internal organs
    - The skull protects the brain.
    - The rib cage protects the heart and lungs.
    - The lower ribs protect most of the liver and spleen.
    - The spinal canal protects the spinal cord.

Maximum bone strength and thickness is reached at about age 30. After age 30, the rate at which old bone is removed slowly begins to exceed the rate at which new bone is formed.

Bones are living, growing tissues that are made up mostly of collagen and calcium. Collagen is a protein that provides a soft framework. Calcium is a mineral that strengthens and hardens the framework. New bone is constantly added to the skeleton and old bone is removed. Bones become large, heavy, and thick during childhood and teenage years because new bone is added faster than old bone is removed.

You Should Know

Osteoporosis is a condition that develops when the rate of old bone removal occurs too quickly or if old bone replacement occurs too slowly. As a result, the bones of a person with osteoporosis become brittle and tend to break easily. Too little calcium over a person's lifetime is thought to play a major role in contributing to the development of osteoporosis.

The axial skeleton is made up of 80 bones. The appendicular skeleton consists of 126 bones.

The skeletal system is divided into the axial and appendicular skeletons (Figure 11-1). The **axial skeleton** includes the skull, spinal column, sternum, and ribs (Table 11-1). The **appendicular skeleton** is made up of the upper and lower extremities (arms and legs), the shoulder girdle, and the pelvic girdle (Table 11-2). The **shoulder girdle** is the bony arch formed by the collarbones (clavicles) and shoulder blades (scapulae). The **pelvic girdle** is made up of bones that enclose and protect the organs of the pelvic cavity. It provides a point of attachment for the lower extremities and the major muscles of the trunk. It also supports the weight of the upper body.

The skull is made up of cranial bones. These bones house and protect the brain, the upper jaw (the maxilla), the lower jaw (the mandible), the facial bones, and the cheekbones (zygomatic bones). The skull is supported by the neck, which receives its strength from the vertebrae.

The vertebral column is made up of 7 cervical (neck) vertebrae; 12 thoracic vertebrae; 5 lumbar vertebrae; 5 fused vertebrae, which form the sacrum; and 3 or 4 fused vertebrae, which form the coccyx (tailbone). The vertebral column gives rigidity to the body while allowing movement. It also encloses the spinal cord. It extends from the base of the skull to the coccyx.

FIGURE 11-1 ▶ The human skeleton is made up of the axial skeleton, which consists of the skull, vertebral column, sternum, and ribs. The appendicular skeleton (blue) is attached and includes the shoulder and pelvic girdles as well as the limb bones.

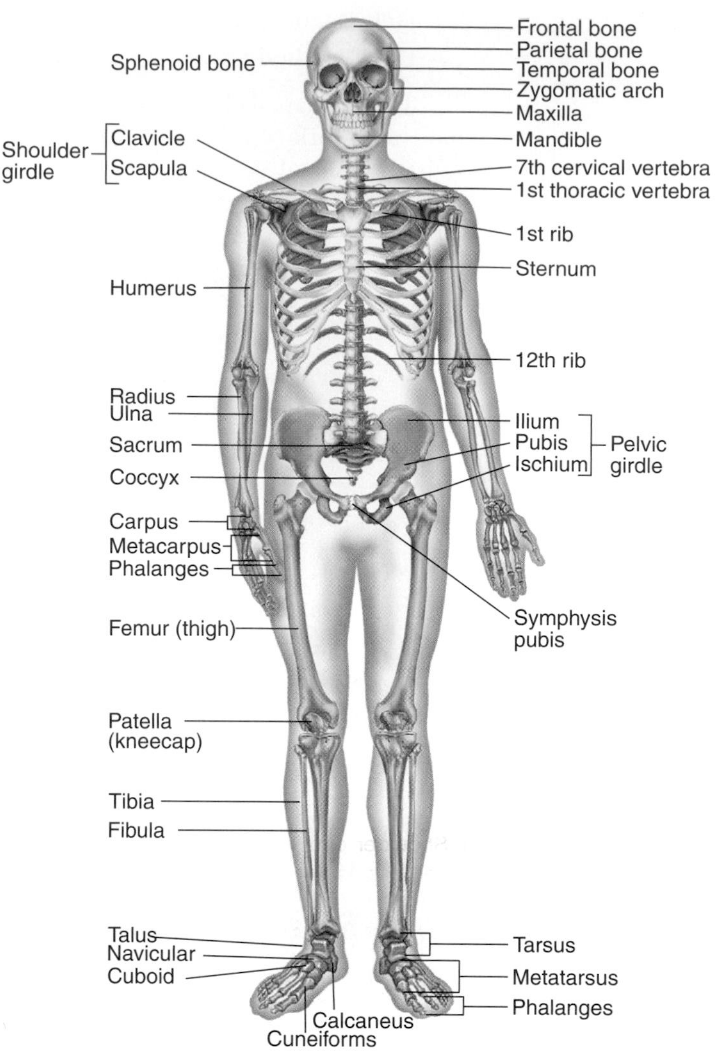

TABLE 11-1 The Axial Skeleton

Bone	Purpose
Skull (cranium)	Houses and protects the brain Serves as a rigid container
Face (eye sockets, cheeks, upper nose, and upper and lower jaw)	Houses and protects the brain and sensory organs (the structures that provide sight, smell, and taste) Provides shape and unique features
Spinal column	Protects the spinal cord Provides a center axis of support
Sternum (breastbone) and ribs	Protect the heart, lungs, and major blood vessels in the chest

The chest (thorax) is made up of the 12 thoracic vertebrae, 12 pairs of ribs, and the breastbone (sternum). These structures form the thoracic cage, which protects the organs within the thoracic cavity (for example, the heart, lungs, and major blood vessels). All of the ribs are attached posteriorly by ligaments to the thoracic vertebrae.

The sternum (breastbone) consists of three sections:

1. The **manubrium** is the uppermost (superior) portion; it connects with the clavicle and the first rib.
2. The body is the middle portion.
3. The **xiphoid process** is a piece of cartilage that makes up the lowermost (inferior) portion.

The uppermost portion of the sternum is attached to the clavicles, which joins the axial skeleton to the appendicular skeleton.

The upper extremities are made up of the bones of the shoulder girdle, the arms, the forearms, and the hands. The **humerus** is the upper arm bone.

TABLE 11-2 The Appendicular Skeleton

Bone	Purpose
Upper Extremities	
Shoulder girdle (collarbone and shoulder blade)	Provide structural support and movement/leverage
Upper arm bone (humerus)	
Forearm bones (radius and ulna)	
Wrist bones (carpals)	
Hand bones (metacarpals)	
Fingers (phalanges)	
Lower Extremities	
Pelvic girdle	Protects the bladder, female reproductive organs, and major blood vessels Provides a point of attachment for the legs and major muscles of the trunk Supports the weight of the upper body
Thigh (femur)	Provides structural support
Kneecap (patella)	Provides joint protection and support
Shin (tibia and fibula)	Provides structural support
Ankle (tarsals)	Provides structural support and movement/leverage
Foot (metatarsals)	Provides structural support and movement/leverage
Toes (phalanges)	Provide structural support and movement/leverage

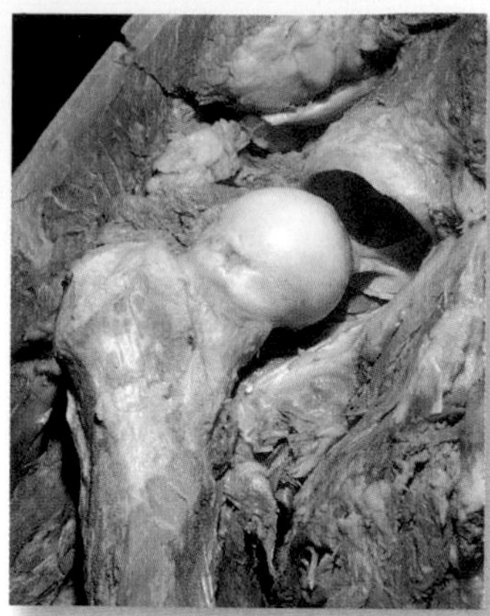

FIGURE 11-2 ▲ The hip joint is an example of a ball-and-socket joint. © The McGraw-Hill Companies, Inc./Rebecca Gray, photographer/Don Kincaid dissections.

Skeletal muscles have a rich supply of blood vessels and nerves. In most cases, an artery and at least one vein accompany each nerve in a skeletal muscle.

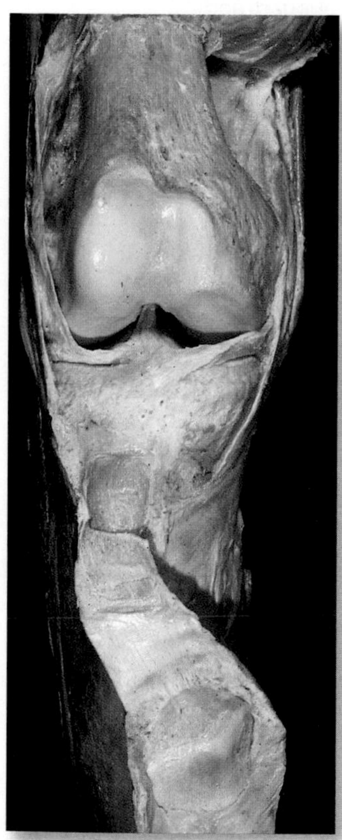

FIGURE 11-3 ▲ The knee joint is an example of a hinge joint. © The McGraw-Hill Companies, Inc./Rebecca Gray, photographer/Don Kincaid dissections.

The biceps and triceps muscles are attached here, allowing the shoulder to rotate, flex, and extend. The forearm contains two bones, the **radius** (lateral/thumb side), and the **ulna** (medial side). The elbow is the joint where the humerus connects with the radius and the ulna. The forearm is connected to the wrist **(carpals),** then to the hand **(metacarpals)** and fingers **(phalanges).**

The lower extremities are made up of the bones of the pelvis, the upper legs, the lower legs, and the feet. The **pelvis** is a bony ring formed by three separate bones that fuse to become one bone in an adult. The lower extremities are attached to the pelvis at the hip joint. The hip joint is formed by the socket of the hip bone and the upper end of the thighbone **(femur).**

The knee is protected anteriorly by the kneecap **(patella),** and it attaches the femur to the two lower leg bones, the **tibia** (shinbone) and **fibula.** The lower leg attaches to the foot by the ankle. The **tarsals** make up the back part of the foot and heel. The **metatarsals** make up the main part of the foot. The toes (phalanges) are the foot's equivalent of the fingers.

The skeletal system includes many joints. A **joint** is a place where two bones come together. Some bone ends are covered with cartilage. Cartilage provides cushioning between bones. Joints are held in place by ligaments. Ball-and-socket joints allow movement in all directions (Figure 11-2). The only ball-and-socket joints in the body are the hip joint (pelvic bone and femur) and shoulder joint (scapula and humerus). A hinge joint allows only flexion and extension. Examples include the elbow (humerus and ulna) and knee (femur and tibia; Figure 11-3).

The Muscular System

The human body has more than 600 muscles (Figure 11-4). Muscles are bundles of tiny fibers that expand and contract. Muscle fibers shorten (contract) when stimulated. They shorten by converting energy obtained from food (chemical energy) into movement (mechanical energy).

Skeletal muscles produce movement of the bones to which they are attached. Skeletal muscles also produce heat, which helps maintain a constant body temperature. They also maintain posture. Skeletal muscle fibers are surrounded by connective tissue. The connective tissue covering supports and protects the delicate fibers. It also provides a pathway through which blood vessels and nerves can pass. A skeletal muscle fiber must receive a signal from a nerve before it can contract. When the signal is received, skeletal muscles produce rapid, forceful contractions.

Most skeletal muscles are attached to bones by means of **tendons.** Tendons create a pull between bones when muscles contract. The tendons of many muscles cross over joints, which contributes to the stability of the joint. Tendons can be damaged from overextension or overuse.

Ligaments connect bone to bone.

A skeletal muscle has three main parts (Figure 11-5):

1. The **origin** is the stationary attachment of the muscle to a bone.
2. The **insertion** is the movable attachment to a bone.
3. The **body** is the main part of the muscle.

Musculoskeletal Injuries

Mechanism of Injury

Injuries to bones and joints can be caused by direct forces, indirect forces, and twisting forces (Figure 11-6). A direct force causes injury at the point of impact, such as being struck in the face by a baseball. Indirect forces cause injury at a site other

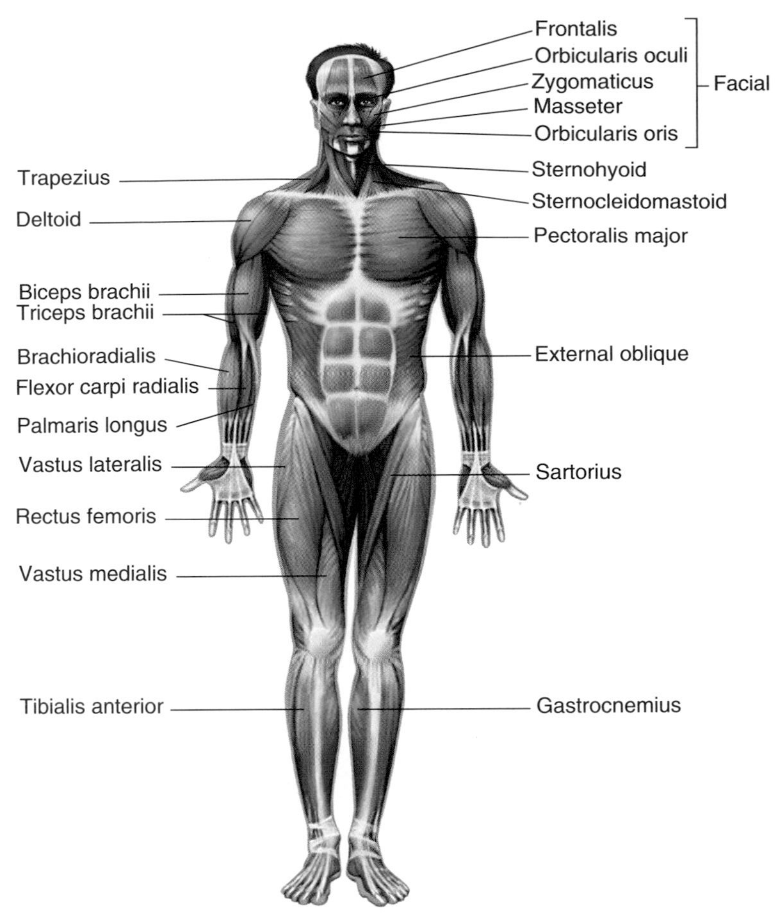

FIGURE 11-4 ▶ The human body has more than 600 skeletal muscles. A few of them are identified here.

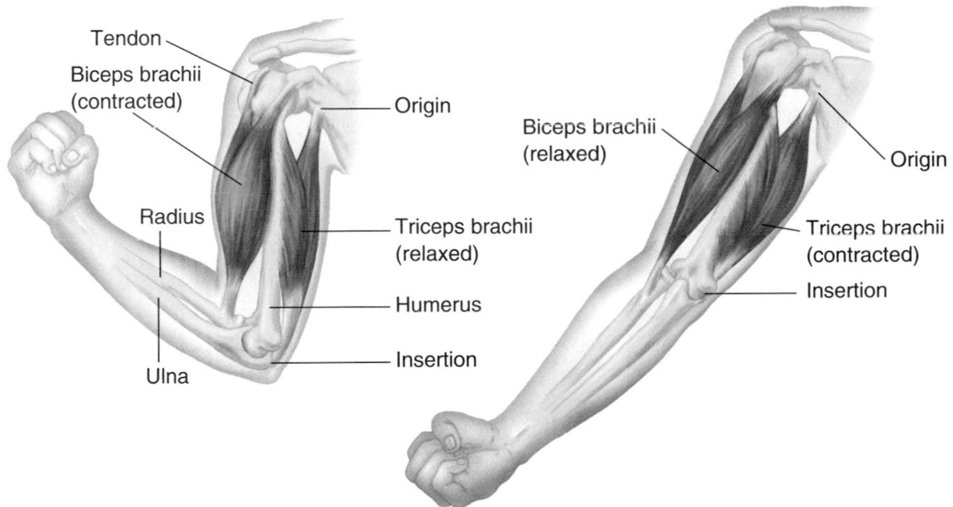

FIGURE 11-5 ▶ The origin of a skeletal muscle is the stationary attachment of the muscle to a bone. The insertion is the movable attachment to a bone. The body is the main part of the muscle.

than the point of impact. For example, if your hand strikes the ground (direct force) during a fall, the energy travels up your arm and may result in an injury near your elbow, shoulder, or clavicle (indirect force). A twisting force causes one part of an extremity to remain in place while the rest twists, such as twisting your ankle while playing basketball. Twisting injuries commonly affect the joints, such as ankles, knees, and wrists. Twisting forces cause ligaments to stretch and tear.

FIGURE 11-6 ► (a) Direct force injury. (b) Indirect force injury. (c) Twisting force injury.

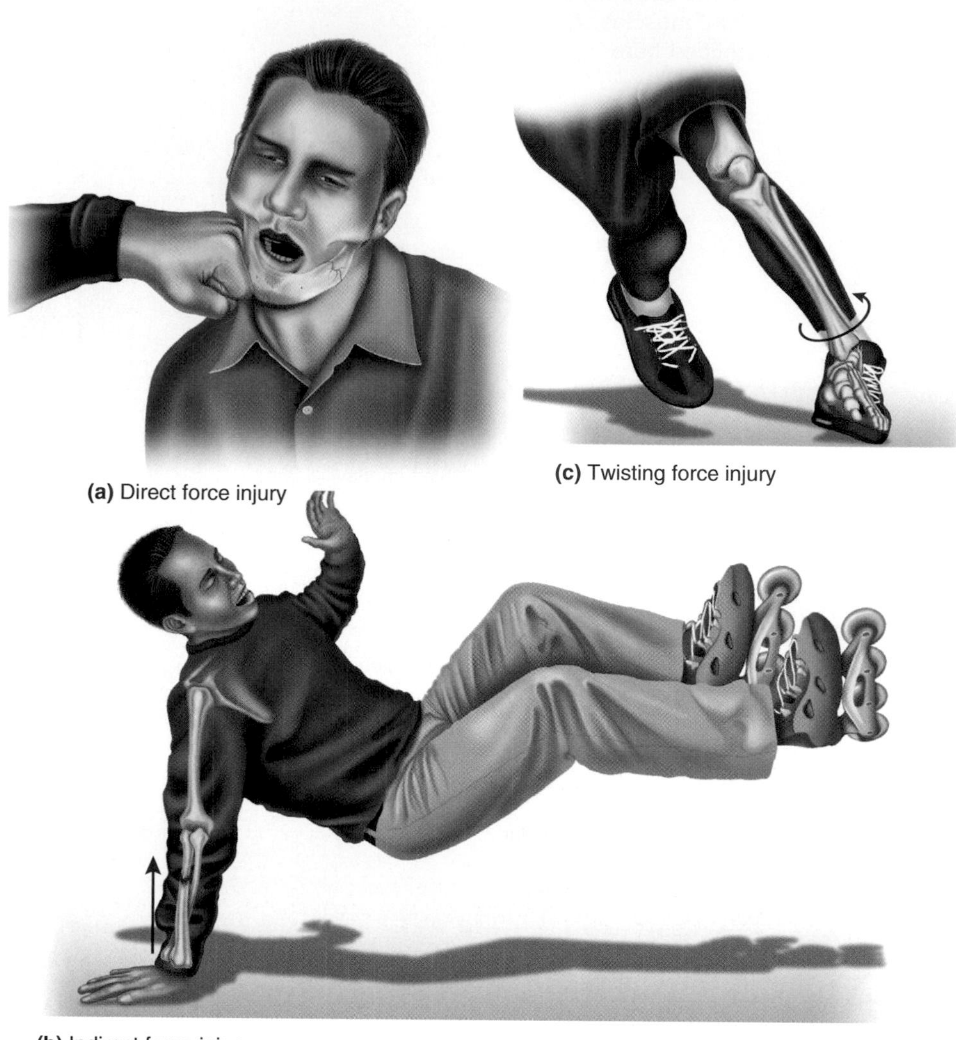

(a) Direct force injury

(c) Twisting force injury

(b) Indirect force injury

Types of Musculoskeletal Injuries

Objective 2 ►

Injuries to bones and joints may be open or closed. In an open injury, the skin surface is broken. The bone may protrude through the wound or may pull back inside the body from muscle contraction. These injuries can result in serious blood loss. An open injury also increases the risk of contamination and infection. In closed bone and joint injuries, the skin surface is not broken. In any case, an open or a closed bone or joint injury is often painful, swollen, and deformed.

Because they are treated in the same way, it is not important for you to know if an injury is a particular type of fracture or if the injury involves a muscle or bone.

A **fracture** is a break in a bone. If a bone is broken, chipped, cracked, or splintered, it is said to be fractured. Figure 11-7 shows some types of fractures. The bones of a child are more flexible than those of an adult and tend to bend more without breaking. This characteristic explains the greenstick fracture that is seen in children. A greenstick fracture occurs when the bone breaks on one side but not the other, like bending a green tree branch. In children and adolescents, an area of growing tissue called the **growth plate** (epiphyseal plate) can be found near each end of a long bone (Figure 11-8). During adolescence, the growth plates are replaced by solid bone when growth is complete. In a child, the growth plate is the weakest part of the skeleton. The growth plate is even weaker than the surrounding ligaments and tendons. An injury to the growth

FIGURE 11-7 ▶ Some types of fractures.

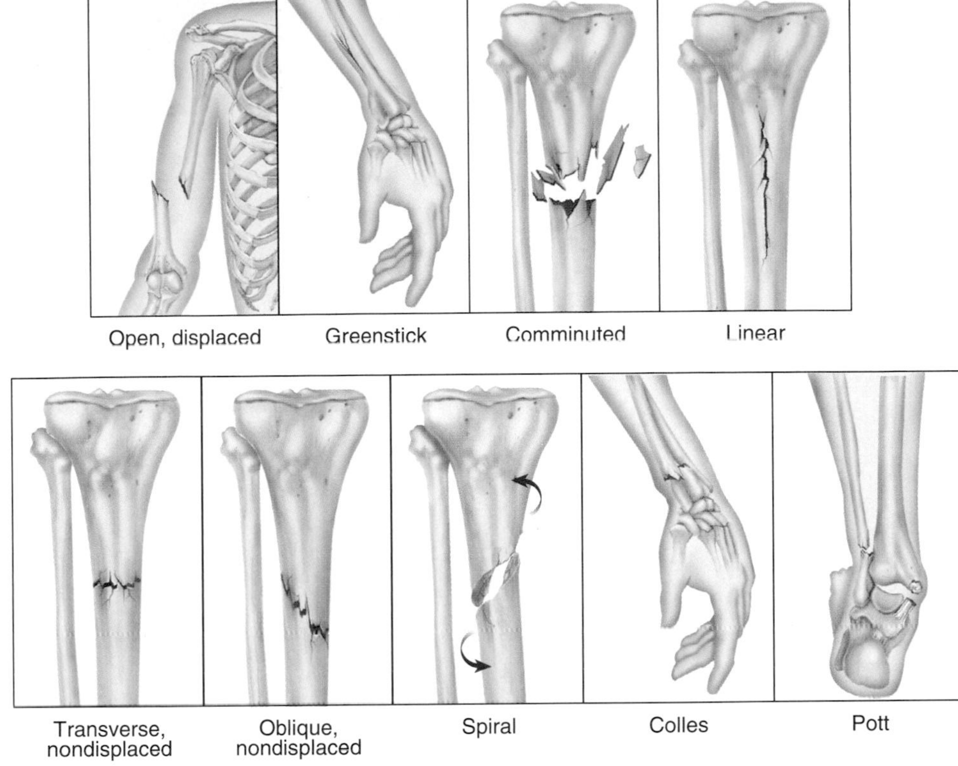

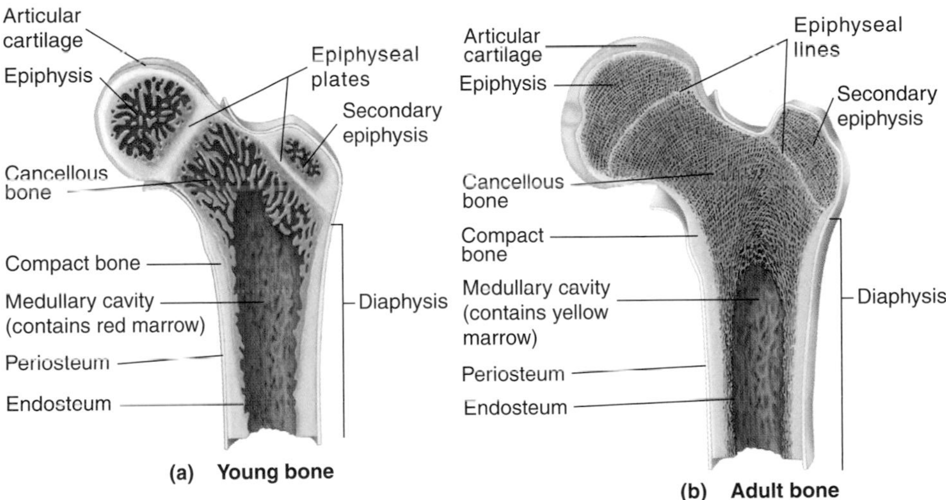

FIGURE 11-8 ▶ (a) The femur (thigh bone) of a child showing the growth plate (epiphyseal plate). (b) Adult long bone.

plate is a fracture. Most growth plate injuries are caused by falls. Growth of the bone can be affected if a fracture in or around the growth plate causes the blood supply to it to be cut off. The healing of this type of injury is watched closely by the child's doctor.

An open fracture may result from bone ends or fragments tearing out through the skin (Figure 11-9). It may also be caused by a penetrating injury that has damaged a bone and the surrounding soft tissues, such as a gunshot wound. Although closed fractures have no opening through the skin, these injuries can result in serious internal bleeding. For example, a broken femur (thighbone) can result in the loss of up to 1 liter of blood. If the fracture is closed, the blood will have no place to go except to the surrounding tissue. As bleeding continues, the blood vessels and

FIGURE 11-9 ▶ An open femur fracture.
Trauma.org Image

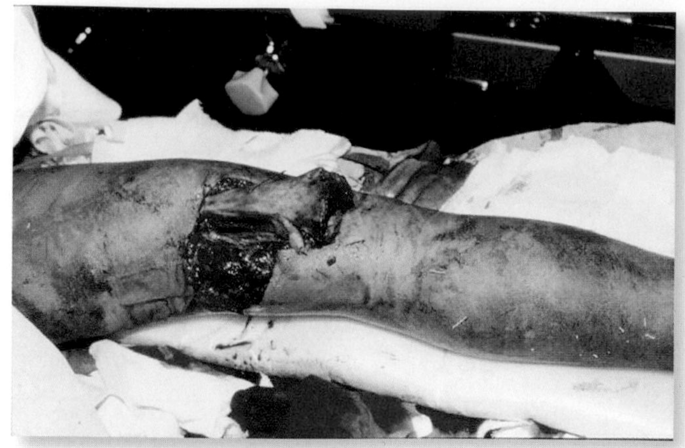

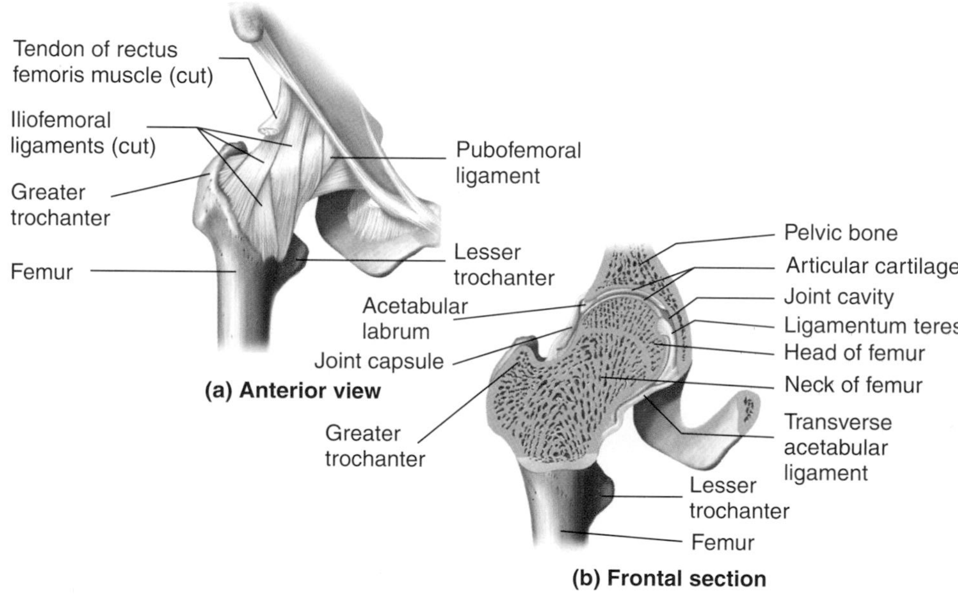

FIGURE 11-10 ▶ Dislocation of the right hip joint. (a) Anterior view. (b) Frontal section.

tissues of the thigh become compressed, reducing blood flow throughout the leg. Whether a fracture is open or closed, the movement of sharp bone ends can cause damage to arteries, muscles, and nerves. A suspected fracture should be immobilized to prevent further injury and pain.

A **dislocation** occurs when the ends of bones are forced from their normal positions in a joint (Figure 11-10). A partial dislocation **(subluxation)** means the bone is partially out of the joint. A complete dislocation means it is all the way out. Dislocations and subluxations usually result in temporary deformity of the joint and may result in sudden and severe pain. The surrounding muscles often spasm from the disruption, which worsens the pain. The pain stops almost immediately once the bone is back in place.

Severe damage to nerves and blood vessels can occur if a joint is not put back into place properly.

Dislocations most often occur in major joints, such as the shoulder, hip, knee, elbow, or ankle (Figure 11-11). They can occur in smaller joints, such as the finger, thumb, or toe. Dislocations are usually caused by trauma, such as a fall. They can also be caused by an underlying disease, such as rheumatoid arthritis.

Dislocations and subluxations are dangerous because the change of position of the bone or bones involved can compress or damage the joint and its surrounding muscles, ligaments, nerves, or blood vessels. For this reason, you should not try to reduce (put back into place) a dislocation. A dislocation or subluxation may go back into place by itself. Be sure to let arriving EMS personnel know if this occurs.

A **sprain** is a stretching or tearing of a ligament, the connective tissue that joins the end of one bone with another (Figure 11-12). Sprains are classified as mild,

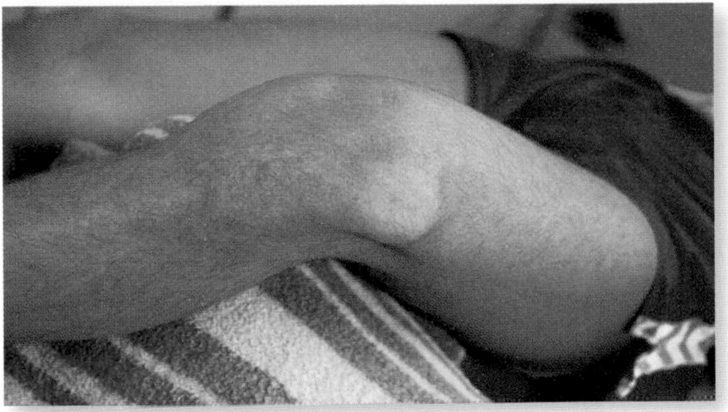

FIGURE 11-11 ▲ Knee dislocation. Trauma.org Image

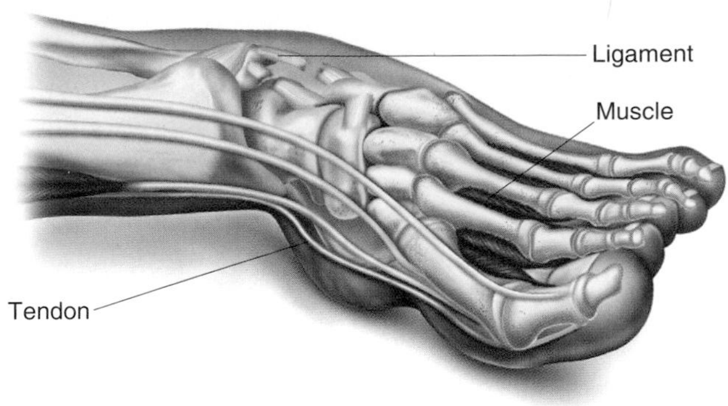

FIGURE 11-12 ▲ A sprain is a stretching or tearing of a ligament. Pain and bruising are usually present with all types of sprains.

FIGURE 11-13 ► A strain is a twist, pull, or tear of a muscle or tendon.

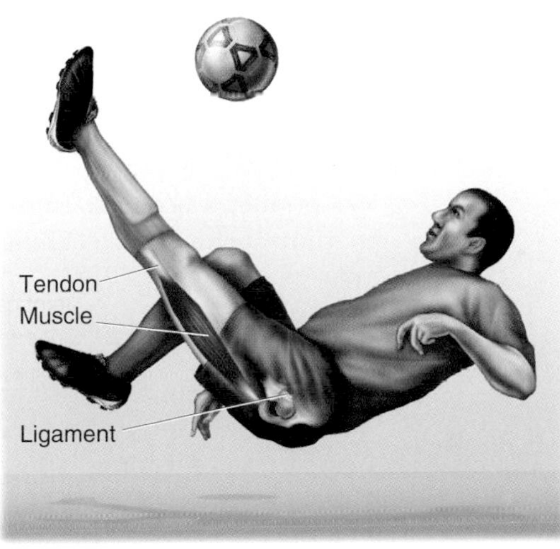

Remember: Ligaments "sprain"; muscles "strain."

moderate, or severe. Pain and bruising are usually present with all categories of sprains. When a sprain occurs, the patient usually feels a tear or pop in the joint. A severe sprain produces excruciating pain at the moment of injury as the ligaments tear completely or separate from the bone. Tearing or separation loosens the joint and makes it nonfunctional. A moderate sprain partially tears the ligament, loosens the joint, and produces some swelling. A ligament is stretched in a mild sprain, but there is no joint loosening.

Muscle injuries are more common than bone injuries.

A **strain** is a twisting, pulling, or tearing of a muscle or tendon (Figure 11-13). A muscle strain usually occurs when a muscle is stretched beyond its limit. A strain often occurs near the point where the muscle joins the tough connective tissue of the tendon. For example, muscles of the lower back may be strained when improper lifting or moving techniques are used. The signs and symptoms of a strain include pain with movement, little or no swelling, and a limited ability to bear weight on the affected extremity. The area around the injury may be tender to the touch. Bruising may be present if blood vessels are broken.

Signs and Symptoms of Musculoskeletal Injuries

The signs and symptoms of musculoskeletal injuries vary depending on the severity and type of injury. The three most common signs and symptoms of a musculoskeletal injury are pain, deformity, and swelling.

You Should Know

Signs and Symptoms of Musculoskeletal Injuries

- Pain or tenderness over the injury site
- Swelling
- Deformity, angulation (the abnormal position of an extremity)
- Crepitation (a grating sensation or sound)
- Limited movement
- Joint locked into position
- Exposed bone ends
- Bruising
- Bleeding
- One extremity appearing to be a different length, shape, or size than the other
- Loss of pulse or sensation below the injury site

Emergency Medical Responder Care of Musculoskeletal Injuries

Objective 3 ▶

To treat a patient with musculoskeletal injuries, use the following steps:

1. Conduct a scene size-up and ensure your safety. Assess the mechanism of injury before approaching the patient. Put on appropriate personal protective equipment (PPE).
2. Form a general impression and determine the urgency of further assessment and care.
3. Perform an initial assessment to identify and treat any life-threatening conditions. Stabilize the cervical spine if needed. If signs of shock are present or if internal bleeding is suspected, treat for shock.
4. Perform a physical examination. *DOTS* is a useful tool to remember what to look and feel for. *DOTS* stands for

   - *D*eformities
   - *O*pen injuries
   - *T*enderness
   - *S*welling

   Look for deformities, open injuries, and swelling. Feel along the length of the extremity for deformities, tenderness, and swelling. Feel and listen for **crepitus,** which is the grating of broken bone ends against each other. Check the *p*ulse, *m*ovement, and *s*ensation (PMS) in each extremity. Compare each extremity to the opposite extremity.

   - Assess the dorsalis pedis pulse (on top of the foot) in each lower extremity. Assess the radial pulse in each upper extremity.
   - If the patient is awake, assess movement of the lower extremities by asking if he can push his feet into your hands. Assess movement of the upper extremities by asking the patient to squeeze your fingers. Compare the strength of his grips and note if they are equal or if one side appears weaker.
   - If the patient is awake, assess sensation by touching the fingers and toes of each extremity and asking him to tell you where you are touching. Assess the patient's thumb or pinky (or great toe or baby toe) to avoid the confusion of having to describe which "middle" digit is being touched. If the patient is unresponsive, assess movement and sensation by pinching each foot and hand. See if the patient responds to pain with facial movements or movement of the extremity.

If you are not sure if a musculoskeletal injury is present, manually stabilize the injured area and then apply a splint. If no life-threatening conditions are present, splint an injured extremity before moving the patient.

Ice reduces blood flow into the affected area, which in turn reduces swelling. Do not apply ice or a cold pack directly to the skin.

5. Take the patient's vital signs and gather the patient's medical history.
6. Cover open wounds with a sterile dressing. If bone ends are visible, do not intentionally reposition or replace them.
7. Splint any bone or joint injuries. This technique is explained in detail in the "Splinting" section.
   - Before applying a splint, manually stabilize the injured extremity. This will require another person, who will use her hands to gently support the extremity. To stabilize an injured bone, support the joints above and below it. For example, if a bone in the lower leg is broken, your assistant should use her hands to stabilize both the ankle and the knee. When a splint is applied, the splint must be long enough to stabilize both of these joints. To stabilize an injured joint, support the bones above and below it. Additional support may be needed underneath the injured area so that it does not sag. Do not release manual stabilization until the injured area has been properly immobilized.
   - Pad a rigid or semi-rigid splint before applying it. Padding helps lessen patient discomfort due to pressure, especially around bony areas. After the extremity is splinted, apply an ice bag or a cold pack. Place a cloth or bandage between the patient's skin and the cold source.
8. Most sprains and strains can be treated with the RICE technique. RICE stands for *R*est, *I*ce, *C*ompression, and *E*levation.
   - *R*est. Using a body part increases blood flow to that area and can increase swelling. Tell the patient to avoid using the injured area while it heals. The length of rest is determined by how severe the injury is.
   - *I*ce. Use a cold pack or place ice in a plastic bag and remove the excess air. Wrap the cold source in a cloth. Apply the ice to the injured area for 20 minutes and then remove it for 40 minutes. Follow this rotation hourly.
   - *C*ompression. Apply an elastic bandage to the injured area. Compression reduces swelling and supports the injured area. It also allows for minor weight bearing and limited function. Use a 2-inch bandage for an injury to the wrist or hand. A 3-inch bandage should be used for the elbow and arm. Use a 4- or 6-inch bandage for an injury to the ankle, knee, or leg. When applying a compression bandage, begin wrapping the bandage below the injury (from the point farthest from the heart; Figure 11-14).

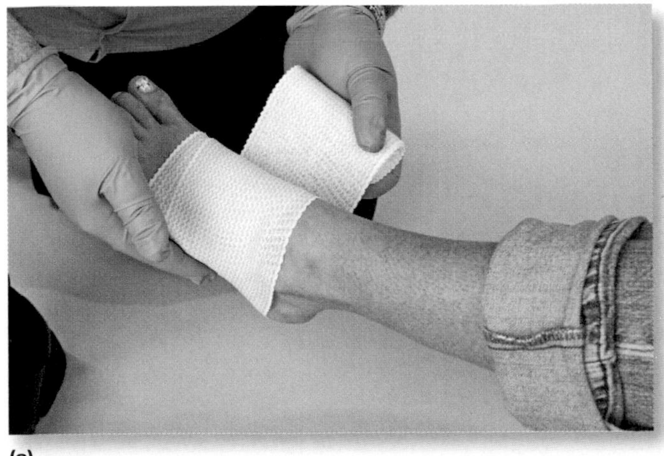
(a)

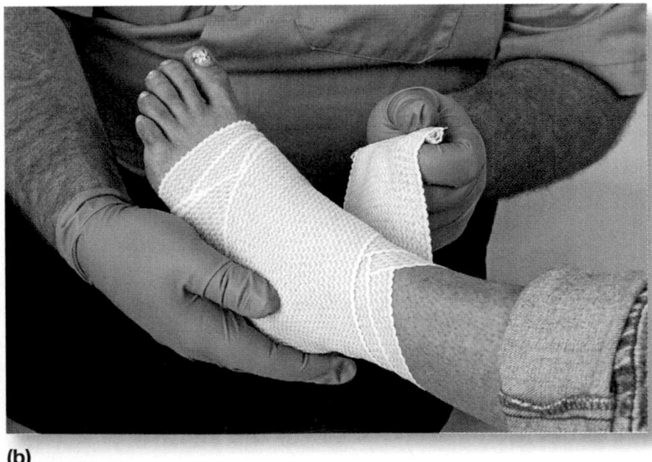
(b)

FIGURE 11-14 ▲ (a) When applying a compression bandage, begin wrapping below the injured area. (b) Wrap the injured area moving toward the heart. Each wrap should overlap about one half the bandage's width.

Wrap the injured area in an upward direction (toward the heart), overlapping about one half of the bandage's width. Make sure that the bandage is not wrapped too tightly. It must be tight enough to provide support but loose enough to allow circulation to the area. Assess pulses, movement, and sensation after applying the bandage. Be sure to document your findings.

- *E*levation. To reduce swelling, keep the injured extremity higher than the patient's heart. This also helps remove waste products from the injured area.

Objective 10 ▶

Objective 12 ▶

9. Comfort, calm, and reassure the patient, family members, and friends of the patient while waiting for EMS personnel. Perform ongoing assessments every 5 minutes if the patient is in shock and every 15 minutes if the patient is stable.

Remember This!

- ***D***eformities
- ***O***pen injuries
- ***T***enderness
- ***S***welling
- ***R***est
- ***I***ce
- ***C***ompression
- ***E***levation
- ***P***ulse
- ***M***ovement
- ***S***ensation

Stop and Think!

- *Always* assess pulses, movement, and sensation in an extremity before and after care of the injury. Compare your findings with the opposite extremity. Be sure to document your findings.
- Make sure to remove any jewelry or tight clothing distal to an extremity injury. Doing so will allow for easy removal without cutting. It will also prevent injury from tissue compression once swelling increases.

Splinting

A **splint** is a device used to limit the movement of (immobilize) an injured arm or leg to reduce pain and further injury. In some situations, the patient will have already splinted the injury by holding the injured part close to his body in a comfortable position. For example, you may find a patient with an injured wrist holding his arm close to his chest. With this type of injury, the patient will usually support the injured arm with his uninjured arm. When the body is used as a splint, it is called a **self-splint** or an **anatomic splint.**

Many types of ready-made splints are available. If a ready-made splint is not available, a splint can be made. Materials commonly used include rolled-up magazines, branches, newspapers, umbrellas, boards, canes, cardboard, broom handles, wooden spoons, and foam sleeping pads. An injured body part is usually secured to a splint with bandages or straps. If these materials are not available, you can substitute for them with bandannas, climbing webbing, or torn pieces of clothing.

You Should Know

Reasons for Splinting

Splinting limits the motion of bone fragments, bone ends, or dislocated joints.

- Lessen the damage to muscles, nerves, or blood vessels caused by broken bones
- Help prevent a closed injury from becoming an open injury
- Lessen the restriction of blood flow caused by bone ends or dislocations compressing blood vessels
- Reduce bleeding due to tissue damage caused by bone ends
- Reduce pain associated with the movement of the bone and the joint
- Reduce the risk of paralysis due to a damaged spine

Remember This!

Hazards of Improper Splinting

- Compressing nerves, tissues, and blood vessels from the splint
- Delaying transport of a patient with a life-threatening injury
- Reducing distal circulation due to the splint's being applied too tightly to the extremity
- Aggravating the musculoskeletal injury
- Causing or aggravating tissue, nerve, vessel, or muscle damage from excessive bone or joint movement

General Rules of Splinting

In most situations, a patient should not be moved before splinting unless he or she is in danger.

Follow these general guidelines when splinting a musculoskeletal injury:

- Take BSI precautions and wear appropriate PPE.
- If possible, remove or cut away clothing to expose the injury. Remove jewelry from the injured area.
- Assess pulses, movement, and sensation distal to the injury before and after applying a splint. You may find it helpful to mark the pulse location lightly with a pen to save time when rechecking pulses. Assess pulses, movement, and sensation every 15 minutes and document your findings.
- Cover open wounds with a sterile dressing.
- Before applying a rigid or semi-rigid splint, pad it to reduce patient discomfort due to pressure, especially around bony areas.
- Splint the area above and below the injury. If a bone is injured, immobilize the joint above and below the injury. If a joint is injured, immobilize the bone above and below the injury.
- Before splinting an injured hand or foot, place it in the **position of function** (Figure 11-15). The natural position of the hand at rest looks as if you were gently grasping a small object, such as a baseball. Use a roll of tape, roller gauze, or a rolled-up sock or glove as the "ball" and place it in the patient's palm before splinting her hand. Do not place the hand or foot in a position of function if you find it in an abnormal position and meet resistance or cause pain when you attempt to place it in the position of function.
- Pad the hollow areas (voids) between the splint and the extremity.

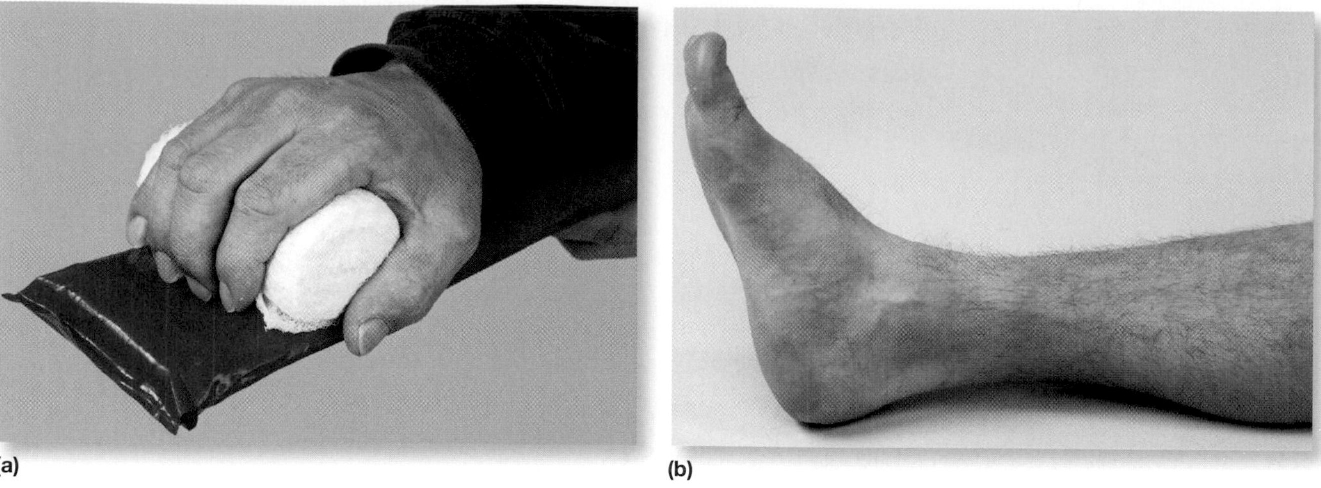

FIGURE 11-15 ▲ (a) Position of function for the hand. (b) Position of function for the foot.

- Do not intentionally replace protruding bones. During the splinting process, bone ends may be drawn back into the wound. This is to be expected and is acceptable.
- Avoid excessive movement of the injured area when applying a splint.
- When securing the splint to the injured area, avoid placing ties or straps directly over the injury.
- Splint the injury before moving the patient unless the patient is in danger or life-threatening conditions exist.
- When in doubt about whether a musculoskeletal injury is present, splint the injury.
- If the patient shows signs of shock, align her in the anatomical position on a long backboard. Treat the patient for shock by raising the foot of the backboard and arrange for transport.

Stop and Think!

If your patient does not have a pulse in an extremity or has lost sensation or the ability to move the fingers or toes of the injured extremity after you have applied a splint, the splint is too tight. Manually immobilize the injured area, loosen the splint, and adjust it. Reassess often and be sure to notify EMS personnel when they arrive.

Remember This!

Warning Signs That a Splint Is Too Tight

- The patient's fingers or toes become cold to the touch in the splinted extremity.
- The patient's fingers or toes begin to turn pale or blue in the splinted extremity.
- The patient is unable to move fingers or toes in the splinted extremity.
- The patient experiences increased pain in the splinted extremity.
- The patient experiences increased swelling below the splint.
- The patient complains of numbness or tingling in the extremity.
- The patient complains of burning or stinging in the splinted extremity.

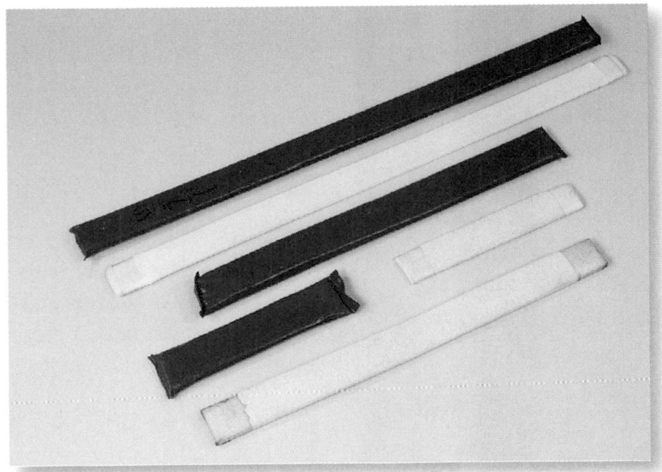

FIGURE 11-16 ▲ Rigid splints.

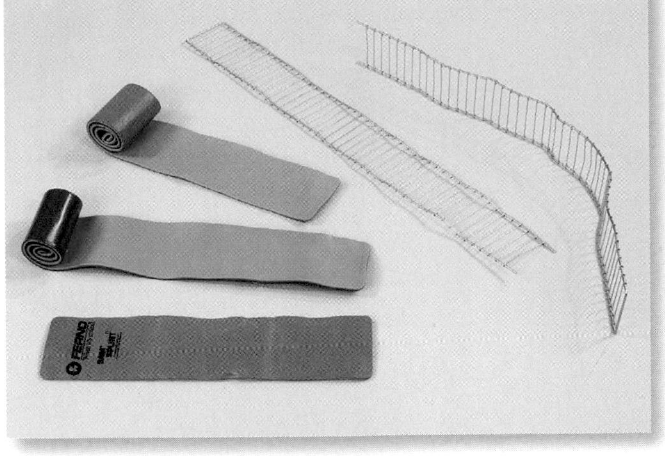

FIGURE 11-17 ▲ Semi-rigid splints.

Types of Splints

A variety of materials and techniques can be used for splinting. You may have to improvise due to the limited availability of splinting materials and/or the patient's position.

Rigid Splints

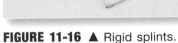

Remember: The splint must be long enough to immobilize the area above and below the injury.

Rigid splints are made of hard material, such as wood, strong cardboard, or plastic (Figure 11-16). They are available in different sizes. Some are preformed to fit certain body areas. Some rigid splints are padded, but others must be padded before they are applied to the patient. This type of splint is useful for immobilizing injuries that occur to the middle portion (midshaft) of a bone. The SAM® Splint and aluminum ladder splints are examples of semi-rigid (flexible) splints. These splints can be molded to the shape of the extremity and are very useful for immobilizing joint injuries (Figure 11-17). They can be used in combination with other splints.

Soft Splints

When a triangular bandage is used to apply a sling, place the knot to either side of the patient's neck. It will be very uncomfortable for the patient if the knot is tied behind the cervical spine.

Soft splints are flexible and useful for immobilizing injuries of the lower leg or forearm. Examples of soft splints include a sling and swathe, blanket rolls, pillows, and towels (Figure 11-18). A sling and swathe is used to immobilize injuries to the shoulder (scapula), collarbone (clavicle), or upper arm bone (humerus). A triangular bandage is often used to make a sling. A **swathe** is a piece of soft material used to secure the injured extremity to the body.

FIGURE 11-18 ► Soft splints.

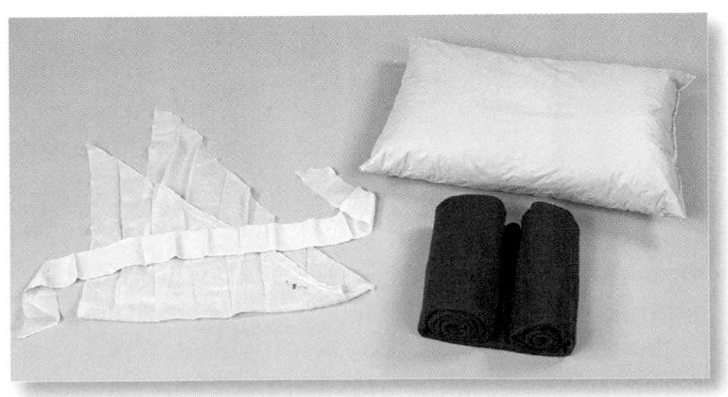

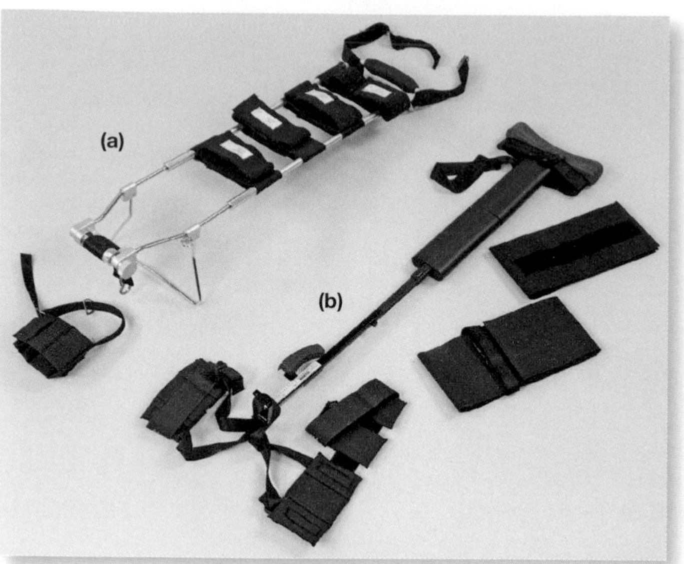

FIGURE 11-19 ▶ Traction splints. (a) Bipolar traction splint. (b) Unipolar traction splint.

Roller gauze can be used as a swathe.

The patient may have difficulty breathing if chest movement is restricted.

- To make a swathe, unwrap a triangular bandage and place it on a flat surface. Grab the point of the shorter end of the triangle and fold it toward the longer end, like a bandanna.
- The swathe must be tight enough to limit movement of the arm but not so tight that chest movement is restricted. Make sure the patient's fingers remain exposed, so that you can assess the pulse, movement, and sensation.

Traction Splints

Two emergency care professionals are needed to apply a traction splint. Use this type of splint only if you have been trained to use it and are allowed to do so.

A **traction splint** is a device used to immobilize a closed fracture of the femur (thighbone) (Figure 11-19). When applied, this type of splint maintains a constant, steady pull (traction) on the femur. A traction splint decreases muscle spasm and pain. It also keeps broken bone ends in a near-normal position. A unipolar traction splint has one pole that provides external support for the injured leg. A bipolar traction splint uses two external poles, one on each side of the injured leg, to provide external support.

You Should Know

Contraindications to the Use of a Traction Splint

- An injury to the hip, knee, or ankle joints or a fracture within 1-2 inches of a joint
- An injury to the lower leg
- An injury to the pelvis
- An injury that is close to the knee
- A partial amputation or avulsion with bone separation (in this circumstance, the distal limb is connected only by marginal tissue and traction would risk separation)

Pneumatic Splints

The pressure within a pneumatic splint can vary with temperature and altitude.

A pneumatic splint requires air to be pumped into or suctioned out of it. An air splint, a vacuum splint, and the pneumatic antishock garment (PASG) are examples of pneumatic splints (Figure 11-20). A pneumatic splint is placed around the injured area and is inflated (air splint or PASG) or deflated (vacuum splint)

FIGURE 11-20 ► Pneumatic splints.

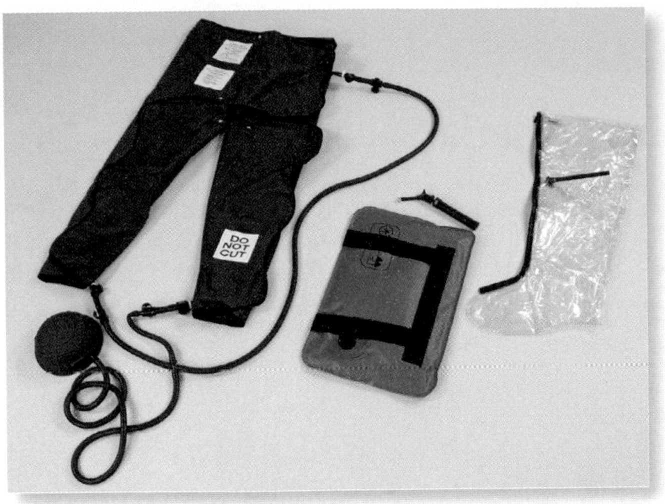

until it becomes firm. When using an air splint, inflate it until you can make a slight dent in the splint with your fingers.

Pneumatic splints are also called air splints, vacuum splints, or pressure splints.

If permitted by local protocol, a PASG may be used to stabilize a pelvic fracture and closed fractures of the lower extremities. Remember that the PASG has three compartments that can be inflated: the abdomen, the left leg, and the right leg. If there is a closed injury to one leg, that leg compartment is inflated. If both legs are injured, both leg compartments are inflated. All three compartments are inflated if there is an injury to the pelvis. The abdominal compartment is *never* used without inflating both leg compartments. When the PASG is positioned on the patient, the top edge of the garment must be below the patient's lowest ribs. If the garment is positioned higher on the patient, the pressure caused by inflating the abdominal compartment can hamper the patient's breathing.

Remember This!

Apply padding to any splint that is hard or does not precisely fit the area to which you will be applying it. Secure the padding to the splint to keep it from bunching up *before* placing the splint against the patient.

The Care of Specific Musculoskeletal Injuries

Upper-Extremity Injuries

Upper-extremity injuries include injuries to the shoulder (clavicle, scapula, and humerus), upper arm (humerus), elbow, forearm (radius and ulna), wrist, and hand.

Injuries to the Shoulder

The sling forms a pouch and is used to support the weight of the arm. The swathe is used to immobilize the injury by securing the patient's arm to his or her chest.

A shoulder injury typically involves three bones: the collarbone (clavicle), the shoulder blade (scapula), and the upper arm bone (humerus). The patient will usually hold her arm in a position of comfort. Immobilize the injury in this position. Because the entire upper extremity must be immobilized to limit shoulder movement, a sling and swathe is usually used for this type of injury (Skill Drill 11-1).

If ready-made materials are not available, fold up the bottom of the patient's shirt and pin or tape it in place for a sling. The arms of a long-sleeved shirt can be tied to one side of the patient's neck and the rest of the shirt used as a sling.

Skill Drill 11-1

Immobilization of a Shoulder Injury

STEP 1 ▶
- Immobilize a shoulder injury using a sling and swathe. After assessing for a pulse, movement, and sensation in the injured arm, drape one end of a triangular bandage under the injured arm.
- Drape the other end over the opposite shoulder and around the patient's neck.

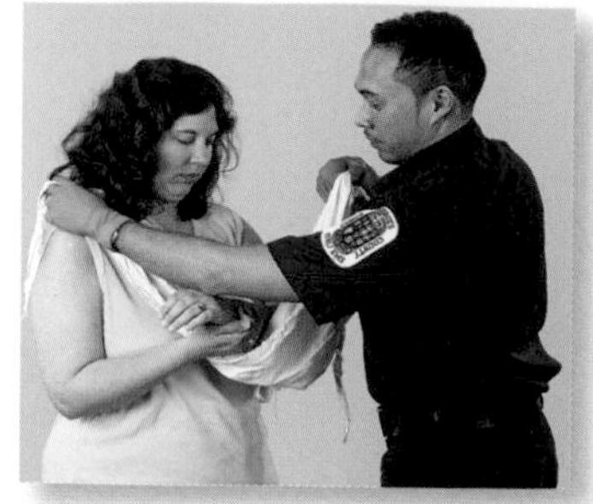

STEP 2 ▶ Pull the end of the bandage that is under the injured arm up to the patient's neck.

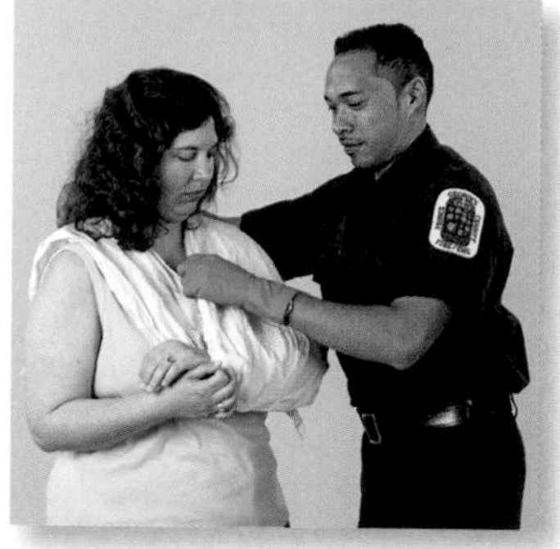

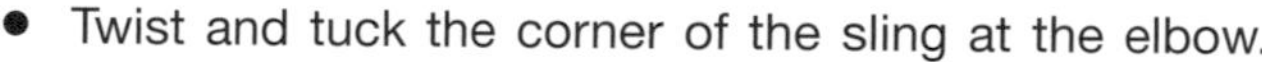

STEP 3 ▶
- Tie the two ends of the bandage to one side of the patient's neck.
- Twist and tuck the corner of the sling at the elbow.

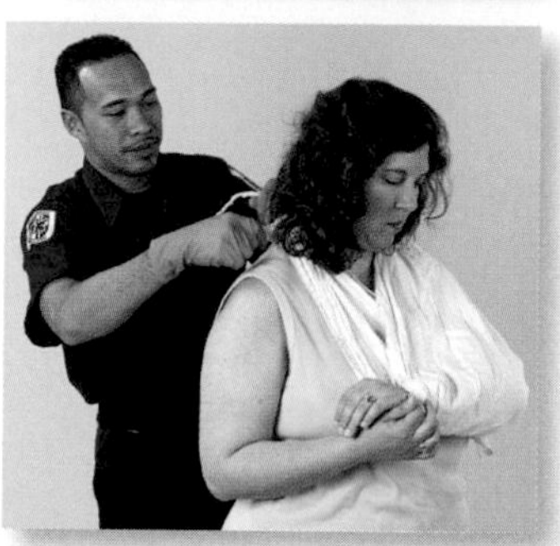

STEP 4 ▶ Use another bandage as a swathe and secure the arm to the chest.

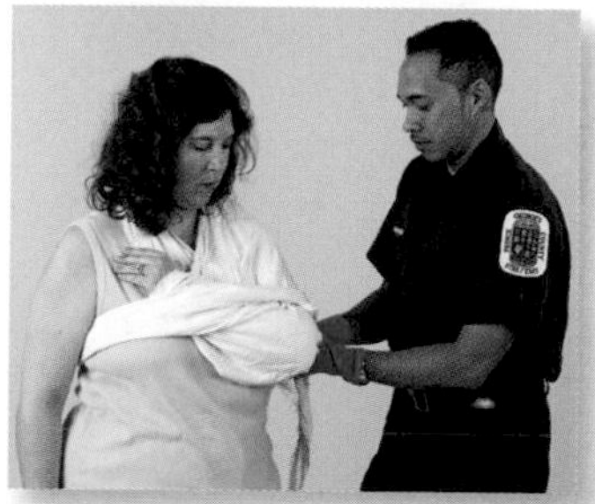

STEP 5 ▶ Reassess pulse, movement, and sensation in the injured arm.

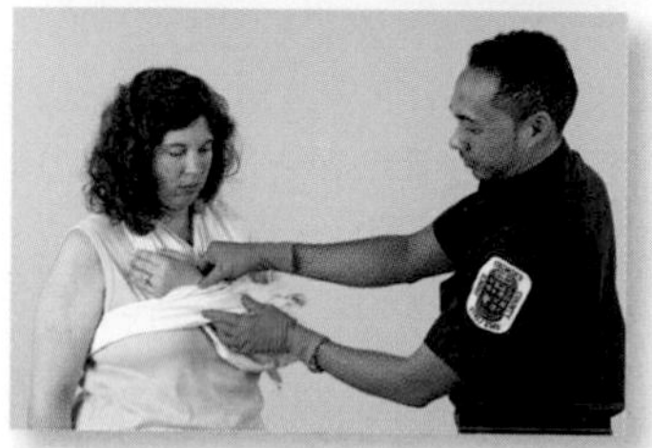

The swathe should not be placed directly on top of the injury. It should be positioned either above or below the fracture site.

A jacket that is zipped closed or wide strips cut from a sheet (or from the bottom of the patient's shirt) can be used as a swathe.

If the patient is holding her arm away from her body, provide support for the injured area using a pillow, rolled towels, or similar material to fill the gap between the patient's arm and her chest. Secure the patient's arm and any support material to the patient's chest with a swathe. Ask the patient to hold her uninjured arm out to the side. Wrap the swathe around her chest and the injured extremity. Secure the swathe in place with a knot.

Injuries to the Upper Arm (Humerus)

The upper arm bone (humerus) extends from the shoulder to the elbow. It is most often fractured at its upper end near the shoulder or in the middle of the bone. Fractures of the upper end of the bone typically occur in elderly patients who fall on an outstretched hand. The middle of the bone is more often fractured in young adults. An upper arm injury should be immobilized from the shoulder (the joint above) to the elbow (the joint below). This type of injury is usually best immobilized with a sling and swathe. A padded splint or a SAM® Splint formed around the upper arm and held in place with roller gauze can be used to provide additional support (Figure 11-21).

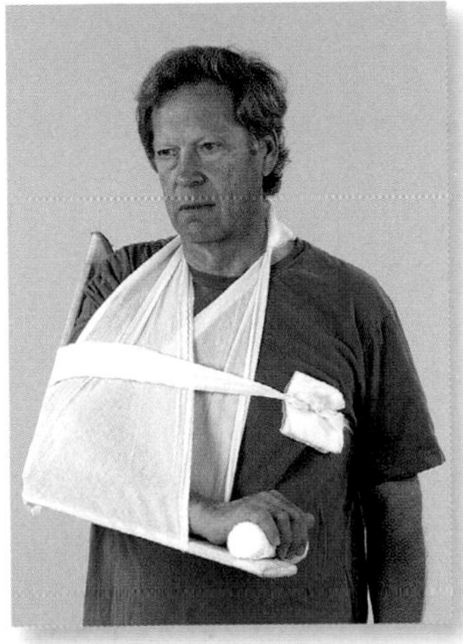

(a)

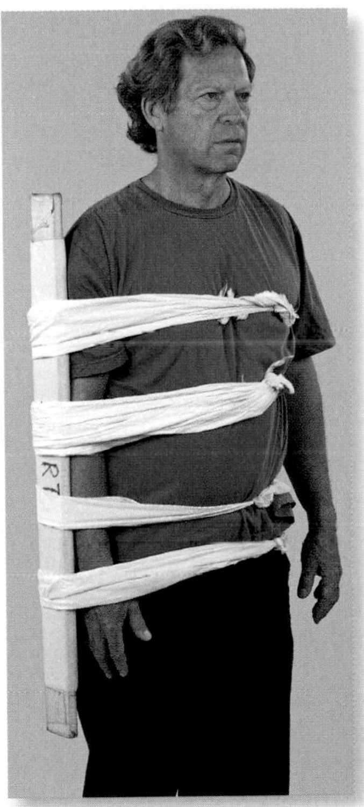

(b)

FIGURE 11-21 ▲ An upper arm injury is usually best immobilized with a sling and swathe. A padded splint can be used to provide additional support. (a) Humerus injury immobilized with the elbow bent. (b) Humerus injury immobilized with the elbow straight.

Making a Difference

Splinting a Long Bone

Follow these steps to immobilize a closed, non-angulated fracture of the humerus, radius, ulna, femur, tibia, or fibula:

1. Take BSI precautions and wear appropriate PPE. Remove or cut away clothing to expose the injury. Remove jewelry from the injured area.
2. Ask an assistant to manually support the injured extremity using one hand above the injury and one hand below the injury.
3. Assess pulses, movement, and sensation below the injured area.
4. Select a splint and measure it for proper length against the uninjured extremity. Make sure that the bones above and below the injured area will be immobilized. Pad a rigid or semi-rigid splint.
5. Apply the splint, immobilizing the injured joint and the bones above and below the injury. When possible, immobilize the injured hand or foot in a position of function. Avoid excessive movement of the injured area when applying the splint.
6. Pad the hollow areas between the extremity and the splint. Secure the entire injured extremity.
7. Assess pulses, movement, and sensation every 15 minutes and document your findings.

Injuries to the Elbow

The elbow is formed by the joining of the upper arm bone (humerus) and the two forearm bones (radius and ulna). Because there are many nerves and blood vessels in the elbow area, consider an elbow injury a serious injury. Splinting an elbow injury requires immobilizing the humerus (the bone above the injury) and the radius and ulna (the bones below the injury).

If you find the patient with her elbow in a bent position, consider using a semi-rigid or vacuum splint to immobilize the injury. These splints will conform to the shape of the arm, despite its odd position. You might also use a padded splint.

After you have applied a splint, use a sling and swathe to further limit movement if the patient's condition allows her to be placed in a sitting or semi-sitting position.

If the arm is straight, use a soft or rigid splint that extends from the armpit to the wrist. Secure the injured arm to the body to prevent movement (Figure 11-22). Arrange for immediate transport.

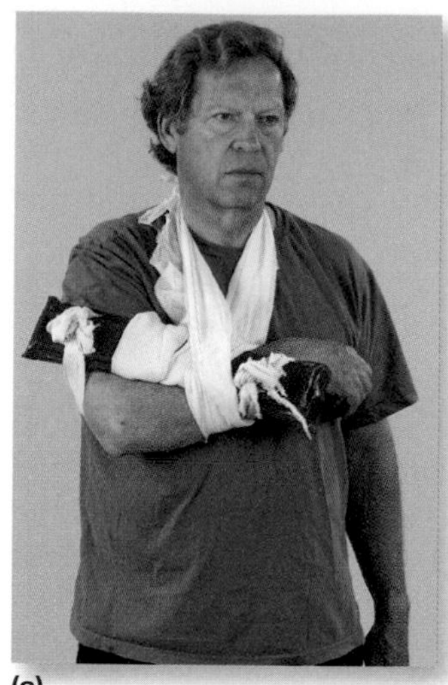

(a)

(b)

FIGURE 11-22 ▲ (a) Elbow injury immobilized with the elbow bent. (b) Elbow injury immobilized in a straight position.

Making a Difference

Splinting a Joint

Follow these steps to immobilize a closed, non-angulated injury to the elbow or knee:

1. Take BSI precautions and wear appropriate PPE. Remove or cut away clothing to expose the injury. Remove jewelry from the injured area.
2. Ask an assistant to manually support the injured extremity using one hand above and one hand below the injury.
3. Assess pulses, movement, and sensation below the injured area.
4. Select a splint and measure it for proper length against the uninjured extremity. Make sure that the bones above and below the injured area will be immobilized. Pad a rigid or semi-rigid splint.
5. Apply the splint, immobilizing the injured joint and the bones above and below the injury. When possible, immobilize an injured hand or foot in a position of function. Avoid excessive movement of the injured area when applying the splint.
6. Pad the hollow areas between the extremity and the splint. Secure the entire injured extremity.
7. Assess pulses, movement, and sensation every 15 minutes and document your findings.

Injuries to the Forearm, Wrist, and Hand

The forearm, wrist, and hands contain many bones and are commonly injured. These areas can sustain serious injury with or without any visible deformity. Some wrist fractures may present with gross deformity and hand displacement. Immobilize the extremity in the position found with a soft, rigid, or pneumatic splint.

When immobilizing an injury of the forearm, wrist, or hand with a rigid, semi-rigid, or soft splint, place the splint underneath the forearm. Remember that the joints above and below the injury site must be immobilized. Therefore, the splint must extend from the elbow (the joint above) to beyond the hand (the joint below). An injured forearm or wrist should be placed in a sling and secured to the body with a swathe (Figure 11-23). A hand injury can be immobilized using a variety of materials. Before applying the splint, place the hand in a position of function unless there is gross deformity or displacement (Figure 11-24).

If a finger is injured, you can use an anatomic splint by taping the injured finger to an uninjured finger next to it. Provide additional support for the injured finger by placing padding between it and the finger next to it (Figure 11-25). If more than one finger is injured, immobilize the entire hand.

The forearm extends from the elbow to the wrist.

When possible, remember to leave the fingers exposed to check color, movement, and sensation.

Taping fingers (or toes) together is also called buddy taping.

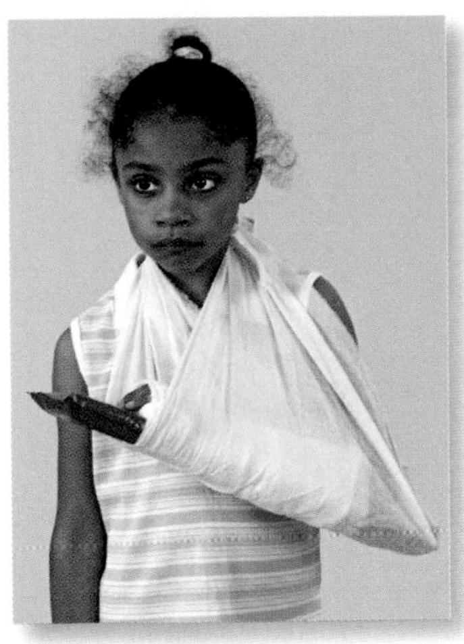

FIGURE 11-23 ▲ Immobilization of an injury to the forearm or wrist.

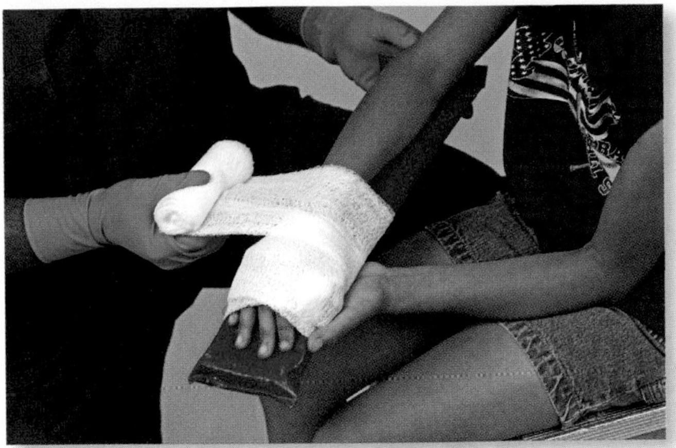

FIGURE 11-24 ▲ Immobilization of an injured hand.

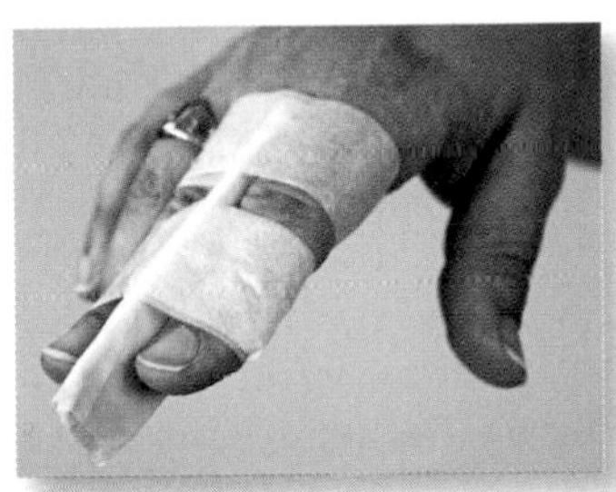

FIGURE 11-25 ▲ Immobilization of a finger injury.

Remember This!

A patient who has an isolated arm injury is often most comfortable in a sitting or semi-sitting position. If a patient's condition requires that he be positioned on his back, the weight of the patient's arm and splint on his chest and upper abdomen can hamper chest movement. If a patient *must* be positioned on her back and the arm must be immobilized with the elbow bent, try to splint the patient's arm so that the weight of the arm and splint will be supported on the patient's upper legs, rather than on her chest or abdomen.

Lower-Extremity Injuries

Lower-extremity injuries involve the pelvis, hip, thigh (femur), knee, lower leg (tibia and fibula), ankle, foot, and toes.

Injuries to the Pelvis and Hip

Objective 11 ▶

An injury to the pelvis can result in massive, life-threatening internal bleeding. Swelling and obvious deformity may not be easy to see because the pelvis is protected by many muscles and soft tissues. Call for advanced EMS personnel immediately. Keep in mind that a force strong enough to cause an injury to the pelvis demands spinal stabilization as well.

Treat the patient for shock if an injury to the pelvis is present.

The hip joint is formed by the socket of the hip bone and the upper end of the thighbone (femur). In a hip dislocation, the upper end of the thighbone is popped out of its socket. As the bone is pushed out of its socket, blood vessels and nerves can be damaged. The patient usually complains of severe pain and is unable to move the affected leg. If nerve damage is present, the patient may not have any feeling in the foot or ankle area. You may see that one leg is shorter than the other, and the affected leg may be turned inward or outward. These signs suggest a hip fracture; however, they are not always present.

Approximately 50% of patients with a hip dislocation have other injuries, such as injuries to the pelvis, legs, back, or head.

In most hip dislocations, the head of the thighbone is pushed out and back (a posterior dislocation). This most often occurs due to a motor vehicle crash, when a front-seat occupant strikes the dashboard with his or her knees. The energy from the impact is transmitted along the femur to the hip joint. In a posterior dislocation, the hip is in a fixed position, bent and twisted in toward the middle of the body.

In an anterior hip dislocation, the upper end of the thighbone slips out of its socket and moves forward. With this type of injury, the hip is usually only slightly bent and the leg twists out and away from the middle of the body. An anterior dislocation is much less common than a posterior dislocation.

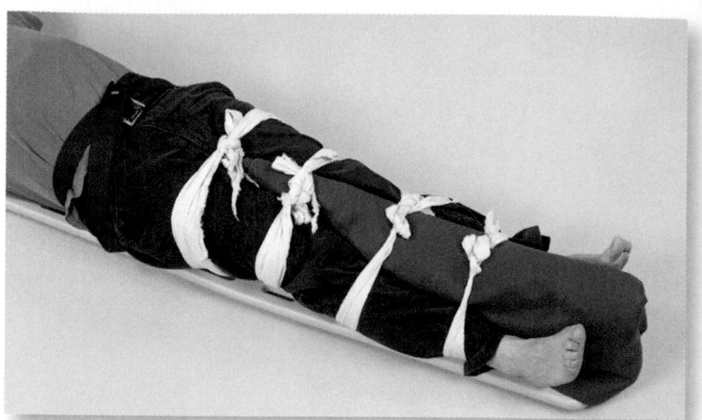

FIGURE 11-26 ▲ Immobilization of an injury to the pelvis or hips.

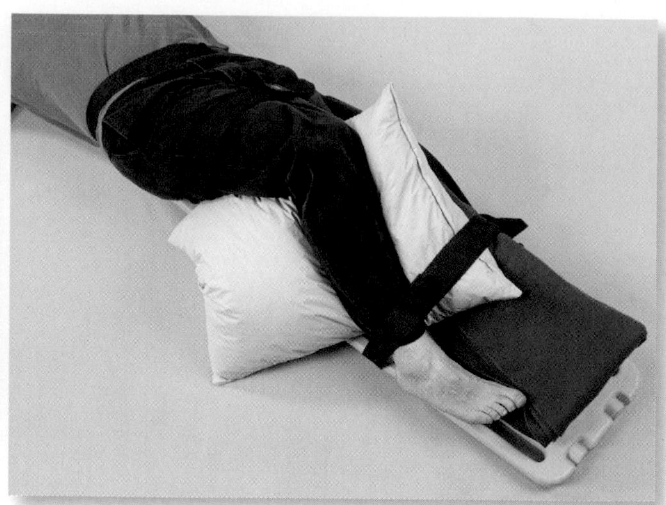

FIGURE 11-27 ▲ Immobilization of a hip injury.

Immobilizing the pelvis or hip requires the use of a splint that extends from the level of the lower back and past the knee on the affected side. A long backboard is usually used for this purpose. A blanket or similar padding is placed between the patient's legs. The injured leg is secured to the uninjured leg and the patient's entire body is secured to the backboard (Figure 11-26). When splinting the legs together, move the good leg to the injured leg. If possible, *do not move the injured leg to the good leg.* Secure the legs together using straps, triangular bandages, or roller gauze secured in four places on the legs—two above the knee and two below. Ties are usually placed just above the ankles, at the calves, just above the knees, and at the thighs. Make sure the knots are secured over the padded material between the patient's legs, so that they do not rub against the patient. Additional straps or triangular bandages should be used around the pelvis to secure it to the backboard and limit movement.

In many cases, a patient with a hip injury will not be able to move the affected leg into a straight position. In these situations, support the affected leg with pillows and rolled blankets between and under the legs. Secure the patient's hips and legs to a long backboard with straps, triangular bandages, or roller gauze to limit movement (Figure 11-27). An injury to the pelvis can also be immobilized with a PASG or pelvic sling. These devices may be used *only* if you have received special training in how to use them and are allowed to do so. Check with your instructor or medical director.

Injuries to the Upper Thigh (Femur)

Most femur fractures involve the middle or upper end of the bone.

Because the femur (thighbone) is protected by large muscles, a great deal of force is required to break it. A broken femur can occur in activities such as skiing, cycling, falls from a great height, and motor vehicle crashes. It can also occur as a result of child abuse. The injured leg will often appear shorter than the other leg. In addition, the injured leg is often rotated. A broken femur is a true emergency because a patient can easily lose more than a liter of blood internally. Call for advanced EMS personnel immediately. Bone fragments can cause damage to blood vessels, nerves, and soft tissues. Life-threatening bleeding may be present if both femurs are broken.

A traction splint may be used *only* if you have received special training in how to use it and are allowed to do so.

A fracture of the upper third of the femur is treated as a hip fracture. A closed fracture of the middle third of the femur is best immobilized with a traction splint (Skill Drills 11-2 and 11-3). Applying traction helps stabilize the bone ends and reduces pain. It also reduces the likelihood of a closed fracture becoming an open one and reduces further soft-tissue damage.

Applying a Unipolar Traction Splint

STEP 1 ▶
- Expose the fracture site and make sure the injury is a closed, non-angulated midshaft femur fracture.
- Remove the patient's shoe and assess distal pulses, movement, and sensation in the injured leg.

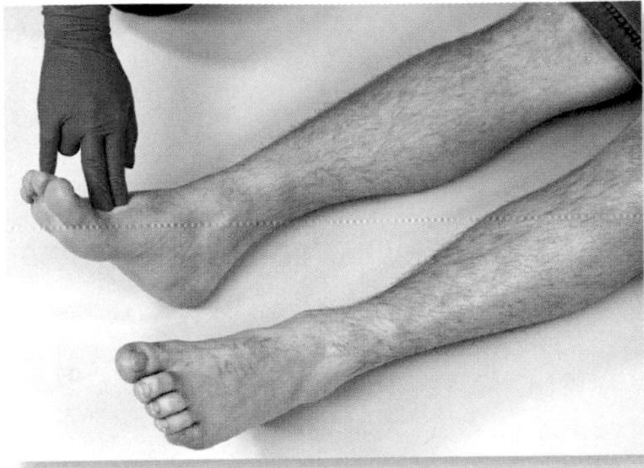

STEP 2 ▶ Place the splint next to the patient's injured leg and adjust the length so that the wheel is even with the patient's heel.

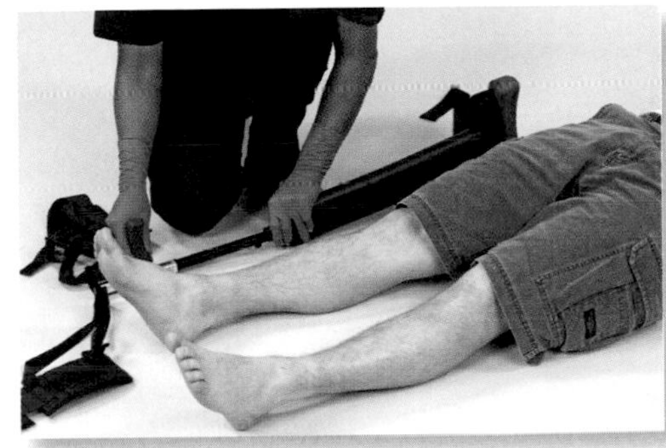

STEP 3 ▶ Place the splint along the inside of the patient's injured leg. Slide the thigh strap up under the thigh. Secure the strap snugly across the thigh.

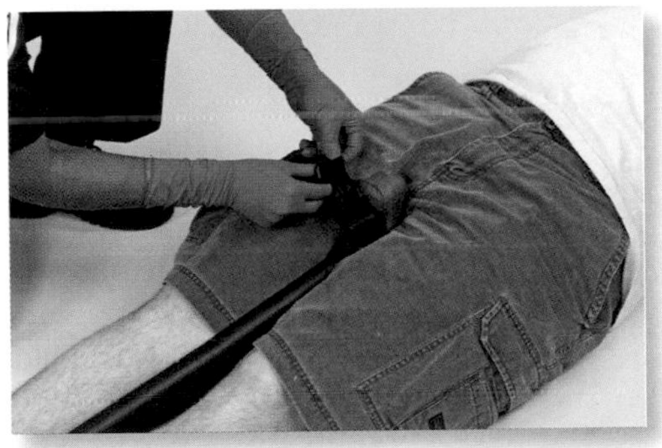

STEP 4 ▶ Apply the ankle hitch to the patient's ankle.

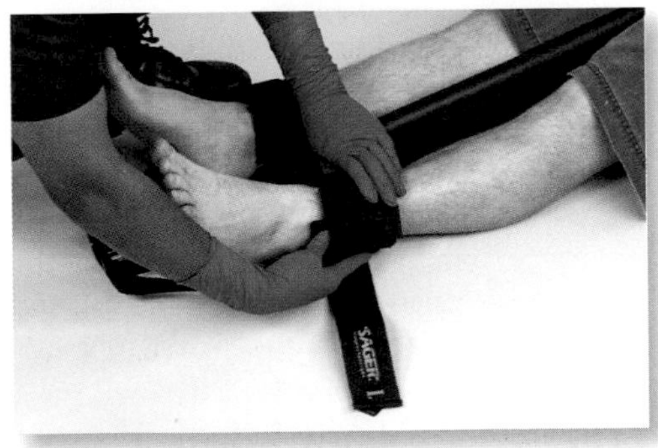

Continued on next page

Skill Drill 11-2

Applying a Unipolar Traction Splint *(continued)*

STEP 5 ▶ Apply traction by lengthening the splint. Traction should be applied that is approximately 10% of the patient's body weight, not to exceed 15 pounds of traction.

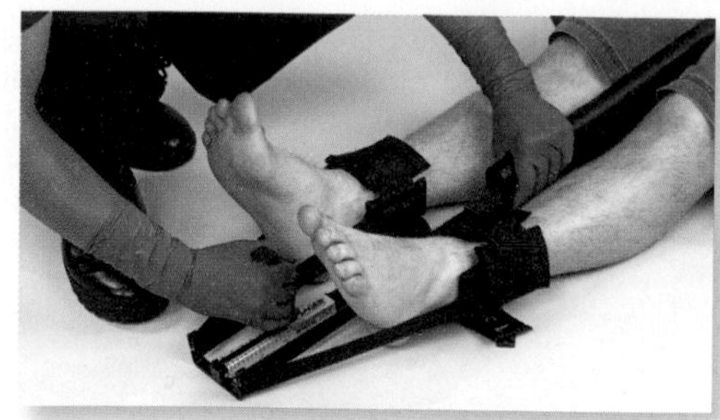

STEP 6 ▶ Fasten the leg straps to secure the leg to the splint. Position the longest strap as high as possible on the thigh. Position the other straps around the knees and lower leg.

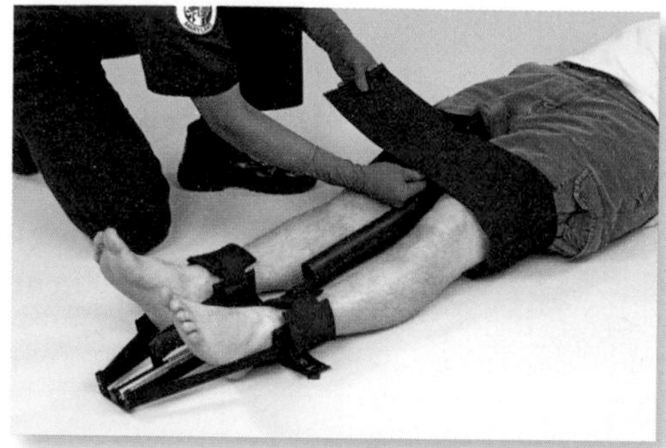

STEP 7 ▶ Reassess distal pulses, movement, and sensation.

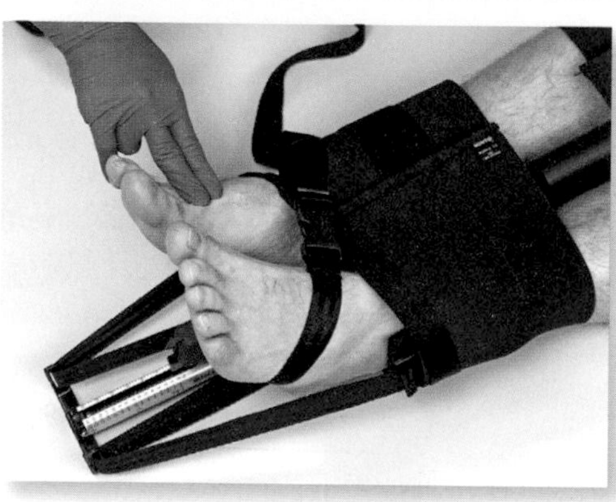

STEP 8 ▶ Place the patient on a long backboard and secure the patient to the board.

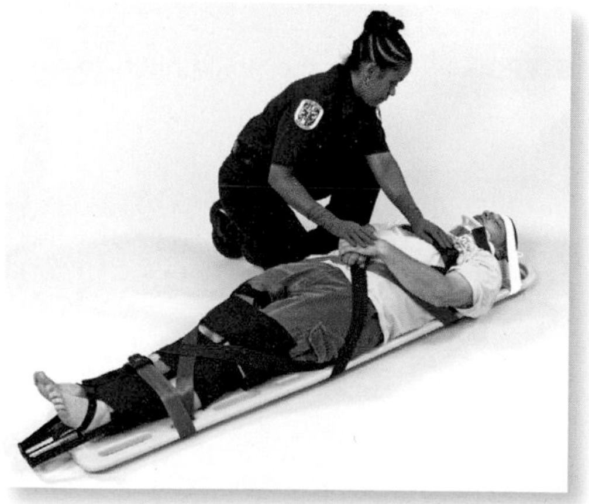

Applying a Bipolar Traction Splint

STEP 1 ▶
- Adjust the traction splint to the proper length. Position the splint next to the patient's uninjured leg using the bony prominence of the buttock as a landmark. Extend the splint 6–12 inches beyond the patient's uninjured heel. Lock the splint in position.
- Position the support straps at the midthigh, above the knee, below the knee, and above the ankle. Open the straps and fasten them under the splint.

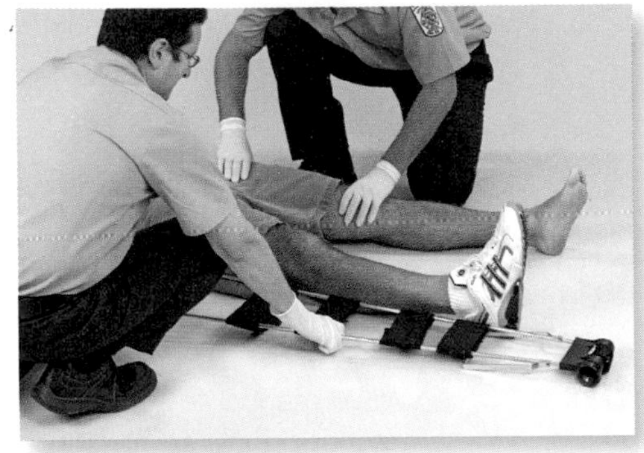

STEP 2 ▶ Stabilize the injured leg so that it does not move while an assistant fastens the ankle hitch around the patient's foot and ankle.

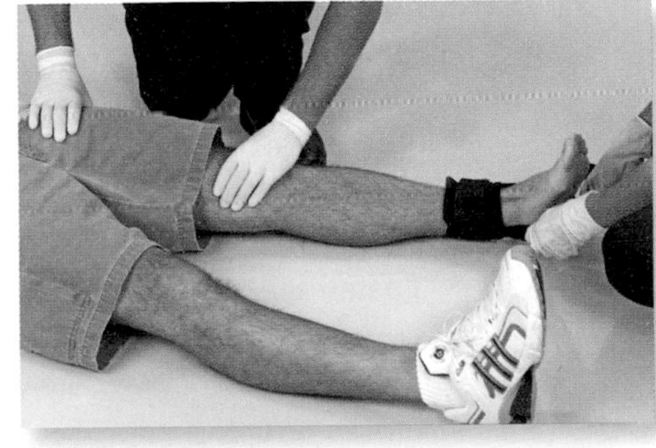

STEP 3 ▶
- While your assistant continues to apply gentle manual traction, position the splint under the injured leg. The ischial pad should rest against the bony prominence of the buttocks.
- Raise the heel stand after the splint is in position.

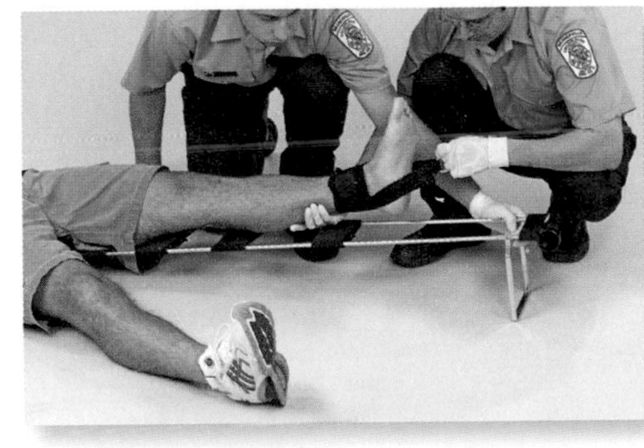

STEP 4 ▶
- Pad the groin area.
- Attach the ischial strap. Secure the strap over the groin and thigh.

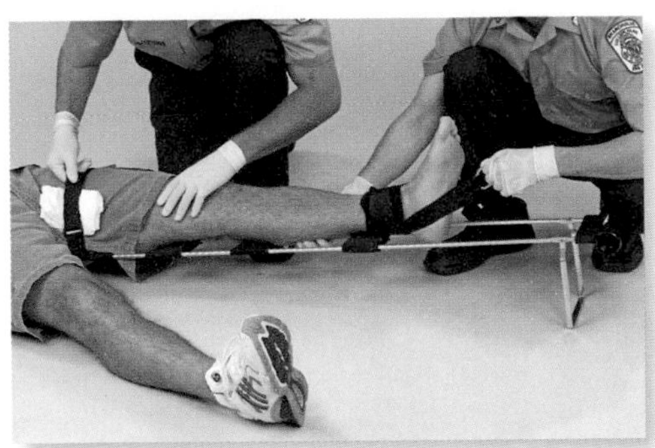

Continued on next page

Skill Drill 11-3

Applying a Bipolar Traction Splint *(continued)*

STEP 5 ▶ While your assistant continues to apply gentle manual traction, attach the S hook of the splint to the D ring of the ankle hitch.

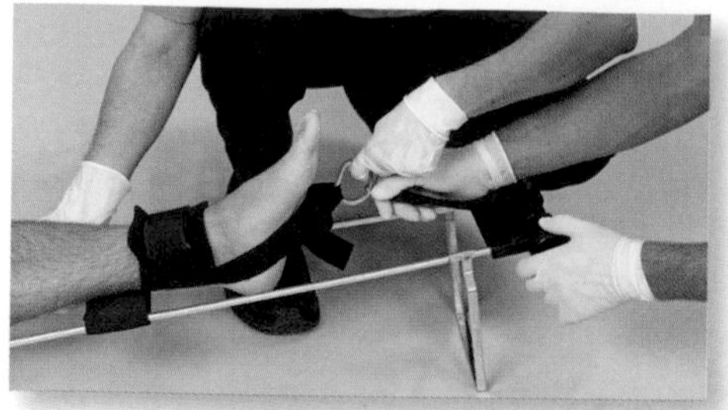

STEP 6 ▶
- While manual traction continues, begin tightening the ratchet on the splint to apply mechanical traction.
- Continue tightening until mechanical traction is equal to the manual traction and the patient's pain and muscle spasms are reduced. If the patient is unconscious, continue tightening until the length of the injured leg equals that of the uninjured leg.

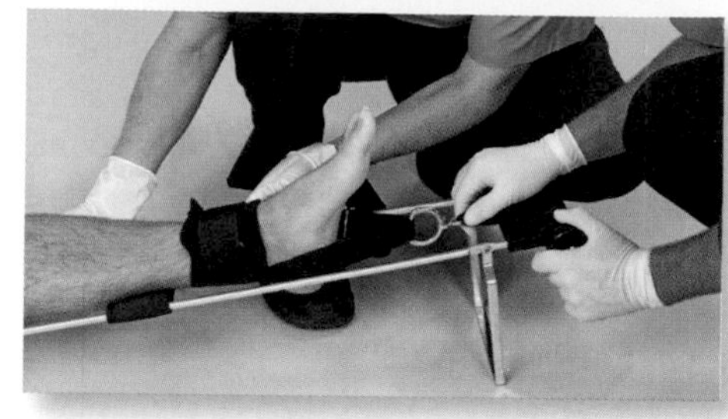

STEP 7 ▶
- Fasten the leg support straps over the injured leg.
- Recheck the ischial strap and ankle hitch. Make sure both are fastened securely.

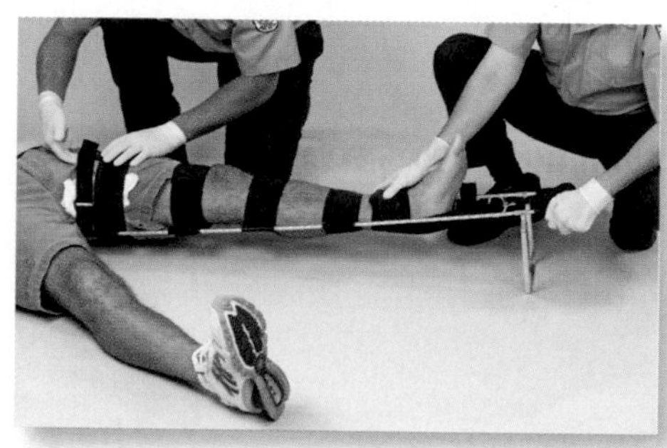

STEP 8 ▶ Reassess distal pulses, movement, and sensation.

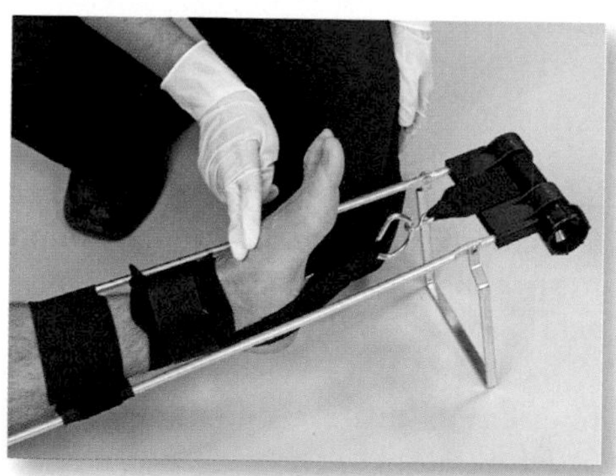

STEP 9 ▶
- Place the patient on a long backboard.
- Secure the leg and splint in place. Place padding between the splint and the uninjured leg.

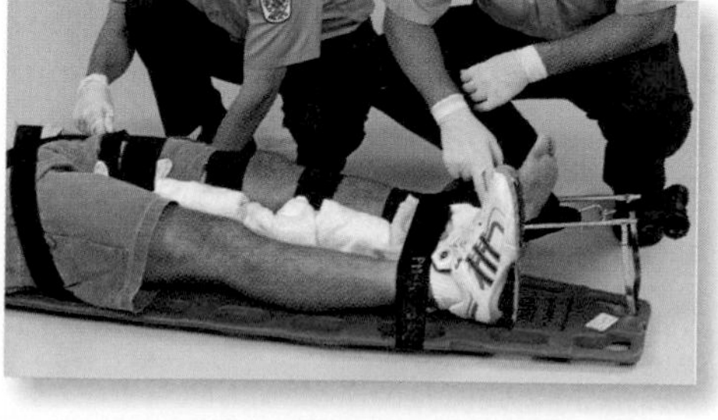

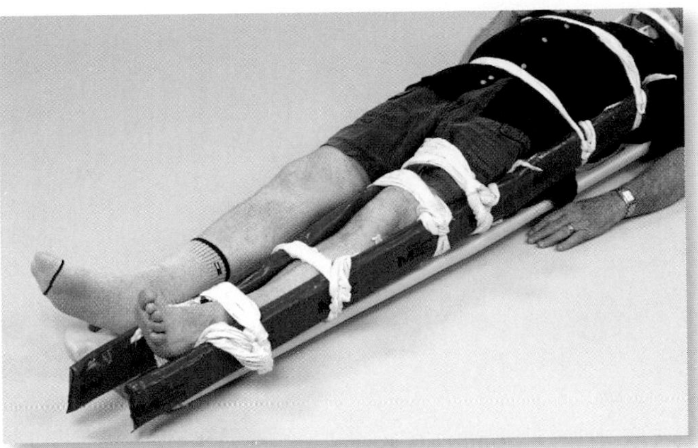

FIGURE 11-28 ▲ Immobilization of a femur fracture.

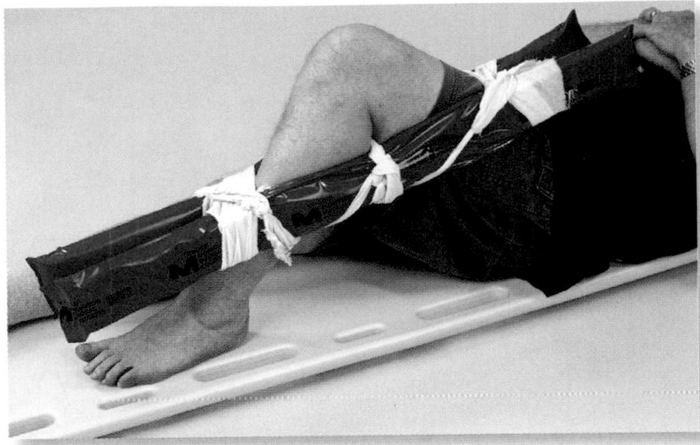

FIGURE 11-29 ▲ Immobilization of the knee in a bent position.

A femur fracture can also be immobilized using two long boards (Figure 11-28). Use a board on the outside of the leg that extends from the patient's armpit to below the bottom of the foot. Use a board on the inside of the leg that extends from the patient's groin to below the bottom of the foot. Be sure to pad any hollow areas and then secure the boards to the patient using straps, triangular bandages, or roller gauze. Secure the boards under the patient's arms, at the hips, just above the knees, at the calves, and just above the ankles. Be sure the knots are secured on the outside of the boards. Additional straps or triangular bandages must be used when securing the patient to a long backboard.

Injuries to the Knee

The knee joint is formed by the lower end of the femur (thighbone), the upper end of the tibia (shinbone), and the patella (kneecap). The kneecap is frequently dislocated from injuries such as a fall. This type of injury usually appears as a lump on the lateral side of the knee. You will often find the patient complaining of pain, with the leg in a bent position at the knee. Distal pulses are usually present.

Check distal pulses frequently.

A knee dislocation may result from violent direct force, such as the knee hitting the dashboard during a motor vehicle crash. This type of injury is serious, because the popliteal artery behind the knee can be cut or compressed. The patient is often unable to move the leg. The affected leg is usually grossly deformed around the knee. Extensive swelling is usually present and distal pulses may be absent. Call for advanced EMS personnel immediately.

If you find the patient with the knee in a bent position, support the affected knee with a pillow. To limit movement, place a padded board splint on each side of the knee from the thigh to the calf (Figure 11-29). Secure the boards in place with triangular bandages or roller gauze above and below the knee.

If the knee is straight, place a long, padded board splint on each side of the knee (Figure 11-30). The board on the outside of the leg should extend from the patient's hip to the ankle. The board on the inside of the leg should extend from the groin to the ankle. Tie triangular bandages or roller gauze above and below the knee, at the uppermost part of the thigh, and just above the ankle. Be sure the ties are positioned on the outside of the splint.

Injuries to the Lower Leg

A fracture of the tibia is the most common type of long-bone fracture.

The tibia and fibula are the bones of the lower leg. Fractures of the lower leg usually occur as a result of a direct force injury, such as a fall or motor vehicle crash, or a twisting force. A fracture of either the tibia or the fibula can occur by itself. However, a tibia fracture is usually associated with a fibula fracture,

FIGURE 11-30 ▶ Immobilization of the knee in a straight position.

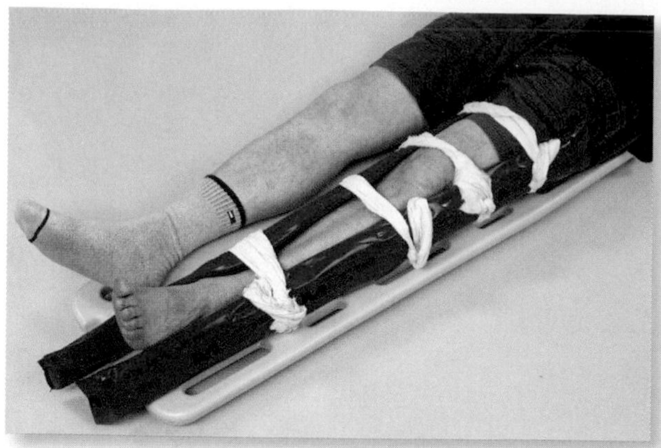

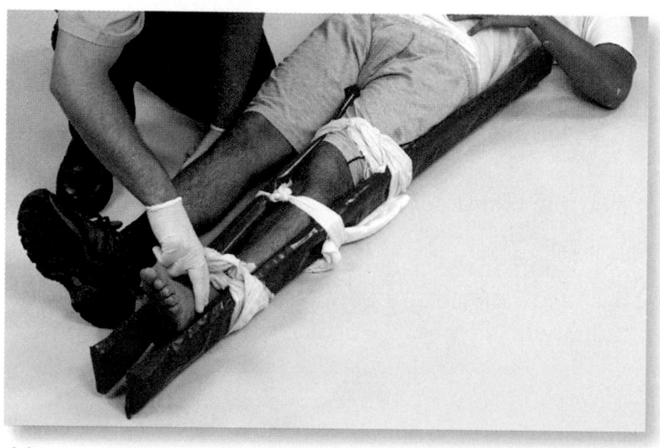

(a)

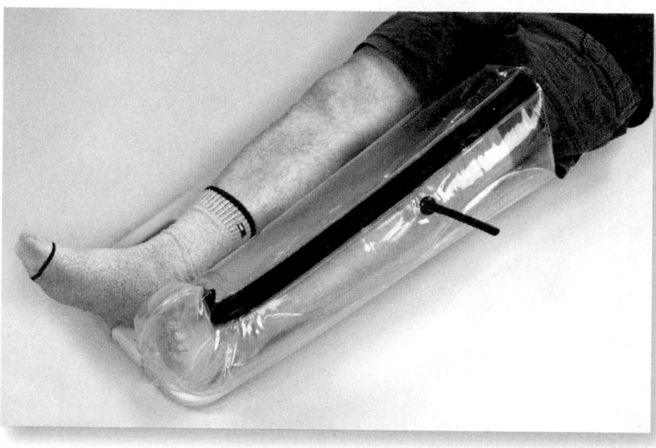

(b)

FIGURE 11-31 ▲ Immobilization of the lower leg. (a) Immobilization using padded boards. (b) Immobilization using an air splint.

because the force that causes the tibia fracture is transmitted to the fibula. Bruising, swelling, and tenderness are usually present over the fracture site. When the tibia is broken, the patient will complain of pain when putting weight on it. Because the tibia lies very close to the skin surface, a large number of fractures involving these bones are open fractures.

Immobilize a fracture of the tibia and fibula with a splint that extends from the hip to the foot. Place a padded board splint on each side of the leg (Figure 11-31). The board on the outside of the leg should extend from the patient's hip to the foot. The board on the inside of the leg should extend from the groin to the foot. Make sure to pad behind the knee to keep it in a position of comfort. Use triangular bandages or roller gauze to secure the boards in place. For a closed injury, an air splint that extends above the knee and covers the entire foot may be used instead of padded boards.

Injuries to the Ankle and Foot

Use the RICE treatment guideline for these injuries.

The ankle is formed by the lower ends of the tibia and the fibula (the shinbones) and the many smaller bones of the foot. It is difficult to tell when an ankle or a foot injury is a fracture or a sprain, because it is very painful and swells a great deal. An ankle or a foot injury is best immobilized with a preformed lower leg splint; a soft splint, such as a pillow or blanket; or an air splint (Figure 11-32).

The splints that can be used for various bone and joint injuries are listed in Table 11-3.

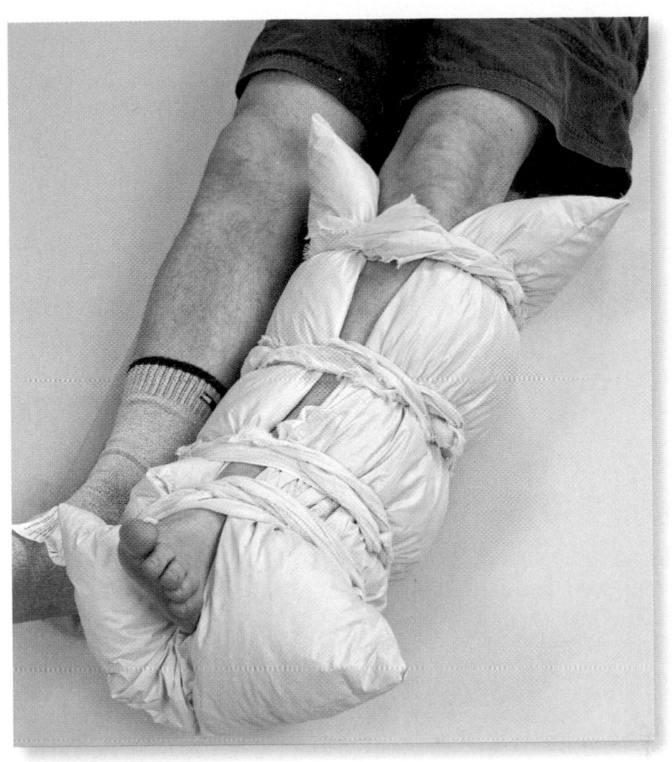

FIGURE 11-32 ▶ Immobilization of an ankle or a foot injury.

TABLE 11-3 Possible Splints for Bone and Joint Injuries

Site of Injury	Possible Splints
Shoulder	Sling and swathe
Upper arm (humerus)	Padded board splint, padded wire ladder splint, sling and swathe, SAM® Splint
Elbow	Padded board splint, padded wire ladder splint, air splint, vacuum splint, sling and swathe, SAM® Splint
Forearm (radius, ulna)	Padded board splint, padded wire ladder splint, air splint, vacuum splint, sling and swathe, SAM® Splint
Wrist, hand	Padded board splint, padded wire ladder splint, air splint, vacuum splint, sling and swathe, SAM® Splint
Pelvis	Long backboard, scoop stretcher, PASG, pelvic sling
Hip	Long backboard with blanket or pillow between the legs, scoop stretcher, PASG
Thigh (femur)	Traction splint, long padded board splints, other leg used as a splint
Knee	Pillow, padded board splint, SAM® Splint, air splint, vacuum splint, other leg used as a splint
Lower leg (tibia, fibula)	Padded board splint, SAM® Splint, air splint, vacuum splint, other leg used as a splint
Ankle, foot	Preformed lower leg splint, pillow or blanket, air splint, vacuum splint

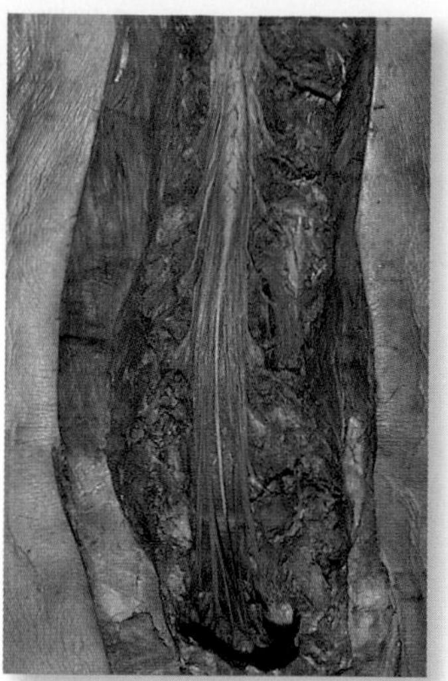

FIGURE 11-33 ▲ A dissected spinal cord and roots of the spinal nerves.

Injuries to the Spine

The spinal cord is made up of long tracts of nerves that join the brain with all body organs and parts (Figure 11-33). It is the center for many reflex activities of the body. The spinal cord is well protected by the spinal column in the back. Injuries associated with a lot of force are usually necessary to cause damage to the spinal cord.

Motor nerves carry responses from the brain and spinal cord, stimulating a muscle or an organ. Sensory nerves send signals to the brain about the activities of the different parts of the body relative to their surroundings. For example, when you want a finger to move, the message "Attention, finger! Move!" is sent down the spinal cord and through the nerve of the finger, and your finger moves. At about the same time, the finger sends a reply to the brain saying, "Mission complete." If the spinal cord is severely damaged, nerve signals cannot get from the brain to the parts of the body below the injury. The patient's signs and symptoms will depend on the type and location of the injury (Figure 11-34).

Because your initial treatment of a patient with a possible injury to the spine can prevent further injury, you must know when to suspect this type of injury and how to provide appropriate care.

You Should Know

Every day in the United States, 30 people experience a spinal cord injury. The most common causes of this injury are motor vehicle crashes, sports accidents, falls, penetrating trauma, and industrial mishaps. Of these individuals, 60% are 30 years of age or younger.

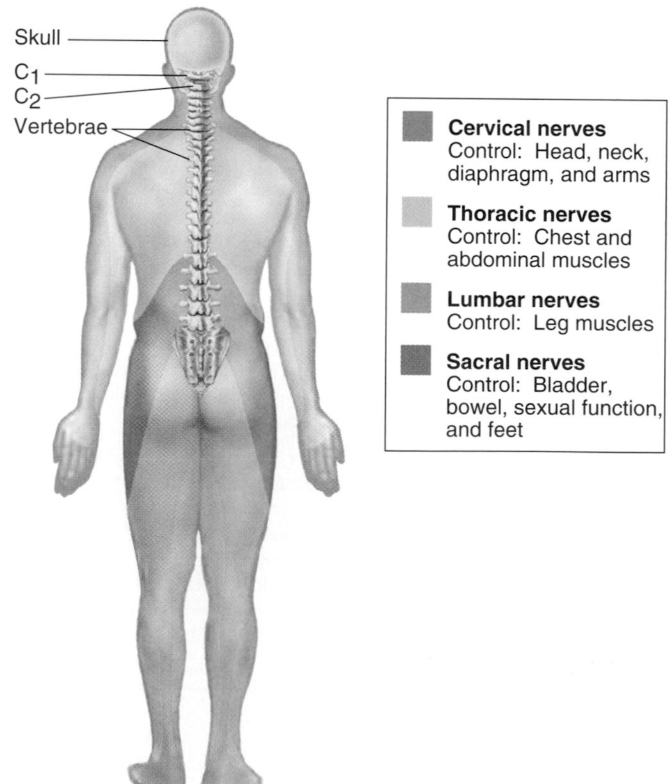

FIGURE 11-34 ► If the patient has a spinal cord injury, the signs and symptoms will depend on the location of the injury.

Mechanism of Injury

Objective 4 ▶

You should have a high index of suspicion for a spinal injury in situations involving any of the following mechanisms of injury:

- Motor vehicle crashes
- Blunt trauma (such as an assault)
- Ejection or fall from a transportation device (such as a bicycle, motorcycle, motorized scooter, snowmobile, skateboard, or rollerblades)
- Electrical injuries, lightning strike
- Involvement in an explosion
- Unresponsive trauma patients
- Hangings
- Any fall, particularly in an elderly patient
- Any shallow-water diving accident
- Any injury in which a helmet is broken (including a sports helmet, a motorcycle helmet, and an industrial hardhat)
- Any injury that penetrates the head, neck, or torso
- Any pedestrian-vehicle crash
- Any high-impact, high-force, or high-speed condition involving the head, spine, or torso

Children and the elderly are most likely to suffer an injury to the spinal cord without damage to the vertebrae.

Most spinal injuries occur to the cervical spine. The next most commonly injured areas are the thoracic and lumbar spine. The spinal column normally allows a limited amount of movement in a forward, backward, and side-to-side direction. Movement beyond this normal range can result in damage to the spinal column and possibly to the spinal cord. A spinal *column* injury (bony injury) can occur with or without a spinal *cord* injury. A spinal *cord* injury can also occur with or without an injury to the spinal *column.* The spinal cord does not have to be severed for a loss of function to occur. In most people with a spinal cord injury, the spinal cord is intact but the damage to it results in a loss of function.

A compression injury of the spine can drive the weight of the head into the neck or the pelvis into the torso (Figure 11-35).

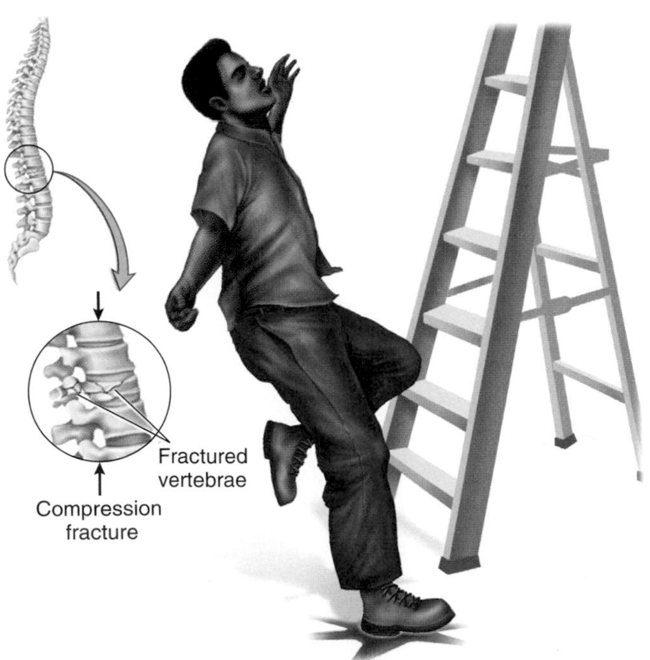

FIGURE 11-35 ▶ A compression injury of the spine can result from a fall from a significant height onto the head or legs. The force of the injury can drive the weight of the head into the neck or the pelvis into the torso.

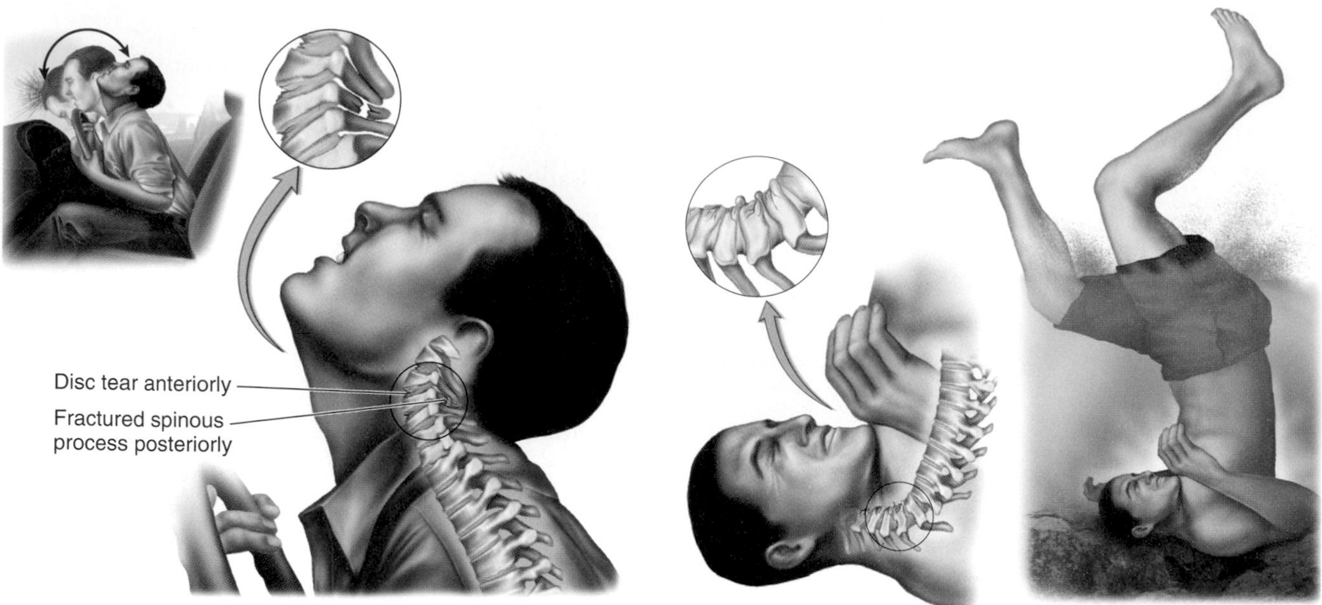

FIGURE 11-36 ▲ Severe backward movement of the head can result if the face hits the windshield in a motor vehicle crash.

FIGURE 11-37 ▲ Severe forward movement of the head onto the chest can result from diving into shallow water.

Compression injuries can result from any of the following:

- Contact sports
- Motor vehicle crashes with unrestrained occupants
- Dives into shallow water
- Falls from moving vehicles
- Falls from a significant height onto the head or legs

Compression fractures of the spine result in weakened vertebrae. A compression fracture can occur with or without a spinal cord injury.

Severe backward movement (extension) of the head can result from diving into shallow water, banging the face into the windshield in a motor vehicle crash, or falling and striking the face or chin (usually seen in an elderly person; Figure 11-36). Severe forward movement (flexion) of the head onto the chest can result from diving into shallow water, the sudden slowing down a motor vehicle, or being thrown from a horse or motorcycle (Figure 11-37). Severe rotation of the torso or head and neck can move one side of the spinal column against the other. A rotation injury can result from a motorcycle crash or a rollover motor vehicle crash. Injuries due to flexion, extension, or rotation can dislocate the disks between the vertebrae, compress the spinal cord, and stretch or tear ligaments in the neck or spine.

Contact sports and T-bone motor vehicle crashes can cause a sudden side impact that moves the torso sideways (lateral bending). The head remains in place until it is moved along by its attachments to the cervical spine. Lateral bending can compress and displace the vertebrae and stretch ligaments (Figure 11-38).

The spine can also be pulled apart (distraction). When the spine is distracted, ligaments and muscles are overstretched or torn and the vertebrae are pulled apart (Figure 11-39). This type of injury occurs in hangings and schoolyard or playground accidents, as well as when a snowmobile or motorcycle is ridden under rope or wire. The spine may also be injured as a result of a penetrating wound to the head, neck, or torso.

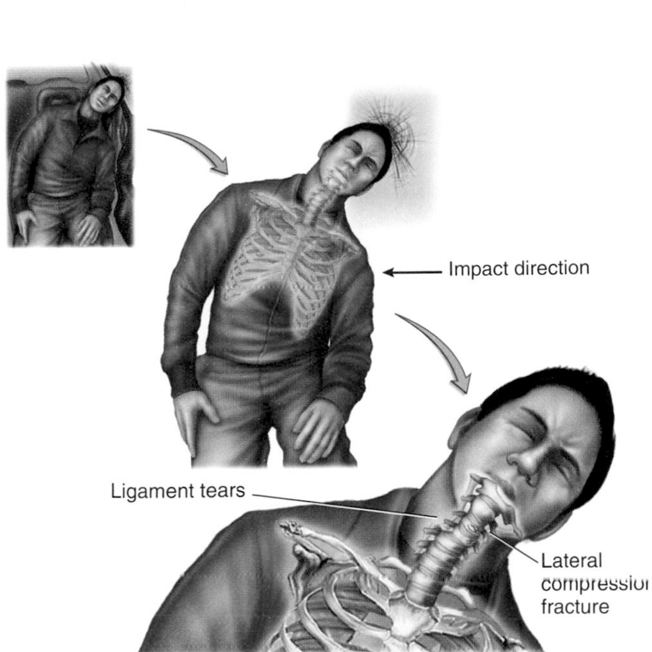

FIGURE 11-38 ▲ T-bone motor vehicle crashes can cause a sudden side impact that moves the torso sideways. The head remains in place until it is moved along by its attachments to the cervical spine.

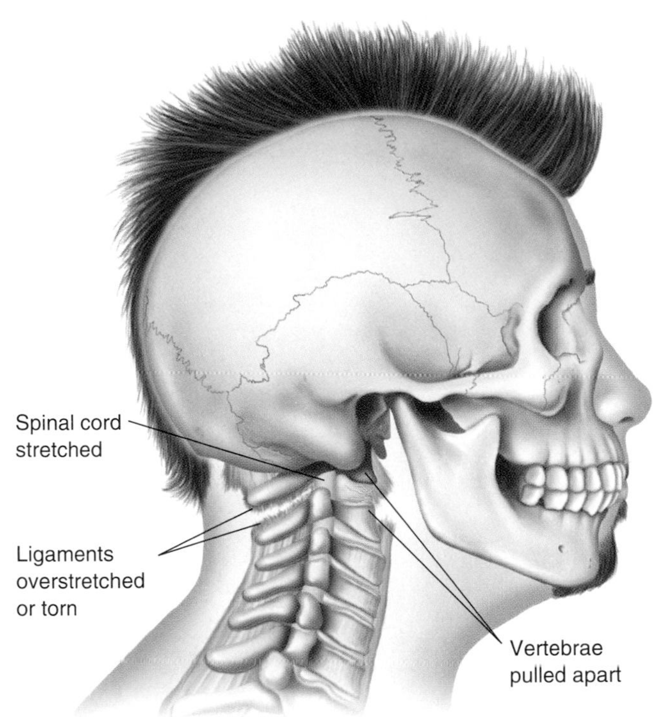

FIGURE 11-39 ▲ Ligaments and muscles are overstretched or torn and the vertebrae are pulled apart when the spine is distracted.

As is evident from the mechanisms of injury mentioned here, a spinal injury is often seen in a patient with injuries to other areas of the body, such as the head, chest, or abdomen. For this reason, it is important to treat every patient with a significant mechanism of injury as if he or she had a spinal injury until it is proven otherwise.

Stop and Think!

The patient's ability to walk, move his or her extremities, and feel sensation, as well as a lack of pain to the spinal column does *not* rule out the possibility of spinal column or spinal cord damage.

Signs and Symptoms of a Spinal Injury

Objective 5 ▶

The most common and devastating spinal injuries occur in the area of the neck (cervical spine).

An injury to the spinal cord may be complete or incomplete. A complete injury occurs when the spinal cord is severed. The patient has no voluntary movement or sensation below the level of the injury. Both sides of the body are equally affected. **Paraplegia** is the loss of movement and sensation in the body from the waist down. Paraplegia results from a spinal cord injury at the level of the thoracic or lumbar vertebrae (Figure 11-40). **Quadriplegia** (also called tetraplegia) is a loss of movement and sensation in both arms, both legs, and the parts of the body below an area of injury to the spinal cord. Quadriplegia results from a spinal cord injury at the level of the cervical vertebrae (Figure 11-41). In paraplegia and quadriplegia, the spinal cord is damaged so severely that nerve signals cannot be sent to areas below the damaged area or back again. About 3% of patients with a complete spinal

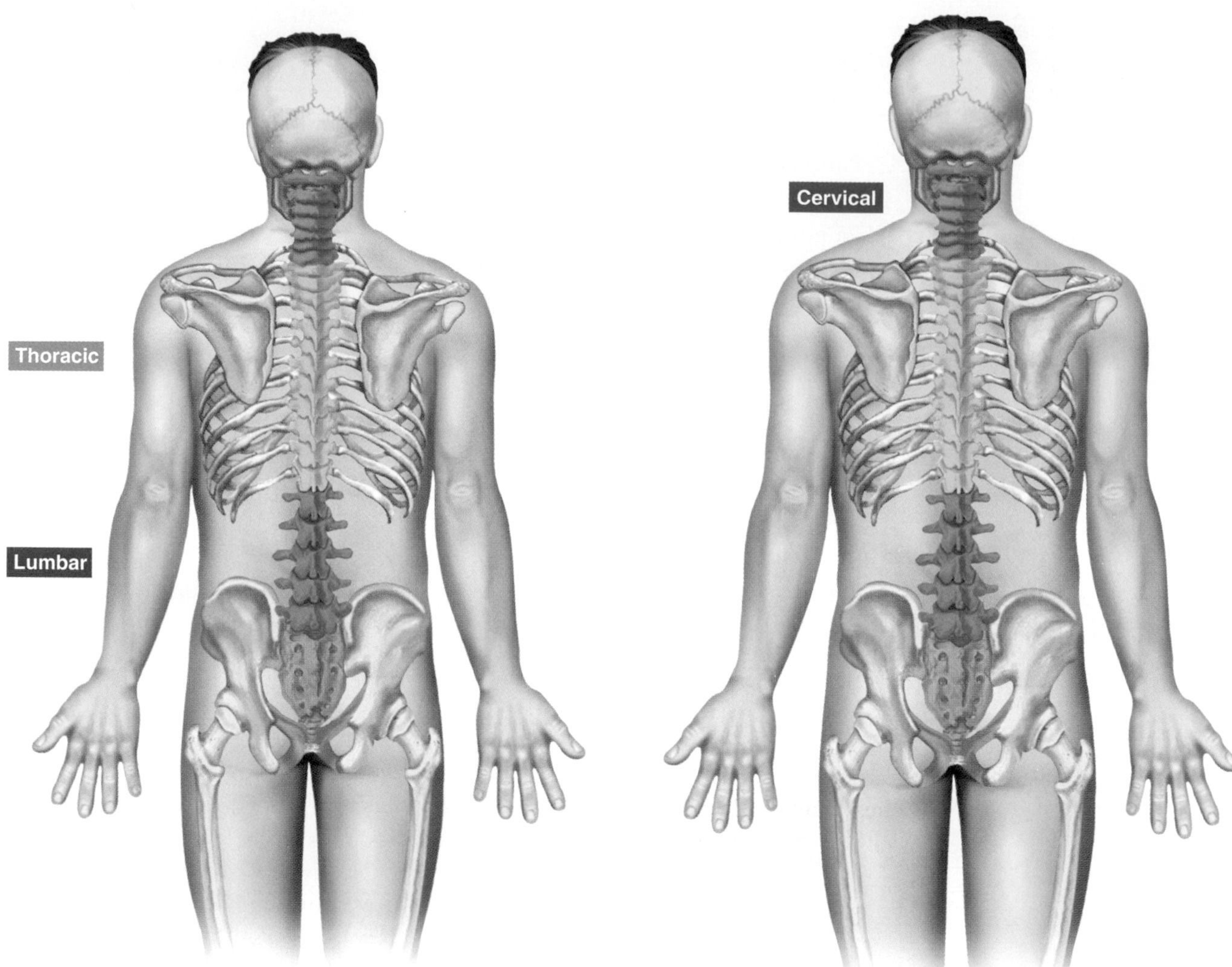

FIGURE 11-40 ▲ Paraplegia results from a spinal cord injury at the level of the thoracic or lumbar vertebrae.

FIGURE 11-41 ▲ Quadriplegia (also called tetraplegia) results from a spinal cord injury at the level of the cervical vertebrae.

cord injury will show some improvement over the first 24 hours after being injured. After 24 hours, improvement is almost never seen.

With an incomplete spinal cord injury, some parts of the spinal cord remain intact. Therefore, the patient has some function below the level of the injury. The patient may be able to move one extremity more than another, may be able to feel parts of the body that cannot be moved, or may have more function on one side of the body than the other. With an incomplete injury, there is a potential for recovery because function may be lost only temporarily.

Remember This!

Spinal cord and spinal column injuries are uncommon in children. However, when they do occur, children younger than eight years of age tend to injure the upper area of the cervical spine (the first and second cervical vertebrae). Adults and older children tend to have cervical spine injuries in the lower area of the cervical spine.

Tell the patient not to move while you are asking questions.

The signs and symptoms of a possible spinal injury include the following:

- Tenderness in the injured area
- Pain associated with movement (do *not* ask the patient to move to see if he or she has pain; do *not* move the patient to test for a pain response)
- Pain independent of movement or palpation along the spinal column
- Pain down the lower legs or into the rib cage
- Pain that comes and goes, usually along the spine and/or the lower legs
- Soft-tissue injuries associated with trauma to the head and neck (cuts, bruises)
- Numbness, weakness, or tingling in the extremities
- A loss of sensation or paralysis below the site of injury
- A loss of sensation or paralysis in the upper or lower extremities
- Difficulty breathing
- A loss of bladder or bowel control
- An inability to walk, move extremities, or feel sensation
- Deformity or muscle spasm along the spinal column

"C3, 4, and 5 keep the diaphragm alive" (cervical vertebrae 3, 4, and 5).

The amount of weakness or loss of sensation your patient has will depend on the extent of the injury. It will also depend on the amount of pressure on the spinal cord or spinal nerves. Be prepared for breathing problems if your patient has an injury to the cervical or thoracic spine. An important nerve that stimulates the diaphragm exits the spinal cord between the third and fifth vertebrae in the neck. If this nerve is severed or compressed, the patient's diaphragm is usually paralyzed. If the diaphragm is paralyzed, you will see shallow abdominal breathing. A spinal cord injury involving the lower neck or upper chest may result in paralysis of the muscles between the ribs. Patients with these injuries will usually need help breathing with a bag-valve-mask device. Give oxygen if it is available and you have been trained to use it.

Making a Difference

Managing a patient with a suspected spinal injury can directly affect the patient's outcome. The early recognition of a spinal injury can help reduce permanent disability and even prevent death. It is *critical* that you have a high index of suspicion for a spinal injury based on the mechanism of injury, even when there are no outward signs of trauma. If the mechanism of injury suggests it, suspect a spinal injury and treat your patient accordingly.

Emergency Medical Responder Care of a Spinal Injury

To treat a patient with a spinal injury, use the following steps:

1. Conduct a scene size-up and ensure your safety. Evaluate the mechanism of injury before approaching the patient. Put on appropriate PPE.
2. Form a general impression and determine the urgency of further assessment and care.
3. Perform an initial assessment to identify and treat any life-threatening conditions. If the mechanism of injury suggests a spinal injury, ask an assistant to stabilize the patient's cervical spine manually while you assess the patient's airway (Figure 11-42.) Maintain manual stabilization of the patient's cervical spine until EMS personnel arrive and assume patient care or until the patient has been completely immobilized on a long backboard.

Ask the patient not to move his or her head while answering questions. Face the patient, so that he or she does not have to turn his or her head to talk with you.

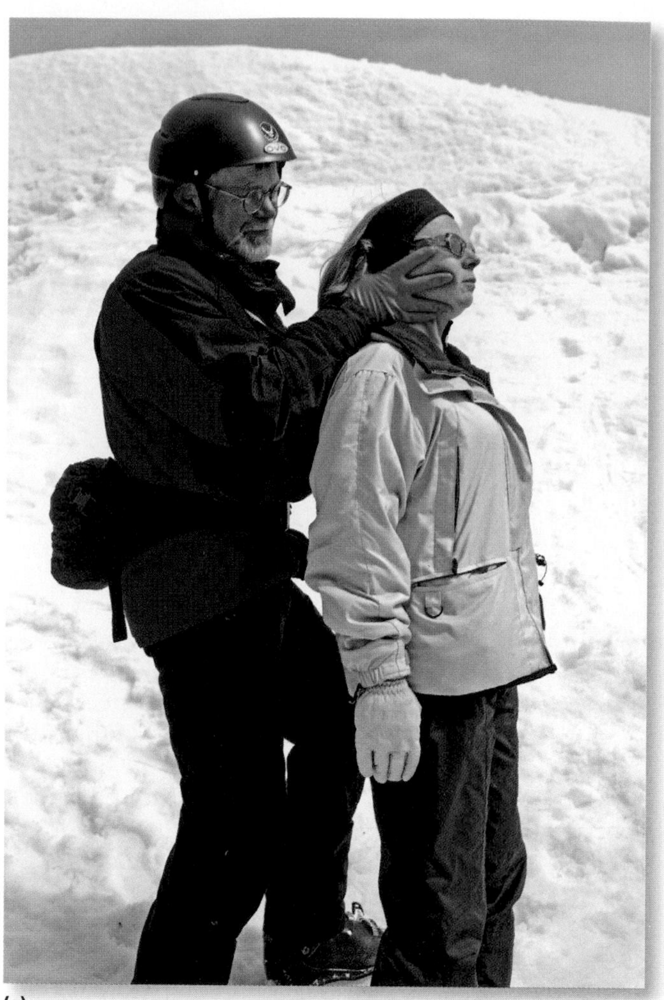

(a)

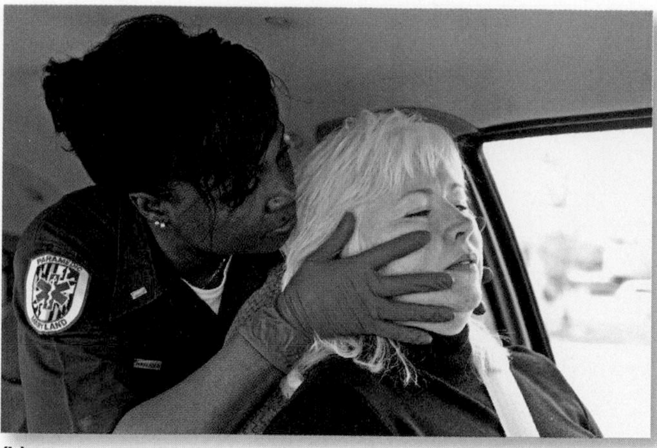

(b)

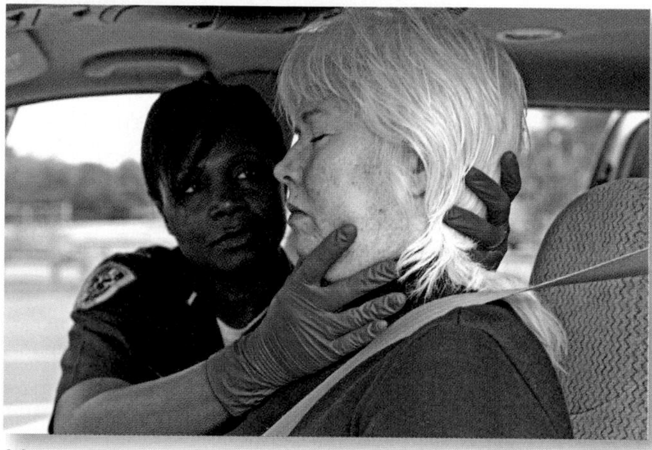

(c)

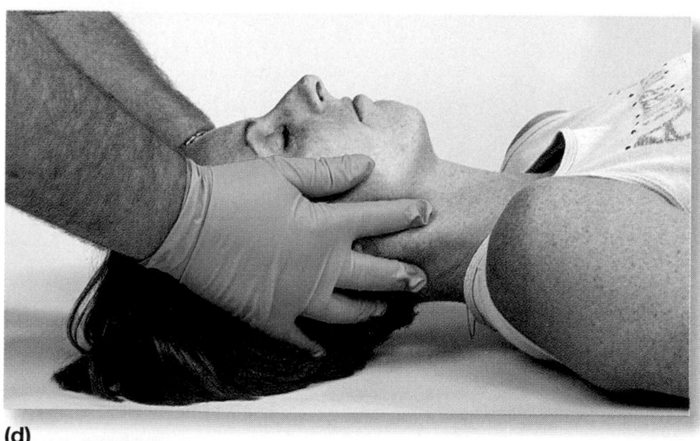

(d)

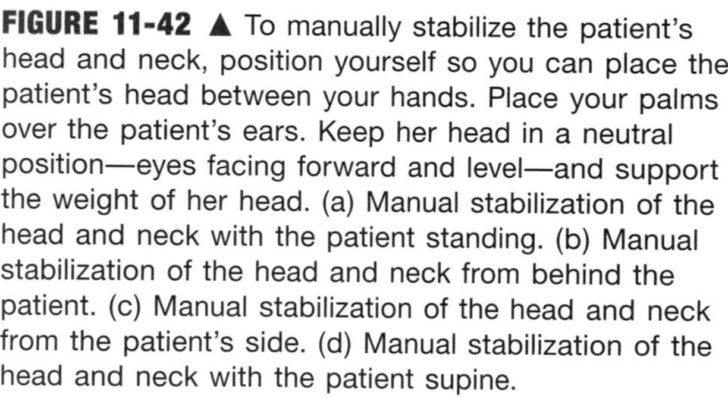

FIGURE 11-42 ▲ To manually stabilize the patient's head and neck, position yourself so you can place the patient's head between your hands. Place your palms over the patient's ears. Keep her head in a neutral position—eyes facing forward and level—and support the weight of her head. (a) Manual stabilization of the head and neck with the patient standing. (b) Manual stabilization of the head and neck from behind the patient. (c) Manual stabilization of the head and neck from the patient's side. (d) Manual stabilization of the head and neck with the patient supine.

- Establish and maintain an open airway. If the patient is unresponsive, remember that a jaw-thrust without head tilt is the only acceptable method for opening the airway in a patient with a suspected spinal injury. Insert an oropharyngeal airway if needed. Suction as necessary.
- If the patient's breathing is inadequate, assist his breathing with a bag-valve-mask device. Provide oxygen if it is available and you have been trained to use it.
- Control bleeding.
- If signs of shock are present or if internal bleeding is suspected, treat for shock.

Objective 6 ▶

4. Perform a physical examination. Check distal pulses, movement, and sensation (PMS) in each extremity. Compare each extremity with the opposite extremity.
   - To assess movement, ask the patient if he can
     - Shrug his shoulders
     - Spread the fingers of both hands
     - Squeeze your fingers and release them
     - Wiggle his toes
     - Push down with each foot against your hand ("gas pedal") and then pull the foot up
   - To assess sensation, touch the fingers and toes of each extremity and ask the patient to tell you where you are touching.
   - If the patient is unresponsive, assess movement and sensation by pinching each foot and hand. See if the patient responds to pain with facial movements or movement of the extremity.
5. Apply a rigid cervical collar (also called a c-collar) if the equipment is available and you have been trained to use it. The technique for applying a cervical collar is discussed in the section "Spinal Immobilization Techniques." If a cervical collar is applied, the patient will need to be immobilized on a backboard.
6. Take the patient's vital signs and gather the patient's medical history. Determine the events leading to the present situation by asking the following questions:
   - What happened?
   - When did the injury occur?
   - Where does it hurt?
   - Does your neck or back hurt?
   - Were you wearing a seat belt?
   - Did you pass out before the accident?
   - Did you move or did someone move you before we arrived?
   - Have your symptoms changed from the time of the injury until the time we arrived?
7. Cover open wounds with a sterile dressing.
8. Splint any bone or joint injuries. If the mechanism of injury suggests the patient has experienced an injury to the spine, the spine must be immobilized. You may be expected to immobilize the patient yourself or assist arriving EMS personnel in doing so. Immobilization techniques are discussed in the section "Spinal Immobilization Techniques."

Stop and Think!

You can use a backboard in specific situations without using a cervical collar. But you must never use a cervical collar without a backboard. For example, a patient in shock from a medical cause may be placed on a backboard. In this situation, a cervical collar is not necessary. However, if you apply a cervical collar because the mechanism of injury warrants it, then the patient needs to be immobilized on a backboard.

Objective 9 ▶

8. Comfort, calm, and reassure the patient while waiting for EMS personnel. Keep in mind that injuries to muscles and bones are painful. Your patient may be worried about a permanent loss of function of the injured area or possible disfigurement. Listen to your patient and do your best to comfort him. Perform ongoing assessments every 5 minutes if the patient is in shock and every 15 minutes if the patient is stable.

Making a Difference

Manual Stabilization of the Head and Neck

Manual stabilization of the head and neck is also called in-line stabilization. Manual stabilization of the head and neck helps prevent further injury to the spine.

- To manually stabilize the patient's head and neck, position yourself so that you can place the patient's head between your hands. You must be able to hold that position comfortably for a significant length of time. Place your palms over the patient's ears. Spread your fingers on each side of the patient's head for added stability. Keep the head in a neutral position and support the weight of the head.
  - When the head and neck are in a neutral (in-line) position, they are in an anatomically correct position. The eyes are facing forward and level, and the patient's nose is in line with the navel.
- Do *not* excessively move the head forward, backward, or from side to side. Do *not* pull on the patient's head or neck. If the patient is lying on his or her back, place your forearms on the ground for support. If the patient is sitting or standing, support your forearms by placing them on the patient's back or chest.
- If an attempt to move the patient's head and neck into a neutral position results in any of the following, *stop* any movement and stabilize the head in the position in which it was found:
  - Airway obstruction
  - Difficulty breathing
  - Neck muscle spasm
  - Increased pain
  - Onset or worsening of numbness or tingling, loss of movement
  - Resistance that is felt when moving the head to a neutral position

Use rolled towels or blanket rolls secured with tape or triangular bandages to stabilize the head and neck in the position in which it was found.

- Continue manual stabilization of the patient's cervical spine until either a cervical collar has been applied and the patient is fully immobilized on a long backboard or additional EMS resources have arrived and have assumed patient care.

A cervical collar cannot be applied to the patient in these situations.

Spinal Immobilization Techniques

You may be expected to immobilize or assist with immobilizing a patient with a suspected spinal injury. The equipment used for spinal immobilization includes

- A cervical collar, large towels, a blanket, or a commercial device to secure the head (such as a head block)
- A long backboard
- Straps, tape, triangular bandages, or 4-inch roller gauze

Some of the more common techniques used for spinal immobilization are discussed in this section.

Cervical Collars

After assessing the front and back of the patient's neck, apply a rigid cervical collar (c-collar) if the equipment is available and you have been trained to use it. When used alone, a rigid cervical collar does not immobilize. For effective immobilization, a rigid collar must be used with manual stabilization or a spinal immobilization device, such as a backboard. A rigid collar is used to

- Temporarily splint the head and neck in a neutral position
- Limit movement of the cervical spine
- Support the weight of the patient's head while she is in a sitting position
- Help maintain the cervical spine in a neutral position when the patient is lying on her back
- Remind the patient and other healthcare professionals that the mechanism of injury suggests a possible spinal injury

The technique for applying a cervical collar is shown in Skill Drill 11-4.

If a cervical collar is not available or does not fit the patient, the patient's head and neck can be stabilized using a long backboard, rolled towels, or a blanket (Figure 11-43).

You should apply a rigid cervical collar *only* if it fits properly:

- If the collar is too tight, it can apply pressure on the blood vessels in the patient's neck and reduce blood flow.
- If the collar is too loose, it can cover the patient's chin and mouth, causing an airway obstruction. If it is too loose, it will also not adequately stabilize the head and neck.
- A collar that is too short will not provide adequate stabilization because the patient's head can move forward.

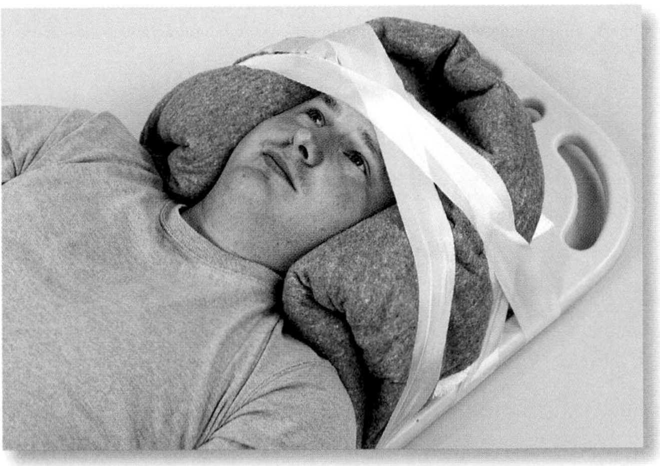

FIGURE 11-43 ► If a cervical collar is not available or does not fit the patient, the patient's head and neck can be stabilized using a long backboard and rolled towels or a blanket.

Skill Drill 11-4

Applying A Cervical Collar

STEP 1 ▶
- Ask an assistant to maintain manual stabilization of the patient's head and neck in a neutral position.
- Assess distal pulses, movement, and sensation.
- Measure the width of the patient's neck by placing your fingers between the patient's lower jaw and shoulder.

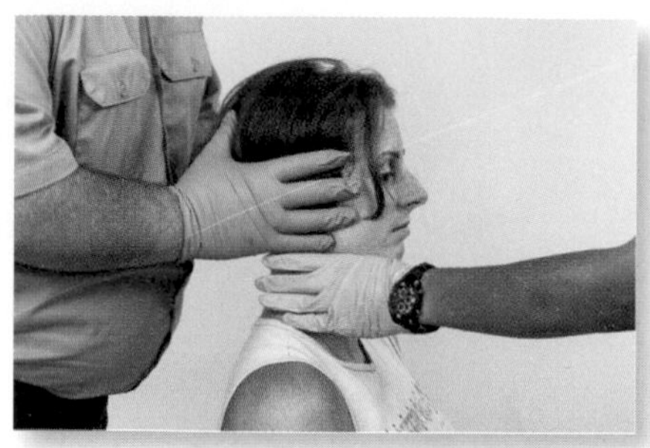

STEP 2 ▶ Select a rigid cervical collar and measure the device. Adjust the size of the collar to fit the patient's measurements as necessary.

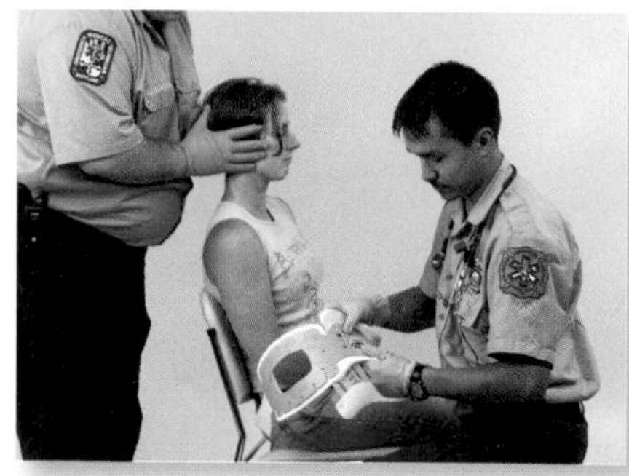

STEP 3 ▶
- Apply the cervical collar to the patient.
- Check to make sure the collar fits according to the manufacturer's instructions.
- Continue manual stabilization of the patient's head and neck until the patient is fully immobilized to a long backboard.
- Remember to check distal pulses, movement, and sensation after applying the collar.

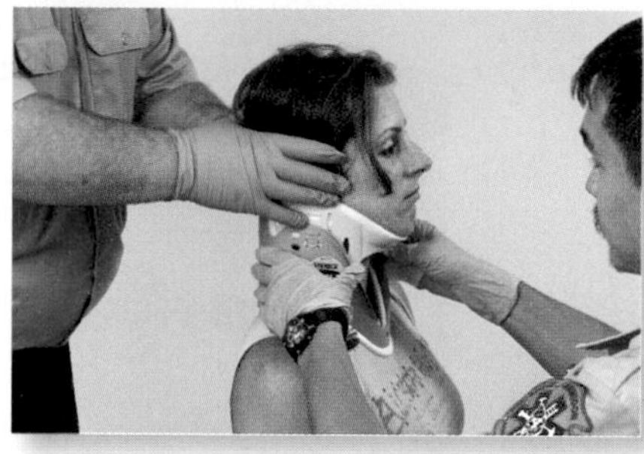

- A collar that is too tall will not provide adequate stabilization because the patient's head will be moved backward by the collar. The collar can also force the jaw closed, limiting access to the airway.

Two-Person or Three-Person Log Roll

You may encounter situations in which you find an unresponsive patient who is lying face down. If the scene suggests that the patient has experienced a trauma, such as a fall or a blow to the body, you should assume a spinal injury exists. A **log roll** is a technique used to move a patient from a face-down to a face-up position while keeping the head and neck in line with the rest of the body. This technique is also used to place a patient with a suspected spinal injury on a backboard. The steps to perform a three-person log roll are shown in Skill Drill 11-5. If you have log-rolled the patient from a face-down to a face-up position but a backboard is not available, provide care to the patient in the position he or she is in until EMS personnel arrive.

Three-Person Log Roll

STEP 1 ▶
- Take appropriate BSI precautions.
- Rescuer #1 kneels at the patient's head, maintaining manual in-line immobilization of the patient's head and neck. This rescuer will direct the move.

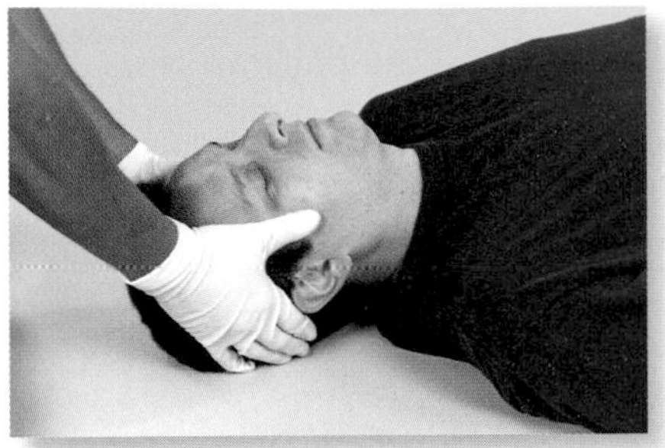

STEP 2 ▶ Rescuer #2 sizes and applies a rigid cervical collar.

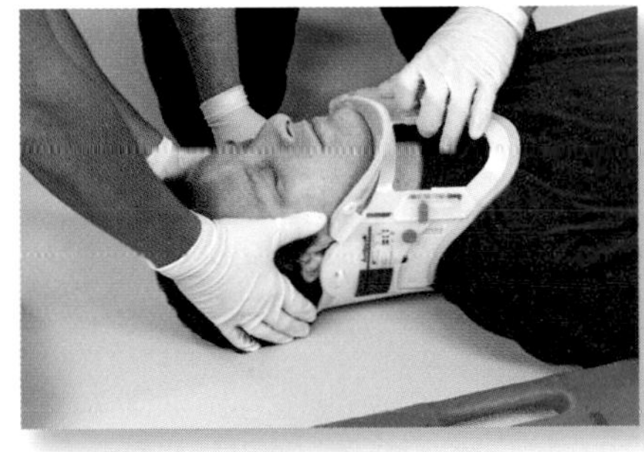

STEP 3 ▶
- Rescuers #2 and #3 position a long backboard at one side of the patient.
- The patient is positioned with his legs and arms straight out at his or her sides, palms facing in.
- Rescuer #2 is positioned at the patient's midchest with his hands placed on the patient's far shoulder and hip.
- Rescuer #3 is positioned at the patient's upper legs with her hands placed on the patient's hip and hand as well as his lower leg.
- If the patient has an injury to the chest or abdomen, he should be rolled onto his uninjured side if possible.

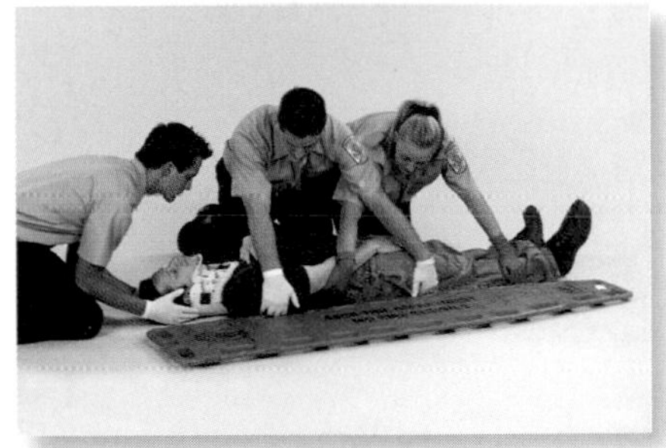

STEP 4 ▶
- When everyone is ready, Rescuer #1 gives the order to roll the patient.
- Rescuer #1 maintains manual stabilization of the patient's head and neck.
- Rescuers #2 and #3 roll the patient onto his side toward them. The patient's head, shoulders, and pelvis are kept in line during the roll.

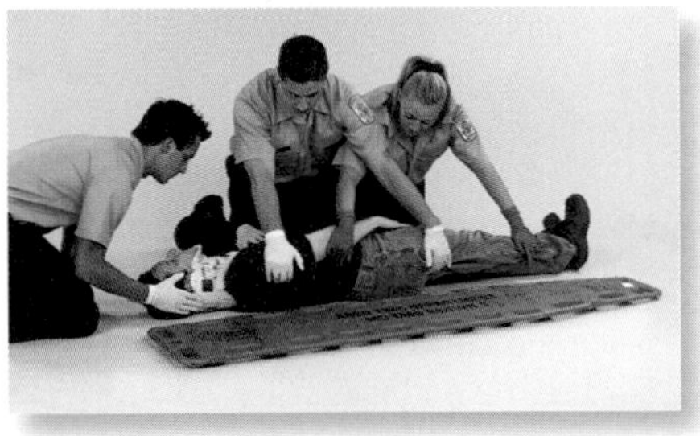

Continued on next page

Skill Drill 11-5

Three-Person Log Roll *(continued)*

STEP 5 ▶ The patient's back is quickly assessed. A long backboard is positioned under the patient.

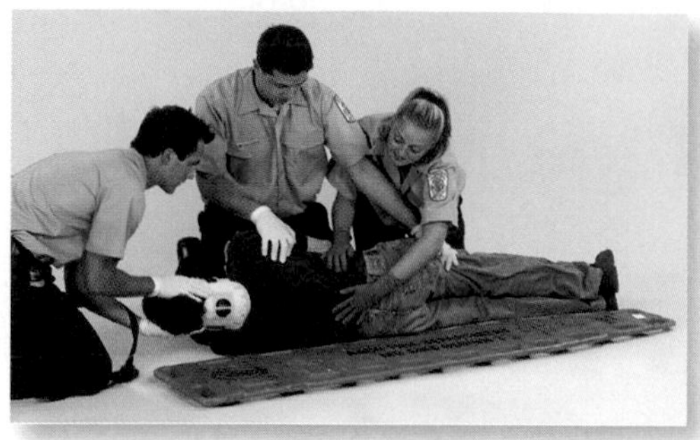

STEP 6 ▶
- When everyone is ready, Rescuer #1 gives the order to roll the patient onto the backboard. If the backboard was angled, the patient and the backboard are lowered to the ground together.
- Manual stabilization of the patient's head and neck is continued until the patient is fully immobilized to the backboard.

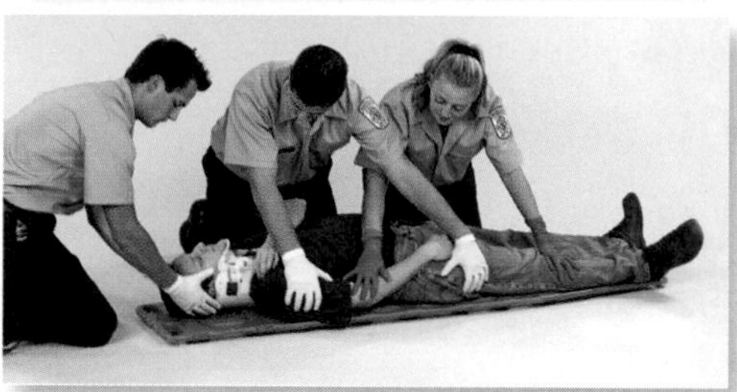

Making a Difference

Remember: Once the patient has been immobilized on the long backboard, he or she will have limited sight. Explain all movements before starting them so that the patient will not be frightened.

Immobilization of a Supine Patient on a Long Backboard

Long backboards help stabilize the head, neck and torso, pelvis, and extremities. They are used to immobilize patients found in a lying, standing, or sitting position.

If your patient is a woman, place the chest strap above her breasts and under her arms, not across the breasts.

After a patient has been log-rolled onto a long backboard, she must be secured to it. To maintain an adult's head and neck in a neutral position, place 1–2 inches of padding on the board under the patient's head (Figure 11-44). Be careful to avoid extra movement. To maintain the head of an infant or a child younger than three years in a neutral position, you may need to place padding under the infant's or child's torso. The padding should extend from the shoulders to the pelvis. It should be thick enough for the child's shoulders to be in line with her ear canal (Figure 11-45). An older child may not require padding to obtain a neutral position.

Pad any hollow areas (spaces) between the patient and the board as necessary. These spaces include the small of the back and under the patient's knees. Immobilize the patient's torso to the board. Immobilize the upper torso to the board with one strap over the chest or, preferably, with two straps placed in an "X" fashion. Make sure that the straps are tight enough to limit patient movement, but not so tight that they restrict breathing.

Immobilize the pelvis to the board with a strap centered over the patient's hips. Secure the patient's upper legs to the board with a strap across the legs above the knees. Secure the lower legs with a strap across the legs below the knees. Secure the

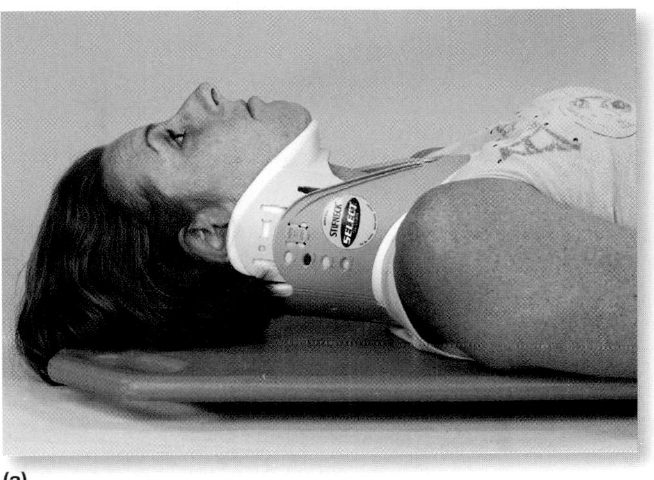

(a)

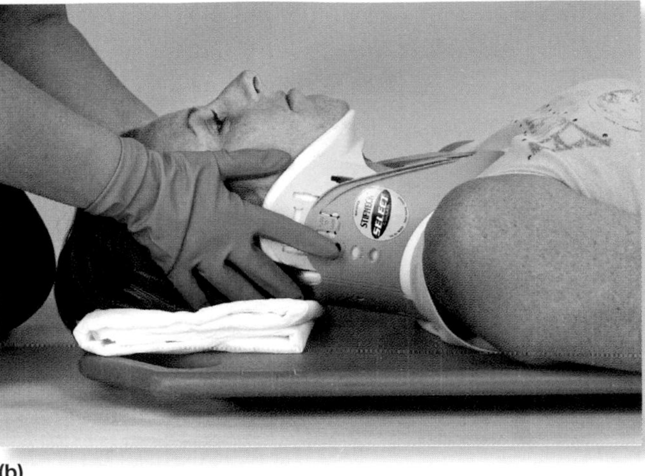

(b)

FIGURE 11-44 ▲ (a) Head and neck stabilization of an adult without padding. (b) Head and neck stabilization of an adult with 1–2 inches of padding on the board under the patient's head.

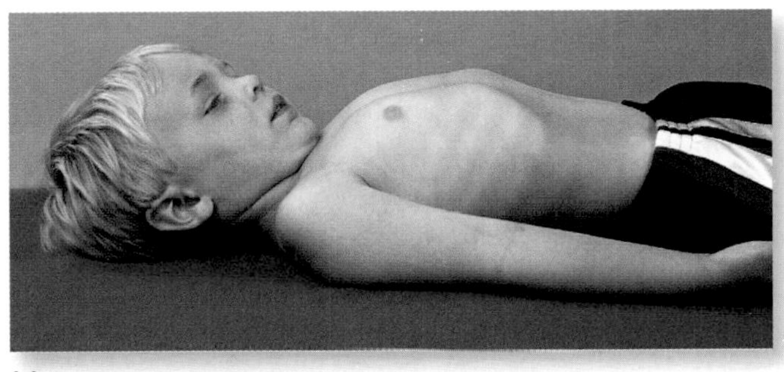

(a)

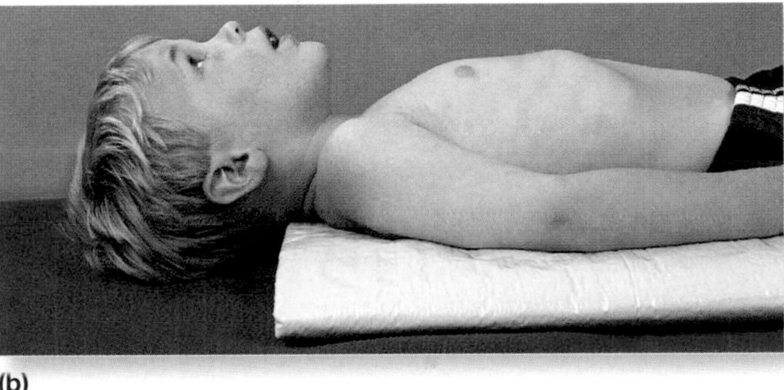

(b)

FIGURE 11-45 ▲ (a) Infants and young children have large heads, which causes the head to move forward when placed on a flat surface. (b) To maintain the head in a neutral position, you may need to place padding under the child's torso. The padding should extend from the shoulders to the pelvis and be thick enough so that the child's shoulders are in line with the ear canal.

The head is secured to the board *last*. You must maintain manual stabilization of the head and neck until the head and the rest of the body are secured to the board.

patient's arms to the board. Secure the patient's head to the board with a ready-made head immobilizer, rolled towels, or blanket rolls. Place a strap or tape snugly across the patient's lower forehead. Place another strap or tape snugly across the front portion of the cervical collar. Reassess the security of the straps. Reassess pulses, movement, and sensation in all extremities (Figure 11-46).

Stop and Think!

Once a patient has been fully immobilized on a backboard, a healthcare professional must remain with the patient *at all times*. Because immobilization will restrict the patient's ability to keep the airway open, a healthcare professional must assume this responsibility. If the patient vomits, turn the board and patient together as a unit and clear the airway.

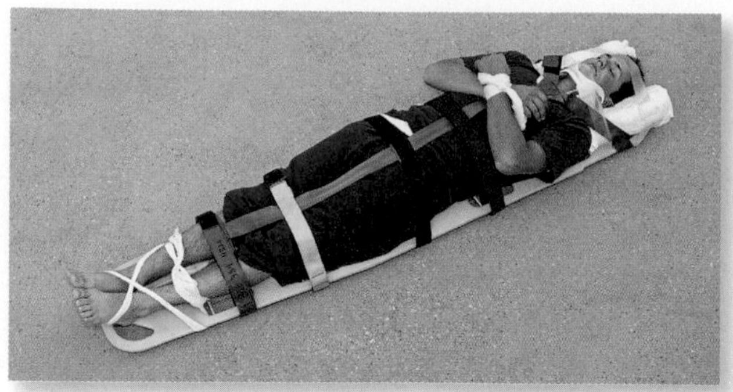

FIGURE 11-46 ▶ A patient fully immobilized to a long backboard.

Short Backboard Immobilization

There are several types of short backboard immobilization devices, including vest-type devices and a rigid short backboard. Short backboards help immobilize a patient's head, neck, and torso. A short backboard is used for the following purposes:

- To immobilize a seated patient who has a suspected spinal injury and stable vital signs
- To immobilize a patient in a confined space
- To be used as a long backboard for a small child

In most areas, vest-type devices are used primarily for extrication. They feature straps to secure the patient's head, chest, and legs. Once the patient has been extricated, the patient should remain in the device and be secured to a long backboard. The steps used to apply a vest-type device are shown in Skill Drill 11-6.

Helmet Removal

It can be a challenge to properly assess a patient wearing a helmet. There are two main types of helmets: sports helmets and motorcycle helmets. Sports helmets usually open in the front and provide easy access to the patient's airway once the face guard is removed. The face guard can be unclipped, unsnapped, removed with a screwdriver, or cut off using rescue scissors. Some sports helmets, such as those used in football and ice hockey, are custom fitted to the individual. Motorcycle helmets usually have a shield that covers the entire face. The face shield can be unbuckled or snapped off to access the patient's airway.

Do not assume that a helmet must be removed. If your patient has a spinal injury, removing the helmet could worsen the injury. To determine if a helmet should be left in place or removed, you should first ask yourself the following questions:

- Can I access the patient's airway?
- Is the patient's airway clear?
- Is the patient breathing adequately?
- Is there room to apply a facemask if it is necessary to assist the patient's breathing?
- How well does the helmet fit?
- Can the patient's head move within the helmet?
- Can the patient's spine be immobilized in a neutral position if the helmet is left in place?

Spinal Immobilization of a Seated Patient

STEP 1
- Rescuer #1 manually stabilizes the patient's head and neck.
- Rescuer #2 assesses the patient's pulses, movement, and sensation in all extremities.
- After the front and back of the patient's neck have been assessed, a rigid cervical collar is applied.

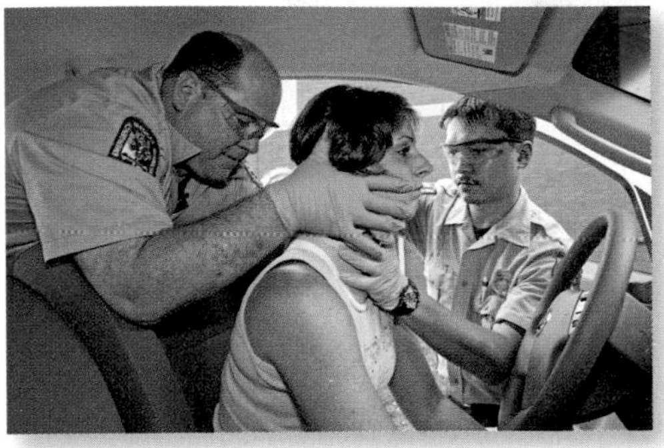

STEP 2 Rescuer #2 positions the vest-type device behind the patient.

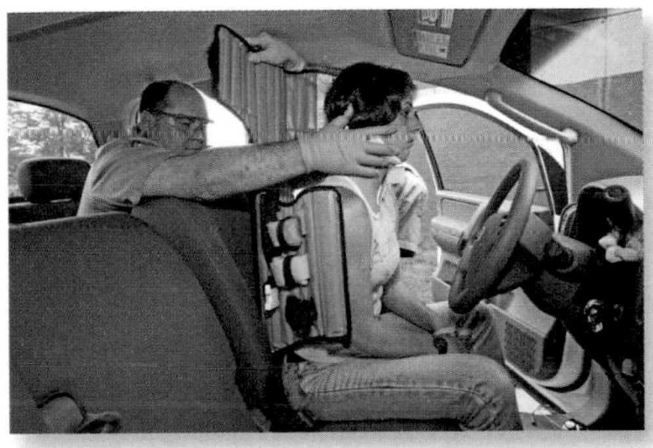

STEP 3
- Rescuer #2 positions the chest panels snugly into the patient's armpits.
- The device is then secured to the patient's torso. Rescuer #2 fastens all chest straps, making sure that the straps are snug but do not interfere with breathing.

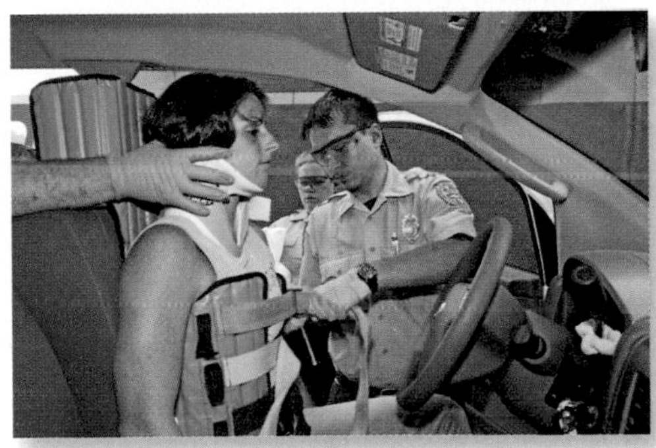

STEP 4
- Rescuer #2 secures the patient's legs next. The leg straps are loosened and wrapped around the leg on the same side. The straps are then fastened and tightened.
- Rescuer #2 evaluates the position of the device and makes sure all straps are secure.

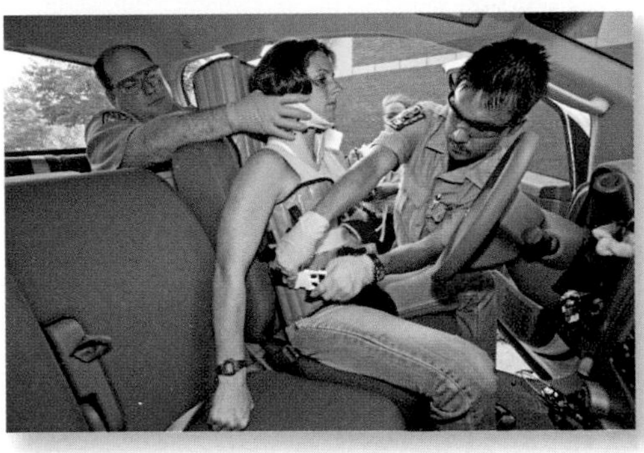

Continued on next page

Skill Drill 11-6

Spinal Immobilization of a Seated Patient *(continued)*

STEP 5 ▶

- To keep the patient's head in a neutral position, Rescuer #2 applies firm padding to any hollow areas between the patient's head and the head-piece of the device.
- Rescuer #2 then positions the head flaps on the side of the patient's head, coordinating with Rescuer #1 to maintain manual stabilization of the head and neck.
- Rescuer #2 then secures the head flaps using elastic straps or wide tape.

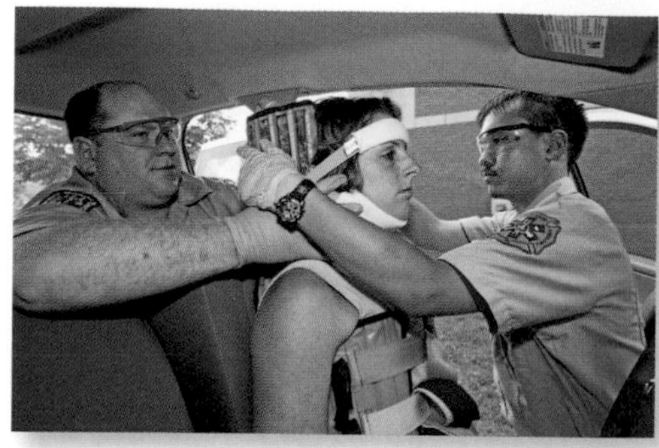

STEP 6 ▶

- After the patient's head is secured to the device, Rescuer #1 releases manual stabilization of the head.
- Rescuer #2 reassesses distal pulses, movement, and sensation in each extremity.

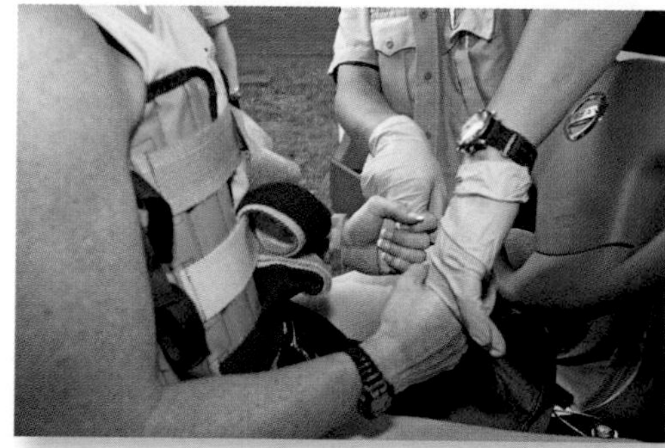

STEP 7 ▶

- The patient is rotated so that her back is to the opening through which the patient will be removed. A long backboard is positioned through the opening and placed under the patient.
- The patient is lowered onto the long backboard and slid into position on the board.

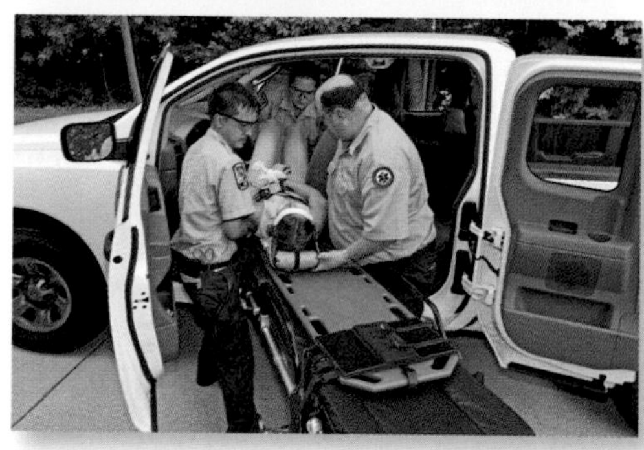

STEP 8 ▶

- The leg straps on the vest-type device are loosened so that the patient can extend her legs out straight. The straps are then retightened.
- The patient is then secured to a long backboard.
- Pulses, movement, and sensation are reassessed in all extremities.

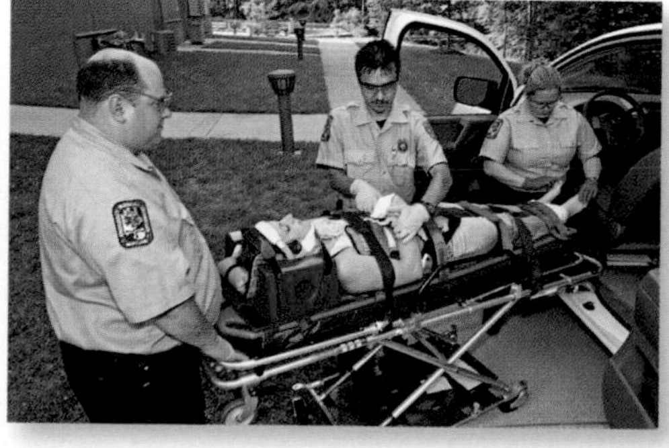

You should *leave a helmet in place* in the following circumstances:

- There are no impending airway or breathing problems.
- The helmet fits well, with little or no movement of the patient's head within the helmet.
- Helmet removal would cause further injury to the patient.
- Proper spinal immobilization can be performed with the helmet in place.
- The presence of the helmet does not interfere with your ability to assess and reassess airway and breathing.

You should *remove a helmet* in these circumstances:

- You are unable to assess and/or reassess the patient's airway and breathing.
- The helmet limits your ability to adequately manage the patient's airway or breathing.
- The helmet does not fit properly, allowing excessive head movement within the helmet.
- You cannot properly immobilize the patient's spine with the helmet in place.
- The patient is in cardiac arrest.

At least two rescuers are needed to remove a helmet. The method used for helmet removal depends on the type of helmet worn by the patient. Skill Drill 11-7 shows the steps for removing a motorcycle helmet from a patient with a possible spinal injury.

Injuries to the Head

Head injuries can be caused by a variety of mechanisms that result in pain, swelling, bleeding, and deformity. These mechanisms of injury are similar to those previously described for spinal injuries. Mechanisms of injury such as motor vehicle crashes and falls often cause the patient to become unresponsive. When a patient loses consciousness, she loses the ability to protect her own airway. Appropriate airway management and breathing support are critical when treating a patient with a head injury.

Injuries to the Scalp

The outermost part of the head is called the scalp. An injury to the scalp may occur because of blunt or penetrating trauma. The scalp contains tissue, hair follicles, sweat glands, oil glands, and a rich supply of blood vessels. When injured, these areas may bleed heavily. In children, the amount of blood loss from a scalp wound may be enough to produce shock. In adults, shock is usually not due to a scalp wound or internal skull injuries. More often, in adults, shock results from an injury elsewhere.

Assess the scalp carefully for cuts because some are not easy to detect. Control bleeding with direct pressure. Do not apply excessive pressure to the open wound if you suspect a skull fracture. Doing so can push bone fragments into the brain.

Injuries to the Skull

Because the brain is protected by a rigid container, called the skull, a scalp injury may or may not cause an injury to the brain.

The skull's job is to protect the brain from injury. However, damage to the skull can cause damage to the brain. Skull injuries may occur from blunt or penetrating trauma. Significant force, such as a severe impact or blow, can result in a skull fracture. The signs of a skull fracture are shown in Figure 11-47.

Skill Drill 11-7

Removing a Motorcycle Helmet

STEP 1 ▶ Rescuer #1 positions him- or herself at the patient's head and removes the face shield from the helmet to assess airway and breathing. If the patient is wearing eyeglasses, they should be removed.

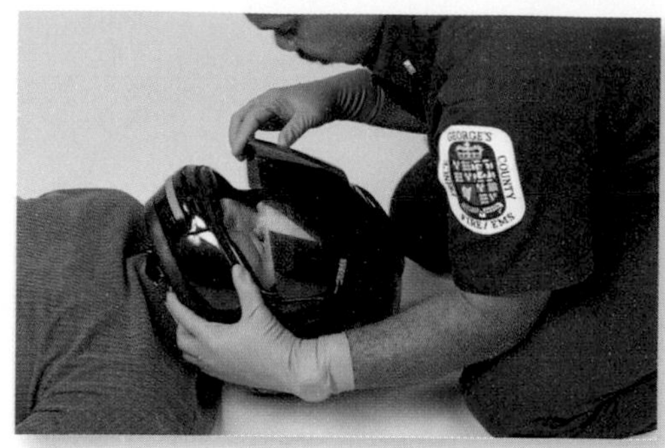

STEP 2 ▶
- Rescuer #1 stabilizes the helmet by placing his or her hands on each side of the helmet. The rescuer's fingers should be on the patient's lower jaw to prevent movement.
- Rescuer #2 loosens the helmet strap.

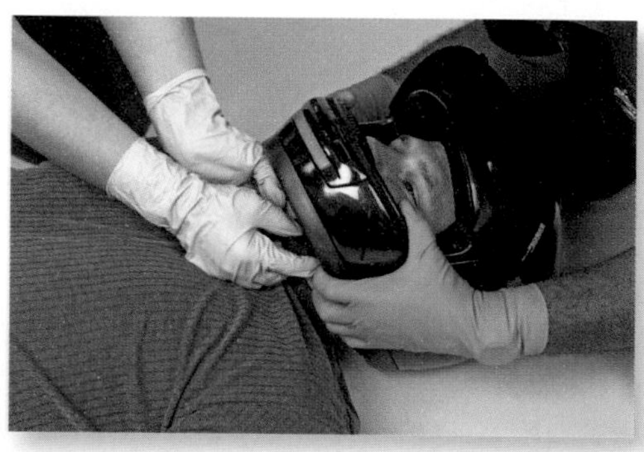

STEP 3 ▶ Rescuer #2 assumes manual stabilization by placing one hand on the patient's lower jaw at the angle of the jaw. The rescuer's other hand should be under the neck and behind the patient's head at the back of the head.

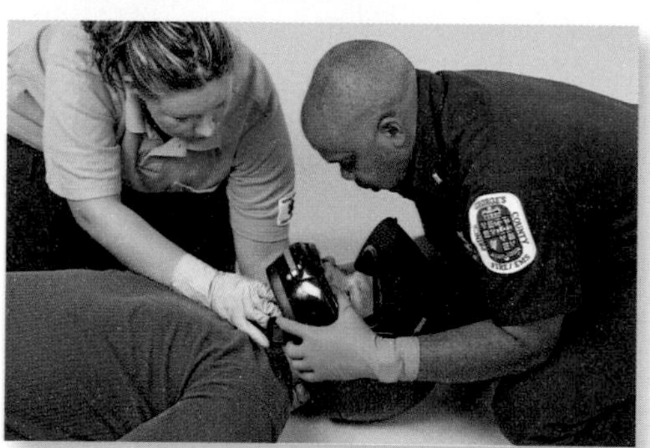

STEP 4 ▶ Rescuer #1 pulls out on the sides of the helmet to clear the patient's ears, gently slips the helmet halfway off the patient's head, and then stops.

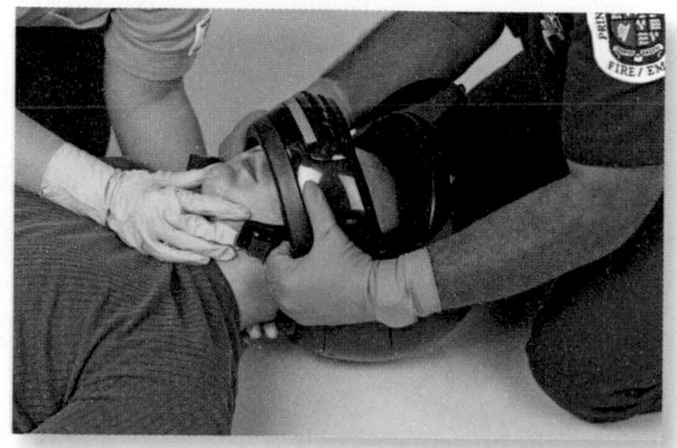

STEP 5 ▶ • Rescuer #2 slides the hand supporting the occiput (the back of the patient's head) toward the top of the patient's head to prevent the head from falling back after complete helmet removal.
• Rescuer #1 tilts the helmet backward to clear the nose and removes the helmet completely.

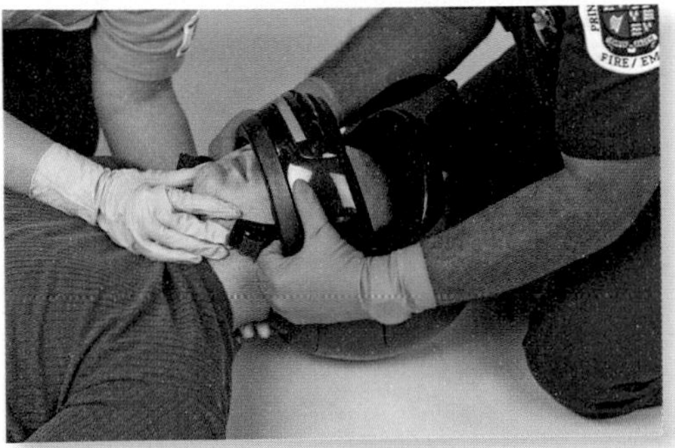

STEP 6 ▶ Manual stabilization is continued until the patient is fully immobilized to a long backboard.

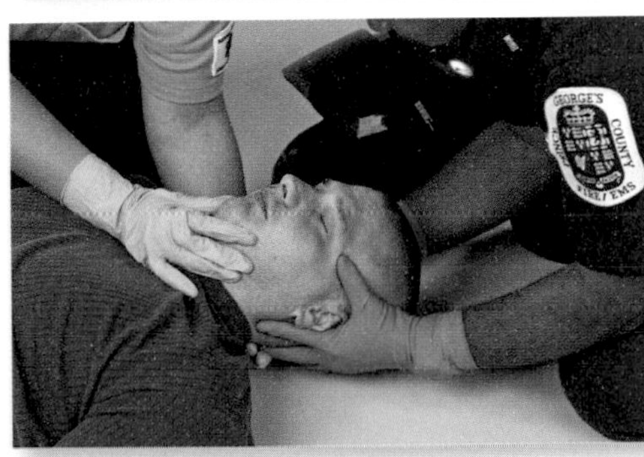

FIGURE 11-47 ▶ Signs of a skull fracture.

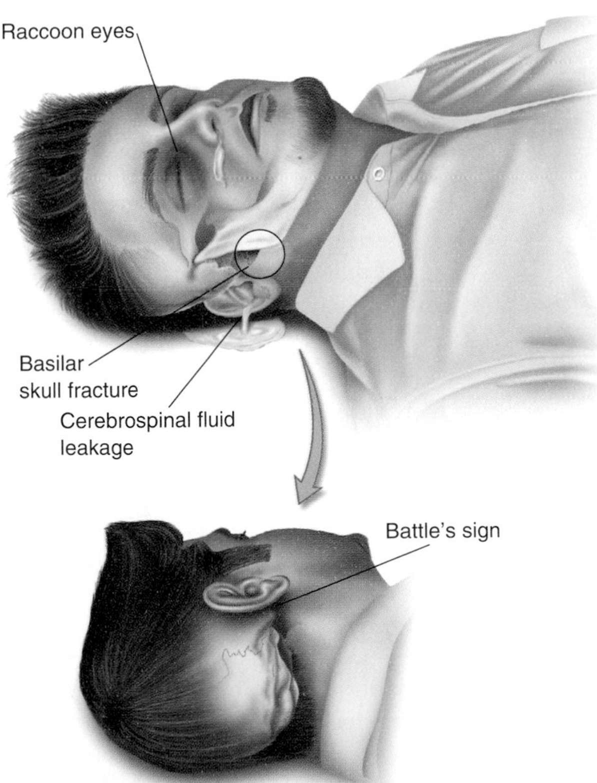

You Should Know

Signs and Symptoms of a Skull Fracture

- Bruises or cuts to the scalp
- Deformity to the skull
- Discoloration around the eyes (raccoon eyes)
- Discoloration behind the ears (Battle's sign)
- Loss of consciousness
- Confusion
- Convulsions
- Restlessness, irritability
- Drowsiness
- Blood or clear, watery fluid (cerebrospinal fluid) leaking from the ears or nose
- Visual disturbances
- Changes in pupils (unequal pupil size or pupils that are not reactive to light)
- Slurred speech
- Difficulties with balance
- Stiff neck
- Vomiting

A head injury may be open or closed. In a closed head injury, the skull remains intact. However, the brain can still be injured by forces or objects that strike the skull. The forces that impact the skull cause the brain to move within the skull. The brain strikes the inside of the skull, which causes injuries to the brain tissue. The impact and shearing forces that affect the brain can cause direct damage to the brain tissue. These forces can also injure the surrounding blood vessels. The skull is a rigid, closed container. If bleeding occurs within the skull, the pressure within the skull increases as the blood takes up more space within the closed container. If the bleeding continues and the pressure continues to rise, the patient can suffer severe brain damage and even death.

In an open head injury, the scalp is not intact and the risk of infection is increased. Broken bones or foreign objects forced through the skull can cut, tear, or bruise the brain tissue itself. If the skull is cracked, the blood and cerebrospinal fluid that normally surrounds the brain and spinal cord can leak through the crack in the skull and into the surrounding tissues. If the forces are strong enough to cause an open head injury, the brain will most likely sustain an injury as well.

Injuries to the Brain

Objective 7 ▶

A **concussion** is a traumatic brain injury that results in a temporary loss of function in part or all of the brain. A concussion occurs when the head strikes an object or is struck by an object (Figure 11-48). The injury may or may not cause a loss of consciousness. A headache, loss of appetite, vomiting, and pale skin are common soon after the injury. A patient who experiences a concussion often appears confused and may not remember what happened. The patient may ask the same questions over and over, such as "What happened? What happened?" This action is called repetitive questioning. If memory loss occurs, maximum memory loss usually happens immediately after the injury and returns as time passes. The signs and symptoms of a concussion are an indication of a brain injury. Although the symptoms of a concussion usually disappear within 48 hours, the patient needs to be evaluated by a physician. Worsening symptoms suggest a more serious injury.

FIGURE 11-48 ► A concussion occurs when the head strikes an object or is struck by an object.

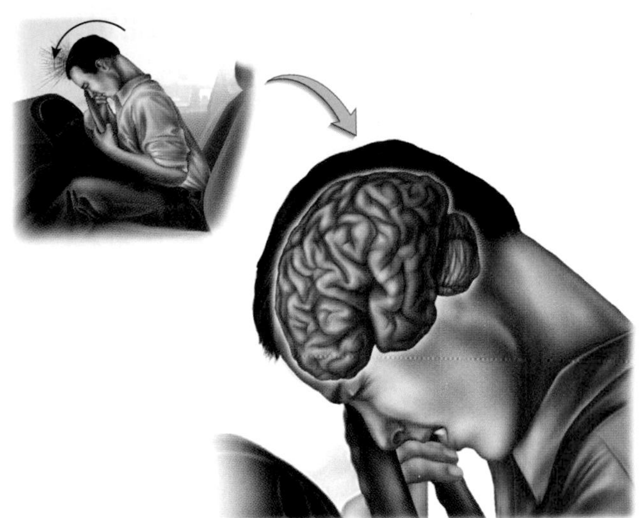

You Should Know

Signs and Symptoms of a Traumatic Head Injury

- Changes in mental status that range from confusion and repetitive questioning to unresponsiveness
- Deep cuts or tears to the scalp or face
- Exposed brain tissue (a very bad sign)
- Penetrating injuries, such as gunshot wounds and impaled objects
- Swelling ("goose eggs"), bruising of the skin
- Edges or fragments of bone seen or felt through the skin
- A deformity of the skull, such as sunken areas (depressions)
- Swelling or discoloration behind the ears (may not be seen for hours after the injury)
- Swelling or discoloration around the eyes (may not be seen for hours after the injury)
- Pupils that are unequal in size, that are irregular in shape, or that do not react to light equally; the dilation of both pupils
- An irregular breathing pattern
- Nausea and/or vomiting
- Possible seizures
- Blood or clear, watery fluid from the ears or nose
- Weakness or numbness of one side of the body
- A deterioration in vital signs
- A loss of bladder or bowel control

Remember This!

An altered or a decreasing mental status is the best indicator of a brain injury.

Brain injuries can occur for reasons other than trauma. For example, a non-traumatic injury may result from clots or hemorrhaging. This type of injury occurs when a patient has a stroke. Non-traumatic brain injuries can cause an altered mental status. Their signs and symptoms are similar to those of traumatic brain injuries.

Emergency Medical Responder Care of Head Injuries

Objective 8 ▶

To treat a patient with a head injury, use the following steps:

Closely monitor the patient's airway, breathing, pulse, and mental status for deterioration.

1. Conduct a scene size-up and ensure your safety. Evaluate the mechanism of injury before approaching the patient. Put on appropriate PPE.
2. Form a general impression and determine the urgency of further assessment and care.
3. Perform an initial assessment to identify and treat any life-threatening conditions.
    - If the mechanism of injury suggests a head or spinal injury, ask an assistant to manually stabilize the patient's head and neck while you continue your assessment. Continue manual stabilization until EMS personnel arrive and assume patient care or until the patient has been completely immobilized on a long backboard.
    - Establish and maintain an open airway. If you must open the patient's airway, use a jaw thrust without head tilt. For an unresponsive patient without a gag reflex, insert an oropharyngeal airway. Suction as necessary.
    - If the patient's breathing is inadequate, assist his breathing with a bag-valve-mask device. Provide oxygen if it is available and you have been trained to use it.
    - Control bleeding.
        - Do not attempt to stop the flow of blood or cerebrospinal fluid from the ears or nose. Cover the area with a loose, sterile dressing to absorb the drainage.
        - Do not remove a penetrating object. Instead, stabilize it in place with bulky dressings.
        - If bleeding is present from an open head wound, apply firm pressure with a clean cloth to control blood loss over a broad area. If blood soaks through the dressing, apply additional dressings on top and continue to apply pressure.
    - If signs of shock are present or if internal bleeding is suspected, treat for shock.
4. Perform a physical examination. Take the patient's vital signs and gather the patient's medical history.
5. Dress and bandage any open wounds.
6. Splint any bone or joint injuries. With any head injury, you must suspect a spinal injury. Immobilize the patient's spine.
7. If a medical condition or non-traumatic injury exists, place the patient on his left side.

Be prepared for changes in the patient's condition, such as seizures.

8. Comfort, calm, and reassure the patient and family members while waiting for EMS personnel. Remember that the patient may ask the same questions over and over because of the injury. Perform ongoing assessments every 5 minutes if the patient is in shock and every 15 minutes if the patient is stable.

On The Scene

Wrap-Up

You apply the cervical collar before the ambulance arrives. The crew chief listens as you give your report. You tell her there are good pulses, movement, and sensation distal to each of the patient's injuries. You and your partner apply a traction splint to care for the suspected femur fracture. The Paramedic fashions a rigid splint to support her upper arm injury. "Pad a formable splint and put it on her right lower arm," the Paramedic instructs you. Your crew carefully reassesses each extremity after the splints are applied to ensure that pulses, movement, and sensation are still present. You apply ice packs to each injured area and move the patient to the life support vehicle. In the ambulance, you reassess her vital signs while the Paramedic starts an IV. After calling in a report to medical direction, she gives the injured woman some medicine to relieve her pain. As you get ready to step off the ambulance, you notice that your patient's eyes close and her face visibly relaxes. ■

Sum It Up

- The mechanism of injury to bones and joints can be caused by direct forces, indirect forces, and twisting forces:
  - A *direct force* causes injury at the point of impact.
  - An *indirect force* causes injury at a site other than the point of impact.
  - A *twisting force* causes one part of an extremity to remain in place while the rest twists. Twisting injuries commonly affect the joints, such as ankles, knees, and wrists. Twisting forces cause ligaments to stretch and tear.
- Injuries to bones and joints may be open or closed:
  - In an *open injury*, the skin surface is broken. An open injury increases the risk of contamination and infection. These injuries can also result in serious blood loss.
  - In *closed injuries* of bones and joints, the skin surface is not broken. The injury is often painful, swollen, and deformed.
- A *fracture* is a break in a bone. If a bone is broken, chipped, cracked, or splintered, it is said to be fractured.
- A *dislocation* occurs when the ends of bones are forced from their normal positions in a joint.
- A *subluxation*, which is a partial dislocation, means the bone is partially out of the joint. A complete dislocation means it is all the way out. Dislocations and subluxations usually result in temporary deformity of the joint and may result in sudden and severe pain.
- A *sprain* is a stretching or tearing of a ligament, the connective tissue that joins the end of one bone with another. Sprains are classified as mild, moderate, or severe.
- A *strain* is a twisting, pulling, or tearing of a muscle. A muscle strain usually occurs when a muscle is stretched beyond its limit. A strain often occurs near the point where the muscle joins the tough connective tissue of the tendon.
- Most sprains and strains can be treated with the *RICE* technique:
  - *R*est
  - *I*ce
  - *C*ompression
  - *E*levation
- In treating musculoskeletal injuries, *DOTS* is a useful tool to remember what to look and feel for:
  - *D*eformities
  - *O*pen injuries
  - *T*enderness
  - *S*welling

- In assessing extremity injuries, check the *p*ulse, *m*ovement, and *s*ensation (PMS) in each extremity.
- A *splint* is a device used to limit the movement of (immobilize) an injured arm or leg to reduce pain and further injury.
  - In some situations, the patient will have already splinted the injury by holding the injured part close to his or her body in a comfortable position. The body used as a splint is called a *self-splint* or an *anatomic splint.*
  - Before splinting an injured hand or foot, place it in the *position of function.* The natural position of the hand at rest looks as if you were gently grasping a small object, such as a baseball.
- *Rigid splints* are made of hard material, such as wood, strong cardboard, or plastic. This type of splint is useful for immobilizing injuries that occur to the middle portion (midshaft) of a bone. Some rigid splints are padded, but others must be padded before they are applied to the patient.
- *Semi-rigid (flexible) splints* are very useful for immobilizing joint injuries. These splints can be molded to the shape of the extremity. Examples include the SAM® Splint and aluminum ladder splints. Semi-rigid splints can be used in combination with other splints.
- *Soft splints* are flexible and useful for immobilizing injuries of the lower leg or forearm. Examples of soft splints include a sling and swathe, blanket rolls, pillows, and towels.
  - A *sling and swathe* is used to immobilize injuries to the shoulder, collarbone, or upper arm bone. A triangular bandage is often used to make a sling. A swathe is a piece of soft material used to secure the injured extremity to the body.
- A *traction splint* is a device used to immobilize a closed fracture of the thighbone. This type of splint maintains a constant, steady pull on the bone. A traction splint keeps broken bone ends in a near-normal position.
  - A *unipolar traction splint* has one pole that provides external support for the injured leg.
  - A *bipolar traction splint* uses two external poles, one on each side of the injured leg, to provide external support
- A *pneumatic splint* requires air to be pumped into or suctioned out of it. An air splint, a vacuum splint, and a pneumatic antishock garment (PASG) are examples of pneumatic splints. A pneumatic splint is placed around the injured area and is inflated (air splint or PASG) or deflated (vacuum splint) until it becomes firm.
- Most spinal injuries occur to the cervical spine. The next most commonly injured areas are the thoracic and lumbar spine. A spinal column injury (bony injury) can occur with or without a spinal cord injury. A spinal cord injury can also occur with or without an injury to the spinal column. The spinal cord does not have to be severed for a loss of function to occur.
- *Compression fractures* of the spine result in weakened vertebrae. A compression fracture can occur with or without a spinal cord injury.
- *Distraction* occurs when the spine is pulled apart. When the spine is distracted, ligaments and muscles are overstretched or torn and the vertebrae are pulled apart.
- An injury to the spinal cord may be complete or incomplete:
  - A *complete spinal cord injury* occurs when the spinal cord is severed. The patient has no voluntary movement or sensation below the level of the injury. Both sides of the body are equally affected.
    - *Paraplegia* is the loss of movement and sensation in the body from the waist down. Paraplegia results from a spinal cord injury at the level of the thoracic or lumbar vertebrae.

- *Quadriplegia* (also called tetraplegia) is a loss of movement and sensation in both arms, both legs, and the parts of the body below an area of injury to the spinal cord. Quadriplegia results from a spinal cord injury at the level of the cervical vertebrae.
- With an *incomplete spinal cord injury*, some parts of the spinal cord remain intact. The patient has some function below the level of the injury. With this type of injury, there is a potential for recovery, because function may be lost only temporarily.

▶ The signs and symptoms of a possible spinal injury include the following:
- Tenderness in the injured area
- Pain associated with movement (do *not* ask the patient to move to see if he or she has pain; do *not* move the patient to test for a pain response)
- Pain independent of movement or palpation along the spinal column
- Pain down the lower legs or into the rib cage
- Pain that comes and goes, usually along the spine and/or the lower legs
- Soft-tissue injuries associated with trauma to the head and neck (cuts, bruises)
- Numbness, weakness, or tingling in the extremities
- A loss of sensation or paralysis below the site of injury
- A loss of sensation or paralysis in the upper or lower extremities
- Difficulty breathing
- A loss of bladder or bowel control
- An inability to walk, move extremities, or feel sensation
- Deformity or muscle spasm along the spinal column

▶ Manual stabilization of the head and neck is also called *in-line stabilization*. Manual stabilization of the head and neck helps prevent further injury to the spine.

▶ As an Emergency Medical Responder, you may need to apply a rigid *cervical collar* (also called a c-collar) in treating a spinal injury. You should use a c-collar only if the equipment is available and you have been trained to use it. When used alone, a rigid cervical collar does not immobilize. For effective immobilization, a rigid collar must be used with manual stabilization or a spinal immobilization device, such as a backboard.

▶ A *log roll* is a technique used to move a patient from a face-down to a face-up position while maintaining the head and neck in line with the rest of the body. This technique is also used to place a patient with a suspected spinal injury on a backboard.

▶ A *long backboard* helps stabilize the head, neck and torso, pelvis, and extremities. It is used to immobilize patients found in a lying, standing, or sitting position.

▶ A *short backboard* helps immobilize a patient's head, neck, and torso. It can also be used as a long backboard for a small child. Examples include vest-type devices and rigid short backboards.

▶ An injury to the scalp may occur because of blunt or penetrating trauma. When injured, the scalp may bleed heavily. In children, the amount of blood loss from a scalp wound may be enough to produce shock.

▶ The skull protects the brain from injury. However, damage to the skull can cause damage to the brain. Skull injuries may occur from blunt or penetrating trauma. Significant force, such as a severe impact or blow, can result in a skull fracture.

▶ A head injury may be open or closed:
- In an *open head injury*, the scalp is not intact and the risk of infection is increased. Broken bones or foreign objects forced through the skull can cut, tear, or bruise the brain tissue itself.

- In a *closed head injury,* the skull remains intact. However, the brain can still be injured by forces or objects that strike the skull. The forces that impact the skull cause the brain to move within the skull. The brain strikes the inside of the skull, which causes injuries to the brain tissue.

▶ A *concussion* is a traumatic brain injury that results in a temporary loss of function in part or all of the brain. A concussion occurs when the head strikes an object or is struck by an object. The injury may or may not cause a loss of consciousness. A headache, loss of appetite, vomiting, and pale skin are common soon after the injury.

▶ An altered or a decreasing mental status is the best indicator of a brain injury.

▶ To treat a patient with a head injury, use the following steps:

1. Conduct a scene size-up, ensure safety, and put on appropriate PPE. Evaluate the mechanism of injury.
2. Form a general impression.
3. Perform an initial assessment.
4. Ask an assistant to manually stabilize the patient's head and neck while you continue your exam.
5. Closely monitor the patient's airway, breathing, pulse, and mental status.
6. Perform a physical examination.
7. Dress and bandage any open wounds.
8. Immobilize the patient's spine.

▶ Tracking Your Progress

After reading this chapter, can you	Page Reference	Objective Met?
• Describe the function of the musculoskeletal system?	384–385	☐
• Differentiate between an open and a closed painful, swollen, deformed extremity?	390–392	☐
• List the emergency medical care for a patient with a painful, swollen, deformed extremity?	394–396	☐
• Relate mechanism of injury to potential injuries of the head and spine?	415–417	☐
• State the signs and symptoms of a potential spine injury?	417–419	☐
• Describe the method of determining if a responsive patient may have a spine injury?	421	☐
• List the signs and symptoms of an injury to the head?	434–435	☐
• Describe the emergency medical care for injuries to the head?	436	☐
• Explain the rationale for the feeling patients who have need for immobilization of the painful, swollen, deformed extremity?	422	☐
• Demonstrate a caring attitude toward patients with a musculoskeletal injury who request Emergency Medical Services?	396	☐
• Place the interests of the patient with a musculoskeletal injury as the foremost consideration when making any and all patient care decisions?	405	☐
• Communicate with empathy to patients with a musculoskeletal injury, as well as with family members and friends of the patient?	396	☐

Chapter Quiz

Multiple Choice

In the space provided, identify the letter of the choice that best completes each statement or answers each question.

____ **1.** The bones of the upper extremity include the

a. tibia, fibula, and femur.
b. tibia, radius, and humerus.
c. femur, humerus, and ulna.
d. humerus, radius, and ulna.

____ **2.** A strain is an injury that usually involves

a. muscles.
b. ligaments.
c. bones.
d. tendons.

____ **3.** A seven-year-old girl has injured her right arm. Your examination reveals a painful, swollen deformity of the middle third of the child's forearm. To immobilize this injury properly, you should apply a splint that stabilizes the

a. hand and wrist.
b. wrist and elbow.
c. knee and ankle.
d. shoulder and elbow.

____ **4.** Which of the following is the largest bone of the arm?

a. radius
b. ulna
c. elbow
d. humerus

____ **5.** Because of the potential for significant blood loss, you should call for advanced EMS personnel *immediately* when your patient has experienced an injury involving the

a. tibia or ankle.
b. pelvis or femur.
c. foot or pelvis.
d. ankle or femur.

____ **6.** Which of the following signs is consistent with a possible head injury?

a. The patient's abdomen is firm to the touch.
b. The patient's breath has a fruity smell.
c. The patient has one pupil that is larger than the other.
d. The patient has bruising and swelling of the left lower leg.

True or False

Decide whether each statement is true or false. In the space provided, write T for true or *F for false.*

____ **7.** Most muscles are attached to bones by tendons.

____ **8.** Ice should be applied to a sprain or strain for 40 minutes and removed for 20 minutes.

____ **9.** Before being applied to a patient, a splint should be padded to prevent pressure and discomfort.

____ **10.** When splinting the legs together, it is best to move the injured leg to the good leg.

Matching

Match the key terms in the left column with the definitions in the right column by placing the letter of each correct answer in the space provided.

____ **11.** Crepitus

____ **12.** Angulation

____ **13.** Splint

____ **14.** Anatomic splint

____ **15.** Swathe

____ **16.** Concussion

____ **17.** Paraplegia

____ **18.** Traction

a. Using the body as a splint

b. Piece of soft material used to secure an injured extremity to the body

c. Maintaining a continuous, steady pull on a bone or an extremity to relieve spasm, pain, or pressure or to align parts

d. Abnormal position of an extremity

e. Traumatic brain injury that results in a temporary loss of function in part or all of the brain

f. Sensation or sound of broken bone ends grating against each other

g. Device used to limit the movement of an injured arm or leg to reduce bleeding

h. Condition that results from a spinal cord injury at the level of the thoracic or lumbar vertebrae

Short Answer

Answer each question in the space provided.

19. List four functions of the musculoskeletal system.

1. ______________________________

2. ______________________________

3. ______________________________

4. ______________________________

20. What is a dislocation?

____

____

____

21. Why is ice used in the treatment of a sprain or strain?

____

____

____

22. RICE is a technique used to treat sprains and strains. Explain the meaning of each of the letters.

R = ______________________________

I = ______________________________

C = ______________________________

E = ______________________________

23. What are the three most common signs and symptoms of a musculoskeletal injury?

1. ______________________

2. ______________________

3. ______________________

24. List four reasons for splinting a musculoskeletal injury.

1. ______________________

2. ______________________

3. ______________________

4. ______________________

25. List three hazards of improper splinting.

1. ______________________

2. ______________________

3. ______________________

26. What is a traction splint?

____

____

____

27. What three things should you assess before and after applying a splint?

1. ______________________

2. ______________________

3. ______________________

28. List three types of splints.

1. ______________________

2. ______________________

3. ______________________

29. List the three areas of the spine that are most commonly injured.

1. ______________________

2. ______________________

3. ______________________

Sentence Completion

In the blanks provided, write the words that best complete each sentence.

30. Cardiac muscle is a(n) ____________________ muscle.

31. The three major parts of a skeletal muscle are the ____________________, the ____________________, and the ____________________.

32. The two main divisions of the skeleton are the ____________________ and the ____________________ skeleton.

33. A shoulder injury typically involves three bones: the ____________________, the __________ __________, and the __________ __________ __________.

34. Splinting an elbow injury requires immobilization of the ____________________ (the bone above the injury) and the ____________________ and ____________________ (the bones below the injury).

Module 6

Childbirth and Children

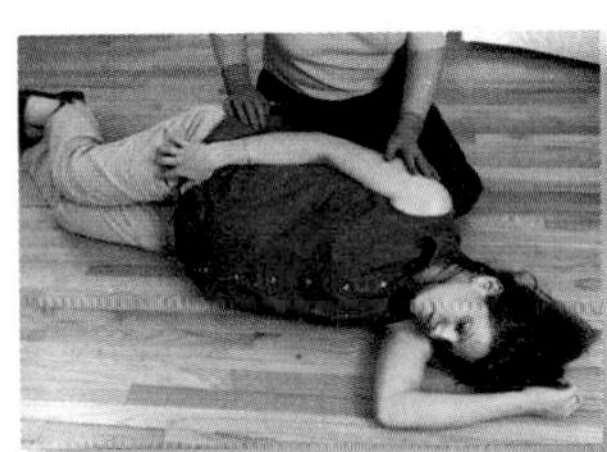

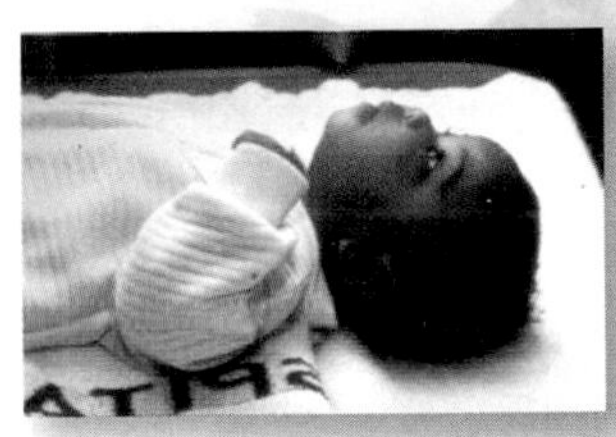

CHAPTER

12 Childbirth

By the end of this chapter, you should be able to

Knowledge Objectives ▶

1. Identify the following structures: birth canal, placenta, umbilical cord, amniotic sac.
2. Define the following terms: crowning, bloody show, labor, abortion.
3. State indications of an imminent delivery.
4. State the steps in the pre-delivery preparation of the mother.
5. Establish the relationship between body substance isolation and childbirth.
6. State the steps to assist in the delivery.
7. Describe care of the baby as the head appears.
8. Discuss the steps in delivery of the placenta.
9. List the steps in the emergency medical care of the mother post-delivery.
10. Discuss the steps in caring for a newborn.

Attitude Objectives ▶

11. Explain the rationale for attending to the feelings of a patient in need of emergency medical care during childbirth.
12. Demonstrate a caring attitude toward patients during childbirth who request Emergency Medical Services.
13. Place the interests of the patient during childbirth as the foremost consideration when making any and all patient care decisions.
14. Communicate with empathy to patients during childbirth, as well as with family members and friends of the patient.

Skill Objectives ▶

DVD Link

15. Demonstrate the steps to assist in the normal cephalic delivery.
16. Demonstrate necessary care procedures of the fetus as the head appears.

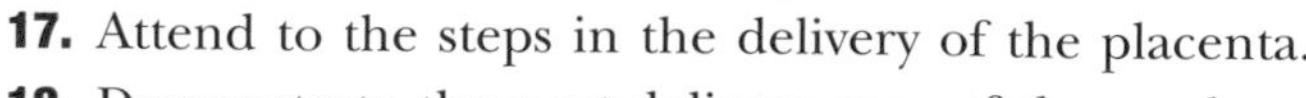

17. Attend to the steps in the delivery of the placenta.
18. Demonstrate the post-delivery care of the mother.
19. Demonstrate the care of the newborn.

On The Scene

It is late in your shift when an emergency page goes out: "Emergency response teams, report to the warehouse." It's clear when you arrive that this is no ordinary emergency. A woman is squatting on the floor, grunting and screaming, "The baby's coming, the baby's coming!" You can tell by the dark stain on her jeans that her bag of waters has broken. The plant supervisor tells you that the ambulance is about 20 minutes away. You put on your goggles, mask, and gloves; ask someone to run to the nurse's office to get the OB kit; and prepare to deliver a baby.

THINK ABOUT IT

As you read this chapter, think about the following questions:

- What questions should you ask the mother to determine if this will be a complicated delivery?
- What equipment will you need?
- How will you assist with the delivery of the baby?
- How will you assess the baby?

Introduction

Caring for Mother and Baby

You may be called to care for a woman in labor. Although childbirth is a natural process and most deliveries occur with no complications, these situations are often stressful for the patient, the patient's family, and emergency care providers. Once the mother delivers, you will be responsible for her care and that of her baby. To provide the best possible care for both patients, you must know how to assist during childbirth and how to provide care for both mother and baby after delivery.

The Anatomy and Physiology of the Female Reproductive System

The female reproductive organs are found in the pelvic cavity. The **ovaries** are paired, almond-shaped organs located on each side of the uterus (Figure 12-1). The ovaries perform two main functions: produce eggs and secrete hormones, such as estrogen and progesterone. Each ovary contains thousands of follicles. About once a month during a woman's reproductive years, a follicle matures to release an egg (ovulation). The **fallopian tubes** (also called *uterine tubes*) extend from an ovary to the uterus. They receive and transport the egg to the uterus after ovulation. Fertilization normally takes place in the upper third of the fallopian tube.

The **uterus** (also called the **womb**) is a pear-shaped, hollow, muscular organ located in the pelvic cavity. It prepares for pregnancy each month of a woman's reproductive life. If pregnancy does not occur, the inner lining of the uterus sloughs off and is discarded. This discharge of blood and tissue from the uterus is called **menstruation.** It is often referred to as a woman's "period." If pregnancy does occur, the developing fetus (unborn infant) implants in the uterine wall and develops there. The uterus stretches throughout pregnancy to adjust to the

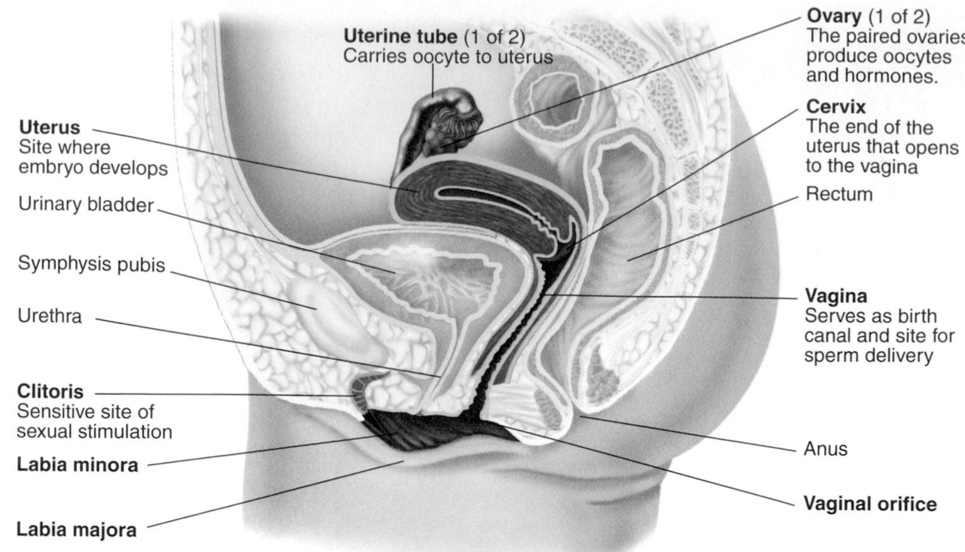

FIGURE 12-1 ▶ Structures of the female reproductive system.

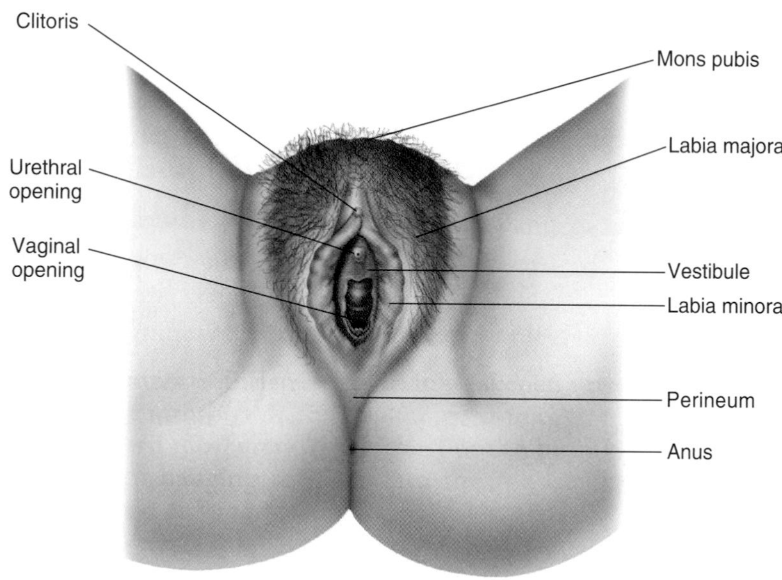

FIGURE 12-2 ▶ External female reproductive structures.

increasing size of the fetus. During **labor,** the uterus contracts powerfully and rhythmically to expel the infant from the mother's body. After delivery of the infant, the uterus quickly clamps down to stop the bleeding.

Objective 2 ▶

The **cervix** is the narrow opening at the distal end of the uterus. It connects the uterus to the vagina. During pregnancy, it contains a plug of mucus. The mucous plug seals the opening to the uterus, keeping bacteria from entering. When the cervix begins to widen during early labor, the mucous plug, sometimes mixed with blood **(bloody show),** is expelled from the vagina. The **vagina** is also called the **birth canal.** It is a muscular tube that serves as a passageway between the uterus and the outside of the body (Figure 12-2). It receives the penis during intercourse. It also serves as the passageway for menstrual flow and the delivery of an infant. The **perineum** is the area between the vaginal opening and the anus. It is commonly torn during **childbirth.**

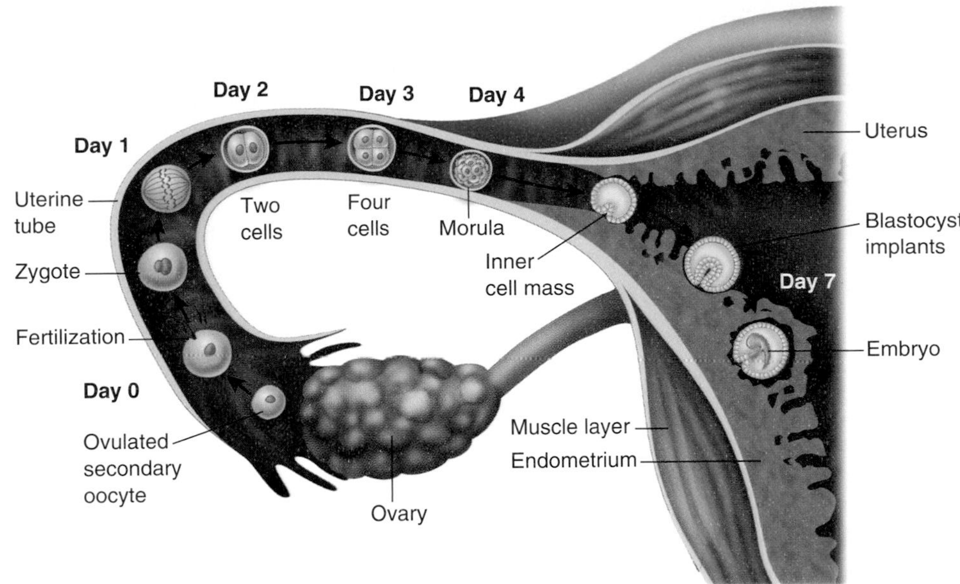

FIGURE 12-3 ▶ Pregnancy begins when an egg joins with a sperm cell (fertilization). The fertilized egg passes from the fallopian tube into the uterus. The egg implants in the wall of the uterus around day 7.

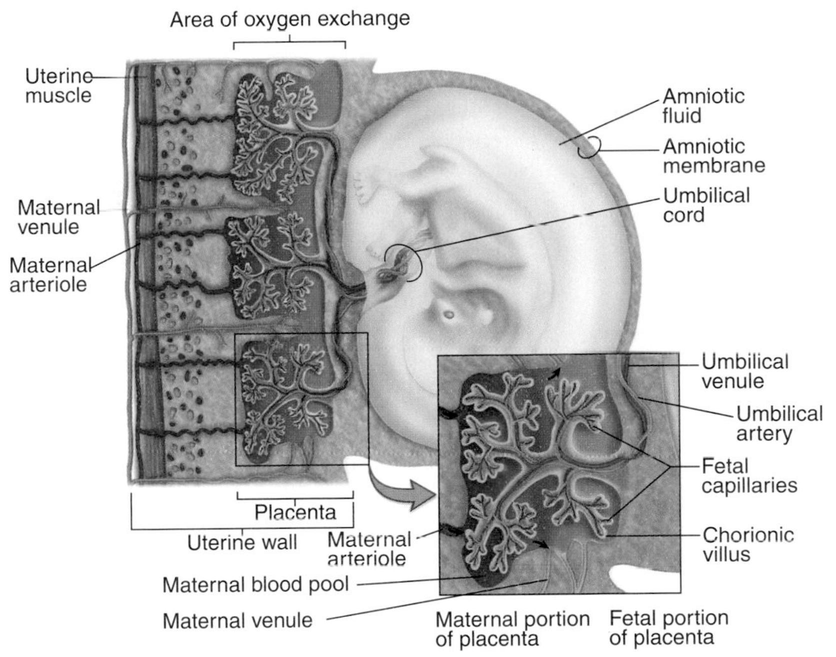

FIGURE 12-4 ▶ In the placenta, nutrients and oxygen pass from the maternal blood to the embryo, while wastes pass in the opposite direction.

Objective 1 ▶

The Structures of Pregnancy

Pregnancy begins when an egg joins with a sperm cell (fertilization). The fertilized egg (ovum) passes from the fallopian tube into the uterus. The ovum implants in the wall of the uterus (implantation; Figure 12-3). During the first three weeks after fertilization, the developing structure is called an *ovum*. From the third to the eighth week, the developing structure is called an *embryo*. From the eighth week until birth, the developing structure is called a *fetus*.

The placenta is also called the *afterbirth* because it is expelled after the baby is born.

The **placenta** is a specialized organ through which the fetus exchanges nourishment and waste products during pregnancy (Figure 12-4). The placenta begins to develop about two weeks after fertilization occurs. It attaches to the mother at the inner wall of the uterus and to the fetus by the umbilical cord. The placenta is responsible for

- The exchange of oxygen and carbon dioxide between the blood of the mother and the fetus (the placenta serves the function of the lungs for the developing fetus)
- The removal of waste products
- The transport of nutrients from the mother to the fetus
- The production of a special pregnancy hormone that maintains the pregnancy and stimulates changes in the mother's breasts, cervix, and vagina in preparation for delivery
- Maintaining a barrier against harmful substances
- The transfer of heat from the mother to the fetus

You Should Know

Although the placenta is an effective protective barrier between the mother and fetus, it does not protect the baby from everything. Some medications and toxic substances pass easily from the mother's blood to the baby. It is very important for a pregnant woman to consult with her doctor before taking any medicine or herbal supplement.

The **umbilical cord** is the lifeline that connects the placenta to the fetus. It contains two arteries and one vein. The umbilical arteries carry blood low in oxygen from the fetus to the placenta. The umbilical vein carries oxygenated blood to the fetus. The umbilical cord attaches to the umbilicus (navel) of the fetus.

The amniotic sac is also called the bag of waters.

The **amniotic sac** is a membranous bag that surrounds the fetus inside the uterus. It contains fluid (amniotic fluid), which helps protect the fetus from injury. The amniotic fluid provides an environment that is at a constant temperature. It also allows the fetus to move and functions much as a shock absorber does. The amniotic sac contains about 1 liter (L) of fluid at term.

Normal Pregnancy

Pregnancy usually takes 40 weeks and is divided into three 90-day intervals called *trimesters.*

The First Trimester

Despite its name, morning sickness can occur at *any* time of day.

During the first trimester (months 1–3), the mother stops menstruating (missed period). Her breasts become swollen and tender. She urinates more frequently and may sleep more than usual. Nausea and vomiting (usually called morning sickness) are usually at its worst during the second month. During the first weeks after conception, the mother's body begins to produce more blood to carry oxygen and nutrients to the fetus. Her heart rate increases by as much as 10–15 beats per minute because her heart must work harder to pump this increased amount of blood. Normal weight gain during the first trimester is only about 2 pounds (approximately 907 grams, or 0.907 kilograms).

During the first 13 weeks of pregnancy, the fetus develops rapidly. Cells differentiate into tissues and organs. The arms, legs, heart, lungs, and brain begin to form. At the end of the first trimester, the fetus is about 3 inches long and weighs about half an ounce.

The Second Trimester

In the second trimester (months 4–6), the signs of pregnancy become more obvious. The uterus expands to make room for the fetus and can be felt above the pubic bone. The mother's abdomen also enlarges and her center of gravity often changes. As a result, she may walk and move differently. The mother begins to feel the fetus move at about the fourth or fifth month. Her circulatory system continues to expand, which lowers her blood pressure. During the first six months of pregnancy, her systolic blood pressure may drop by 5–10 points. Her diastolic blood pressure may drop by 10–15 points. (In her third trimester, her blood pressure gradually returns to its pre-pregnancy level.) The mother may feel dizzy or faint when taking a hot bath or shower or in hot weather. This occurs because heat causes the capillaries in her skin to dilate, temporarily reducing the amount of blood returning to her heart.

During the second trimester (about the 13th to 24th week of pregnancy), the fetus's fingers, toes, eyelashes, and eyebrows are formed. At about the 5th month, the heartbeat of the fetus can be heard with a stethoscope. By the end of this trimester, the heart, lungs, and kidneys are formed. The fetus weighs about 1¾ pounds (approximately 794 grams, or 0.794 kilograms) and is about 13 inches (approximately 33 centimeters) long.

The Third Trimester

Premature labor (also called *preterm labor*) occurs when a woman has labor before her 37th week of pregnancy.

During the third trimester (months 7–9), the mother may complain of a backache because of muscle strain. Stretch marks may appear. The mother urinates frequently, because the weight of the uterus presses on her bladder. She may be short of breath as her uterus expands beneath her diaphragm.

During the third trimester (about the 25th to 40th week of pregnancy), the fetus continues to grow rapidly, gaining about a ½ pound a week and reaching a length of about 20 inches. Fetal movement occurs often and is stronger. Normally, the head of the fetus settles into the pelvis in preparation for delivery.

Complications of Pregnancy

Abortion

An **abortion** is a termination of pregnancy before the fetus is able to live on its own outside the uterus. A therapeutic abortion is an abortion performed for medical reasons, often because the pregnancy poses a threat to the mother's health. An elective abortion is an abortion performed at the request of the mother.

Most miscarriages occur between the 7th and 12th weeks of pregnancy.

A **spontaneous abortion**, also called a miscarriage, is the loss of a fetus due to natural causes. It usually occurs before the 20th week of pregnancy. In most miscarriages, the fetus dies because of a genetic abnormality that is usually unrelated to the mother. During a miscarriage, the mother often experiences lower back pain or cramping abdominal pain, vaginal bleeding, and the passage of tissue or clotlike material from the vagina.

Not all abdominal pain or bleeding that occurs during the early weeks of pregnancy is due to a miscarriage. Bleeding sometimes occurs during early pregnancy and the mother is still able to carry the fetus to full term. The patient needs to be evaluated by a physician. Arrange for transport to the hospital. Provide oxygen if it is available and you have been trained to use it. Treat the patient for shock if signs are present. Keep the patient warm. Collect any tissue or clotlike material passed from the vagina. A clean plastic container with a lid or a biohazard bag can be used for this purpose. Be sure the collected tissue is sent with the patient to the hospital.

Making a Difference

Any situation that involves bleeding during pregnancy is likely to be a very emotional one. Most women associate bleeding during pregnancy with "losing the baby." This may or may not be the case and cannot be determined accurately in the field. Grief is a very normal reaction to the threatened loss of the pregnancy. While treating your patient's physical condition, remember to provide her with emotional support as well.

Ectopic Pregnancy

An ectopic pregnancy that occurs in a fallopian tube is called a tubal pregnancy. An ectopic pregnancy is a medical emergency.

Once conception occurs, the fertilized egg normally travels through the fallopian tube to the uterus. The fertilized egg implants in the uterine lining and begins to grow. This process usually takes four to nine days. An **ectopic pregnancy** occurs when a fertilized egg implants outside the uterus. The most common site where this occurs is inside a fallopian tube (Figure 12-5). Less commonly, the egg implants in the abdomen, the cervix, or an ovary. In an ectopic pregnancy, the growing fetus bursts through the tissue in which it has implanted. Severe bleeding can occur due to ruptured blood vessels.

The initial signs and symptoms of an ectopic pregnancy include a missed menstrual period or small amounts of vaginal bleeding that occur irregularly over six to eight weeks. The patient may complain of mild cramping on one side of the pelvis, nausea, lower back pain, and lower abdominal or pelvic pain.

If rupture occurs, the patient often complains of a sudden onset of severe pain on one side of the lower abdomen. Vaginal bleeding may or may not be present. She may feel faint or may actually faint. In addition, the patient may complain of severe pain in the back of the shoulder (referred pain). Severe internal bleeding may be present. The patient may have signs of shock, such as decreasing blood pressure, an increased heart rate, and cool, clammy skin.

Arrange for immediate transport to the closest appropriate facility. Provide oxygen if it is available and you have been trained to use it. Treat the patient for shock if signs are present. Keep the patient warm. Provide emotional support for the patient and family.

Remember This!

Although there are many causes of abdominal pain, you must consider lower abdominal pain in any woman of childbearing age to be due to an ectopic pregnancy until proven otherwise.

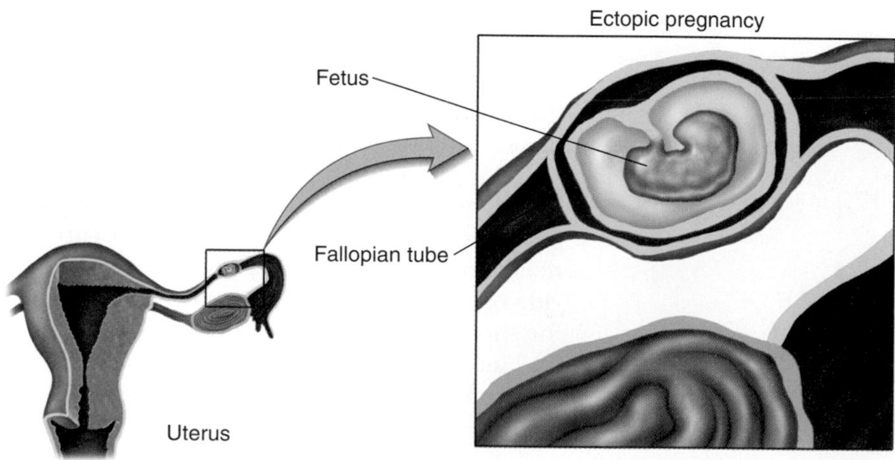

FIGURE 12-5 ► An ectopic pregnancy occurs when a fertilized egg implants outside the uterus, usually inside a fallopian tube.

Preeclampsia and Eclampsia

Preeclampsia is also called *pregnancy-induced hypertension* or *toxemia*. The cause of preeclampsia is not known.

Preeclampsia is a disorder of pregnancy that causes blood vessels to spasm and constrict. Blood vessel constriction results in high blood pressure. It also decreases blood flow to the mother's organs, including the placenta. Less blood flow to the placenta usually means that less oxygenated blood and fewer nutrients reach the baby. In some cases, the baby may need to be delivered early to protect the mother's health. Preeclampsia also causes changes in the blood vessels. These changes cause the mother's capillaries to leak fluid into her tissues. This results in swelling.

Preeclampsia usually occurs during the third trimester of pregnancy. It tends to occur in young mothers during their first pregnancy and in women whose mothers or sisters had preeclampsia. The risk for preeclampsia is higher in women older than 40, in women carrying multiple babies, and in teenage mothers. Women who had high blood pressure, diabetes, or kidney disease before they became pregnant are also at risk for preeclampsia.

If your patient complains of blurred vision, nausea, a severe headache, and pain in the right upper quadrant of the abdomen, she may be very close to having a seizure.

The signs and symptoms of preeclampsia include the following:

- Weight gain of more than 2 pounds per week or a sudden weight gain over one to two days
- Visual disturbances, such as blurred vision, or the appearance of flashing lights or spots before the eyes
- Swelling of the face and hands that is present on arising
- Headaches
- Right upper quadrant abdominal pain
- Increased blood pressure (more than 140/90 mm Hg)

Eclampsia is associated with a significant risk of death for the mother and fetus.

If untreated, preeclampsia may progress to eclampsia. **Eclampsia** is the seizure phase of preeclampsia. Be sure to have suction readily available. Provide oxygen if it is available and you have been trained to use it. Keep the patient calm and position her on her left side. Avoid any stimulus that might trigger a seizure, such as bright lights and siren noise. Dim the lights. Arrange for prompt transport without lights or siren. If the patient has a seizure, protect her from injury and watch her breathing closely. When the seizure is over, make sure her airway is clear and give oxygen if it is available and you have been trained to use it.

Remember This!

It is not necessary for you to determine the cause of vaginal bleeding. However, it is important for you to recognize that the patient needs immediate transport and evaluation by a physician.

Vaginal Bleeding in Late Pregnancy

All third-trimester bleeding should be considered a life-threatening emergency.

Vaginal bleeding may occur late in pregnancy (third trimester). It may or may not be accompanied by pain. The possible causes of vaginal bleeding in late pregnancy include *placenta previa, abruptio placenta,* and a ruptured uterus.

Placenta previa occurs when the placenta attaches low in the wall of the uterus instead of at its top or sides. In this position, the placenta may cover all or part of the cervix (the entrance to the birth canal; Figure 12-6). If the placenta covers the cervical opening during the early months of pregnancy, it will often shift position as the uterus grows, moving away from the cervical opening. If the placenta does not shift from the cervical opening as the pregnancy progresses, then *placenta previa* exists.

FIGURE 12-6 ▶
Placenta previa. (a) In a total *placenta previa*, the placenta completely covers the cervix. (b) In a partial *placenta previa*, the placenta partially covers the cervix.

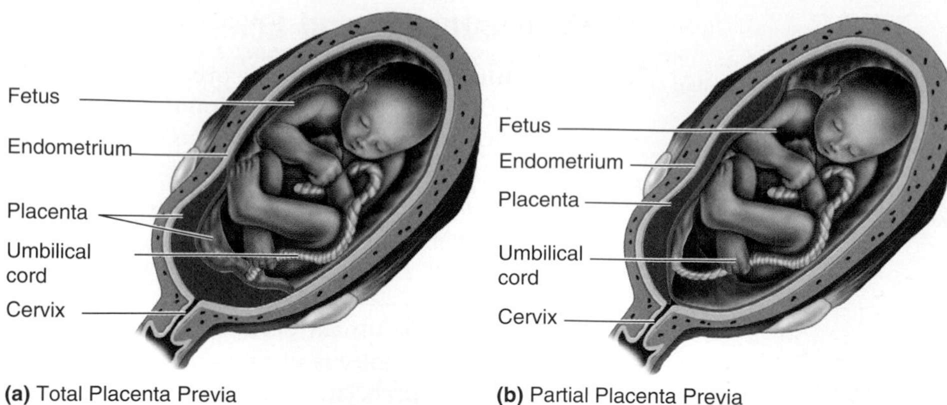

FIGURE 12-7 ▶
(a) *Abruptio placenta* occurs when a normally implanted placenta separates prematurely from the wall of the uterus (endometrium) during the last trimester of pregnancy. Vaginal bleeding may be absent (concealed, or hidden, bleeding).
(b) Vaginal bleeding that is visible may be moderate to severe and is usually dark red.

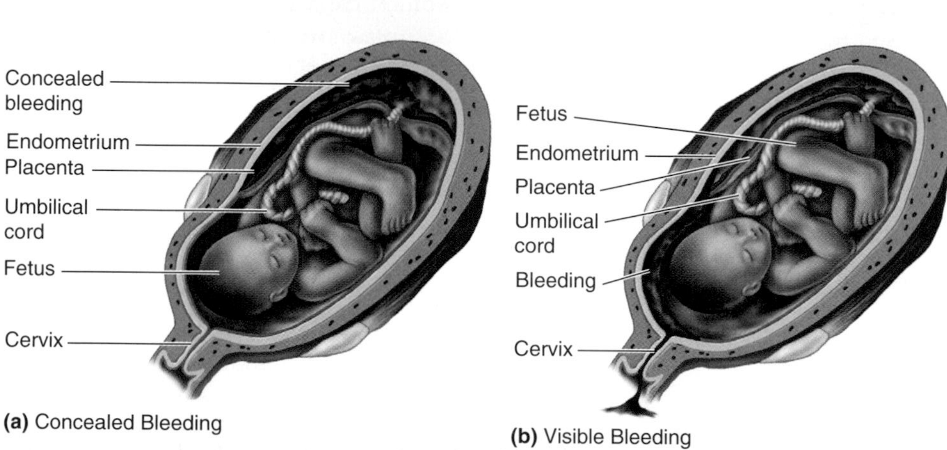

Placenta previa is the cause of most cases of severe bleeding in the third trimester of pregnancy.

Abruptio placenta is also called placental abruption.

Because exposure to blood is possible, be sure to wear appropriate PPE.

Normally, the cervix begins to widen and thin out in the third trimester of pregnancy. This is the body's way of preparing for labor. If the mother has *placenta previa*, vaginal bleeding can occur, because placental blood vessels that are implanted in the wall of the uterus are torn as the cervix widens and thins out. The more the placenta covers the cervical opening, the greater the risk of bleeding.

Abruptio placenta occurs when a normally implanted placenta separates prematurely from the wall of the uterus (endometrium) during the last trimester of pregnancy. If the placenta begins to peel away from the wall of the uterus, bleeding occurs from the blood vessels that transfer nutrients to the fetus from the mother. The larger the area that peels away, the greater the amount of bleeding. The placenta may separate partially or completely (Figure 12-7). Partial separation may allow time for treatment of the mother and fetus. Complete separation often results in the death of the fetus.

A ruptured uterus is the tearing (rupture) of the uterus. Uterine rupture can occur when the patient has been in strong labor for a long time, which is the most common cause. It can also occur when the patient has sustained abdominal trauma, such as a severe fall or a sudden stop in a motor vehicle collision.

A patient with any of these conditions needs Advanced Life Support care and immediate transport to the closest appropriate facility. Treat the patient for shock while waiting for EMS personnel to arrive. Keep the patient warm and provide oxygen if it is available and you have been trained to use it. Monitor the patient's vital signs every five minutes.

Table 12-1 lists some of the causes, signs, and symptoms of vaginal bleeding in late pregnancy.

TABLE 12-1 Causes, Signs, and Symptoms of Vaginal Bleeding in Late Pregnancy

Signs and Symptoms	*Placenta Previa*	*Abruptio Placenta*	Uterine Rupture
Vaginal bleeding	• Sudden • Bright red	• May be absent (concealed or hidden) • If seen, may be moderate to severe; usually dark red	• May or may not be present
Abdominal pain	• Usually none (*p*ainless = *Previa*)	• Sudden, severe	• Sudden, severe • Abdomen tender, rigid • Possible contractions
Signs of shock	• Likely	• Yes; may seem out of proportion to the amount of blood loss seen	• Yes
Fetal movement	• Usually present	• Decreased • May be absent	• Absent

Making a Difference

A woman late in her second trimester or in her third trimester of pregnancy should be positioned on her left side. When a woman in late pregnancy is placed on her back, the weight of the fetus compresses major blood vessels, such as the inferior vena cava and the aorta (Figure 12-8). This compression decreases the amount of blood returning to the mother's heart and lowers her blood pressure. As a result, the amount of oxygen and nutrients delivered to the fetus is decreased.

Positioning the patient on her left side shifts the weight of her uterus off the abdominal vessels. If the patient is immobilized to a backboard, tilt the board slightly to the left by placing a rolled towel, a small pillow, a blanket, or another type of padding under the right side of the board. Doing so will shift the weight of the patient's uterus and decrease the pressure on the abdominal blood vessels.

Trauma and Pregnancy

Trauma is more likely to cause the death of the mother than any other complication of pregnancy. The effects of trauma on the fetus depend on

- The length of the pregnancy (the age of the fetus)
- The type and severity of the trauma
- The severity of blood flow and oxygen disruption to the uterus

Direct or indirect trauma to a pregnant uterus can cause injury to the uterine muscle. This can cause the release of chemicals that cause uterine contractions, perhaps inducing premature labor.

You Should Know

Causes of Trauma in Pregnancy

- Motor vehicle crashes
- Gunshot wounds
- Stabbings
- Domestic violence
- Falls
- Burns

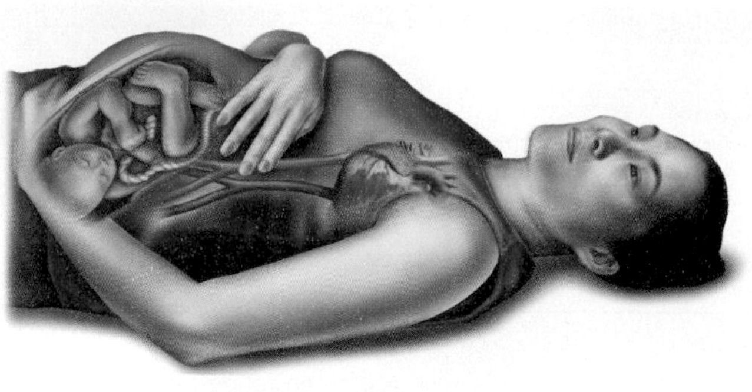

(a)

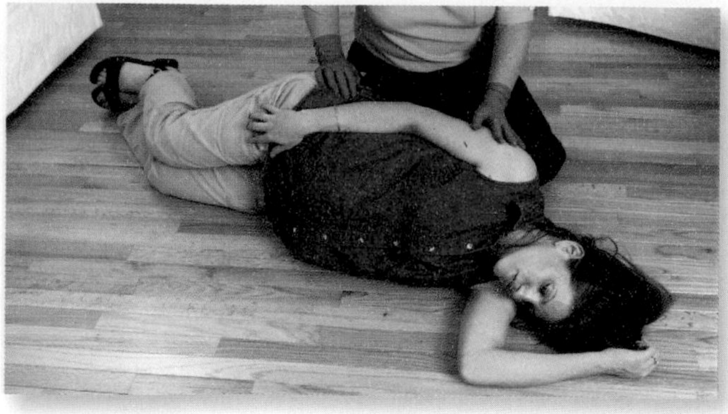

(b)

FIGURE 12-8 ▲ (a) When a woman in late pregnancy is placed on her back, the weight of the fetus compresses major blood vessels in the abdomen, such as the inferior vena cava and the aorta. This decreases the amount of blood returning to the mother's heart and lowers her blood pressure. (b) To relieve pressure on the abdominal blood vessels, place the pregnant patient on her left side.

Motor vehicle crashes (MVCs) are the most common cause of serious blunt trauma in pregnancy. *Abruptio placenta, placenta previa,* and uterine rupture are often seen in MVCs. These conditions increase the risk of fetal distress or death. Gunshot wounds and stab wounds to the abdomen of a pregnant patient do not usually result in the mother's death. However, the likelihood of fetal death is high.

Of women who are battered, 25–45% are battered during pregnancy.

For some women, pregnancy is a time when physical abuse starts. Physical abuse can result in the following conditions:

- Blunt trauma to the abdomen
- Severe bleeding
- Uterine rupture
- Miscarriage
- Premature labor
- Premature rupture of the amniotic sac

One in four pregnant women experiences falls during pregnancy.

During pregnancy, a woman's center of gravity shifts as the size of her abdomen increases and her pelvic ligaments loosen. As a result, a pregnant woman must readjust her body alignment and balance, which increases her risk for falls and injury. Some of these falls are a result of walking on slippery floors, hurrying, or carrying objects.

A thermal burn of more than 20% of the mother's body surface area increases the risk of fetal death. In cases of electrical burns, the likelihood of fetal death is high, even with a rather low electrical current. This is most likely because the fetus is floating in amniotic fluid and has a low resistance to the current.

Assessment of the Pregnant Patient

Blood flow to the fetus may be significantly decreased before signs of shock are obvious in the mother.

The assessment of a pregnant patient is the same as that of other patients. However, due to the normal changes in vital signs that occur with pregnancy, the patient's vital signs may not be as helpful as they are in a nonpregnant patient. For example, the pregnant patient's heart rate is normally slightly faster than usual. Her breathing rate is also slightly faster and more shallow than normal. Her blood pressure is often slightly lower than normal until the third trimester. It is important to take vital signs in all patients. However, you will need to pay special attention to the pregnant patient's history and look for other signs that may suggest a potential problem. For example, a patient with a history of vaginal bleeding for three hours who has cold, pale, clammy skin is probably in shock—even if her vital signs appear normal.

Despite a significant amount of internal or external bleeding, young, healthy pregnant patients can maintain relatively normal vital signs for a significant time and then develop signs of shock very quickly. For example, a pregnant patient may lose as much as 1½ liters of blood before you will see a decrease in blood pressure.

The signs of early shock are difficult to detect in a pregnant patient. As blood is lost due to trauma or complications of pregnancy, available blood is shunted away from the uterus and to the mother's heart and brain. This change compromises blood flow to the fetus. You can increase blood flow to the fetus by placing the pregnant patient on her left side.

Obtaining a SAMPLE History

Obtain a SAMPLE history to gather information about the pregnant patient's medical history.

- *Signs and symptoms.* The signs and symptoms that may indicate a possible complication of pregnancy include
  - Seizures
  - Weakness
  - Dizziness
  - Faintness
  - Signs of shock
  - Lightheadedness
  - Vaginal bleeding
  - Altered mental status
  - Passage of clots or tissue
  - Swelling of the face and/or extremities
  - Abdominal cramping or pain; may be constant or may come and go
- *Allergies.* Ask if the patient has any allergies to medications or other materials, such as latex.
- *Medications.* Examples of questions to ask about medications include the following:
  - Do you take any prescription medications? What is the medication for? When did you last take it? Are you taking prenatal vitamins? Have you taken fertility medications?
  - Do you take any over-the-counter medications, such as aspirin, allergy medications, cough syrup, or vitamins? Do you take any herbs?
  - Have you recently started taking any new medications? Have you recently stopped taking any medications?
  - Do you use any recreational drugs (crack, heroin, methadone, cocaine, marijuana)?
- *Pertinent past medical history.* Ask the patient the following questions:
  - Have you been seeing a doctor during your pregnancy?
  - Do you have a history of heart problems, respiratory problems, high blood pressure, diabetes, epilepsy, or any other ongoing medical conditions?
  - Do you smoke? Do you use alcohol?
- *Last oral intake.* When did you last have something to eat or drink?
- *Events leading to the injury or illness.* Find out about the events leading to the present situation by asking specific questions.
  - If the patient is complaining of abdominal pain, ask the following questions:
    - Are you sexually active? Is it possible that you are pregnant?
    - Do you use birth control?
    - When was your last menstrual period? Was it a normal period? Are your periods usually regular? Did you have any bleeding after that period?
    - Where is your pain exactly? (Ask the patient to point to the location.) What is it like (constant, comes and goes, dull, sharp, cramping)?
    - Have you had any vaginal bleeding or discharge? What color was it?

If childbirth is likely while the patient is in your care, the patient's answers to your questions about drugs are *very* important. For example, if the patient admits to heroin use within the past four hours, you must anticipate that her baby will need resuscitation when it is delivered.

Remember to use *OPQRST* to help identify the type and location of the patient's pain.

Stop and Think!

You must consider the possibility of pregnancy in any woman of childbearing age—especially if the patient is complaining of abdominal pain.

- If the patient is having vaginal bleeding, ask the following questions:
  - How long have you been bleeding?
  - What color is it?
  - How much are you bleeding? (How many pads have you used?)
  - Have you passed any clots?
- If the patient is pregnant, ask the following questions:
  - Do you know your due date?
  - Is this your first pregnancy?
  - How many children do you have? Were your children delivered vaginally? Did you have any problems with any of those pregnancies (such as premature labor, large babies, hemorrhage, cesarean section, miscarriage, abortion)?
  - Have you had any prenatal care?
  - Have you had any problems with this pregnancy?

If the patient is having contractions, ask specific questions to determine if delivery is about to happen. These questions are covered in the section "Pre-Delivery Considerations."

Perform a physical exam. Keep in mind that your patient may be anxious about having her clothing removed and having an examination performed by a stranger. Be certain to explain what you are about to do and why it must be done. Remember to properly drape or shield an unclothed patient from the stares of others. Conduct the examination professionally and efficiently, and talk with your patient throughout the procedure.

If possible, include a female attendant or rescuer in your examination.

As an Emergency Medical Responder, you must not visually inspect the vaginal area unless major bleeding is present or you anticipate that childbirth is about to occur. In these situations, it is best to have another healthcare professional or law enforcement officer present. The vaginal area is touched *only* during delivery and when another healthcare professional or law enforcement officer is present.

Remember This!

When caring for a pregnant patient, keep in mind that the well-being of the fetus is entirely dependent on the well-being of the mother.

Emergency Medical Responder Care of Pregnancy Complications

When you arrive at the scene, first consider your personal safety. During the scene size-up, evaluate the mechanism of injury or the nature of the illness before approaching the patient.

An **obstetric emergency** (an emergency related to pregnancy or childbirth) is frequently associated with bleeding.

- Take BSI precautions and put on appropriate PPE. In addition to gloves, you should wear eye protection, a mask, and a gown. During childbirth, blood and amniotic fluid are expected and may splash.
- Determine the total number of patients. If a delivery is about to happen, there is going to be another patient. Call for additional help to the scene to assist you in caring for both mother and baby.

- After the scene size-up, form a general impression by pausing a short distance from the patient to determine if the patient appears "sick" or "not sick." Determine the urgency of further assessment and care.
- Perform an initial assessment to identify and treat any life-threatening conditions.
    - As with all patients, your initial attention must be directed at making sure the patient has an open airway, adequate breathing, and adequate circulation.
    - Manually stabilize the patient's head and neck if trauma is suspected.
    - Control any obvious external bleeding. If vaginal bleeding is present, apply external vaginal pads as necessary. As the pad becomes blood-soaked, replace it with a new one. Place all blood-soaked clothing and pads in a biohazard container and send them to the hospital with the patient. These items will be used to estimate the patient's blood loss.
    - Treat for shock if indicated. Give oxygen if it is available and you have been trained to use it. Maintain the patient's body temperature. Use blankets or sheets as needed to prevent heat loss.
- Perform a physical exam. Take the patient's vital signs and gather her medical history.
- If a spinal injury is suspected, immobilize the patient on a long backboard. Remember to tilt the board slightly to the left by placing a rolled towel, a small pillow, a blanket, or another type of padding under the right side of the board.
- Arrange for transport to the nearest appropriate hospital. If possible, update the EMS unit responding to the scene with a brief report by phone or radio. Provide emotional support to the patient and family members while awaiting the arrival of EMS personnel.
- If the patient is stable, perform ongoing assessments every 15 minutes. If the patient is unstable, perform ongoing assessments every 5 minutes.

Stop and Think!

If the mother suffers a cardiac arrest, continue CPR. If the mother is more than 24 weeks pregnant, the fetus may be able to survive outside the uterus. Update the EMS personnel responding to the scene so that they can notify the hospital that will receive the patient. On arrival at the hospital, special equipment will be used to assess the condition of the fetus.

Normal Labor

Labor is the time and process in which the uterus repeatedly contracts to push the fetus and placenta out of the mother's body. It begins with the first uterine muscle contraction and ends with delivery of the placenta. **Delivery** is the birth of the baby at the end of the second stage of labor.

The Stages of Labor

Before labor begins, the head of the fetus normally settles into the pelvis. The mother may feel she can "breathe easier" but will also feel the need to urinate frequently. The cervix begins to open (dilate) and thin out (efface). In addition, the mucous plug may be expelled (bloody show).

The First Stage of Labor

The bag of waters (amniotic sac) often bursts during this stage.

The first stage of labor begins with the first uterine contraction. This stage ends with a complete thinning and opening of the cervix. Contractions usually begin as regular, cramplike pains that gradually increase in strength. They usually last from 30–60 seconds and occur every 5–15 minutes. In a woman who has not previously given birth, this stage of labor lasts about 8–16 hours. It lasts about 6–8 hours in a woman who has previously given birth.

You Should Know

Timing Contractions

You will need to know how far apart your patient's contractions are and how long each contraction lasts. Place the fingertips of one hand high on the patient's uterus. When you feel the patient's abdomen become hard under your fingers, the contraction has started. When the hardness is gone, the contraction has ended.

Using a watch that shows seconds, begin timing at the start of a contraction. End timing at the beginning of the next contraction. This measure tells you how far apart the contractions are. You will need to time a series of contractions, such as four or five contractions in a row, to see if they are regular or irregular.

To determine how long a contraction is, begin timing at the start of a contraction and end timing when the same contraction is over.

The Second Stage of Labor

The second stage of labor begins with the full dilation (opening) of the cervix and ends with the delivery of the infant. The contractions during this stage are stronger. They last 45–60 seconds and occur every 2–3 minutes.

During this stage, the fetus begins its descent into the birth canal. The **presenting part** is the part of the infant that comes out of the birth canal first. Normally, the first part of the infant that descends into the birth canal is the head. This is called a **cephalic (head) delivery** or presentation. If the buttocks or feet descend first, it is called a **breech delivery** or presentation.

Toward the end of this stage of labor, the mother experiences an urge to bear down, or push, with each contraction. The presenting part will appear and disappear at the vaginal opening between contractions. As the presenting part presses on the rectum, the mother will feel an urge to move her bowels. Eventually, the presenting part will remain visible at the vaginal opening between contractions. This is called **crowning**. This stage of labor averages 1–2 hours in a woman who has not previously given birth. In a woman who has given birth in the past, this stage of labor lasts 20–30 minutes.

The Third Stage of Labor

This stage of labor normally lasts five minutes to an hour.

The third stage of labor begins with the delivery of the infant and ends with the delivery of the placenta (Figure 12-9). The placenta peels away from the wall of the uterus, leaving tiny blood vessels exposed. The uterus normally contracts to close these blood vessels. The placenta usually delivers within 15–30 minutes of the infant's birth.

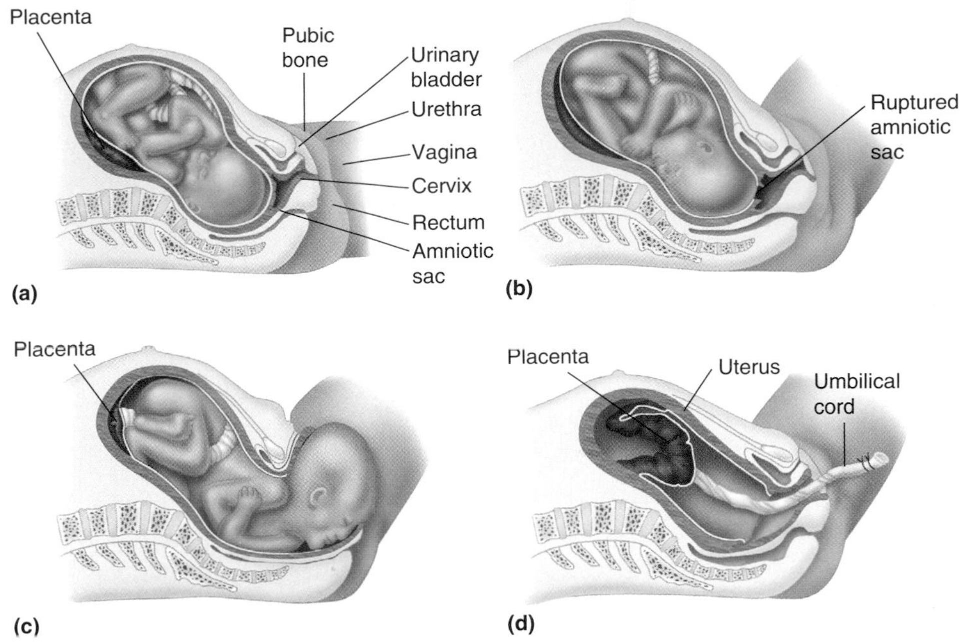

FIGURE 12-9 ▶ The stages of labor. (a) The relationship of the fetus to the mother. (b) Stage 1 begins with the onset of uterine contractions and ends with the complete thinning out and opening of the cervix. (c) Stage 2 begins with full dilation of the cervix and ends with the delivery of the baby. (d) Stage 3 begins with the delivery of the baby and ends with the delivery of the placenta.

Remember This!

The Stages of Labor

Stage 1. Begins with the onset of uterine contractions; ends with complete thinning and opening of the cervix

Stage 2. Begins with opening of the cervix; ends with delivery of the infant

Stage 3. Begins with delivery of the infant; ends with delivery of the placenta

You Should Know

False Labor

Many women have false labor pains about two to four weeks before delivery. False labor pains are called Braxton Hicks contractions. These contractions help prepare the woman's body for delivery by softening and thinning her cervix. It is sometimes difficult to tell the difference between false labor and true labor. Table 12-2 lists the differences between the contractions of true and false labor.

TABLE 12-2 True and False Labor Contractions

True Labor Contractions	False Labor Contractions
• Occur regularly • Get closer together • Become stronger as time passes; each lasts about 30–60 seconds • Continue despite the patient's activity	• Usually are weak, irregular • Do not get closer together over time • Do not get stronger • May stop or slow down when the patient walks, lies down, or changes position

Normal Delivery

Pre-Delivery Considerations

Generally, you should transport a woman in labor to the hospital unless delivery of the baby is expected within a few minutes. You must determine if there is time for the mother to reach the hospital or if preparations should be made for delivery at the scene. To make this decision, ask the patient the following questions:

- Is this your first pregnancy?
  - Labor with a first pregnancy is usually longer than that of subsequent deliveries.
- When is your due date?
  - Knowing the due date will help you determine if the baby is premature or full-term.
- Has your bag of waters broken? When? What was the color of the water?
  - Labor usually begins shortly after the bag of waters breaks. The greater the length of time since the bag of waters has broken until the start of labor, the greater the risk of fetal infection. The fetus usually needs to be delivered within 18–24 hours after the bag of waters has ruptured. Some women may not be sure if their water has broken or not. Some will tell you there was a "big gush of water." Others will describe a steady trickle of water when their water breaks. In others, the bag of waters may not break until well into the labor process. The fluid from the amniotic sac should be clear. If the mother tells you that the color of the water was brownish-yellow or green (like pea soup), expect the baby's airway to need special care after delivery.
- Have you experienced any vaginal bleeding or discharge? How long ago? Did you have any pain with the bleeding?
  - A discharge of mucus mixed with blood (bloody show) is a sign that labor has begun. If excessive bleeding is present, the mother is at risk for shock and the baby's well-being is also at risk.
- Are you having any contractions? When did they start? How close are they now?
  - Contractions that are strong and regular, last 45–60 seconds, and are 1–2 minutes apart indicate that delivery will happen soon.
- Do you feel the need to push or bear down?
  - The urge to push, bear down, or have a bowel movement occurs as the baby moves down the birth canal and presses on the bladder and rectum. Delivery will occur soon.
- How many babies are there?
  - If delivery is to occur at the scene, this information will help you determine the additional resources you may need to call to help you. It will also help you determine the equipment you need to gather to assist with the delivery.

Additional questions that are important to ask include the following:

- Have you taken any medications or drugs?
  - Some medications or drugs taken by the mother will affect her baby. If the mother has taken narcotics within four hours of delivery, the baby's breathing may be very slow at delivery.
- Has your doctor told you if the baby is coming head first or feet first?
  - Normally, the baby's head presents first in the birth canal. If the mother has been told that her baby is coming feet first (breech delivery) and the baby will be delivered on the scene, call for additional help.

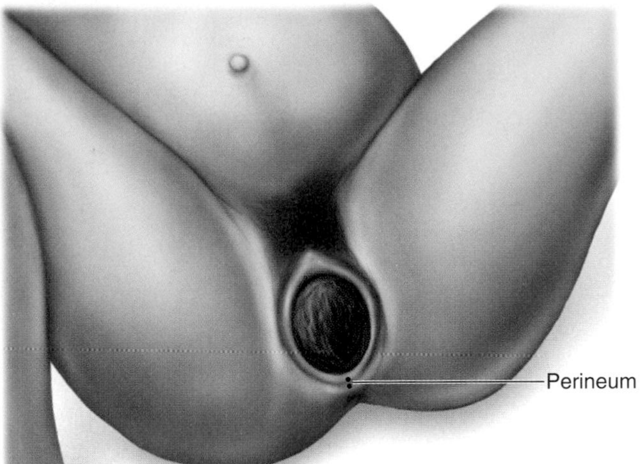

FIGURE 12-10 ▶ To check for crowning, look at the patient's perineum while she is having a contraction. If you see bulging or the baby's head beginning to emerge from the birth canal, prepare for immediate delivery.

Signs of Imminent Delivery

Consider delivering at the scene in the following three circumstances:

Objective 3 ▶

Objective 5 ▶

1. Delivery can be expected in a few minutes.
   - A woman in late pregnancy feels the urge to push, bear down, or have a bowel movement.
   - Crowning is present. To determine if crowning is present, you will need to look at the patient's perineum (Figure 12-10). Take appropriate BSI precautions, such as gloves, mask, gown, and eye protection. Position the patient on her back and remove her undergarments. Place padding under her hips to elevate them. Ask the patient to bend her knees and spread her thighs apart. Look at the patient's perineum while she is having a contraction. If you see bulging or the baby's head beginning to emerge from the birth canal, prepare for immediate delivery. After visually examining the perineum, remember to cover the area with a towel or sheet to protect the patient's modesty.
   - Contractions are regular, last 45–60 seconds, and are 1–2 minutes apart.
2. No suitable transportation is available.
3. The hospital cannot be reached due to heavy traffic, bad weather, a natural disaster, or a similar situation.

If there is time to transport the patient to the hospital, remove any undergarments that might obstruct delivery. Place the patient on her left side. Arrange for prompt transport.

Preparing for Delivery

Objective 11 ▶

If you decide that the delivery will occur on the scene, you will need to prepare yourself and the patient. As you make preparations for the delivery, keep in mind that the mother-to-be is doing all the work. Your job is to help the mother and newborn. For most women, the pain of labor and delivery is one of the things that worries them the most about having a baby. Although some women have labor with relatively little pain, most women experience considerable pain that worsens as labor progresses. The amount of pain varies from woman to woman. Even if your patient has previously given birth, the pain she experiences may be different with each delivery.

Objective 12 ▶

Although you may be nervous about helping with the delivery, it is important that you appear calm and confident. Reassure the mother-to-be that you will not leave her alone and that you are there to help her. Because labor and delivery are

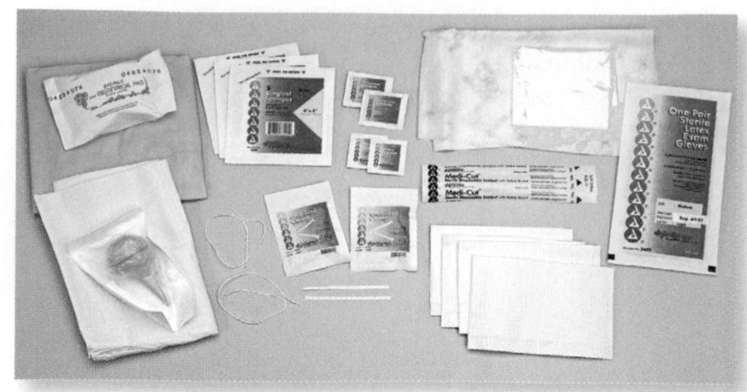

FIGURE 12-11 ▶ Contents of a ready-made childbirth delivery kit.

Objective 13 ▶
Objective 14 ▶

very hard work, she may become tired and quite cranky. If she is irritable, do not take any comments she makes personally. Help her through her labor by offering words of support, such as "You're doing great!" Coach her to breathe slowly in through her nose and out through her mouth. As she tires, she may become less and less receptive to your instructions. You may need to repeat these instructions often. Repeat them as often as needed, without appearing frustrated. As you prepare the patient and surroundings for the baby's arrival, remember to explain what you are doing to the patient and any family members that are present.

Objectives 5, 6 ▶

Because blood and amniotic fluid are expected during childbirth and may splash, you must use BSI precautions, including gloves, mask, eye protection, and a gown. You will need a ready-made childbirth delivery kit (also called an obstetrics, or OB, kit; Figure 12-11). If a ready-made kit is not available, substitute the items in the following list with similar items that will serve the same purpose:

- Scissors (used to cut the umbilical cord)
- Hemostats or cord clamps (used to clamp the umbilical cord) or umbilical tape (used to tie the umbilical cord instead of clamping it)
  - If these items are not available, you can use thick string, gauze, or clean shoelaces to tie off the umbilical cord.
- A bulb syringe (used to clear secretions from the infant's mouth and nose)
- Gauze sponges or towels (used to wipe and dry the infant)
- Sterile gloves (for protection from infection during delivery)
- A baby blanket (used to wrap and warm the infant)
- Sanitary pads (used to absorb vaginal drainage after delivery)
- A plastic bag or large plastic container with a lid (used to transport the placenta to the hospital)
- A sterile sheet, sterile towels, or barrier drapes (to create a sterile field around the vaginal opening).
  - If these items are not available, you can use clean towels or clothing, a plastic sheet, or newspapers to provide a clean surface.

Objective 4 ▶

Position your patient on her back, with her head and back raised (Figure 12-12). Support her head and back with pillows. This position allows gravity to help when she pushes. Remove the patient's clothing and undergarments from the waist down. Gather clean, absorbent materials, such as towels, sheets, blankets, clean clothing, or paper barriers. Place some of the absorbent material under the patient's buttocks. Make sure there is enough room in front of the mother's buttocks to provide a firm surface to support the infant after delivery. Have the patient bend her knees and spread her thighs apart. Place a towel, folded sheet, or paper barrier over the patient's abdomen and another across the inside of the patient's thighs. Remember not to touch the patient's vaginal area except during delivery and when another healthcare professional or law enforcement officer is present.

Remember: Positioning the mother flat on her back compresses major blood vessels. This can lower her blood pressure and decrease blood flow to the uterus. It is also very hard for the patient to push well when lying flat.

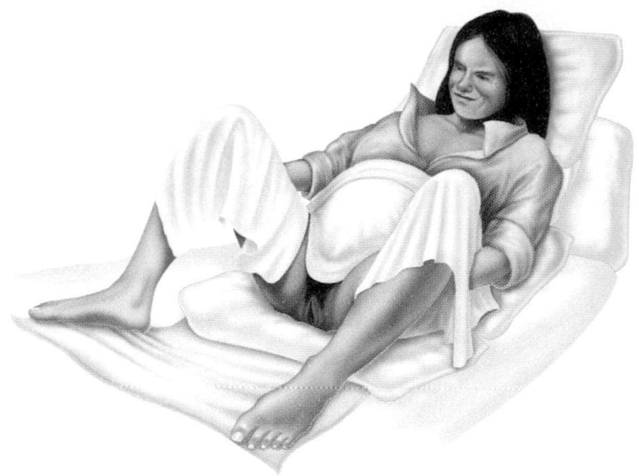

FIGURE 12-12 ▶ To prepare the mother for delivery, position her on her back, with her head and back raised, supported with pillows.

Your patient may tell you she feels as if she needs to have a bowel movement. Do not let her go to the bathroom. This sensation is caused by the presenting part of the infant in the birth canal pressing against the walls of the patient's rectum. If the mother urinates or has a bowel movement during a contraction, remove the material completely with a pad or washcloth and replace the soiled absorbent materials with clean ones. Do not hold the mother's legs together or attempt to delay or restrain delivery in any way.

Delivery Procedure

When the mother's cervix is completely open, she will feel an almost involuntary need to push. Pushing is done only with uterine contractions. When a contraction begins, tell the mother to take in a deep breath and blow it out. Have her take another deep breath, hold it while you or a family member quickly counts to 10, and bear down as if she is straining to have a bowel movement. Your patient will be holding her breath for about 6 seconds (not 10), but a quick count of 10 will be helpful to her. At the end of the count of 10, tell her to breathe out and quickly take another breath in, holding for another count of 10. Most contractions are long enough to permit 2 or 3 attempts at this. Once the contraction is over, she should blow out any remaining air and begin restful breathing. Encourage her to relax completely to conserve energy and recover for the next contraction.

At this point, it is common for patients to say, "I just can't do this anymore." Offer your patient words of encouragement. Praise her on the progress she is making. You may notice more bloody show during this stage of labor. This is normal as the patient's cervix stretches open and some of the tiny blood vessels break.

Objective 7 ▶

When the infant's head appears, cup your gloved fingers over the bony part of the infant's crowning head. Apply very gentle pressure to prevent the baby's head from coming out too fast and tearing the perineum (an explosive delivery; Figure 12-13). Do not apply pressure to the infant's face or the soft spots on the baby's head (fontanelles). If the bag of waters does not break or has not broken, use your gloved fingers to tear it. Push the sac away from the infant's head and mouth as they appear.

As the baby's head is being born, check the infant's neck to see if a loop of the umbilical cord is wrapped around it. If the cord is around the neck, gently loosen the cord and try to slip it over the baby's shoulder or head. If the umbilical cord is wrapped tightly around the baby's neck and cannot be loosened or is wrapped around the neck more than once, immediately notify the responding EMS unit. If your EMS protocols allow it, remove the cord. To do this, place two umbilical clamps or ties on the cord about 3 inches apart (Figure 12-14). Carefully cut the cord between the two clamps. Remove the cord from the baby's neck.

Babies breathe mostly through their noses. Suction the baby's mouth first to be sure there is nothing for the baby to suck into the lungs if the baby should gasp when you suction the nose.

Do not pull on the baby's head.

As the baby's head is delivered and before delivery of the shoulders, support the head with one hand and clear the infant's airway. Squeeze the bulb of a bulb syringe and then gently insert the narrow end of the syringe into the baby's mouth (Figure 12-15). To apply suction, slowly release pressure on the bulb. Remove the syringe from the baby's mouth and squeeze the syringe several times to remove secretions from it. Suction the mouth two or three times. Do not apply suction for more than three to five seconds per attempt. Be careful not to touch the back of the baby's throat with the bulb syringe. This can cause severe slowing of the baby's heart rate. After clearing the mouth, suction each nostril. If a bulb syringe is not available, use a clean gauze pad or a cloth to wipe secretions from the baby's mouth and nose.

Once the baby's head is delivered, its head will usually turn to line up with its shoulders. This allows the baby's shoulders and the rest of the body to pass through the birth canal. Gently guide the head downward to deliver the top shoulder. Gently guide the head upward to deliver the bottom shoulder (Figure 12-16). Tell the mother not to push during this time.

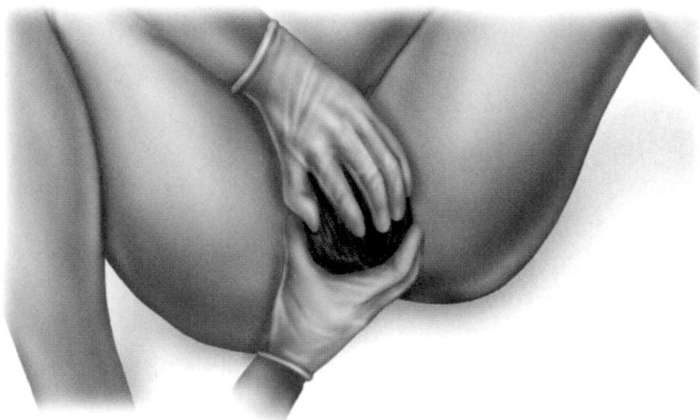

FIGURE 12-13 ▲ When the infant's head appears during crowning, cup your gloved fingers over the bony part of the infant's skull. Exert very gentle pressure to prevent the baby's head from coming out too fast and tearing the perineum.

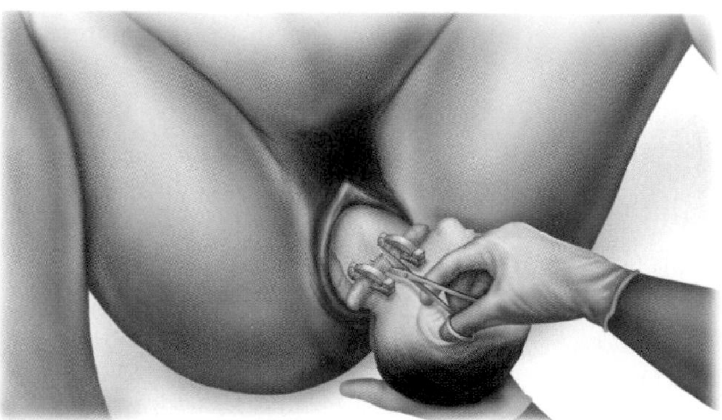

FIGURE 12-14 ▲ If the umbilical cord is wrapped tightly around the baby's neck and cannot be loosened, you will need to remove it. To do this, place two umbilical clamps or ties on the cord, approximately 3 inches apart. Carefully cut the cord between the two clamps. Remove the cord from the baby's neck.

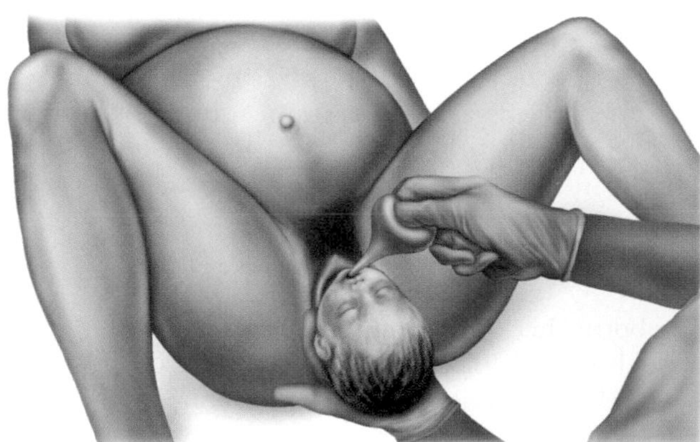

FIGURE 12-15 ▲ As the baby's head is delivered and before delivery of the shoulders, support the baby's head with one hand and clear the airway using a bulb syringe.

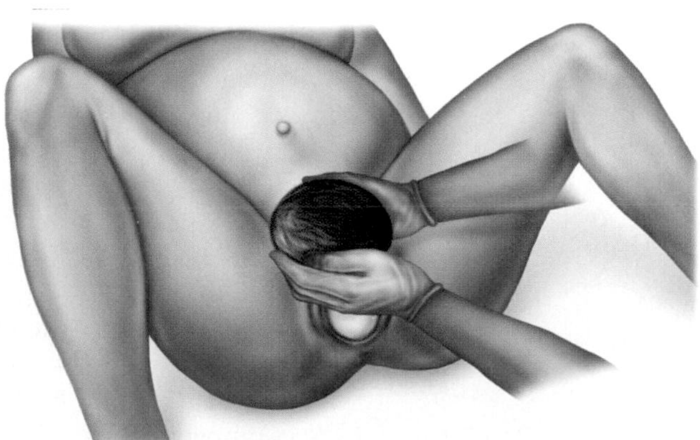

FIGURE 12-16 ▲ Gently guide the baby's head upward to deliver the bottom shoulder.

After the shoulders are delivered, the rest of the baby's body should slip right out. Because the baby will be covered with blood and amniotic fluid, he or she will be wet and very slippery. You may find it helpful to use a clean towel to hold onto the baby. As the baby's chest and abdomen are born, support the newborn with both hands. As the feet are born, grasp them. Try to remember to note the time the baby was born. Keep the baby at or around the same level as the mother's vaginal opening until it is time to clamp the umbilical cord.

Remember This!

It is important to keep the baby at or around the same level as the mother's vaginal opening until the umbilical cord has been clamped. This is because blood can continue to flow between the newborn and the placenta. If you position the baby above the level of the mother's vaginal opening, such as on the mother's abdomen or chest, blood may drain from the baby's circulation into the placenta. This will decrease the amount of blood in the baby's circulation. If you place the baby below the level of the mother's vaginal opening, blood may drain from the placenta into the baby's circulation. This may cause thickening of the baby's blood.

Emergency Medical Responder Care of the Newborn and Mother

Once the baby is born, you will have two patients—the newborn and the mother. First provide care for the newborn. If possible, position the baby between you and the mother so that you can periodically observe the mother while providing care for her baby.

Caring for the Newborn

Objective 10 ▶

Quickly dry the baby's body and head to remove blood and amniotic fluid (Figure 12-17). Immediately remove the wet towel or blanket from the infant and then quickly wrap the baby in a clean, warm blanket. Place the baby on his or her back or side, with the neck in a neutral position. Wipe blood and mucus from the baby's mouth and nose. Suction the mouth and then the nose again. This suctioning will often cause the baby to begin crying and breathing. Cover the baby's body and head to prevent heat loss, keeping the face exposed.

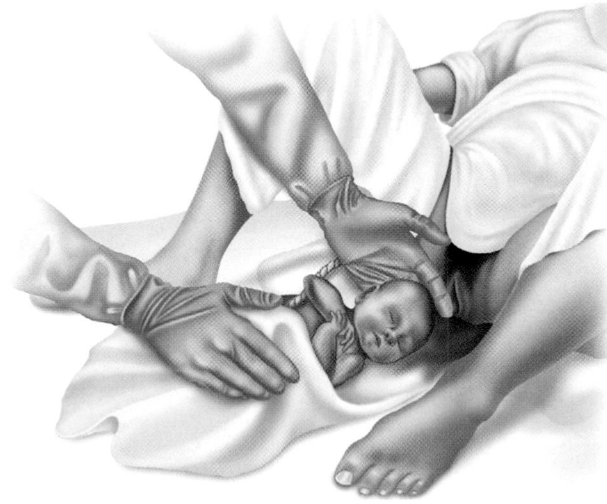

FIGURE 12-17 ▶ Keep the baby at or around the same level as the mother's vaginal opening until it is time to clamp the umbilical cord. Quickly dry the baby's body and head to remove blood and amniotic fluid.

Provide warmth, position the baby, clear the airway as necessary, dry, stimulate, and reposition. These actions should take 30 seconds or less to accomplish.

Remember This!

It is very important to keep a newborn warm. Newborns lose heat very quickly because they are wet and suddenly exposed to an environment that is cooler than that inside the uterus. Most body heat is lost through the head and is due to evaporation. Therefore, immediately dry the baby and cover the head as soon as possible.

Airway and Breathing

A full-term baby's respiratory rate is normally between 30 and 60 breaths per minute in the first 12 hours of life. After that, a newborn's normal respiratory rate is 30–50 breaths per minute.

You should begin to assess the newborn immediately after birth. Focus on the baby's breathing rate and effort, the heart rate, and skin color. Most babies will begin crying and breathing as a result of the stimulation provided during warming, suctioning, and drying. If the baby has not begun to breathe or is breathing very slowly, stimulate the baby. Do this by rubbing his or her back, chest, or extremities or by tapping or flicking the bottom of the feet (Figure 12-18). These methods may be tried for 5–10 seconds to stimulate breathing.

If the baby's breathing is adequate, assess the heart rate. If there is no improvement after 5–10 seconds, help the baby breathe using mouth-to-mask breathing or a BVM. Breathe at a rate of 40–60 breaths per minute (slightly less than 1 breath per second). Use 100% oxygen if it is available and you have been trained to use it. Use just enough pressure to see a gentle chest rise. If you use too much pressure, you will force air into the baby's stomach, which will compromise breathing. Recheck the baby's breathing, heart rate, and color after 30 seconds. If there is no improvement, continue breathing for the baby. Reassess often.

Heart Rate

A full-term baby's heart rate is normally 100–180 beats per minute in the first 12 hours of life. After that, a newborn's normal heart rate is 120–160 beats per minute.

Assess the baby's pulse by feeling the brachial pulse on the inside of the upper arm. Count the heart rate for 6 seconds and multiply by 10 to estimate the beats per minute. Because a baby's heart rate is usually very fast, it may be helpful to tap out the heart rate as you count it. If the baby's heart rate is more than 100 beats per minute, assess the baby's skin color. If the heart rate is less than 100 beats per minute, immediately breathe for the baby using mouth-to-mask breathing or a bag-valve mask. Reassess the baby's breathing, heart rate, and color after 30 seconds. If there is no improvement and the baby's heart rate is less than 60 beats per minute, begin chest compressions. If the baby's heart rate is more than 60 beats per minute but breathing is inadequate, continue breathing for the baby using mouth-to-mask breathing or a BVM. Reassess in 30 seconds.

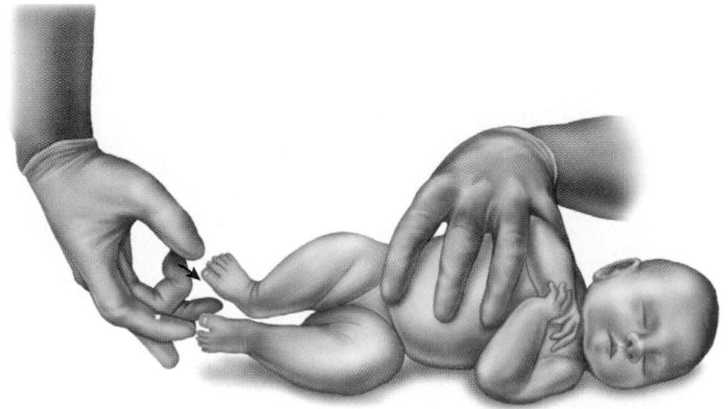

FIGURE 12-18 ► If the baby has not begun to breathe or is breathing very slowly, stimulate the baby by rubbing the back, chest, or extremities or by tapping or flicking the bottom of the feet.

Skin Color

Do not blow oxygen directly into the baby's face.

Look at the color of the baby's face, chest, or inside the mouth. A bluish tint in these areas is called central cyanosis. The skin of a newborn's extremities is often blue (acrocyanosis) immediately after delivery. This finding is common and should quickly improve if the baby is breathing adequately and is kept warm. If the baby is breathing adequately and has a heart rate of more than 100 beats per minute but central cyanosis is present, give blow-by oxygen if available. To do this, cup your hand around the oxygen tubing. Hold the tubing close to the baby's nose and mouth. The oxygen source should be set to deliver at least 5 liters per minute.

Caring for the Mother

Objective 9 ▶

Because the umbilical cord will tear easily, always handle it very gently.

When the umbilical cord stops pulsating, clamp or tie the umbilical cord in two places between the mother and the baby. The cord usually stops pulsating 3–5 minutes after delivery of the baby. Place the first clamp or tie approximately 4–6 inches from the baby's belly. Place the second clamp or tie approximately 2–3 inches distal to the first clamp (farther away from the baby). If the clamps or ties are firmly in place, cut the cord between the two clamps with scissors if your EMS system permits you to do so (Figure 12-19). If you are not permitted to cut the cord, EMS personnel will do this when they arrive. If the cord is cut, periodically check the cut ends for bleeding. If the cut end of the cord attached to the baby is bleeding, clamp (or tie) the cord proximal to the existing clamps or ties. Do not remove the first clamp or tie.

Objective 8 ▶

Gently wipe away any blood and amniotic fluid from the mother's perineum. Watch for delivery of the placenta. The placenta is usually delivered within 30 minutes of the baby. The signs that indicate the separation of the placenta from the uterus include

It is not necessary to wait for the placenta to deliver before transporting the mother and infant.

- A gush of blood
- A lengthening of the umbilical cord
- A contraction of the uterus
- An urge to push

Encourage the mother to push to help deliver the placenta. Wrap the placenta in a towel. If the cord was cut, place the placenta in an appropriate

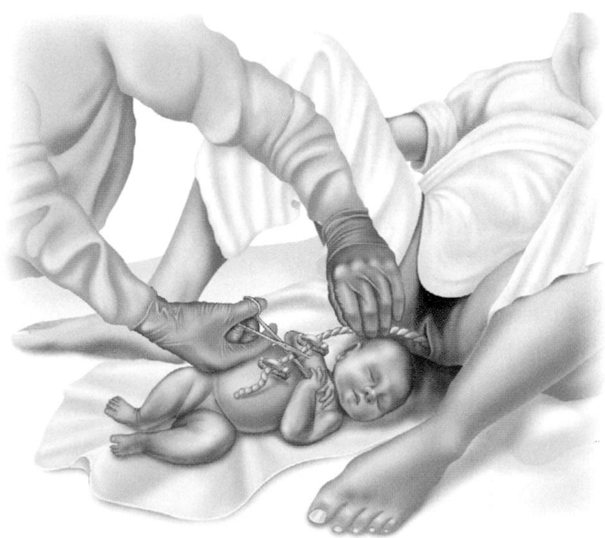

FIGURE 12-19 ▶ If your EMS system permits you to do so, cut the umbilical cord when it stops pulsating. Clamp or tie the umbilical cord in two places between the mother and the baby. Place the first clamp or tie approximately 4–6 inches from the baby's belly. Place the second clamp approximately 2–3 inches distal to the first. If the clamps/ties are firmly in place, cut the cord between the two clamps with scissors.

biohazard container. If you clamped but did not cut the cord, place the wrapped placenta next to the baby.

Stop and Think!

Never pull on the umbilical cord to speed delivery of the placenta. Pulling or tugging on the cord can cause the uterus to turn inside out. Shock often follows.

If you have not already done so, record the time of delivery.

After delivery of the placenta, check the mother's perineum for bleeding. During delivery, the perineum can tear as it stretches to make room for the baby's head and body. This tearing can result in bleeding. Use a sanitary pad to apply pressure to any bleeding tears. Be careful not to touch the side of the pad that will be placed against the patient. Do not place anything inside the vagina.

When looking at the mother's vaginal area for bleeding, keep in mind that it is normal for the mother to lose up to 500 mL (1/2 L) of blood during childbirth. This amount of blood loss will not negatively affect most healthy, young women. If the mother appears alarmed or concerned about the amount of blood, reassure her that this is normal. Place a sanitary pad over the vaginal opening, lower the mother's legs, and help her hold them together. While the patient is in your care, reassess her often to be sure she does not lose too much blood.

Uterine massage is painful. Try to understand your patient's complaints of pain if you must perform this procedure. Explain what you are doing and why.

If blood loss appears excessive, give oxygen to the mother by nonrebreather mask if it is available and you have been trained to use it. Stimulate the uterus to contract by performing uterine massage. With your fingers fully extended, place one hand horizontally across the abdomen, just above the pubic bone. This positioning is very important. It helps prevent downward shifting of the uterus during the massage. Cup your other hand around the uterus. Massage the area using a kneading motion. Continue massaging until the uterus feels firm, like a ball (Figure 12-20). Bleeding should lessen as the uterus becomes firm. Recheck the patient every five minutes. If bleeding continues to appear excessive, reassess your massage technique and treat the patient for shock. If possible, update EMS personnel en route to the scene about the patient's condition.

Encourage the mother to breast-feed her baby. Breast-feeding stimulates the uterus to contract. When the uterus contracts, blood vessels within the walls of the uterus constrict, decreasing bleeding. Make sure the placenta is transported to the hospital with the mother. Hospital staff will look closely at the placenta for completeness. If pieces of the placenta stay in the uterus, the mother will have ongoing bleeding.

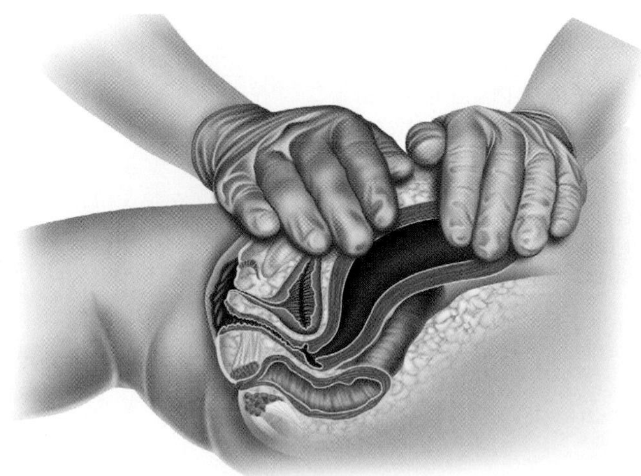

FIGURE 12-20 ▶ Stimulate the uterus to contract by performing uterine massage. With the fingers fully extended, place one hand horizontally across the abdomen, just above the pubic bone. Doing so helps prevent downward displacement of the uterus during the massage. Cup your other hand around the uterus. Massage the area using a kneading motion. Continue massaging until the uterus feels firm, like a ball.

While awaiting transport of the mother and baby to the hospital, continue to provide supportive care. This care should include the following:

- Taking the patient's vital signs often
- Helping the mother to a position of comfort
- Keeping the mother warm
- Rechecking the amount of vaginal bleeding, replacing sanitary pads with clean ones as needed
- Replacing any soiled sheets and blankets with fresh ones
- Carefully placing all soiled items in an appropriate biohazard container

On The Scene

Wrap-Up

The woman tells you that she already has seven children and that the last one came in 30 minutes. You place a hand on her abdomen and can tell that her contractions last about a minute, with only two minutes between them. As you open the OB kit, she begins to grunt and her eyes bulge as she strains. The supervisor clears the area. When you remove the patient's jeans, you can see the baby's head protruding from her vagina. "Pant," you tell her as you grab a blanket and a bulb syringe. With the next contraction, the baby's head is delivered. You quickly suction the baby's mouth and nose. With one more push from the mother, you guide the baby's body out, one shoulder at a time, into your waiting hands.

You hang on carefully to the slippery little infant, suctioning the little boy and taking a breath only when you see the baby's face scrunch into a grimace and you hear a hearty cry. You note the time as you glance at your watch to check his pulse. The baby's pulse is fine at 160 beats per minute. After drying him off, you place a dry blanket around him, taking care to cover his head. When the pulsation in the cord stops, you apply the clamps securely and then carefully cut it. You note that the baby's hands are a little blue, but the rest of his body is pink. He is crying and moving around.

You make sure that the baby is covered and then turn your attention to his mother. You can see the umbilical cord move up and down slightly and hear the mother moan. A moment later there is a small gush of blood and the placenta is delivered. At that moment, the ambulance crew enters the warehouse, takes your report, and assesses the mother and her newborn. As they wheel their patients toward the ambulance, one of the Paramedics turns to you with a grin on her face and says, "Great job, but I don't know why you called us—you've already done all the hard work." ■

Sum It Up

- ▶ The *vagina* is also called the *birth canal.* It is a muscular tube that serves as a passageway between the uterus and the outside of the body.
- ▶ The *placenta* is a specialized organ through which the fetus exchanges nourishment and waste products during pregnancy. It attaches to the mother at the inner wall of the uterus and to the fetus by the umbilical cord. The placenta begins to develop about 2 weeks after fertilization occurs.
- ▶ The *umbilical cord* is the lifeline that connects the placenta to the fetus. It contains two arteries and one vein. The umbilical vein carries oxygen-rich blood to the fetus. The umbilical cord attaches to the umbilicus (navel) of the fetus.

- The *amniotic sac* is a membranous bag that surrounds the fetus inside the uterus. It contains fluid (amniotic fluid), which helps protect the fetus from injury. The amniotic fluid provides an environment that is at a constant temperature. It also allows the fetus to move and functions much as a shock absorber does.
- The *first trimester* is the first three months of pregnancy.
  - The mother stops menstruating (missed period). She urinates more frequently and may sleep more than usual. Nausea and vomiting (usually called "morning sickness") are usually at its worst during the second month.
  - The fetus develops rapidly. Fetal cells differentiate into tissues and organs. The arms, legs, heart, lungs, and brain begin to form. At the end of the first trimester, the fetus is about 3 inches long and weighs about ½ ounce.
- The *second trimester* is months 4–6 of the pregnancy.
  - The uterus expands to make room for the fetus. The mother's abdomen enlarges and her center of gravity often changes. The mother begins to feel the fetus move at about the fourth or fifth month. Her circulatory system continues to expand, which lowers her blood pressure.
  - The fetus's fingers, toes, eyelashes, and eyebrows are formed. At about the fifth month, the heartbeat of the fetus can be heard with a stethoscope. By the end of this trimester, the heart, lungs, and kidneys have formed. The fetus weighs about 1¾ pounds and is about 13 inches long.
- The *third trimester* is months 7–9 of the pregnancy.
  - The mother may experience a backache due to muscle strain. Stretch marks may appear. The mother urinates frequently because the weight of the uterus presses on the bladder. She may be short of breath as her uterus expands beneath the diaphragm.
  - The fetus continues to grow rapidly, gaining about ½ pound a week and reaching a length of about 20 inches. Fetal movement occurs often and is stronger. Normally, the head of the fetus settles into the pelvis in preparation for delivery.
- An *abortion* is a termination of pregnancy before the fetus is able to live on its own outside the uterus.
  - A *therapeutic abortion* is an abortion performed for medical reasons, often because the pregnancy poses a threat to the mother's health.
  - An *elective abortion* is an abortion performed at the request of the mother.
  - A *spontaneous abortion,* also called a *miscarriage,* is a loss of a fetus due to natural causes. It usually occurs before the 20th week of pregnancy. In most miscarriages, the fetus dies because of a genetic abnormality that is usually unrelated to the mother. During a miscarriage, the mother experiences lower back pain or cramping abdominal pain, vaginal bleeding, and the passage of tissue or clotlike material from the vagina.
- An *ectopic pregnancy* occurs when a fertilized egg implants outside the uterus. The most common site where this occurs is inside a fallopian tube. In an ectopic pregnancy, the growing fetus bursts through the tissue in which it has implanted. Severe bleeding can occur due to ruptured blood vessels.
- *Preeclampsia* is a disorder of pregnancy that causes blood vessels to spasm and constrict. Blood vessel constriction results in high blood pressure. It also decreases blood flow to the mother's organs, including the placenta. Less blood flow to the placenta usually means that less oxygenated blood and fewer nutrients reach the baby. Preeclampsia usually occurs during the third trimester of pregnancy.
- If untreated, preeclampsia may progress to *eclampsia.* Eclampsia is the seizure phase of preeclampsia. In treating eclampsia, you should have suction readily

available. Provide oxygen if it is available and you have been trained to use it. Keep the patient calm and position her on her left side. Avoid any stimulus that might trigger a seizure, such as bright lights and siren noise.

- *Placenta previa* occurs when the placenta attaches low in the wall of the uterus instead of at its top or sides. In this position, the placenta may cover all or part of the cervix (the entrance to the birth canal). *Placenta previa* can cause sudden, painless, bright red vaginal bleeding.
- *Abruptio placenta* occurs when a normally implanted placenta separates prematurely from the wall of the uterus (endometrium) during the last trimester of pregnancy. If the placenta begins to peel away from the wall of the uterus, bleeding occurs from the blood vessels that transfer nutrients to the fetus from the mother. The placenta may separate partially or completely. Partial separation may allow time for treatment of the mother and fetus. Complete separation often results in the death of the fetus.
- A *ruptured uterus* is the tearing (rupture) of the uterus. Uterine rupture can occur when the patient has been in strong labor for a long time, which is the most common cause. It can also occur when the patient has sustained abdominal trauma, such as a severe fall or a sudden stop in a motor vehicle collision.
- Due to the normal changes in vital signs that occur with pregnancy, assessing the patient's vital signs may not be as useful as it is with a nonpregnant patient. A pregnant patient's heart rate is normally slightly faster than usual. Her breathing rate is also slightly faster and more shallow than normal. Her blood pressure is often slightly lower than normal until the third trimester. It is important to take vital signs in all patients. However, you will need to pay special attention to the pregnant patient's history and look for other signs that suggest a potential problem.
- In treating a pregnant patient, you should obtain a SAMPLE history to gather information about the patient's medical history:
  - *S*igns and symptoms
  - *A*llergies
  - *M*edications (prescribed, herbal, or recreational drug use)
  - (Pertinent) *p*ast medical history (prenatal care and preexisting illness)
  - *L*ast oral intake
  - *E*vents leading to the injury or illness
- As an Emergency Medical Responder, you must not visually inspect the vaginal area unless major bleeding is present or you anticipate that childbirth is about to occur. In these situations, it is best to have another healthcare professional or a law enforcement officer present. The vaginal area is touched *only* during delivery and when another healthcare professional or a law enforcement officer is present.
- An *obstetric emergency* is an emergency related to pregnancy or childbirth. It is frequently associated with bleeding. During childbirth, blood and amniotic fluid are expected and may splash. Therefore, in caring for a patient with an obstetric emergency, you should take BSI precautions and put on appropriate PPE. In addition to gloves, you should wear eye protection, a mask, and a gown.
- *Labor* is the time and process in which the uterus repeatedly contracts to push the fetus and placenta out of the mother's body. It begins with the first uterine muscle contraction and ends with delivery of the placenta. *Delivery* is the birth of the baby at the end of the second stage of labor.
- Before labor begins, the head of the fetus normally settles into the pelvis. The cervix begins to open (dilate) and thin out (efface). In addition, the mucous plug may be expelled (bloody show).

- The *first stage of labor* begins with the first uterine contraction. This stage ends with a complete thinning and opening of the cervix. Contractions usually last 30–60 seconds and occur every 5–15 minutes. In a woman who has not previously given birth, this stage of labor lasts about 8–16 hours. It lasts about 6–8 hours in a woman who has previously given birth.
- The *second stage of labor* begins with the opening of the cervix and ends with the delivery of the infant. The contractions during this stage are stronger. They last 45–60 seconds and occur every 2–3 minutes. This stage of labor averages 1–2 hours in a woman who has not previously given birth. In a woman who has given birth, this stage of labor lasts 20–30 minutes.
  - During this stage, the fetus begins its descent into the birth canal. The *presenting part* is the part of the infant that comes out of the birth canal first. Normally, the first part of the infant that descends into the birth canal is the head. This type of delivery is called a *cephalic (head) delivery.* If the buttocks or feet descend first, it is called a *breech delivery.* Eventually, the presenting part will remain visible at the vaginal opening between contractions, which is called *crowning.*
- The *third stage of labor* begins with delivery of the infant and ends with delivery of the placenta. The placenta peels away from the wall of the uterus, leaving tiny blood vessels exposed. The uterus normally contracts to close these blood vessels. The placenta usually delivers within 15–30 minutes of the infant's birth. This stage of labor normally lasts 5 minutes to an hour.
- Women often have *false labor pains* about 2–4 weeks before delivery. False labor pains are called *Braxton Hicks contractions.* These contractions help prepare the woman's body for delivery by softening and thinning her cervix.
- As an Emergency Medical Responder, you should transport a woman in labor to the hospital unless delivery of the baby is expected within a few minutes. You must determine if there is time for the mother to reach the hospital or if preparations should be made for delivery at the scene. Consider delivering at the scene in the following three circumstances:
  1. Delivery can be expected in a few minutes.
     - A woman in late pregnancy feels the urge to push, bear down, or have a bowel movement.
     - Crowning is present.
  2. No suitable transportation is available.
  3. The hospital cannot be reached due to heavy traffic, bad weather, a natural disaster, or a similar situation.

Tracking Your Progress

After reading this chapter, can you	Page Reference	Objective Met?
• Identify the following structures: birth canal, placenta, umbilical cord, amniotic sac?	449–450	☐
• Define the following terms: crowning, bloody show, labor, abortion?	448	☐
• State indications of an imminent delivery?	463	☐
• State the steps in the pre-delivery preparation of the mother?	464–465	☐
• Establish the relationship between body substance isolation and childbirth?	463–464	☐
• State the steps to assist in the delivery?	464	☐

• Describe care of the baby as the head appears?	465	☐
• Discuss the steps in delivery of the placenta?	469	☐
• List the steps in the emergency medical care of the mother post-delivery?	469	☐
• Discuss the steps in caring for a newborn?	467	☐
• Explain the rationale for attending to the feelings of a patient in need of emergency medical care during childbirth?	463	☐
• Demonstrate a caring attitude toward patients during childbirth who request Emergency Medical Services?	463	☐
• Place the interests of the patient during childbirth as the foremost consideration when making any and all patient care decisions?	464	☐
• Communicate with empathy to patients during childbirth, as well as with family members and friends of the patient?	464	☐

Chapter Quiz

Multiple Choice

In the space provided, identify the letter of the choice that best completes each statement or answers each question.

_____ **1.** The ovaries are responsible for
- **a.** stretching to adapt to the increasing size of a fetus.
- **b.** contracting to expel an infant from its mother's body.
- **c.** receiving and transporting the egg to the uterus.
- **d.** producing eggs and secreting hormones.

_____ **2.** Which of the following statements is true?
- **a.** There are five stages of labor.
- **b.** Stage 2 of labor begins with delivery of the infant.
- **c.** Stage 3 of labor ends with delivery of the infant.
- **d.** Stage 1 of labor begins with the onset of uterine contractions.

_____ **3.** The fetus normally develops in the
- **a.** birth canal.
- **b.** uterus.
- **c.** fallopian tube.
- **d.** perineum.

_____ **4.** A 27-year-old woman is in labor with her first baby. She states she has seen a doctor regularly throughout her pregnancy. Her due date is next Friday. All of the following questions pertain to this scenario. Which of the following is normally seen when the cervix begins to widen during early labor?
- **a.** bloody show
- **b.** a large amount of painless, bright red bleeding
- **c.** a large amount of dark, "coffee-ground" colored blood
- **d.** a gush of fluid that looks like pea soup

_____ **5.** A normal term of pregnancy is considered
- **a.** 29 weeks.
- **b.** 34 weeks.
- **c.** 40 weeks.
- **d.** 44 weeks.

_____ **6.** Labor for a first pregnancy typically lasts
a. 4–6 hours.
b. 6–12 hours.
c. 8–16 hours.
d. 24–48 hours.

_____ **7.** A sign that indicates that delivery is about to occur is
a. contractions that are regular and occurring 5–6 minutes apart.
b. contractions that the mother rates a 9 on a 0–10 pain scale.
c. the bag of waters breaks.
d. crowning.

_____ **8.** Which of the following items should you use when assisting with this delivery?
a. gloves and mask only
b. gloves, mask, and gown only
c. gloves, mask, and protective eyewear only
d. gloves, gown, mask, and protective eyewear

_____ **9.** When the infant's head appears during crowning, where should you place your gloved fingers to prevent the baby's head from coming out too fast?
a. on the soft spots on the baby's head
b. over the bony part of the baby's skull
c. on the baby's face
d. on each side of the baby's neck

_____ **10.** When should you suction the baby's airway?
a. as the baby's head is delivered and before delivery of the shoulders
b. after the baby's chest has delivered but before delivery of the feet
c. only after the baby's chest and abdomen are born
d. only after the baby has been completely delivered

_____ **11.** To deliver the baby's upper shoulder, you should
a. gently guide the baby's head upward.
b. gently pull on the baby's head.
c. gently turn the baby's head sideways.
d. gently guide the baby's head downward.

_____ **12.** Until the umbilical cord is clamped or tied, you should position the baby
a. above the level of the mother's vaginal opening.
b. below the level of the mother's vaginal opening.
c. at or around the same level as the mother's vaginal opening.
d. in any position—it does not matter where the baby is positioned.

_____ **13.** Where should you check the baby's pulse?
a. at the wrist
b. on the inside of the upper arm
c. in the groin
d. on either side of the neck

True or False

Decide whether each statement is true or false. In the space provided, write T for true or F for false.

_____ **14.** The well-being of the fetus is entirely dependent on the well-being of the mother.

_____ **15.** When clearing a newborn's airway, suction the baby's nose first and then the mouth.

Matching

Match the key terms in the left column with the definitions in the right column by placing the letter of each correct answer in the space provided.

_____ **16.** Placenta

_____ **17.** Crowning

_____ **18.** Labor

_____ **19.** Abortion

_____ **20.** Bloody show

_____ **21.** Birth canal

_____ **22.** Amniotic sac

_____ **23.** Umbilical cord

a. Bag of fluid that surrounds the fetus inside the uterus

b. Termination of pregnancy before the fetus is able to live on its own outside the uterus

c. Extension of the placenta, through which the fetus receives nourishment while in the uterus

d. Vagina and lower part of the uterus

e. Mucous and blood that may come out of the vagina as labor begins

f. Stage of birth when the presenting part of the baby is visible at the vaginal opening

g. Specialized organ through which the fetus exchanges nourishment and waste products during pregnancy

h. Time and process beginning with the first uterine muscle contraction until delivery of the placenta

Short Answer

Answer each question in the space provided.

24. List three functions of the placenta.

1. ______________________________

2. ______________________________

3. ______________________________

25. Explain why a woman in late pregnancy should not lie flat on her back.

____

____

____

26. An infant's head is crowning. You see that the bag of waters has not broken. What should you do?

____

____

____

____

27. Why is it very important to keep a newborn warm?

____

____

____

28. List three signs that suggest the placenta is about to be delivered.

1. ______________________________

2. ______________________________

3. ______________________________

Sentence Completion

In the blanks provided, write the words that best complete each sentence.

29. A full-term baby's respiratory rate is normally between ____________ and ____________ breaths per minute.

30. A full-term baby's heart rate is normally between ____________ and ____________ beats per minute.

31. A breech birth occurs when the baby's ____________ or ____________ comes out of the uterus first.

CHAPTER

13 Infants and Children

By the end of this chapter, you should be able to

Knowledge Objectives ▶

1. Describe differences in anatomy and physiology of the infant, child, and adult patient.
2. Describe assessment of the infant or child.
3. Indicate various causes of respiratory emergencies in infants and children.
4. Summarize emergency medical care strategies for respiratory distress and respiratory failure/arrest in infants and children.
5. List common causes of seizures in the infant and child patient.
6. Describe management of seizures in the infant and child patient.
7. Discuss emergency medical care of the infant and child trauma patient.
8. Summarize the signs and symptoms of possible child abuse and neglect.
9. Describe the medical-legal responsibilities in suspected child abuse.
10. Recognize the need for an Emergency Medical Responder debriefing following a difficult infant or child transport.

Attitude Objectives ▶

11. Attend to the feelings of the family when dealing with an ill or injured infant or child.
12. Understand the provider's own emotional response to caring for infants or children.
13. Demonstrate a caring attitude toward infants and children with illness or injury who require Emergency Medical Services.
14. Place the interests of the infant or child with an illness or injury as the foremost consideration when making patient care decisions.
15. Communicate with empathy to infants and children with an illness or injury, as well as with family members and friends of the patient.

Skill Objectives ▶

16. Demonstrate assessment of the infant and child.

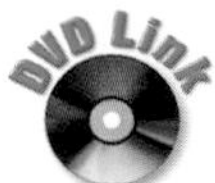

On The Scene

You are dispatched to a cottage in the village for a "child with difficulty breathing." As you walk into the room, it is obvious that a four-year-old girl is struggling to catch her breath. She is pale, she is leaning forward on the edge of her bed, and her nostrils flare open with each breath. A high-pitched whistle is audible without even using your stethoscope. "She has asthma," her father tells you, "but we're on vacation and we ran out of her inhalers." You count her breathing at 40 breaths per minute. Her radial pulse is 146 beats per minute. When you lift her shirt, you can see the skin between her ribs pull in with each breath. ■

THINK ABOUT IT

As you read this chapter, think about the following questions

- Which signs of respiratory distress have you observed in this child?
- Are her vital signs within normal limits?
- What treatment could you consider until the ambulance arrives?
- Which signs or symptoms would indicate that her condition is worsening?

Introduction

Caring for Infants and Children

Children are not just small adults. Children have unique physical, mental, emotional, and developmental characteristics that you must consider when assessing and caring for them. You may be anxious when treating a child due to your lack of experience in treating children, a fear of failure, or identifying the patient with your own child. If you understand the expected physical and developmental characteristics of infants and children of different ages, you will be able to more accurately assess your patient and provide appropriate care.

The key to working with children is "Keep it simple." Children respond very well to basic management skills.

You Should Know

Age Classifications of Infants and Children

Life Stage	Age
Newly born infant	Birth to several hours following birth
Neonate	Birth to 1 month
Infant	1 to 12 months of age • Young infant: 0 to 6 months of age • Older infant: 6 months to 1 year of age
Toddler	1 to 3 years of age
Preschooler	4 to 5 years of age
School-age child	6 to 12 years of age
Adolescent	13 to 18 years of age

You Should Know

Depending on the state you reside in or the pediatric hospital in your area, the upper age limit for a pediatric patient may be 14, 18, or 21 years. Be sure to check with your instructor to find out the upper age limit for a pediatric patient in your area.

The Anatomical and Physiological Differences in Children

Objective 1 ▶

Head

A child's head is proportionately larger and heavier than an adult's is until about four years of age. It takes several months for a child to develop neck muscles that are strong enough to support his or her head. Because the back of a child's head (occiput) sticks out and a child's forehead is large, these areas are susceptible to injury. It is not unusual for children to have multiple forehead bruises from hitting their heads on tables and floors.

Trauma to the head may result in flexion and extension injuries.

The necks of infants and toddlers are flexed when they are lying flat because the back of the skull is large. The chin is then angled toward the chest. Proper positioning of an infant's or a toddler's head is an important factor when managing the airway (Figure 13-1).

Appropriate positioning of the head will be one of the most important techniques that you will use when managing children.

The bones of an infant's head are soft and flexible to allow for growth of the brain. On both the top and back of the head are small, triangular openings called fontanels ("soft spots"). These areas will not completely close until about 6 months of age for the rear fontanel and 18 months for the top one. You should assess the fontanels of an infant and a toddler for bulging or a depression. The soft spots of an infant or a toddler are normally nearly level with the skull. Coughing, crying, or lying down may cause the soft spots to bulge temporarily. Bulging in a quiet patient suggests increased pressure within the skull, such as fluid or pressure on the brain. A depression suggests that the patient is dehydrated.

Face

The tongue of an infant or a child fills the majority of the space in his or her mouth.

A child's nasal passages are very small, short, and narrow. It is easy for children to develop obstruction of these areas with mucus or foreign objects. Newborns are primarily nose breathers. A newborn will not automatically open his mouth to breathe when his nose becomes obstructed. As a result, any obstruction of the nose will lead to respiratory difficulty. You must make sure the newborn's nose is clear to avoid breathing problems.

Although the opening of the mouth is usually small, a child's tongue is large in proportion to the mouth. The tongue is the most common cause of upper airway obstruction in an unconscious child because the immature muscles of the lower jaw (mandible) allow the tongue to fall to the back of the throat.

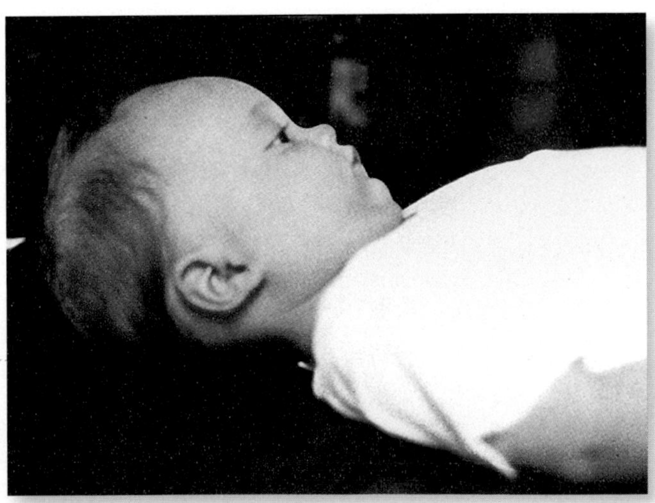

FIGURE 13-1 ▶ Proper positioning of an infant's or a toddler's head is an important consideration during airway management. EMSC Slide Set (CD-ROM). 1996. Courtesy of the Emergency Medical Services for Children Program, administered by the U.S. Department of Health and Human Service's Health Resources and Services Administration, Maternal and Child Health Bureau.

Airway

In children, the opening between the vocal cords (glottic opening) is higher in the neck and more toward the front than in an adult. As we grow, our necks get longer and the glottic opening drops down. The flap of cartilage that covers this opening, the epiglottis, is larger and floppier in children. Therefore, any injury to or swelling of this area can block the airway.

The windpipe (trachea) is the tube through which air passes from the mouth to the lungs. In children, this area is softer, is more flexible, and has a smaller diameter and shorter length than in adults. The trachea has rings of cartilage that keep the airway open. In children, this cartilage is soft and collapses easily, which can then obstruct the airway. Extending or flexing the neck too far can result in crimping of the trachea and a blocked airway. To avoid blocking the airway, place the head of an infant or a young child in a neutral or "sniffing" position. This position is covered in more detail in the section "A is for Airway."

Breathing

The amount of oxygen a child requires is about twice that of an adolescent or adult.

Because the muscles between the ribs are not well developed, a child cannot keep up a rapid rate of breathing for very long.

A child's ribs are soft and flexible because they are made up mostly of cartilage. Bone growth occurs with time, filling in the cartilaginous areas from the center out to the ends. Because the rib cage is softer than in an adult, trauma to the chest will be transmitted to the lungs and other internal structures more easily.

The muscles between the ribs (intercostal muscles) help lift the chest wall during breathing. Because these muscles are not fully developed until later in childhood, the diaphragm is the primary muscle of breathing. As a result, the abdominal muscles move during breathing. During normal breathing, the abdominal muscles should move in the same direction as the chest wall. If they are moving opposite each other, this is called "see-saw" breathing and is abnormal. A child's respiratory rate is faster than an adult's and decreases with age (Table 13-1).

The stomach of an infant or a child often fills with air during crying. Air can also build up in the stomach if rescue breathing is performed. As the stomach swells with air, it pushes on the lungs and diaphragm. This action limits movement and prevents good ventilation. Because infants and young children depend on the diaphragm for breathing, breathing difficulty results if movement of the diaphragm is limited.

TABLE 13-1 Normal Respiratory Rates in Children at Rest

Life Stage	Age	Breaths per Minute
• Newborn	• Birth to 1 month	• 30–50
• Infant	• 1 to 12 months	• 20–40
• Toddler	• 1 to 3 years	• 20–30
• Preschooler	• 4 to 5 years	• 20–30
• School-age child	• 6 to 12 years	• 16–30
• Adolescent	• 13 to 18 years	• 12–20

Circulation

Children breathe faster than adults do, and their hearts beat harder and faster. Infants and young children have a relatively small blood volume (80 milliliters per kilogram [mL/kg]). A sudden loss of 1/2 liter (500 mL) of the blood volume in a child and 100–200 mL of the blood volume in an infant is considered serious. For example, a one-year-old child has a blood volume of approximately 800 mL; thus, a loss of 150 mL is considered a major blood loss. A child's heart rate will increase due to shock, fever, anxiety, and pain. It will also increase as she loses body fluid (hypovolemia). This condition can occur because of bleeding, vomiting, or diarrhea. Most of an infant's body weight is water, so vomiting and diarrhea can result in dehydration. Blood loss due to broken bones and soft-tissue injuries may quickly result in shock. The system of an infant or a child tries to make up for a loss of blood or fluid through an increase in heart rate and a constriction of the skin's blood vessels. These actions help deliver as much blood and oxygen as possible to the brain, heart, and lungs.

In children, circulatory problems often develop due to respiratory problems.

A child's rate and effort of breathing will increase when the amount of oxygen in the blood is decreased (as in late shock). This helps make up for a lack of oxygen. As the child tires and the blood oxygen level becomes very low, the heart muscle begins to pump less effectively. As a result, the child's heart rate slows. If the lack of oxygen is not corrected, the child will stop breathing (respiratory arrest). A child will often survive a respiratory arrest as long as his oxygen level is maintained sufficiently so that the heart does not stop. The normal heart rates for children at rest are shown in Table 13-2.

If you have the necessary equipment and have been trained to do so, measure the blood pressure in children older than three years of age. The blood pressure of a child is normally lower than that of an adult.

Infants and young children are susceptible to changes in temperature. A child has a large body surface area, compared with his weight. The larger the body surface area that is exposed, the greater the area of heat loss.

An infant's skin is thin, with few fat deposits under it. This condition contributes to an infant's sensitivity to extremes of heat and cold. Infants have poorly developed temperature-regulating mechanisms. For example, newborns are unable to shiver in cold temperatures. In addition, their sweating mechanism is immature in warm temperatures. Because infants and children are at risk for hypothermia, it is very important to keep them warm.

The tissue in the mouth of a healthy child should be pink and moist, regardless of the child's race.

The skin of an infant or a child will show changes related to the amount of oxygen in the blood. Pale (whitish) skin may be seen in shock, fright, or anxiety. A bluish (cyanotic) tint, often seen first around the mouth, suggests inadequate

TABLE 13-2 Normal Heart Rates in Children at Rest

Life Stage	Age	Beats per Minute
• Newborn	• Birth to 1 month	• 120–160
• Infant	• 1 to 12 months	• 80–140
• Toddler	• 1 to 3 years	• 80–130
• Preschooler	• 4 to 5 years	• 80–120
• School-age child	• 6 to 12 years	• 70–110
• Adolescent	• 13 to 18 years	• 60–100

breathing or poor perfusion. This is a critical sign that requires immediate treatment. The skin may appear blotchy (mottled) in shock, hypothermia, or cardiac arrest. Flushed (red) skin may be caused by fever, heat exposure, or an allergic reaction. Most children should feel slightly warm to the touch. Their skin should be tight but not dry or flaky.

The Developmental Stages of Children

Infants (Birth to One Year of Age)

Infants are completely dependent on others for their needs (Figure 13-2). They cry for many reasons, including pain, hunger, extremes in temperature, or a dirty diaper. Young infants (birth to six months of age) are unafraid of strangers and have no modesty. Older infants (six months to one year of age) do not like to be separated from their caregivers (separation anxiety). They may be threatened by direct eye contact with strangers. They show little modesty.

When providing care for an infant, watch the baby from a distance before making contact. If possible, assess the baby on the caregiver's lap. Avoid loud noises, bright lights, and quick, jerky movements. Smile and use a calm, soothing voice. Allow the baby to suck on a pacifier for comfort. Be sure to handle an infant gently but firmly, always supporting the head and neck if the baby is not on a solid surface.

An infant must be kept warm and covered as much as possible, particularly the head. The head is the largest body surface area in infants and young children. Heat loss from this area significantly cools the rest of the body. Make sure your hands and stethoscope are warmed before touching the infant.

Stop and Think!

The risk of a foreign body airway obstruction begins at approximately six months of age. Be careful not to leave small objects within an infant's reach.

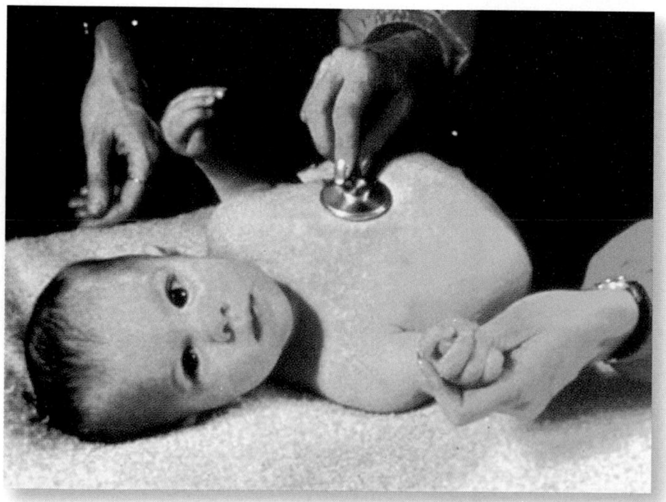

FIGURE 13-2 ► Infants are completely dependent on others for their needs. EMSC Slide Set (CD-ROM). 1996. Courtesy of the Emergency Medical Services for Children Program, administered by the U.S. Department of Health and Human Service's Health Resources and Services Administration, Maternal and Child Health Bureau.

You Should Know

Shaken Baby Syndrome is a severe form of head injury. It occurs when an infant or a child is shaken by the arms, legs, or shoulders with enough force to cause the baby's brain to bounce against the skull. This shaking can cause bruising, swelling, and bleeding of the brain. It can lead to severe brain damage or death.

Just two to three seconds of shaking can cause bleeding in and around the brain. *Never shake or jiggle an infant or a child.*

Toddlers (One to Three Years of Age)

A toddler is always on the move. A toddler's eye-hand coordination improves, and sitting, standing, and walking begin. As a result, toddlers are prone to injury (Figure 13-3). A toddler responds appropriately to an angry or a friendly voice. When separated from their primary caregivers, most toddlers experience strong separation anxiety.

A toddler can answer simple questions and follow simple directions. However, you cannot reason with a toddler. A toddler is likely to be more cooperative if given a comfort object, such as a blanket, stuffed animal, or toy.

Toddlers understand "soon," "bye-bye," "all gone," and "uh-oh." A toddler's favorite words are *no* and *mine,* so avoid asking questions that can be answered with a yes or no. If you ask questions that begin with "May I," "Can I," or "Would you like to," a toddler will probably say, "No." If you then do whatever you asked him or her, anyway, you will immediately lose the toddler's trust and cooperation.

Toddlers view illness and injury as punishment.

Toddlers are distrustful of strangers. They are likely to resist examination and treatment. When touched, they may scream, cry, or kick. Toddlers do not like having their clothing removed and do not like anything on their faces. They are afraid of being left alone, monsters, interruptions in their usual routine, and getting hurt (such as from a fall or cut).

Try a game such as counting toes or fingers to enlist the child's cooperation.

Encourage the child's trust by gaining the cooperation of the caregiver. By talking with the caregiver first, the child may be more at ease if she sees that the adult is not threatened. When possible, allow the child to remain on the caregiver's lap. If this is not possible, try to keep the caregiver within the child's line of vision. Approach the child slowly and address her by name. Talk to her at eye level, using simple words and short phrases. Speak to her in a calm,

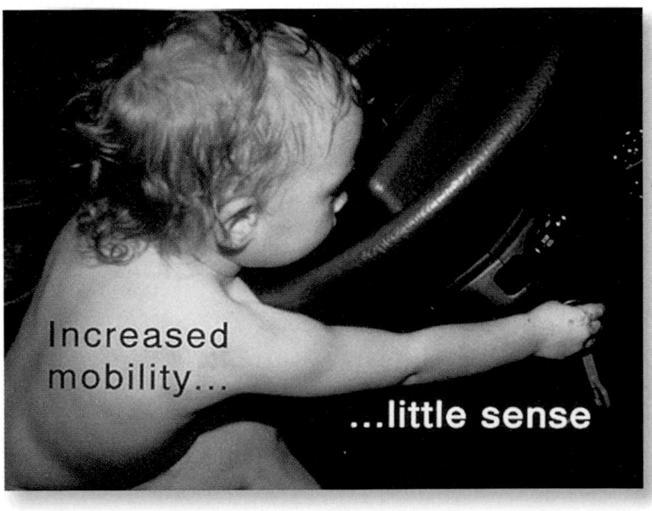

FIGURE 13-3 ► A toddler is always on the move. As a result, they are prone to injury. EMSC Slide Set (CD-ROM). 1996. Courtesy of the Emergency Medical Services for Children Program, administered by the U.S. Department of Health and Human Service's Health Resources and Services Administration, Maternal and Child Health Bureau.

reassuring tone of voice. Although the child may not understand your words, she will respond to your tone. Assess the child's head last. Start with either her trunk or her feet and move upward. Respect the child's modesty by keeping her covered. When it is time to remove an item of clothing, if possible, ask the child's caregiver to do so. Replace clothing promptly after assessing each body area. Be sure to praise the child for cooperative behavior.

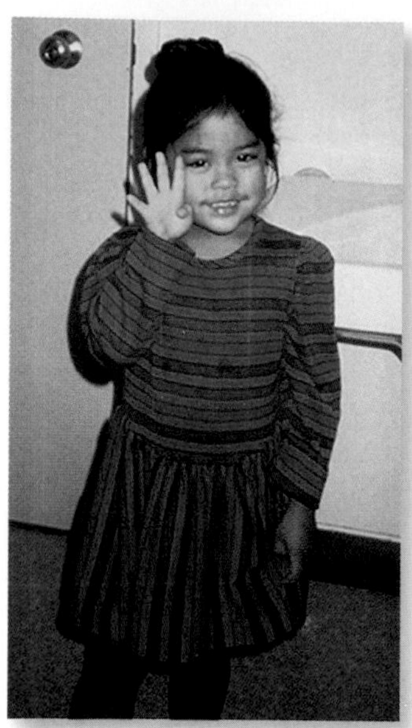

FIGURE 13-4 ▲
Preschoolers are highly imaginative and may think their illness or injury is punishment for bad behavior or thoughts. EMSC Slide Set (CD-ROM). 1996. Courtesy of the Emergency Medical Services for Children Program, administered by the U.S. Department of Health and Human Service's Health Resources and Services Administration, Maternal and Child Health Bureau.

Remember This!

Do not tell a child he or she cannot cry or that he or she needs to be strong. Instead, reassure the child that it is okay to cry, be angry or frightened, and express emotion. However, you can remind the child that hitting, kicking, and biting are not allowed.

Preschoolers (Four to Five Years of Age)

Preschoolers are afraid of the unknown, the dark, being left alone, and adults who look or act mean. They may think their illness or injury is punishment for bad behavior or thoughts (Figure 13-4). Approach the child slowly and talk to her at eye level. Use simple words and phrases and a reassuring tone of voice. Assure the child that she was not bad and is not being punished.

A preschooler may feel vulnerable and out of control when lying down. Assess and treat the child in an upright position when possible. Preschoolers are modest. They do not like being touched or having their clothing removed. When assessing a child, keep in mind that she has probably been told not to let a stranger touch her. Remove the clothing, assess the child, and then quickly replace the clothing. Allow the caregiver to remain with the child whenever possible.

Preschoolers are curious and like to "help." Encourage the child to participate. Tell the child how things will feel and what is to be done just before doing it. For example, a preschooler may fear being suffocated by an oxygen mask. It may be helpful to use a doll or stuffed animal to explain the procedure. The child may want to hold or look at the equipment first.

Preschoolers are highly imaginative. When talking with a preschooler, choose your words carefully. Avoid baby talk and frightening or misleading terms. For example, avoid words such as *take, cut, shot, deaden,* or *germs.* Instead of saying, "I'm going to take your pulse," you might say, "I'm going to see how fast your heart is beating." Instead of saying, "I'm going to take your blood pressure," you might say, "I'm going to hug your arm" or "I'm going to see how strong your muscles are." Because preschoolers are afraid of blood, dress and bandage wounds right away.

Depending on the child's age, you may find that distracting them is helpful. Remember that children are self-centered—they imagine that the world revolves around them. Paying attention to their world and needs will improve your ability to assess and care for your pediatric patients.

You Should Know

Distractions

- Ask a child about his or her favorite foods, games, cartoon characters, movies, or computer game.
- Ask the child to visually locate an item in the area.
- Ask the child to sing a song or tell you about school.
- Use a stuffed animal as a distraction or comfort item.

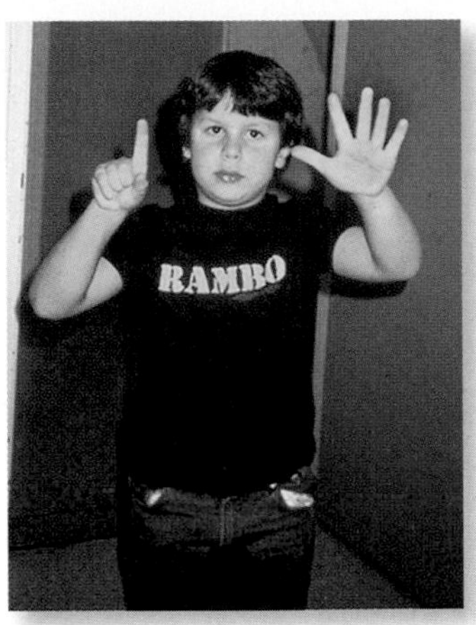

FIGURE 13-5 ▲ School-age children are usually cooperative. EMSC Slide Set (CD-ROM). 1996. Courtesy of the Emergency Medical Services for Children Program, administered by the U.S. Department of Health and Human Service's Health Resources and Services Administration, Maternal and Child Health Bureau.

School-Age Children (6–12 Years of Age)

School-age children are less dependent on their caregivers than are younger children. They are usually cooperative (Figure 13-5). They fear pain, permanent injury, and disfigurement. They are also afraid of blood and prolonged separation from their caregivers. A school-age child is very modest and does not like his body exposed to strangers. A child of this age may still view his illness or injury as punishment. Reassure the child that how he feels or what is happening to him is not related to being punished.

When caring for a school-age child, approach him in a friendly manner and introduce yourself. Talk directly to the child about what happened, even if you also obtain a history from the caregiver. Explain procedures before carrying them out. Because school-age children often view things in concrete terms, choose your words carefully. For example, the phrase "I am going to take your pulse" will concern a school-age child. He will wonder why you are taking it away and when he will get it back. Allow the child to see and touch equipment that may be used in his care.

Honesty is very important when interacting with school-age children. If you are going to do something to the child that may cause pain, warn the child just before you do it. Give a simple explanation of what will take place and do it just before the procedure so that he does not have long to think about it. For example, if a child has a possible broken leg and you must move the leg to apply a splint, warn the child just before you move the leg. Do not threaten the child if he is uncooperative.

Adolescents (13–18 Years of Age)

Adolescents often show inconsistent and unpredictable behavior. They expect to be treated as adults (Figure 13-6). Talk to an adolescent in a respectful, friendly manner, as if speaking to an adult. If possible, obtain a history from the patient instead of a caregiver. Expect an adolescent to have many questions and want detailed explanations about what you are planning to do or what is happening to him. Explain things clearly and honestly. Allow time for questions. Do not bargain with an adolescent in order to do what you need to do. Recognize the tendency for adolescents to overreact. Do not become angry with an emotional or hysterical adolescent.

Adolescents fear pain and permanent damage to their bodies that results in a change in appearance, scarring, or death. They may go back and forth between modesty and open displays of their bodies. Try to have an adult of the same gender present while you examine them. Allow the caregiver to be present

FIGURE 13-6 ► Adolescents expect to be treated as adults. EMSC Slide Set (CD-ROM). 1996. Courtesy of the Emergency Medical Services for Children Program, administered by the U.S. Department of Health and Human Service's Health Resources and Services Administration, Maternal and Child Health Bureau.

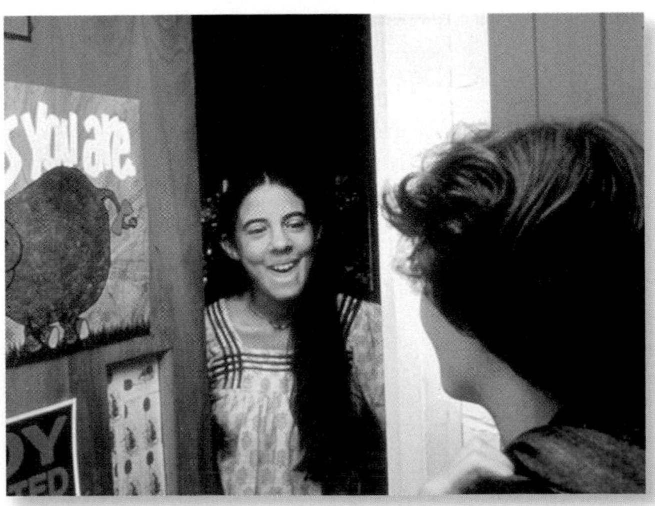

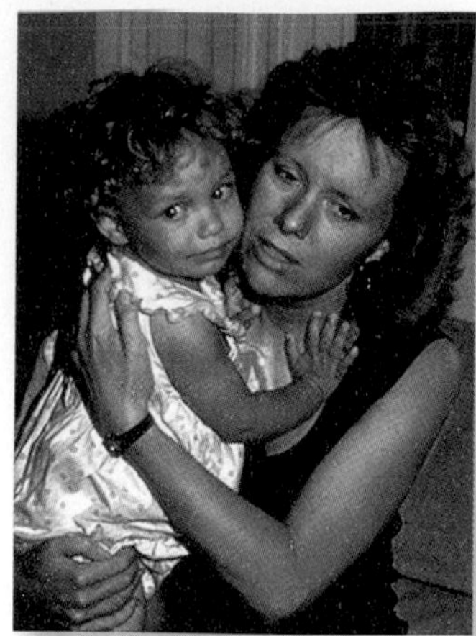

FIGURE 13-7 ▲ Quickly determine if the emergency is due to trauma or a medical condition. If the emergency is due to trauma, determine the mechanism of injury. EMSC Slide Set (CD-ROM). 1996. Courtesy of the Emergency Medical Services for Children Program, administered by the U.S. Department of Health and Human Service's Health Resources and Services Administration, Maternal and Child Health Bureau.

during your assessment if the patient wishes. However, some adolescents may prefer to be assessed privately, away from their caregivers.

Peers are a major influence in the life of an adolescent. When you are providing care, an adolescent may prefer to have a peer close by for reassurance. When caring for an adolescent, do not tease or embarrass her—particularly in front of her peers.

Assessment of Infants and Children

Scene Size-Up

When you are called for an emergency involving a child, quickly determine if the emergency is due to trauma or a medical condition. If the emergency is due to trauma, determine the mechanism of injury (Figure 13-7). If the emergency is due to a medical condition, determine the nature of the illness. This information can be obtained from the patient, family members, or bystanders, as well as from your observations of the scene.

Survey the patient's environment for clues to the cause of the emergency. Note any hazards or potential hazards. For example, open pill bottles or cleaning solutions may indicate a possible toxic ingestion. Look at the child's environment. Does it appear clean and orderly? Do other children appear healthy and well cared for? Determine if you need additional resources, including law enforcement personnel. Remember to wear appropriate PPE before approaching the patient.

Initial Assessment

Objective 12 ▶ Any incident that involves children will cause some degree of anxiety and stress for every person present. Your emotional response in these situations will play an important part in how effective you can be. Your emotional response may be related to a limited exposure to children as a healthcare professional and/or caregiver. Alternately, caring for an ill or injured child who is the same age as a member of your own family may also affect your response.

Objective 11 ▶ In most situations, your approach to an ill or injured infant or child should include the patient's caregiver. Watch the interaction between the caregiver and the child. Does the caregiver appear concerned? Or is he or she angry or indifferent? Keep in mind that an agitated caregiver equals an agitated child. A calm caregiver equals a calm child. If the child's caregiver is adding to the child's anxiety, give the adult something to do. For example, you might ask the caregiver to locate the child's favorite comfort object. Including the caregiver in the child's care reassures both the child and caregiver. It also allows the adult a chance to take part in the child's recovery.

Objective 15 ▶

General Impression

Objective 2 ▶ Your assessment of an infant or a child should begin from across the room. When forming a general impression of an infant or a child, look at his or her appearance, breathing, and circulation. Quickly determine if the child appears "sick" or "not sick."

- *Appearance.* A child should be alert and responsive to his surroundings. Is the child awake and alert? Does the child behave appropriately for his age? Does he recognize his caregiver? Is the child playing or moving around, or does he appear drowsy or unaware of his surroundings? Does the child show interest in what is happening? Does the child appear agitated or irritable? Does he appear confused or combative? If the child appears agitated, restless, or limp, or if he appears to be asleep, proceed immediately to the initial assessment.

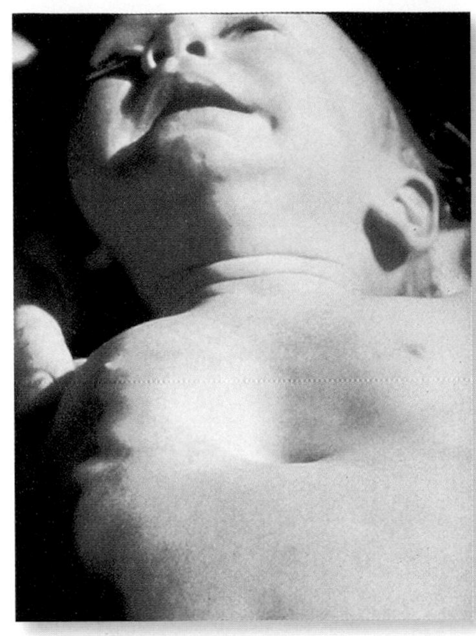

FIGURE 13-8 ▶ Retractions are a sign of an increased work of breathing. EMSC Slide Set (CD-ROM). 1996. Courtesy of the Emergency Medical Services for Children Program, administered by the U.S. Department of Health and Human Service's Health Resources and Services Administration, Maternal and Child Health Bureau.

- *(Work of) breathing.* With normal breathing, both sides of the chest rise and fall equally. Breathing is quiet, is painless, and occurs at a regular rate. Is the child sitting up, lying down, or leaning forward? Can you hear abnormal breathing sounds, such as wheezing, stridor (a high-pitched sound), or grunting? Do you see retractions (sucking in around the ribs and collarbones), nasal flaring, or shoulder hunching (Figure 13-8)? Is the child's breathing rate faster or slower than expected? Is his head bobbing up and down toward his chest? If the child appears to be struggling to breathe, has noisy breathing, moves his chest abnormally, or has a rate of breathing that is faster or slower than normal, proceed immediately to the initial assessment.
- *Circulation.* The visual signs of circulation relate to skin color, obvious bleeding, and moisture. What color is the child's skin? Is it pink, pale, mottled, flushed, or blue? Do you see any bleeding? If bleeding is present, where is it coming from? How much blood is there? Does the child look sweaty? Or do the child's lips look dry and flaky? If the child's skin looks pale, mottled, flushed, gray, or blue, proceed immediately to the initial assessment.

Once your general impression is complete, perform a hands-on assessment. In a responsive infant or child, use a toes-to-head or trunk-to-head approach. This approach should help reduce the infant's or child's anxiety.

Remember This!

During your initial assessment, find the answers to these five questions:

1. Is the child awake and alert?
2. Is the child's airway open?
3. Is the child breathing?
4. Does the child have a pulse?
5. Does the child have severe bleeding?

Level of Responsiveness and Cervical Spine Protection

After forming a general impression, you must assess the pediatric patient's level of responsiveness (mental status) and the need for cervical spine protection.

Level of Responsiveness (Mental Status)

Is the child awake and alert?

An alert infant or young child (younger than three years of age) smiles, orients to sound, follows objects with his eyes, and interacts with those around him. As the infant or young child's mental status decreases, you may see the following changes (in order of decreasing mental status):

- The child may cry but can be comforted.
- The child may show inappropriate, constant crying.
- The child may become irritable and restless.
- The child may be unresponsive.

An infant or a child who does not recognize your presence is sick.

Assessing the mental status of a child older than three years of age is the same as assessing that of an adult. Most children will be agitated or resist your assessment. A child who is limp, allows you to perform any assessment or skill, or does not respond to her caregiver is sick. If the patient is a child with special healthcare needs, the child's caregiver will probably be your best resource. The caregiver will be able to tell you what "normal" is for the child regarding her mental status, vital signs, and level of activity.

Unresponsiveness in an infant or a child usually indicates a life-threatening condition.

Depending on the child's age, you may ask the child or caregiver, "Why did you call 9-1-1 today?" If the child appears to be asleep, gently rub his shoulder and ask, "Are you okay?" or "Can you hear me?" If the child does not respond, ask the family or bystanders to tell you what happened while you continue your assessment.

Cervical Spine Protection

If the child complains of pain or if you meet resistance when moving the child's head and neck to a neutral position, stop and maintain the head and neck in the position in which they were found.

If you suspect trauma to the head, neck, or back, or if the child is unresponsive with an unknown nature of illness, take spinal precautions. If the child is awake and you suspect trauma, face her, so that she does not have to turn her head to see you. Tell her not to move her head or neck. Use your hands to manually stabilize the child's head and neck in line with her body. Once begun, manual stabilization must be continued until the child has been secured to a backboard with her head stabilized.

A Is for *Airway*

Is the child's airway open?

A child who is talking or crying has an open airway. If the child is responsive and the airway is open, assess the child's breathing. If the child is responsive but unable to speak, cry, cough, or make any other sound, the airway is completely obstructed. If the child has noisy breathing, such as snoring or gurgling, he has a partial airway obstruction. A responsive child may have assumed a position to maintain an open airway. Allow the child to maintain this position as you continue your assessment. For example, in cases of serious upper airway obstruction, the child may instinctively assume a sniffing position (Figure 13-9). In this position, the child is seated, with his head and chin thrust slightly forward, as if sniffing a flower. In cases of severe respiratory distress, the child may assume a tripod position. In this position, the child is seated and leaning forward (Figure 13-10).

Using irregularly shaped or insufficient padding, or placing padding only under the shoulders can result in movement or misalignment of the spine.

If the child is unresponsive and no trauma is suspected, use the head tilt–chin lift maneuver to open the airway. If trauma to the head or neck is suspected, use the jaw thrust without head tilt to open the airway. Do not hyperextend the neck. Doing so can cause an airway obstruction. To help maintain the proper positioning of the patient's head and neck, you may need to place padding under the torso of an infant or small child. The padding should be firm and evenly shaped and should

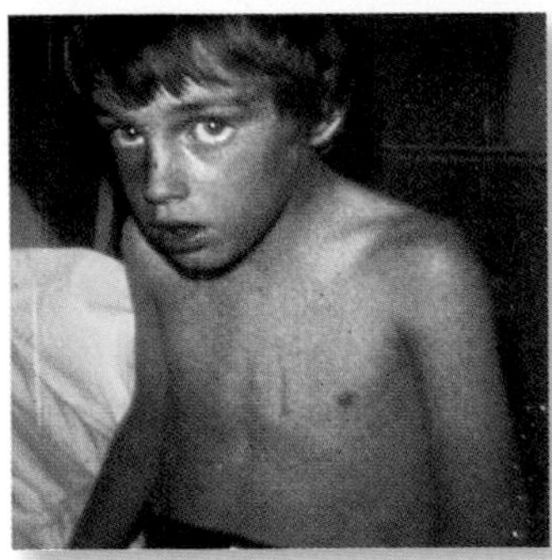

FIGURE 13-9 ▲ In cases of serious upper airway obstruction, the child may instinctively assume a sniffing position. In this position, the child is seated, with his or her head and chin thrust forward slightly. EMSC Slide Set (CD-ROM). 1996. Courtesy of the Emergency Medical Services for Children Program, administered by the U.S. Department of Health and Human Service's Health Resources and Services Administration, Maternal and Child Health Bureau.

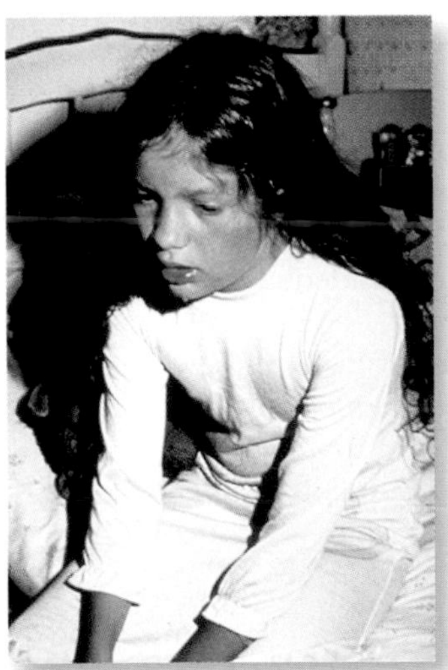

FIGURE 13-10 ▲ In cases of severe respiratory distress, the child may assume a tripod position. In this position, the child is seated and leaning forward. EMSC Slide Set (CD-ROM). 1996. Courtesy of the Emergency Medical Services for Children Program, administered by the U.S. Department of Health and Human Service's Health Resources and Services Administration, Maternal and Child Health Bureau.

extend from the shoulders to the pelvis. The padding should be thick enough that the child's shoulders are in alignment with the ear canal (Figure 13-11).

After opening the airway, look in the mouth of every unresponsive child. To do this, open the child's mouth with your gloved hand. Look for an actual or a potential airway obstruction, such as a foreign body, blood, vomitus, teeth, or the child's tongue. If you see a foreign body in the child's mouth, attempt to remove it with your gloved fingers. If there is blood, vomitus, or other fluid in the airway, clear it with suctioning.

Clearing the Airway

The recovery position, finger sweeps, and suctioning may be used to clear the child's airway. If the child is unresponsive, uninjured, and breathing adequately, you can place her on her side. In this position, gravity allows fluid to flow from the child's mouth. You must continue to monitor the child until additional EMS personnel arrive and assume care.

If you see foreign material in an unresponsive child's mouth, remove it using a finger sweep:

- If the child is uninjured, roll him to his side.
- Wipe any liquids from the airway using your index and middle fingers covered with a cloth.
- Remove solid objects using a gloved finger positioned like a hook. Use your little finger when performing a finger sweep in an infant or a child.

Remember: Blind finger sweeps are *never* performed in an infant or a child.

Suctioning may be needed if the recovery position and finger sweeps are not effective in clearing the patient's airway. It may also be necessary if trauma is suspected and the patient cannot be placed in the recovery position. Use a rigid suction catheter to remove secretions from the child's mouth. Remember that the catheter should be inserted into the child's mouth no deeper than the base of the tongue.

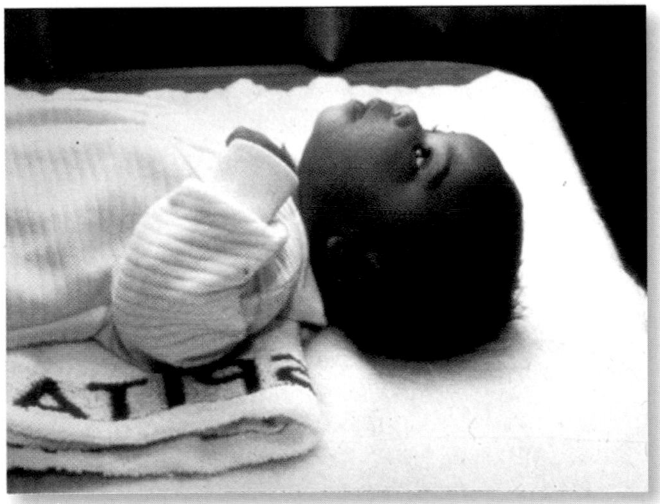

FIGURE 13-11 ▲ To assist in maintaining the proper positioning of the patient's head and neck, it is often necessary to place padding under the torso of an infant or a small child. EMSC Slide Set (CD-ROM). 1996. Courtesy of the Emergency Medical Services for Children Program, administered by the U.S. Department of Health and Human Service's Health Resources and Services Administration, Maternal and Child Health Bureau.

If both the mouth and the nose need to be suctioned, always suction the mouth first and then the nose.

A bulb syringe is used to remove secretions from an infant's mouth or nose. To use a bulb syringe, squeeze the bulb before inserting it into the baby's mouth. With the bulb depressed, insert the syringe into the mouth. Release the bulb. Remove the syringe from the infant's mouth and empty the contents. Gentle suctioning is usually enough to remove secretions.

Do not suction a newborn for more than 3–5 seconds per attempt. When suctioning an infant or a child, do not apply suction for more than 10 seconds at a time. The child's heart rate may slow or become irregular due to a lack of oxygen or because the tip of the device stimulates the back of the tongue or throat. If the patient's heart rate slows, stop suctioning and provide ventilation. Give oxygen between each suctioning attempt if it is available and you have been trained to use it.

Airway Adjuncts

An oral airway may be used to help keep the airway open in an unresponsive child. Remember that this airway is used only if the patient does not have a gag reflex. If the child gags, coughs, chokes, or spits out the airway, do not use it. Nasal airways are not used in children by Emergency Medical Responders.

B Is for *Breathing*

Is the child breathing?

After you have made sure that the child's airway is open, assess her breathing. To do this, you must be able to see her chest or abdomen. Watch and listen to the child as she breathes. Look for the rise and fall of the chest. Does the chest rise and fall equally? Count the child's respiratory rate for 30 seconds. Double this number to determine the breaths per minute.

Listen for air movement. Determine if breathing is absent, quiet, or noisy. Stridor is a high-pitched sound that is heard when the upper airway passages are partially blocked. Wheezing is heard when the lower airway passages are narrowed. Listen for a change in the child's voice or cry. Hoarseness may be caused by a foreign body or an inflamed upper airway. Look for signs of increased breathing effort, such as nasal flaring (widening of the nostrils), retractions, head bobbing, seesaw respirations, and the use of accessory muscles. Feel for air movement from the child's nose or mouth against your chin, face, or palm.

If breathing is present, quickly determine if breathing is adequate or inadequate. If the child's breathing is inadequate or absent, you must begin breathing for her immediately. If the chest does not rise, assume the airway is blocked. The three methods you can use to clear a patient's airway are the recovery position, finger sweeps, and suctioning. The patient's situation will dictate which technique is most appropriate. The procedures for clearing an airway obstruction are discussed in Chapter 6.

C Is for *Circulation*

Does the child have a pulse? Is severe bleeding present?

In infants and children, it is important to compare the pulse of the central blood vessels (such as the femoral artery) with those found in the peripheral areas of the body (such as the feet). For example, locate the dorsalis pedis pulse on top of the foot. Then place your other hand in the child's groin area. Compare the strength and rate of the pulses in these areas. They should feel the same. If they do not, a circulatory problem is present. For example, a weak central pulse can be a sign of late shock.

Use the carotid artery to assess the pulse in an unresponsive child older than 1 year of age. Feel for a brachial pulse in an unresponsive infant. Feel for a pulse for about 10 seconds. If there is no pulse, you must begin chest compressions.

If severe bleeding is present, control it by using direct pressure. Assess the child's skin temperature, color, and moisture. Determine if the skin is warm, hot or cold, moist or dry, and loose or firm. When you have completed your initial assessment, update the EMS unit responding to the scene with a brief report by phone or radio, if possible.

Common Problems in Infants and Children

Airway Obstruction

There are many causes of an airway obstruction, including

- Foreign body
- Mucus plug
- Blood or vomitus
- The tongue
- Trauma to the head or neck
- Infection, such as croup and pneumonia

If a child is unable to speak, cry, cough, or make any other sound, his airway is completely obstructed. If the child has noisy breathing, such as snoring or gurgling, he has a partial airway obstruction. A child with a partial airway obstruction and good air exchange is typically alert and sitting up. You may hear stridor or a crowing sound and see retractions when the child breathes in. The child's skin color is usually normal and a strong pulse is present. You should allow an older child to assume a position of comfort. Assist a younger child in sitting up. Do not allow him to lie down. He may prefer to sit on his caregiver's lap.

Do not agitate the child. If the child has a foreign body in his airway, agitation could cause the object to move into a position that completely blocks the airway. Encourage the child to cough and allow him to continue his efforts to clear his own airway. Continue to watch the child closely.

You will need to intervene if the child has a complete airway obstruction. You will also need to intervene if the child has a partial airway obstruction that is accompanied by any of the following signs of poor air exchange:

- Ineffective cough
- Increased respiratory difficulty accompanied by stridor
- Loss of responsiveness
- Altered mental status

Clear the child's airway using the techniques described in Chapter 6 for the removal of a foreign body airway obstruction.

Respiratory Emergencies

Objective 3 ▶

Respiratory emergencies are the most common medical emergencies encountered in children. There are many causes of respiratory emergencies in children. Some conditions affect the upper airway, some affect the lower airway, and some affect both. Upper airway problems usually occur suddenly. Lower airway problems usually take longer to develop. A patient with an upper airway problem is more likely to worsen during the time you are providing care than is a patient with a lower airway problem. You must watch closely for changes in the patient's condition and adjust your treatment as needed.

There are three levels of severity of respiratory problems: (1) respiratory distress, (2) respiratory failure, and (3) respiratory arrest. Most children will present with either respiratory distress or respiratory failure. **Respiratory distress** is an increased work of breathing (respiratory effort). **Respiratory failure** is a condition in which there is not enough oxygen in the blood and/or ventilation to meet the demands of body tissues. Respiratory failure is evident when the patient becomes tired and can no longer maintain good oxygenation and ventilation. **Respiratory arrest** occurs when a patient stops breathing.

Respiratory distress is associated with several signs that you will be able to spot. These signs reflect an increased work of breathing (respiratory effort). The child works harder than usual to breathe in order to make up for the low level of oxygen in his or her blood.

You Should Know

Signs of Respiratory Distress

- Alertness, irritability, anxiousness, restlessness
- Noisy breathing (stridor, grunting, gurgling, wheezing)
- A breathing rate that is faster than normal for the patient's age
- An increased depth of breathing
- Nasal flaring
- A mild increase in heart rate
- Retractions
- Head bobbing
- See-saw respirations (abdominal breathing)
- The use of neck muscles to breathe
- Changes in skin color

Remember This!

Give oxygen to *every* infant and child who is experiencing a respiratory problem, if it is available and you have been trained to use it. There is no medical reason to avoid giving oxygen to an infant or a child. Attempts to deliver oxygen should not delay transport.

You will see signs of respiratory failure as the child tires and can no longer maintain good oxygenation and ventilation. A child in respiratory failure looks very sick. The child becomes limp, peripheral pulses become weak, her color worsens, and her heart rate slows down. The breathing rate slows to below 20 breaths per minute in an infant and 10 breaths per minute in a child. A slow heart rate in a child with respiratory failure is a red flag. Cardiopulmonary arrest will occur soon if the child's oxygenation and ventilation are not corrected quickly.

You Should Know

Signs of Respiratory Failure

- Sleepiness or agitation
- Combativeness
- Limpness; the patient may be unable to sit up without help
- A breathing rate that is initially fast, with periods of slowing and then eventual slowing
- An altered mental status
- A shallow chest rise
- Nasal flaring
- Retractions
- Head bobbing
- Pale, mottled, or bluish skin
- Weak peripheral pulses

Making a Difference

When providing care for any patient with a respiratory problem, reassess the patient's condition frequently.

Objective 4 ▶

You can assist a child with respiratory distress by doing the following:

- Help the child into a position of comfort.
- Reposition the child's airway for better airflow if necessary.
- Provide oxygen if it is available and you have been trained to use it.

A child with respiratory distress is usually most comfortable in a sitting position. Do not place a child in a sitting position if you suspect trauma.

If the child shows signs of respiratory failure or respiratory arrest, assist the child's breathing with a BVM. If a BVM is not available, assist breathing using a mouth-to-mask device. Bag-valve-mask or mouth-to-mask breathing is also appropriate if you are uncertain about the child's degree of respiratory difficulty. If the child resists your efforts to ventilate him, he is probably not sick enough to need it. On the other hand, if he does not resist your efforts, he most likely does need your help. Deliver each breath over 1 second for an infant or a child. Watch for the rise and fall of the patient's chest with each breath. Stop ventilation when an adequate chest rise is observed. Allow the patient to exhale between breaths. Breathe at a rate of 12 to 20 breaths per minute for infants and children (1 breath every 3 to 5 seconds). Breathe at a rate of 12 to 20 breaths per minute for adolescents (1 breath every 5 to 6 seconds). Check the child's pulse about every 1–2 minutes to see if chest compressions need to be started.

Cardiopulmonary Failure

When a person stops breathing, a respiratory arrest occurs. When a person's heart stops, a cardiac arrest occurs. When the heart and lungs stop working, a cardiopulmonary arrest results. When respiratory failure occurs together with shock, **cardiopulmonary failure** results. Cardiopulmonary failure is the result of inadequate oxygenation, inadequate ventilation, and poor perfusion (Figure 13-12).

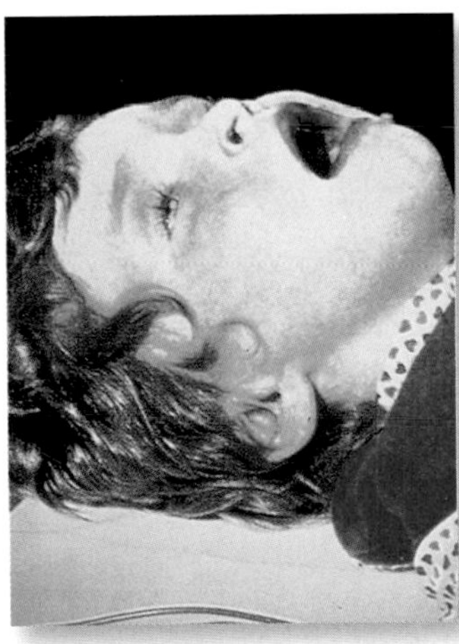

FIGURE 13-12 ▲ Inadequate oxygenation, inadequate ventilation, and poor perfusion can all result in cardiopulmonary failure. EMSC Slide Set (CD-ROM). 1996. Courtesy of the Emergency Medical Services for Children Program, administered by the U.S. Department of Health and Human Service's Health Resources and Services Administration, Maternal and Child Health Bureau.

In adults, cardiopulmonary failure and arrest are often the result of underlying heart disease. In children, cardiopulmonary failure and arrest are usually the result of an uncorrected respiratory problem. Some illnesses and injuries are associated with a high risk of cardiopulmonary failure.

You Should Know

Conditions Associated with a High Risk of Cardiopulmonary Failure

- Traumatic injuries
- Burns
- Severe dehydration
- Severe asthma, (reactive airway disease)
- Near drowning
- An upper airway obstruction
- Seizure
- Coma

The signs and symptoms of cardiopulmonary failure are

- Mental status changes
- A weak respiratory effort
- Slow, shallow breathing

- Pale, mottled, or bluish skin
- A slow pulse rate
- Weak central pulses and absent peripheral pulses
- Cool extremities
- A delayed capillary refill

Cardiopulmonary failure will progress to cardiopulmonary arrest unless it is recognized and treated promptly. If your patient is showing signs of cardiopulmonary failure, make sure the patient's airway is open. If trauma is suspected, take spinal precautions as necessary. Assist the child's breathing with a bag-valve-mask or mouth-to-mask device. Perform chest compressions if necessary.

Seizures

Objective 5 ▶

A **seizure** is a temporary change in behavior or consciousness caused by abnormal electrical activity in one or more groups of brain cells. **Status epilepticus** is a seizure that lasts longer than 30 minutes. Alternately, it is a series of seizures that occurs over a 30-minute period in which the patient remains unresponsive between seizures. Status epilepticus is a medical emergency that can cause brain damage or death if it is not treated.

Seizures are common in children. Seizures, including those caused by fever (febrile seizures), should be considered potentially life-threatening. Seizures from fever are most common in children under the age of five. It is the rapid rise of the child's temperature in a short period—not how high the temperature is—that causes the seizure. Many conditions can cause seizures. It is not necessary for you to determine the cause of a seizure in order to manage a patient who is having one.

You Should Know

Causes of Seizures

- Low blood oxygen level
- Low blood sugar
- Brain tumor
- Poisoning
- Head injury
- Previous brain damage
- Seizure disorder
- Fever
- Infection
- Abnormal heart rhythm
- Inherited factors
- Unknown cause

Seizures generally last about 30–45 seconds but can continue for minutes to hours. During the seizure, the child may have an altered mental status, changes in behavior, uncontrolled muscle movements, and a loss of bowel or bladder control. Depending on the seizure's severity, injuries can occur during a seizure. Injuries include biting of the tongue or cheek, injury to the head, bruises, and broken bones.

When you arrive on the scene, perform a scene size-up before starting emergency medical care. If the scene is safe, approach the child and perform an initial assessment. Complete a physical exam as needed.

Objective 6 ▶

It is most likely that once you have arrived the seizure will be over. Obtaining a good history is very important when treating these patients. Is this the child's first seizure? If the child has a history of seizures, is he or she on a seizure medication? Is this the child's normal seizure pattern? What did the caregiver do for the child during the seizure? Could the child have ingested any medications, household products, or any potentially toxic item? How long did the seizure last? Does the child have a fever?

If the patient is actively seizing when you arrive, look to see if she has bitten her tongue or hit her head during the seizure. If you witness the seizure, you will need to be able to describe what it looked like to responding EMS personnel. Important information includes how long the seizure lasted and if the seizure involved full body jerking or movement of only an arm or a leg. If the seizure has stopped, look for clues to the cause. Check for a medical identification device. Look for evidence of burns or suspicious substances that indicate poisoning or a toxic exposure. Are there signs of recent trauma?

Comfort, calm, and reassure the patient while waiting for additional EMS personnel to arrive. Protect the patient's privacy. Ask bystanders (except the caregiver) to leave the area. During the seizure, protect the child from harm by moving hard or sharp objects out of the way. Never attempt to restrain a child having a seizure. Do not put anything in the patient's mouth. Make sure suction is available because the child may vomit during or after the seizure.

As soon as the seizure is over, make sure the child's airway is open. Place the child in the recovery position if there is no possibility of spinal trauma. Loosen tight clothing. Gently suction the child's mouth if secretions are present. Provide oxygen if it is available and you have been trained to use it. If the child's skin appears blue, assist his breathing with a bag-valve-mask or mouth-to-mask device. Report your assessment findings to the EMS personnel arriving at the scene.

The period after a seizure is called the **postictal phase.** During this recovery period, the child often appears limp, has shallow breathing, and has an altered mental status. This altered mental status may appear as confusion, sleepiness, memory loss, unresponsiveness, or difficulty talking. The postictal phase may last minutes to hours.

Altered Mental Status

Altered mental status is also called altered level of consciousness (ALOC).

An **altered mental status** is a change in a patient's level of awareness. For example, a person may be awake and know her name but may be unable to answer questions about where she is or what happened to her. In order for you to determine if there has been a change in the patient's behavior, you must find out what the patient's normal behavior is. The patient's caregiver is usually the best person to provide this information. In fact, the child's caregiver is often the person who calls 9-1-1 because he or she has noticed that the child "isn't acting right." A patient with an altered mental status may appear agitated, combative, sleepy, difficult to awaken, or unresponsive.

There are many causes of altered mental status. The most common causes in a pediatric patient are a low level of oxygen in the blood (hypoxia), head trauma, seizures, infection, low blood sugar, and drug or alcohol ingestion.

You Should Know

Causes of Altered Mental Status

- A low blood oxygen level (hypoxia)
- Head trauma
- Seizures
- Infection
- Shock
- Low blood sugar
- Drug or alcohol ingestion
- Abuse
- Fever
- Respiratory failure

Any patient with an altered mental status is in danger of an airway obstruction. The patient may lose the ability to keep his or her own airway open because the soft tissues of the airway and the base of the tongue relax. The tongue falls into the back of the throat, blocking the airway. The patient may also have depressed gag and cough reflexes. A blocked airway can result in low blood oxygen levels, respiratory failure, or respiratory arrest. Many causes of an altered mental status may be associated with vomiting. Anticipate the need to place the patient in the recovery position (if no trauma is suspected). Be prepared to clear the patient's airway with suctioning. Remember to comfort, calm, and reassure the patient while waiting for additional EMS help to arrive.

Sudden Infant Death Syndrome (SIDS)

SIDS can be diagnosed only by autopsy.

The National Institute of Child Health and Human Development defines **sudden infant death syndrome (SIDS)** as "the sudden and unexpected death of an infant that remains unexplained after a thorough case investigation, including performance of a complete autopsy, examination of the death scene, and review of the clinical history."

Approximately 90% of all SIDS deaths occur during the first six months of life. Most deaths occur between the ages of two and four months. SIDS occurs in apparently healthy infants. Boys are affected more often than girls. Most SIDS deaths occur at home, usually during the night after a period of sleep. The baby's death is most often discovered in the early morning.

The cause of SIDS is not clearly understood. Research is ongoing. The number of SIDS deaths has decreased significantly since 1992, when caregivers were first told that infants should sleep on their backs and sides, rather than on their stomachs.

Although not present in all cases, common physical exam findings include an unresponsive baby who is not breathing and has no pulse. The skin often appears blue or mottled. There may be frothy sputum or vomitus around the mouth and nose. The underside of the baby's body may look dark and bruised due to pooled blood (dependent lividity). General stiffening of the body (rigor mortis) may be present.

Check with your instructor about your local protocols regarding obvious death.

Unless signs of obvious death are present, you should begin resuscitation. Rigor mortis is an obvious sign of death. Dependent lividity is considered an obvious sign of death only when there are extensive areas of reddish-purple discoloration of the skin on the underside of the body of an unresponsive, breathless, and pulseless patient. In some EMS systems, both lividity and rigor mortis must be present to be considered signs of obvious death.

Whether or not resuscitation is performed, you must find out about the events leading up to the call for help. Ask questions as tactfully as possible. Start by asking the caregiver the baby's name. Once the baby's name is given to you, refer to the baby by name. Do not use nonspecific words, such as *the baby* or *it*. Carefully document what you see at the scene and the caregiver's responses to your questions. Avoid any comments or a tone of voice that seems to point blame at the caregiver.

One of the most important skills you can perform on the scene of a SIDS patient is to provide emotional support for the baby's caregiver. The caregiver will usually be very distressed. You may observe crying, screaming, yelling, a stony silence, or physical outbursts.

The caregiver's feelings of guilt are often enormous.

If the infant is obviously dead, you will need to tell the caregiver. Speak slowly in a quiet, calm voice. Begin by saying, "This is hard to tell you, but . . ." Explain that the baby is dead. Use the word *dead* or *death*. Do not use phrases such as "passed on" or "no longer with us." Explain that there was nothing the caregiver could have done to prevent the baby's death. Pause frequently and ask the caregiver if he or she understands what you are saying. You may need to repeat information several times.

Before leaving the scene, make sure a friend, relative, member of the clergy, or grief support personnel are available to provide grief support for the family. Remain with the family until law enforcement personnel assume responsibility for the body and grief support personnel are on the scene.

Objective 10 ▶

After the call, make sure to assess your own emotional needs. It may be helpful for you and other personnel involved in the call to discuss the feelings that normally follow the death of an infant or a child.

Trauma

Injuries are the leading cause of death in infants and children. Blunt injury is the most common mechanism of serious injury in pediatric patients.

You Should Know

Causes of Common Blunt Trauma Injuries

- Falls
- Bicycle-related injuries
- Motor vehicle–related injuries (restrained and unrestrained passengers)
- Car-pedestrian incidents
- Drowning, near drowning
- Sports-related injuries
- Abuse and neglect

The injury pattern seen in a child may be different from that seen in an adult. In a motor vehicle crash, an unrestrained infant or child will often have head and neck injuries. Restrained passengers often have abdominal and lower spine injuries. Child safety seats are often improperly secured, resulting in head and neck injuries. If a child is struck while riding a bicycle, a head injury, a spinal injury, and/or an abdominal injury often results. If a child is struck by a vehicle, he or she may experience an abdominal injury with internal bleeding, a head injury, and/or a possible fracture of the thigh. Head and neck injuries may occur when a child falls from a height or dives into shallow water. Sports injuries are also associated with injuries to the head and neck.

Head Trauma

Children are prone to head injuries because their heads are large and heavy when compared with their body size. The younger the child, the softer and thinner the skull is. The force of injury is more likely to be transferred to the underlying brain instead of fracturing the skull. The blood vessels of the face and scalp bleed easily. Even a small wound can lead to major blood loss. When the head is struck, it jars the brain. The brain bounces back and forth, causing multiple bruised and injured areas.

Airway and breathing problems are common with head injuries. Vomiting and inadequate breathing are common. You must make sure that the child's airway is open and that his breathing is adequate. In an unresponsive child with a head injury, the single most important maneuver you can perform is to make sure the airway is open. You should use the jaw thrust without head tilt.

Chest, Abdominal, and Pelvic Trauma

> The presence of a rib fracture in a child suggests that major force caused the injury.

> Abdominal trauma is the most common cause of unrecognized fatal injury in children.

Signs of blunt trauma to the chest and abdomen may be hard to see on the body surface. The younger the patient, the softer and more flexible her ribs are. Therefore, rib fractures are less common in children than in adults. However, the force of the injury can be transferred to the internal organs of the chest, resulting in major damage. Bruising of the lung (pulmonary contusion) is one of the most frequently observed chest injuries in children. This injury is potentially life-threatening.

The abdomen is a more common site of injury in children than in adults. The abdomen is often a source of hidden injury. The abdominal organs of an infant or a child are prone to injury because the organs are large and the abdominal wall is thin. As a result, the organs are closer to the surface of the abdomen.

In infants and young children, the liver and spleen extend below the lower ribs. Their location gives them less protection and makes them more susceptible to injury. A swollen, tender abdomen is a cause for concern.

Pelvic fractures are uncommon in children. However, when they do occur, they are often the result of the child's being struck by a moving vehicle. Because the pelvis contains major blood vessels, you must be alert for signs of internal bleeding and shock.

Extremity Trauma

Extremity trauma is common in children. The younger the child, the more flexible his bones are. When a child has multiple injuries, fractures are often missed. Assessing non-displaced fractures in young children can be difficult because they cannot verbalize well. If a child is not walking on an injured extremity or using an upper extremity during normal activity, suspect a fracture until proven otherwise. Fractures of both thighs can cause a major blood loss, resulting in shock. Extremity injuries in children are managed in the same way as for adults.

Objective 7 ▶

When arriving on the scene, complete a scene size-up before beginning emergency medical care. Consider the mechanism of injury and form your general impression of the patient. Remember to complete an initial assessment of all patients. Comfort, calm, and reassure the patient while waiting for additional EMS resources.

If the child is not alert or the mechanism of injury suggests that the child experienced trauma to the head or neck, stabilize the child's spine. Making sure the child's airway is open and clear of secretions is the most important step in managing a trauma patient. Suction the airway as needed with a rigid suction catheter. If the child is unresponsive, open the child's airway using the jaw thrust without head tilt. Insert an oral airway to help keep the airway open. If the child's breathing is inadequate or there is no air movement, assist breathing with bag-valve-mask or mouth-to-mask ventilation. Give oxygen if it is available and you have been trained to use it.

Control obvious bleeding if present. Check for signs of shock by assessing the child's mental status, heart rate, and skin color. If the child is younger than six years old, assess capillary refill. Remember to keep the child warm.

Extremity injuries should be stabilized by immobilizing the joint above and below the fracture site. Remember to assess pulses, motor function, and sensation in the affected extremity before and after immobilization. Update the EMS unit responding to the scene with a brief report of the child's condition by phone or radio, if possible.

Child Abuse and Neglect

These definitions are from the National Clearinghouse on Child Abuse and Neglect and the National Child Abuse and Neglect Data System Glossary.

Child maltreatment is an act or a failure to act by a parent, a caregiver, or another person as defined by state law that results in physical abuse, neglect, medical neglect, sexual abuse, and/or emotional abuse. It is also defined as an act or a failure to act that presents an impending risk of serious harm to a child (Figure 13-13). State laws define the specific acts that make up the various forms of abuse. These laws vary from state to state.

Physical abuse refers to physical acts that have caused or could have caused physical injury to a child. Examples of physical abuse are burning, hitting, punching, shaking, kicking, beating, or otherwise harming a child. **Neglect** is the failure to provide for a child's basic needs. Neglect can be medical, physical, educational, or emotional (Figure 13-14). **Medical neglect** is a type of maltreatment caused by a caregiver's failure to provide for the appropriate healthcare

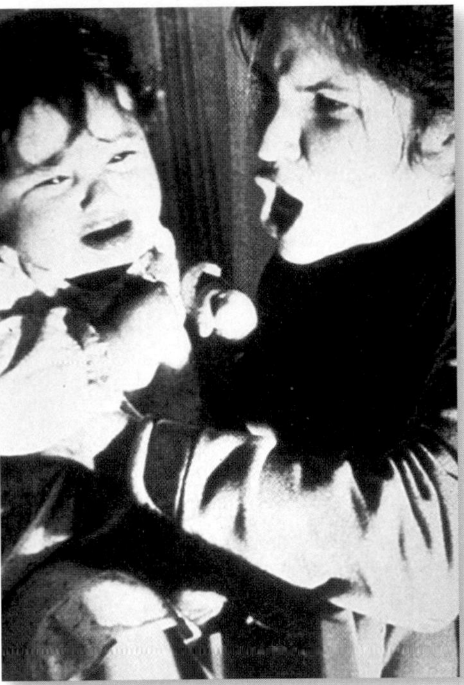

FIGURE 13-13 ▲ *Never* shake or jiggle a baby. EMSC Slide Set (CD-ROM). 1996. Courtesy of the Emergency Medical Services for Children Program, administered by the U.S. Department of Health and Human Service's Health Resources and Services Administration, Maternal and Child Health Bureau.

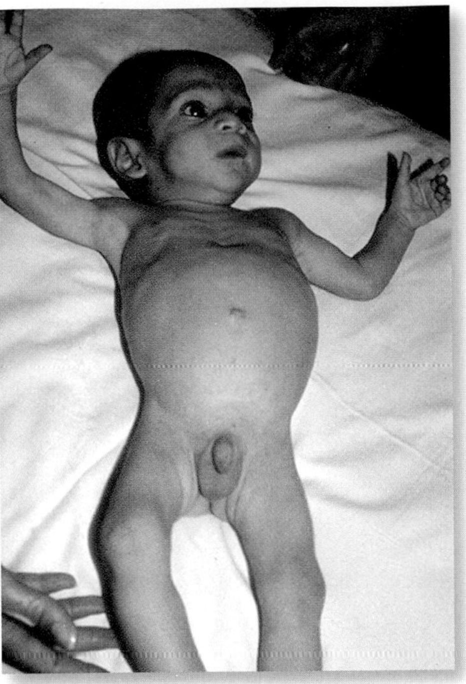

FIGURE 13-14 ▲ Neglect is the failure to provide for a child's basic needs. Neglect can be medical, physical, educational, or emotional. EMSC Slide Set (CD-ROM). 1996. Courtesy of the Emergency Medical Services for Children Program, administered by the U.S. Department of Health and Human Service's Health Resources and Services Administration, Maternal and Child Health Bureau.

of the child although financially able to do so. The signs of neglect that you may see in the child's environment include

- Untreated chronic illness (such as a diabetic or an asthmatic child with no medication)
- Untreated soft-tissue injuries
- A home that is bug- or rodent-infested
- A lack of adult supervision
- A lack of food or basic necessities
- A child who appears to be malnourished
- Stool or urine present on items in the home
- An unsafe living environment
- The presence of drugs or alcohol paraphernalia

Sexual abuse is inappropriate adolescent or adult sexual behavior with a child. To be considered child abuse, these acts have to be committed by a person responsible for the care of a child (for example a babysitter, parent, or daycare provider) or a person related to the child. If a stranger commits these acts, it is considered sexual assault and is handled solely by the police and criminal courts. **Psychological maltreatment** is a pattern of caregiver behavior that conveys to children that they are worthless, flawed, unloved, unwanted, endangered, or only of value in meeting another's needs. This type of maltreatment includes verbal abuse, emotional abuse or neglect, psychological abuse, and mental injury.

As a healthcare professional, you must be aware of these conditions and be able to recognize them. Physical abuse and neglect are the two forms of child maltreatment that you are most likely to detect. As an Emergency Medical Responder, you may be the only trained healthcare professional in the child's environment. You will be able to see things that other healthcare professionals will never see. Your eyes and ears will help them complete the puzzle of suspected abuse.

You Should Know

Physical Signs That May Indicate Abuse

- Multiple bruises in various stages of healing
- Human bite marks
- Inflicted burns—stockinglike burns with no associated splash marks, usually present on the buttocks, genitalia, or extremities
- Circular burns from a cigarette or cigar
- Rope burns on the wrists
- Burns in the shape of a household utensil or appliance, such as a spoon or an iron
- Fractures
- Head, face, and oral injuries
- Abdominal injuries
- An injury inconsistent with the history or developmental level of the child

Objective 8 ▶

According to the National Clearinghouse on Child Abuse and Neglect, you should consider the possibility of physical abuse when the *child*

- Has unexplained burns, bites, bruises, broken bones, or black eyes
- Has fading bruises or other marks noticeable after an absence from school
- Seems frightened of the caregiver and protests or cries when it is time to go home
- Shrinks at the approach of adults
- Reports injury by a parent or another adult caregiver

You should consider the possibility of physical abuse when the *parent or another adult caregiver*

- Offers conflicting, unconvincing, or no explanations for the child's injury
- Describes the child as "evil" or in some other very negative way
- Uses harsh physical discipline with the child
- Has a history of abuse as a child

You should consider the possibility of neglect when the *child*

- Is frequently absent from school
- Begs or steals food or money
- Lacks needed medical or dental care, immunizations, or glasses
- Is consistently dirty and has severe body odor
- Lacks sufficient clothing for the weather
- Abuses alcohol or drugs
- States that there is no one at home to provide care

You should consider the possibility of neglect when the *parent or another adult caregiver*

- Appears to be indifferent to the child
- Seems apathetic or depressed
- Behaves irrationally or in a bizarre manner
- Is abusing alcohol or drugs

Do not confront or accuse any caregiver of abuse. Accusation and confrontation delay transportation. Keep in mind that the caregiver with the child at the scene may not be the abuser.

Objective 9 ► Reporting known or suspected child abuse is required by law in most states. Individuals who are typically required to report abuse have frequent contact with children. Some states require all citizens to report suspected abuse or neglect, regardless of their profession. It is your responsibility to know what the requirements are in your area.

Report what you see and hear. Do not comment on what you think.

Carefully document your physical exam findings as well as your observations of the child's environment. Document the caregiver's comments exactly as stated and enclose them in quotation marks. Make sure that your documentation reflects the facts, not your opinion of what may or may not have occurred. Report your findings to the EMS personnel responding to the scene.

Objective 13 ► Providing care for an infant or a child who is ill or injured due to neglect or abuse is stressful for most healthcare professionals. Show a professional and caring attitude as you care for the patient. You must make the interests of an ill or injured infant or child your main concern when making patient care decisions. **Objective 14 ►** After the call, assess your own emotional needs. A discussion with other personnel involved in the call may be helpful.

On The Scene

Wrap-Up

You apply an oxygen mask to your small patient while calmly reassuring her that it will help her. Luckily, the ambulance crew walks in a few moments later. They quickly assess her and begin treating her with an inhaled medicine. The whistling sounds quiet and you notice that, within a few minutes of starting the drug, her breathing is slowing. The ambulance crew is concerned because her wheezing is still significant and they call medical direction. Following their advice, the ambulance crew members start an IV and give another breathing treatment. You assist the crew to secure the patient in the ambulance. Then you stay with your patient until the ambulance pulls away on the 30-mile trip to the hospital. ■

Sum It Up

► As an Emergency Medical Responder, you should be familiar with the anatomical and physiological differences between children and adults.

- A child's head is proportionately larger and heavier than an adult's until about 4 years of age. Because the back of a child's head sticks out and children's foreheads are large, these areas are susceptible to injury, especially bruising.
- The top and back of an infant's head contain small, triangular openings called fontanels ("soft spots"). These areas will not completely close until about 6 months of age for the rear fontanel and 18 months for the top one.

You should assess the fontanels of an infant and a toddler for bulging or a depression. Bulging in a quiet patient suggests increased pressure within the skull, such as fluid or pressure on the brain. A depression suggests the patient is dehydrated.

- The necks of infants and toddlers are flexed when they are lying flat because the back of the skull is large. The chin is then angled toward the chest. Proper positioning of an infant's or a toddler's head is an important factor when managing the airway.
- A child's nasal passages are very small, short, and narrow. Because newborns are primarily nose breathers, a newborn will not automatically open his or her mouth to breathe when his or her nose becomes obstructed. As a result, any obstruction of the nose will lead to respiratory difficulty. You must make sure the newborn's nose is clear to avoid breathing problems.
- Although the opening of the mouth is usually small, a child's tongue is large in proportion to the mouth. The tongue is the most common cause of upper airway obstruction in an unconscious child because the immature muscles of the lower jaw (mandible) allow the tongue to fall to the back of the throat.
- In children, the flap of cartilage that covers the opening between the vocal cords, the epiglottis, is larger and floppier than in adults. Therefore, any injury to or swelling of this area can block the airway.
- The windpipe (trachea) is softer and more flexible, and has a smaller diameter and shorter length than in adults. The trachea has rings of cartilage that keep the airway open. In children, this cartilage is soft and collapses easily, which can then obstruct the airway.
- A child's ribs are soft and more flexible than those of an adult. Therefore, trauma to the chest will be transmitted to the lungs and other internal structures more easily.
- Children breathe faster and their hearts beat harder and faster than those of adults. Infants and young children also have a relatively small blood volume. A sudden loss of 1/2 liter (500 mL) of the blood volume in a child, or 100–200 mL of the blood volume in an infant, is considered serious.
- Most of an infant's body weight is water, so vomiting and diarrhea can result in dehydration.
- Because an infant's skin is thin, with few fat deposits under it, an infant is sensitive to extremes of heat and cold. Infants have poorly developed temperature-regulating mechanisms. They are unable to shiver in cold temperatures and their sweating mechanism is immature in warm temperatures. Because infants and children are at risk for hypothermia, it is very important to keep them warm.
- The age classification of infants and children is the following:
  - Newly born—birth to several hours following birth
  - Neonate—birth to 1 month
  - Infant—1 to 12 months of age
    - Young infant: 0 to 6 months of age
    - Older infant: 6 months to 1 year of age
  - Toddler—1 to 3 years of age
  - Preschooler—4 to 5 years of age
  - School-age child—6 to 12 years of age
  - Adolescent—13 to 18 years of age

► Your assessment of an infant or a child should begin from across the room. Quickly determine if the child appears "sick" or "not sick." Quickly assess

- *Appearance.* A child should be alert and responsive to the surroundings.

- *(Work of) breathing.* With normal breathing, both sides of the chest rise and fall equally. Breathing is quiet, is painless, and occurs at a regular rate.
- *Circulation.* The visual signs of circulation relate to skin color, obvious bleeding, and moisture. If the child's skin looks pale, mottled, flushed, gray, or blue, proceed immediately to the initial assessment.

▶ Once your general impression is complete, perform a hands-on assessment. In a responsive infant or child, use a toes-to-head or trunk-to-head approach. This approach should help reduce the infant's or child's anxiety.

▶ During your initial assessment, find the answers to these five questions:

1. Is the child awake and alert?
2. Is the child's airway open?
3. Is the child breathing?
4. Does the child have a pulse?
5. Does the child have severe bleeding?

▶ If a child is unable to speak, cry, cough, or make any other sound, the airway is completely obstructed. If the child has noisy breathing, such as snoring or gurgling, he or she has a partial airway obstruction. Do not agitate the child. If the child has a foreign body in the airway, agitation could cause the object to move into a position that completely blocks the airway. Encourage the child to cough and allow the child to continue his or her efforts to clear his or her own airway. Continue to watch the child closely. You will need to intervene if the child has a complete airway obstruction.

▶ The most common medical emergencies in children are respiratory emergencies. Upper airway problems usually occur suddenly. Lower airway problems usually take longer to develop. A patient with an upper airway problem is more likely to worsen during the time you are providing care than is a patient with a lower airway problem. You must watch closely for changes in the patient's condition and adjust your treatment as needed.

▶ The three levels of respiratory problems are the following:

1. *Respiratory distress* is an increased work of breathing (respiratory effort).
2. *Respiratory failure* is a condition in which there is not enough oxygen in the blood and/or ventilation to meet the demands of body tissues. Respiratory failure becomes evident when the patient becomes tired and can no longer maintain good oxygenation and ventilation.
3. *Respiratory arrest* occurs when a patient stops breathing.

▶ Most children will present with either respiratory distress or respiratory failure. As an Emergency Medical Responder, you must know how to treat both conditions:

- You can assist a child with respiratory distress by doing the following:
  - Help the child into a position of comfort.
  - Reposition the child's airway for better airflow if necessary.
  - Provide oxygen if it is available and you have been trained to use it.
- If the child shows signs of respiratory failure or respiratory arrest, assist the child's breathing with a bag-valve-mask device. If a bag-valve-mask device is not available, assist breathing using a mouth-to-mask device. Bag-valve-mask or mouth-to-mask breathing is also appropriate if you are uncertain about the child's degree of respiratory difficulty.

▶ *Cardiopulmonary arrest* results when the heart and lungs stop working. When respiratory failure occurs together with shock, *cardiopulmonary failure* results. Cardiopulmonary failure will progress to cardiopulmonary arrest unless it is recognized and treated promptly.

- A *seizure* is a temporary change in behavior or consciousness caused by abnormal electrical activity in one or more groups of brain cells. *Status epilepticus* is a seizure that lasts longer than 30 minutes. Alternately, it is a series of seizures that occurs over a 30-minute period in which the child remains unresponsive between seizures. Status epilepticus is a medical emergency that can cause brain damage or death if it is not treated.
- It is most likely that, once you have arrived at the scene, the seizure will be over. Obtaining a good history is very important when treating these patients. If you witness the seizure, you will need to be able to describe what it looked like to responding EMS personnel.
  - Comfort, calm, and reassure the patient while waiting for additional EMS personnel to arrive. Protect the patient's privacy. Do not put anything in the patient's mouth. Make sure that suction is available because the child may vomit during or after the seizure.
  - As soon as the seizure is over, make sure the child's airway is open. Place the child in the recovery position if there is no possibility of spinal trauma. Gently suction the child's mouth if secretions are present. Provide oxygen if it is available and you have been trained to use it. Report your assessment findings to the EMS personnel arriving at the scene.
- The period after a seizure is called the *postictal phase*. During this recovery period, the child often appears limp, has shallow breathing, and has an altered mental status. This phase may last minutes to hours.
- The most common causes of an *altered mental status* in a pediatric patient are a low level of oxygen in the blood, head trauma, seizures, infection, low blood sugar, and drug or alcohol ingestion. Any patient with an altered mental status is in danger of an airway obstruction. Anticipate the need to place the patient in the recovery position (if no trauma is suspected). Be prepared to clear the patient's airway with suctioning.
- *Sudden infant death syndrome (SIDS)* is the sudden and unexpected death of an infant. The cause of SIDS is not clearly understood. Approximately 90% of all SIDS deaths occur during the first 6 months of life. Boys are affected more often than girls. Most SIDS deaths occur at home, usually during the night after a period of sleep.
- Injuries are the leading cause of death in infants and children.
  - When arriving on the scene, complete a scene size-up. Consider the mechanism of injury and form your general impression of the patient. Complete an initial assessment of all patients. Comfort, calm, and reassure the patient while awaiting additional EMS resources.
  - If the child is not alert or the mechanism of injury suggests that the child experienced trauma to the head or neck, stabilize the child's spine. Making sure the child's airway is open and clear of secretions is the most important step in managing a trauma patient.
  - Control obvious bleeding if present. Check for signs of shock by assessing the child's mental status, heart rate, and skin color.
  - Extremity injuries should be stabilized by immobilizing the joint above and below the fracture site. Remember to assess pulses, motor function, and sensation in the affected extremity before and after immobilization. Update the EMS unit responding to the scene with a brief report of the child's condition by phone or radio.
- As an Emergency Medical Responder, you must be aware of the signs of child abuse and neglect:
  - *Child maltreatment* is an act or a failure to act by a parent, a caregiver, or another person as defined by state law that results in physical abuse, neglect, medical

neglect, sexual abuse, and/or emotional abuse. It is also defined as an act or a failure to act that presents an impending risk of serious harm to a child.

- *Physical abuse* refers to physical acts that have caused or could have caused physical injury to a child. Examples of physical abuse include burning, hitting, punching, shaking, kicking, beating, or otherwise harming a child.
- *Neglect* is the failure to provide for a child's basic needs. Neglect can be medical, physical, educational, or emotional. *Medical neglect* is a type of maltreatment caused by a caregiver's failure to provide for the appropriate healthcare of the child although financially able to do so.
- *Sexual abuse* is inappropriate adolescent or adult sexual behavior with a child. To be considered child abuse, these acts have to be committed by a person responsible for the care of a child (for example a babysitter, parent, or daycare provider) or a person related to the child. If a stranger commits these acts, it is considered sexual assault and is handled solely by the police and criminal courts.
- *Psychological maltreatment* is a pattern of caregiver behavior that conveys to children that they are worthless, flawed, unloved, unwanted, endangered, or only of value in meeting another's needs. This type of maltreatment includes verbal abuse, emotional abuse or neglect, psychological abuse, and mental injury.

▶ When providing care for an infant or a child who is ill or injured due to neglect or abuse, show a professional and caring attitude toward the patient. Report known or suspected child abuse as required by law in your state. Carefully document your physical exam findings, as well as your observations of the child's environment. Document the caregiver's comments exactly as stated and enclose them in quotation marks. Your documentation must reflect the facts, not your opinion of what may or may not have occurred. Report your findings to the EMS personnel responding to the scene. After the call, assess your own emotional needs. A discussion with other personnel involved in the call may be helpful.

▶ Tracking Your Progress

After reading this chapter, can you	Page Reference	Objective Met?
• Describe differences in anatomy and physiology of the infant, child, and adult patient?	481–484	☐
• Describe assessment of the infant or child?	488–492	☐
• Indicate various causes of respiratory emergencies in infants and children?	493	☐
• Summarize emergency medical care strategies for respiratory distress and respiratory failure/arrest in infants and children?	495	☐
• List common causes of seizures in the infant and child patient?	496	☐
• Describe management of seizures in the infant and child patient?	496–497	☐
• Discuss emergency medical care of the infant and child trauma patient?	500	☐
• Summarize the signs and symptoms of possible child abuse and neglect?	502–503	☐
• Describe the medical-legal responsibilities in suspected child abuse?	503	☐
• Recognize the need for an Emergency Medical Responder debriefing following a difficult infant or child transport?	498	☐
• Attend to the feelings of the family when dealing with an ill or injured infant or child?	488	☐

• Understand the provider's own emotional response to caring for infants or children?	488	☐
• Demonstrate a caring attitude toward infants and children with illness or injury who require Emergency Medical Services?	503	☐
• Place the interests of the infant or child with an illness or injury as the foremost consideration when making any and all patient care decisions?	503	☐
• Communicate with empathy to infants and children with an illness or injury, as well as with family members and friends of the patient?	488	☐

Chapter Quiz

Multiple Choice

In the space provided, identify the letter of the choice that best completes each statement or answers each question.

_____ 1. You have been called to the scene of a car-pedestrian accident. You can see a young girl lying in the road. She appears to be about four years old. She is lying still and her eyes are closed. You can see that her chest is moving slightly. She looks very pale. Your first concern at the scene must be to

a. look, listen, and feel for breathing.
b. ensure that the scene is safe for you to enter.
c. place the child in the recovery position.
d. check to see if the child has a pulse.

_____ 2. The child in question 1 is unresponsive. What should you do next?

a. Open her airway using a head tilt–chin lift.
b. Open her mouth and perform a blind finger sweep.
c. Look for signs of obvious bleeding.
d. Open her airway using a jaw thrust without head tilt.

_____ 3. You hear gurgling sounds coming from a child's airway. When suctioning this child, you should apply suction for no longer than how many seconds at a time?

a. 10
b. 15
c. 30
d. 60

_____ 4. If a child's heart rate slows during suctioning, you should

a. continue suctioning until the airway is clear.
b. begin chest compressions.
c. stop suctioning and begin ventilation.
d. make sure the tip of the suction catheter is touching the back of the child's throat.

_____ 5. Which of the following statements is *true* regarding pediatric patients?

a. Poisonings are the leading cause of death in infants and children.
b. Airway and breathing problems are common with head injuries.
c. Penetrating trauma is the most common mechanism of serious injury in a pediatric patient.
d. The injury patterns seen in children are identical to those seen in an adult.

_____ 6. You are called for an "ill baby." You arrive to find an unresponsive 5-month-old baby in his crib. The baby's mother is hysterical. She says she put the baby down for a nap an hour ago. She went in to check on him about 10 minutes ago and could not awaken him. The baby is not moving. There are no obvious signs of breathing. His skin has a bluish tint. You should assess the infant's pulse by checking the

a. carotid pulse.
b. dorsalis pedis pulse.
c. brachial pulse.
d. femoral pulse.

_____ 7. Select the correct statement regarding sudden infant death syndrome (SIDS).

a. Although there are many theories, the cause of SIDS is unknown.
b. More girls are affected than are boys.
c. Positioning an infant to sleep on his or her stomach has helped reduce the number of SIDS deaths.
d. Most SIDS deaths occur in infants 6–12 months of age.

Short Answer

Answer each question in the space provided.

8. List three possible causes of an increased heart rate in an infant or a child.

1. _______________
2. _______________
3. _______________

9. List four signs of physical abuse.

1. _______________
2. _______________
3. _______________
4. _______________

10. List five possible causes of an altered mental status.

1. _______________
2. _______________
3. _______________
4. _______________
5. _______________

Module 7

EMS Operations

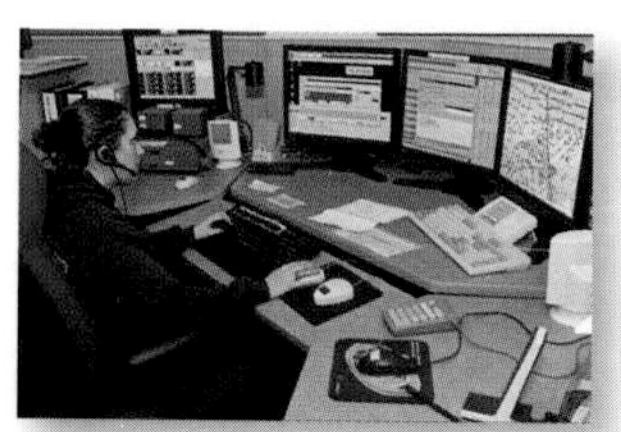

CHAPTER

14 EMS Operations

By the end of this chapter, you should be able to

Knowledge Objectives ▶

1. Discuss the medical and non-medical equipment needed to respond to a call.
2. List the phases of a prehospital call.
3. Discuss the role of the Emergency Medical Responder in extrication.
4. List various methods of gaining access to the patient.
5. Distinguish between simple and complex access.
6. Describe what the Emergency Medical Responder should do if there is reason to believe that there is a hazard at the scene.
7. State the role the Emergency Medical Responder should perform until appropriately trained personnel arrive at the scene of a hazardous materials situation.
8. Describe the criteria for a multiple-casualty situation.
9. Discuss the role of the Emergency Medical Responder in a multiple-casualty situation.
10. Summarize the components of basic triage.

Attitude Objectives ▶

11. Explain the rationale for having the unit prepared to respond.

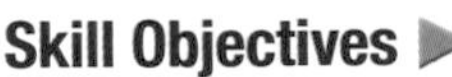

12. Given a scenario of a mass casualty incident, perform triage.

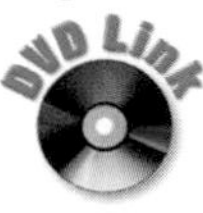

On The Scene

You drive with caution through thick, milky fog to a vehicle collision, thankful you are on the ambulance with a seasoned veteran tonight. As you approach the scene, you can see that this is no ordinary car crash. A car has collided with a train. The car lies crushed in the ditch about 10 feet off the road. Bystanders are pointing you to several patients who are scattered in the area.

You and your partner quickly size up the situation. There were six teens in the car—four were ejected and two remain trapped in the mangled wreckage. You open the airway of a young girl. She is not breathing, so you reopen her airway and look, listen, and feel again; there is still no breathing. You know what you have to do, but it's not easy—you tag her as "black" and move on. The others are breathing, but three are unconscious and the remaining two have signs of shock. Your partner radios for more ambulances and equipment, and you begin the overwhelming task of trying to provide some care for your seriously injured patients as you hear the distant whine of sirens approaching. ■

THINK ABOUT IT

As you read this chapter, think about the following questions:

- How will you categorize the remaining patients?
- How should incoming units protect the scene from another collision while you move your patients across the road to the ambulance?
- Who will remove the trapped patients?

Introduction

Understanding the EMS System

As an Emergency Medical Responder, you are a part of the EMS System. This chapter will provide you with a brief overview of some of the operational aspects of prehospital care. You should be familiar with the medical and non-medical equipment used in patient care. You should also be aware of the phases of an EMS response and your role in each. Although an Emergency Medical Responder is not usually responsible for rescue and extrication (removing persons from a vehicle or confined space), it is important that you understand the process.

Preparing for an EMS Call

Objective 1 ►

As an Emergency Medical Responder, you should have appropriate equipment and supplies with which to assess a patient, provide emergency care, and assist other healthcare professionals:

- Personal protective equipment. PPE should include a minimum of two pairs of latex or other sterile gloves (if you are allergic to latex). It should also include masks and barrier devices for ventilating patients, including high-efficiency particulate air (HEPA) masks, goggles or face shields, and disposable gowns.
- Basic wound care supplies. These supplies should include dressings and bandages, adhesive tape, trauma shears, triangular bandages, roller-type bandages, universal dressings or gauze pads, occlusive dressings (such as petroleum gauze) for making an airtight seal, upper- and lower-extremity splints, a stick (for a tourniquet), an eye protector (such as a paper cup or cone), tweezers, and antiseptic wipes.
- If you are expected to measure blood pressure, you will need a watch that shows seconds, a stethoscope, and a blood pressure cuff (adult and pediatric).
- Consider carrying additional items, such as a blanket, pillow, and disposable chemical cold pack.

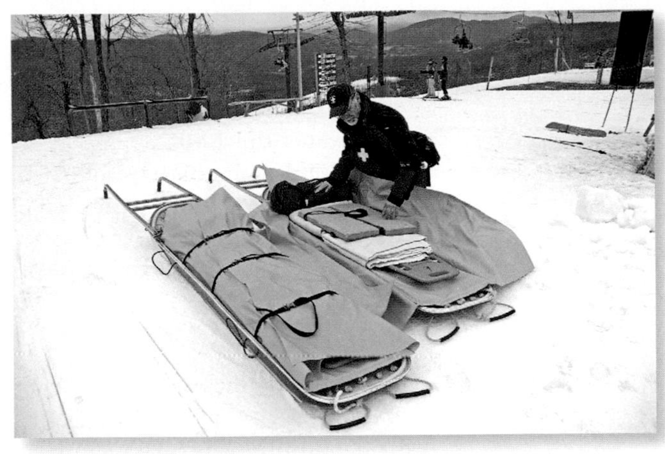

FIGURE 14-1 ► All emergency supplies should be placed in a sturdy bag or case. Make sure to check the contents of your emergency kit regularly and replace items as they become outdated.

All emergency supplies should be placed in a sturdy bag or case (Figure 14-1). Make sure to check the contents of your emergency kit regularly and replace items as they become outdated. You should also have basic extrication tools and devices available. These should include a jack and jack handle, pliers, a hammer, screwdrivers, a knife, and a rope.

Flashlights, planned routes or comprehensive street maps, and flares are some examples of non-medical equipment you may need to respond to a call.

You may want to include additional items in your emergency kit or in a separate kit if you have been trained in their use and are permitted to use them (according to your local protocol):

- Oral airways (adult and pediatric)
- Bag-valve masks (adult and pediatric)
- Biohazard bag
- Flashlight (aluminum; heavy duty)
- Seat belt cutter
- Two-way hand-held radio and/or cellular telephone
- Notebook or clipboard with black ink pen, emergency phone numbers, radio frequencies, and copies of your protocols
- Bag or case for equipment
- Hand-operated suction device
- Obstetrics (OB) kit (for emergency childbirth)
- Raincoat/poncho (for wet weather)
- Safety vest (for visibility)
- Window punch
- Flares and/or chemical light sticks
- Local maps and/or a GPS unit

Phases of a Typical EMS Response

A typical EMS response consists of six phases:

1. Detection of the emergency
2. Reporting the emergency (the call made for assistance) and dispatch
3. Response (medical resources sent to the scene)
4. On-scene care
5. Care during transport
6. Transfer to definitive care

Detection

Objective 2 ▶

In the detection phase of an EMS response, an emergency is recognized, usually by a bystander. In some situations, you may be the person who sees an emergency and activates the EMS system. It is much different when you witness the event and respond immediately than when you are dispatched to a call. Being dispatched gives you the chance to gather your thoughts en route and begin to create a plan. When you witness an emergency, you experience the emotion of the event and must react and respond instantly.

Reporting and Dispatch

In the second phase of an EMS response, the witness reports the emergency by calling 9-1-1 or another emergency number. The call to 9-1-1 goes to a central communications system that is available 24 hours a day. This system links police, fire, and EMS resources. An Emergency Medical Dispatcher (EMD) receives the call and gathers information from the caller. The dispatcher then activates (dispatches) an appropriate EMS response based on the information received (Figure 14-2). The important information the EMD attempts to gather from the caller includes

- The nature of the call
- The name, location, and callback number of the caller
- The location of the patient
- The number of patients and the severity of their illness or injury
- Other special problems that can be identified through the caller

The EMD is also responsible for coordinating logistics. An EMD is knowledgeable about the geography of the area, the emergency medical system's capabilities, and the activities of other public service agencies. In most EMS systems, the EMD is trained to relay instructions to the caller for life-saving procedures that can be performed, if necessary, while waiting for trained medical personnel to arrive. A good EMD can make a big difference on a call. He or she can shave minutes off your response time by getting precise information about the location of your patient. The EMD can keep you safe by asking about hazards on the scene. The EMD can also send you appropriate resources in a timely manner.

Response

The third phase of a typical EMS response is response to the scene of the emergency. Notify dispatch that you are responding to the call. Write down the essential information from the dispatcher, including the nature and location of the call.

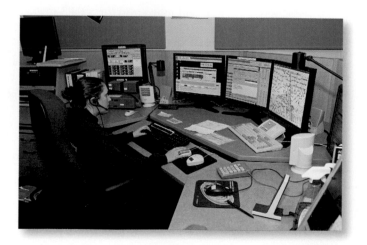

FIGURE 14-2 ▶ An Emergency Medical Dispatcher (EMD) receives an emergency call, gathers information from the caller, and activates an appropriate EMS response based on the information received.

Remember that your own safety is your first priority. If you are responding to the scene in a vehicle, make sure to wear your seat belt. While en route, prepare for the patient and situation based on the information given by the EMD. Consider these factors:

- The number of patients
- The possible problems in gaining access to the patient
- Scene safety
- The potential complications based on the patient's reported illness or injury
- The equipment and supplies that will need to be taken to the patient to begin emergency care

Determine the responsibilities of the crewmembers before arriving on the scene. For example, while you and your partner are en route to the scene, decide who will assess the patient and who will document the call. In most agencies, these responsibilities are determined at the start of a shift instead of on the way to a call.

When you position the emergency vehicle, park it with convenient access to the patient. Consider the effects of traffic flow, the roadway, known hazards, the public, and other agencies. In most cases, you should park in front of or behind a collision. This positioning is done so that you do not block the movement of other emergency vehicles. Avoid parking in a location that will hamper your exit from the scene.

Park at a safe distance from wreckage or hazardous scenes. Park uphill and upwind from leaking hazards. Park a minimum of 100 feet from wreckage or a burning vehicle. Park at least 2,000 feet from a hazardous substance. Use warning lights. Shut off headlights unless there is a need to illuminate the scene.

On-Scene Care

Actions at the scene should be rapid, efficient, and organized.

When you arrive on the scene, notify the EMD of your arrival. Before initiating patient care, take BSI precautions and perform a scene size-up. Determine if the scene is safe by looking for possible hazards. For example, is the emergency vehicle parked in a safe location? Is it safe to approach the patient? Does the patient require immediate movement because of hazards? Identify the mechanism of injury or the nature of the illness, as well as the total number of patients. Request additional help if necessary. If law enforcement personnel are not present on the scene, create a safe traffic environment and then size up the scene.

After making sure the scene is safe, quickly perform a patient assessment. Safely and efficiently provide emergency care until additional EMS help arrives. When more highly trained medical professionals arrive, give them a brief description of the emergency and a summary of the care you have provided before transferring patient care.

Care During Transport

One of your responsibilities as an Emergency Medical Responder is to assess the need for patient transport for further care. If patient transport is needed, help the transport crew prepare the patient for transport. Make sure that dressings and splints, if used, are secure. When they are ready, help the transport crew with lifting and moving the patient to the ambulance, using the techniques discussed in Chapter 5. The lifting and moving method and the device used will depend on the patient's illness or injury. They will also be determined by the safety of the scene, such as an emergency move at an unsafe scene versus the moving of a stable medical patient.

If you will accompany the patient to the hospital and provide care, remember that your safety must be your priority. Wearing a seat belt is one way to ensure your safety. While some people may consider it cumbersome to wear a seat belt during transport, your risk of injury increases if you are not restrained. Notify dispatch when you are leaving the scene. Let the dispatcher know your destination. Follow your local protocol regarding the communication of additional patient information.

Providing care during patient transport is challenging.

Care begun on the scene should be continued throughout patient transport. The frequency of performing ongoing patient assessments during transport will be based on the patient's condition. The patient's condition may improve, remain the same, or worsen during transport. A good rule to follow is that, if the patient is unstable, he should be reassessed every 5 minutes. If the patient is stable, it should be adequate to reassess him every 15 minutes. Reassure the patient throughout the transport.

Complete your prehospital care report (PCR). Contact the receiving facility, if possible, and use a standardized medical reporting format. In most EMS systems, the information that is relayed to the receiving facility includes

- Your unit's name and level of service (Basic Life Support or Advanced Life Support)
- The estimated time of arrival
- The patient's age and gender
- The patient's chief complaint
- A brief, pertinent history of the present illness
- Major past illnesses
- The patient's mental status and baseline vital signs
- Pertinent physical exam findings
- The emergency medical care given (and by whom)
- The patient's response to emergency medical care

Transfer to Definitive Care

Once at the hospital, you must give a verbal report to the hospital staff. As the healthcare professional who provided patient care, you are the only link the hospital staff has to the patient's history and what happened at the scene. Information about how you found the patient, how the scene looked, and what care was given to the patient by family members or bystanders before you arrived will only be available to the hospital staff through your report.

To provide an accurate report, you must pay attention to details at the scene. In some cases, an instant camera is very helpful. For example, many EMS services use instant cameras to take pictures of motor vehicle crash scenes. These photos provide information about the scene. They also give a detailed view of the mechanism of injury.

You should give a verbal report to the appropriate hospital staff member at the patient's bedside. Introduce the patient by name (if known). Summarize the information already provided by radio or telephone to the receiving facility, including

- The patient's chief complaint
- Pertinent patient history that was not previously given
- The emergency medical care given en route and the patient's response to the treatment given
- The vital signs taken en route

Provide any additional information collected en route but not transmitted by telephone or radio. Be sure to let hospital staff know if there was any delay in reaching the patient or if there were any unusual circumstances at the scene.

Objective 11 ▶

Make sure the hospital staff member who listens to your report signs your PCR when you transfer patient care. Leave a copy of your PCR with the hospital staff person. Your report will be included in the patient's hospital medical record. After your report is complete, the emergency vehicle and any equipment used should be cleaned and disinfected as needed. Dispose of contaminated linens properly. Restock disposable supplies and refuel the vehicle to ensure your readiness for the next call.

Air Medical Transport Considerations

When air medical transport is necessary, the scene is usually complex. In most cases, air transportation is used because the condition of one or more patients is critical (Figures 14-3 and 14-4). In these types of scenes, emotions run high and safety considerations can be overlooked. Remember that the goal in any EMS operation is to ensure the safety of every person at the scene.

It is important to identify the need for air transport as early as possible. The mechanisms of injury that may require helicopter transport include

- A vehicle rollover with unrestrained passengers
- An incident in which a vehicle strikes a pedestrian at a speed greater than 10 miles per hour
- Falls from a height greater than 15 feet
- An incident in which a motorcyclist is thrown from the motorcycle at a speed of more than 20 miles per hour
- Multiple victims

Time and distance must also be considered before transporting by helicopter. Helicopter transport should be considered in the following circumstances:

- The transport time to a trauma center is more than 15 minutes by ground ambulance.
- The transport time to a local hospital by ground ambulance is more than the transport time to a trauma center by helicopter.
- The patient is entrapped and extrication will take longer than 15 minutes.
- Using local ground ambulance leaves the local community without ground ambulance coverage.
- The patient needs rapid transport to a specialty center (e.g., a burn center or pediatric center).

You will need to notify the appropriate agency for help in securing a landing zone (LZ). In most cases, the local fire department will be the agency contacted. However, in some cases, police departments assume this role. When more than one agency is on the scene, each agency should have the ability to communicate on a common radio channel. All healthcare professionals who provide care need

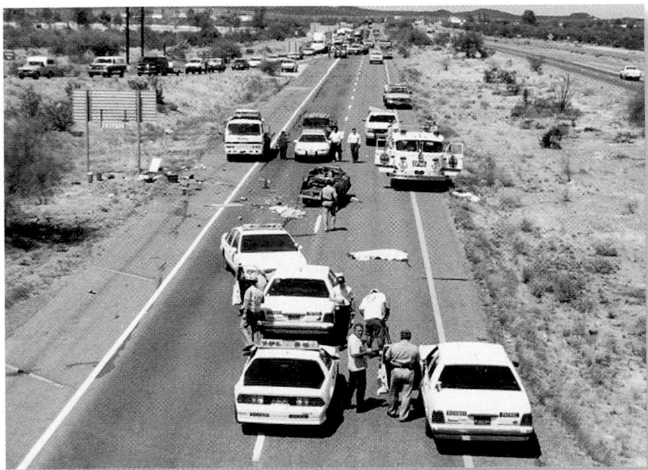

FIGURE 14-3 ▲ When the condition of one or more patients is critical, air medical transportation is often used. © The McGraw-Hill Companies, Inc./Carin Marter/photographer

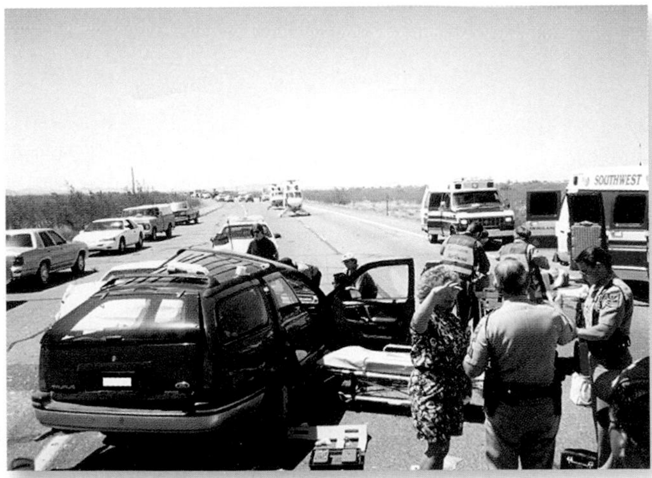

FIGURE 14-4 ▲ Multiple helicopters may be necessary at a multi-patient scene. Courtesy of AirEvac Services, Phoenix, Arizona

to be aware of the location of the landing zone and the helicopter's estimated time of arrival (ETA).

Check with your local helicopter service for landing zone requirements.

If your unit is designated to land the helicopter, you will need to locate a secure landing zone. This means that you must locate an area that is easily controlled for traffic and pedestrians. A good rule to follow is to allow *at least* 100 feet by 100 feet for any helicopter. The area should be free of overhead obstacles, such as wires, trees, and light poles. The area should be free of debris and relatively level. The ground should be clear of rocks and grooves and must be firm enough to support the aircraft. Mark the corners of the landing area with light sticks or cones. Alternately, you can use emergency vehicles with headlights directed toward the landing area (but not at the approaching aircraft). If the landing area is dirt, lightly moisten the area with water if possible. Under no circumstances should anyone be allowed to enter the landing zone after it has been secured.

Constant communication must be maintained throughout the helicopter operation. If you are the ground contact, you may be responsible for relaying important information to the responding flight crew about the patient's condition. All aspects of the landing zone—including hazards, such as light poles, trees, and power lines—must be relayed to the pilot. The pilot should also be told the approximate ground wind conditions.

As the helicopter is landing (or taking off), lower the face shield on your helmet or turn your head momentarily to avoid getting debris in your eyes from the rotor wash.

As the helicopter approaches, it is important to maintain eye contact with the helicopter and pay attention to any visible hazards on the ground at the same time. At any moment it may be necessary to abort the landing. Your assessment of ground conditions could be the key factor in this decision.

Once the helicopter is on the ground, it is very important to pay attention to traffic. The arrival of a helicopter often draws a large crowd, with many bystanders. Pay particular attention to bicycles and motorized vehicles because they can approach the scene quickly and without warning. As the patient is moved toward the helicopter, the flight crew will be focused on loading the patient. They may not see all of the hazards on the ground. Your constant attention to the scene is critical to the safety of the flight crew and all persons on the scene. The rear of a helicopter can be especially dangerous. The tail rotor is often low and invisible when turning. Use extreme caution and follow the crew's instructions when you are close to the aircraft.

Stop and Think!

Working Safely Around Helicopters

- Never move toward a helicopter until signaled by the flight crew.
- Always approach the helicopter from the front, so that the pilot can see you.
- Wear ear and eye protection when approaching the helicopter.
- Never raise your arms or equipment above your head.
- Remove loose items, such as hats, that can be blown around or sucked into the rotors or engines.
- If the aircraft is parked on a slope, always approach and exit from the downhill side.
- When moving from one side of the helicopter to the other, always cross in front of the helicopter.
- Do not open or pull on any part of the aircraft.
- Do not allow vehicles or nonaircraft personnel within 60 feet of the aircraft.

After the patient is loaded into the helicopter, the pilot will radio you when he or she is ready for liftoff. A brief response from you that the scene is still clear will assure the pilot that you have been vigilant about surveying the scene for hazards. As the helicopter leaves the scene, advise your coworkers to keep the landing zone intact for several minutes. This step is done in case the helicopter must return for an emergency landing.

Make sure your dispatcher is aware of all the times associated with helicopter operations. For example, you should notify the EMD when the helicopter has arrived on the scene. You should also notify dispatch when the helicopter has left the scene and its destination. In your prehospital care report, make sure to document the time patient care was transferred to the flight crew, the patient's condition at the time care was transferred, and the patient's destination.

Fundamentals of Extrication

Objective 3 ▶

Extrication is a means of freeing a trapped or otherwise inaccessible patient and getting him or her to a treatment area. **Disentanglement** is the moving or removal of material that is trapping a victim.

The Role of the Emergency Medical Responder

At a vehicle extrication, the rescue crew should always have a safety line (fire hose) at the ready. Extrication is hazardous because fuel and tools that generate sparks are involved.

As an Emergency Medical Responder, you will be responsible for giving necessary care to the patient before extrication. You will also make sure that the patient is removed in a way that minimizes further injury. Some Emergency Medical Responders are also responsible for extrication procedures. A chain of command should be established at the scene to ensure patient care priorities. Patient care takes priority over extrication unless delayed movement would endanger the life of the patient or rescuer.

Equipment

The sounds associated with extrication are much louder inside a vehicle than outside of it.

All persons involved in an extrication operation must wear proper protective clothing. At least one member of the team should be in full protective clothing, including some kind of flash protection (fire gear).

Assess the scene and be alert for possible hazards before beginning the extrication operation (Figure 14-5). Ideally, a safety officer should be present to watch the overall operation and note potential hazards. If a safety officer is not available, it is very important for you to watch for hazards. Possible hazards include the presence of fluid leaking from the vehicle or batteries, airbags that have not deployed, and changes in the stability of the vehicle. Make sure that all hazards are addressed before beginning the operation.

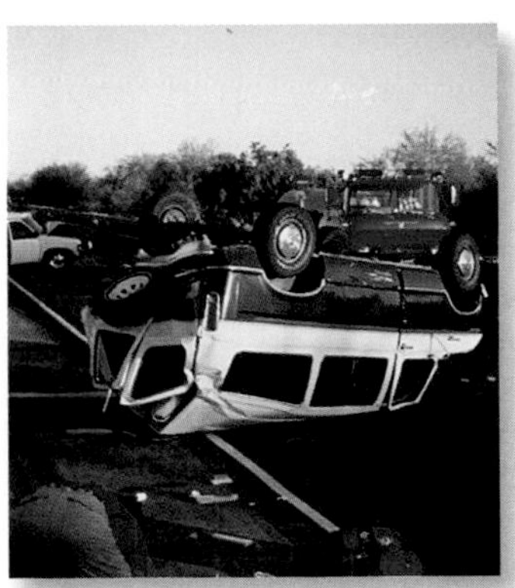

FIGURE 14-5 ▲ Before beginning an extrication operation, assess the scene and be alert for possible hazards. © The McGraw-Hill Companies, Inc./Carin Marter/ photographer

Before beginning the extrication, determine the resources that will be needed. All tools should be in the extrication area before the operation begins. Going to and from a vehicle to get more tools is time-consuming and can cause unnecessary delays.

It is your responsibility to ensure patient safety during extrication. Tell the patient what is going to happen. The patient may become frightened as the operation begins. Constant communication between rescuers and the patient will help the process go smoothly. During disentanglement, protect the patient from broken glass, sharp metal, loud noise, and other hazards, including the environment. Cover, shield, and pad the patient as needed.

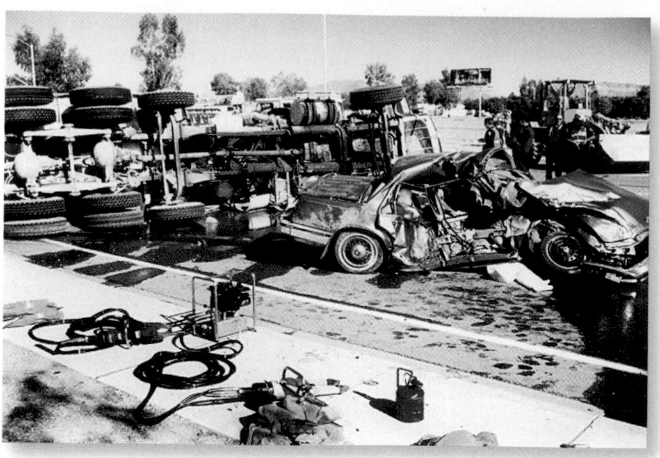

FIGURE 14-6 ▶ Complex access requires special training, equipment, and tools.

Getting to the Patient

Objective 5 ▶

The two types of gaining access to a patient are simple and complex. Simple access does not require equipment. Opening a door, rolling down a window, and having the patient unlock a door are examples of simple access. Complex access requires the use of tools, special equipment, and special training (Figure 14-6).

Complex access may take several minutes and may require the use of tools.

As the operation begins, remember that a power tool should never be used without first checking to see how it will react relative to the patient's location. Make sure to use the right tool for the right job. Call for additional help if necessary.

Remember This!

Extrication is not limited to motor vehicle crashes. There are more complex rescues, such as trench, high-angle, water and ice, and confined space rescue. Each of these situations requires specialized skills, tools, and extensive training. You must be able to identify the types of rescues you are qualified to handle and the situations for which you will need additional resources.

Objective 4 ▶

The route used to reach the patient is not necessarily the route through which the patient will be removed. Use the path of least resistance. Try opening each door. Roll down windows. Have the patient unlock doors. If these methods are unsuccessful, it may be necessary to break a window to gain access. Modern windshields are made of laminated safety glass, which consists of two sheets of plate glass bonded to a sheet of tough plastic. Most modern passenger car side and rear windows are made of tempered glass, which breaks into small, round pieces instead of sharp shards of glass. Cover or shield the patient with a rescue blanket. When intentionally breaking a window for access, use a side or rear window as far from the patient as possible.

Remove wreckage from the patient, not the patient from the wreckage.

As disentanglement progresses, the patient can be prepared for removal. Maintain cervical spine stabilization. Dress and bandage open wounds, splint or stabilize fractures, and stabilize the patient's spine to a short or long backboard as needed. Move the patient, not the immobilization device. Make sure to use sufficient personnel for the move. Choose the path of least resistance when removing the patient. Continue to protect the patient from hazards.

After the patient is extricated, move her away from the incident area to an appropriate treatment area. The rescuers responsible for extrication must communicate with the person in charge of the scene, the Incident Commander. They must continuously update the Incident Commander about the patient's condition and the progress of the extrication. Doing so will aid in overall scene operations. It will also allow the Incident Commander to predict any additional resources that might be needed.

When the extrication is complete, transfer the responsibility for the patient to the crew handling the patient treatment. Replace any fluids and change any batteries that may be needed for your power equipment.

Hazardous Materials

The National Fire Protection Association (NFPA) defines a **hazardous material** as *a substance (solid, liquid, or gas) that, when released, is capable of creating harm to people, the environment, and property.* (Reprinted with permission from NFPA 1991–2005, *Vapor Protective Ensembles for Hazardous Materials Emergencies,* Copyright © 2005 National Fire Protection Association.) Hazardous materials may be found in incidents involving vehicle crashes, railroads, pipelines, storage containers and buildings, chemical plants, and acts of terrorism. Hazardous materials can also be found in the home.

The Role of the Emergency Medical Responder

Objective 6 ▶

In some cases, you will be able to recognize a hazardous material from the information given by the dispatcher. Alternately, you may be the one who activates the EMS system because you have discovered the incident.

Identifying Hazardous Substances

The substance involved in an incident can be identified using a number of resources:

- U.S. Department of Transportation (DOT) *Emergency Response Guidebook*
- United Nations (UN) classification numbers
- NFPA 704 placard system
- UN/DOT placards
- Shipping papers
- Material safety data sheets

DOT Regulations

The U.S. Department of Transportation (DOT) regulates all aspects of transporting hazardous materials in the United States. These regulations include the design of the container, the type of container used, and the means by which hazardous materials are transported. If dangerous materials are being transported, the DOT requires that a placard be displayed on shipping containers and transport vessels (railroad cars, trucks, and ships). The color of the placard tells the class of the hazardous material. The presence of a four-digit number allows more specific identification. This four-digit number is keyed to the DOT's *Emergency Response Guidebook.* This book is a quick reference guide for hazardous materials incidents. Chemicals are listed in the book alphabetically and by their four-digit DOT numbers. Each chemical is given a reference number that corresponds to a set of instructions and precautions, listed in the back of the book, for dealing with that class of chemical.

NFPA's Standard 704

The National Fire Protection Association's Standard 704 designates a hazardous material's classification. The NFPA placard uses a diamond-shaped diagram divided into four different colored sections. The NFPA 704 diagram lists hazards in three categories on a scale of 0 to 4, with 4 being an extremely high hazard.

Material Safety Data Sheets (MSDS)

Material safety data sheets (MSDS) provide detailed information about materials. This information includes the name and physical properties of a substance, fire and explosion hazard information, and emergency first aid treatment. The Occupational Safety and Health Association (OSHA) requires MSDS to be kept on site anywhere chemicals are used.

You Should Know

Hazardous Materials Information Resources

Resources for information about hazardous materials include the following:

- Your local hazardous materials (hazmat) response team
- The Chemical Transportation Emergency Center (CHEMTREC)
  - This organization provides a 24-hour hot line: (800) 424-9300. It can provide product and emergency action information.
- The *Emergency Response Guidebook*, published by the United States Department of Transportation
- Your regional Poison Control Center
  - Your local center can provide detailed information, including decontamination methods and treatment.
- Material Safety Data Sheets (MSDS)

Scene Safety and Reporting

Objective 7 ▶

The first phase of dealing with a hazardous materials incident is recognizing that one exists and recognizing your limitations and those of your crew. Remember that hazardous materials pose a threat to the community. As always, your personal safety is your priority in any emergency scene. Dealing with hazardous materials requires extensive training and proper equipment.

Without the proper equipment, any intervention could put you and your crew at risk.

Stop and Think!

Do not enter a hazardous materials scene unless you are trained to handle hazardous materials and know how to use the necessary protective equipment.

Next, report the incident to an EMD so that the appropriate agencies can be notified. To maximize safety, approach and park uphill and upwind of a hazardous materials scene. In this position, you are less likely to become exposed if the hazardous material becomes airborne or a large spill occurs. Stage (wait for instructions) a minimum of 2,000 feet from a suspected hazardous materials incident. If possible, attempt to identify the material using placards or ID numbers through binoculars while remaining at a safe distance from the area.

Do not enter a hazmat area unless you are trained as a Hazmat Technician.

Avoid contact with the material. If there is no risk to you, remove patients to a safe zone. Hazardous materials scenes are divided into zones according to safety. The safe zone (also called the cold zone) is an area safe from exposure or the threat of exposure. The warm zone is a controlled area for entry into the hot zone. It also serves as the decontamination area after exiting the hot zone. All personnel in the warm zone must wear appropriate protective equipment. The hot zone is the danger zone. The size of the hot zone depends on many factors, including the characteristics of the chemical, the amount released (or spilled or escaped), local weather conditions, the local terrain, and other chemicals in the area.

Mass Casualty Incidents

Objective 8 ▶

A mass casualty incident (MCI) may also be called a multiple-casualty incident or a multiple-casualty situation (MCS). A mass casualty incident is any event that places a great demand on resources—equipment, personnel, or both. An MCI is four patients for some communities but a much larger number for others. No set number of patients defines an MCI.

Triage is used in situations involving more than one patient.

In most EMS situations, emergency care is provided first to the most seriously injured patient(s). In an MCI, the goal is to do the most good for the most people. Priority is given to the most salvageable patients with the most urgent problems. *Triage* is a French word that means "to sort." Triage is sorting multiple victims into priorities for emergency medical care or transportation to definitive care. By quickly sorting the injured patients and identifying the needs of those patients, you are better able to grasp what resources will be needed to care for them.

START Triage System

Objective 10 ▶

Many EMS systems are using the START triage system. START is an acronym for *S*imple *T*riage *A*nd *R*apid *T*reatment." When using the START system, your initial patient assessment and treatment should take less than 30 seconds for each patient. Four areas are evaluated during your initial assessment: (1) the ability to walk (ambulation), (2) respirations, (3) perfusion, and (4) mental status. Based on your assessment findings, you then place the patient into one of four categories:

START was developed by the Newport Beach (California) Fire and Marine Department in cooperation with the staff at Hoag Hospital in Newport Beach.

- Red—immediate
- Yellow—delayed
- Green—minor (ambulatory patients; "walking wounded")
- Black—dead or dying

Color-coded triage tags that correspond with these categories are placed on the patient and used to identify the level of injury sustained.

Triaging patients during an MCI goes against an Emergency Medical Responder's instincts to help everyone he or she encounters. Practice using the START triage system, so that it will be easy to use if you are ever faced with an MCI.

When you begin triaging patients, first identify the patients who are able to walk. Patients who are able to walk are called the "walking wounded." Clear them from the area, so that you can triage the more seriously injured patients. For example, instruct the patients who can walk to go to a predetermined evaluation and treatment area. These patients should be tagged as "green," or "minor." Next, determine the patients who are injured but have adequate respirations, perfusion, and mental status. For example, you might say, "If you can hear me, please raise an arm or leg so we can help you!" These patients should be tagged as "yellow," or "delayed." Proceed to the remaining patients. These patients will be tagged as "red" (immediate) or "black" (dead or dying), depending on your assessment. Start with the patient closest to you.

A rule of triage is to do the greatest good for the greatest number. To make sure you are ready in the event of an MCI, a MCI drill should be a part of regular training for you and your agency.

To assess a patient using the START method, assess his respirations. If the patient is not breathing, open his airway. If he is still not breathing, triage the patient as dead. If opening the patient's airway results in breathing, check his respiratory rate. If he is breathing more than 30 times per minute, triage the patient as immediate (red tag). If the patient is breathing less than 30 times per minute, check perfusion. To assess perfusion, check the patient's radial pulse. If a radial pulse is absent, triage the patient as immediate. If a radial pulse is present, check the patient's mental status. If the patient cannot follow simple commands (he is unresponsive or has an altered mental status), triage the patient as immediate. If the patient can follow simple commands, triage the patient as delayed. If the patient is triaged as immediate, repositioning the airway and controlling severe bleeding are the only initial treatment efforts that are performed before moving on to the next patient. Continue triaging patients until all patients have been assigned a category. However, do not triage the patients once and think you are done. Triage is an ongoing process. In most MCIs, reassessing patients is done in the treatment area and again when they are moved to the transportation area. The patients' triage categories are updated as needed.

JumpSTART Triage System

The START system works very well for adults. However Dr. Lou Romig, a well-known pediatric emergency and EMS physician, identified some weaknesses in the START system when applied to children. As a result, in 1995 she developed a modified START system for use with children. This system is called JumpSTART Triage.

Using the JumpSTART system, you should triage all children who are able to walk in the minor (green) category. Begin assessing children who are not able to walk as you come to them. First, assess the child's breathing. If she is breathing, assess her respiratory rate. If the child is not breathing or has very irregular breathing, open her airway using the jaw thrust without head tilt. If the child begins breathing, triage her as immediate (red) and move on to the next patient. If the child does not begin breathing, check for a pulse. If there is no pulse, triage the patient as dead (black) and move on. If the child does have a pulse, give 15 seconds of mouth-to-mask breathing (about 5 breaths). If the child begins breathing, triage her as immediate (red) and move on. If she does not begin breathing, triage the patient as dead (black) and move on.

If a child is breathing on her own when you find her, quickly check her respiratory rate. If the child is breathing faster than 45 times per minute or slower than 15 times per minute, or if her breathing is irregular, triage her as immediate. If the child is breathing 15–45 times per minute, assess perfusion. If a pulse is present, assess mental status. If no pulse is present in the least injured limb, triage the child as immediate and move on.

Assess mental status using the AVPU scale. If the child is alert, responds to a verbal stimulus, or responds appropriately to pain, triage the child as delayed (yellow) and move on. If the child responds inappropriately to pain or is unresponsive, triage her as immediate (red) and move on. As with adults, children need to be reassessed in the treatment and transportation areas.

Incident Command System

In 2003, President Bush directed the Secretary of Homeland Security to develop and administer a National Incident Management System (NIMS). The purpose of NIMS is to provide a consistent nationwide template that allows all government, private-sector, and nongovernment agencies to work together during domestic incidents. Examples of domestic incidents are acts of terrorism, wildland and urban fires, floods, hazardous materials spills, nuclear accidents, aircraft accidents, earthquakes, tornadoes, hurricanes, typhoons, and war-related disasters.

The Incident Command System (ICS) is an important part of this comprehensive system. The ICS is a standardized system developed to assist with the control, direction, and coordination of emergency response resources. The ICS can be used at an incident of any type and size.

An Incident Commander (IC) is responsible for managing all operations at the incident site. The Incident Commander has three priorities:

- Life safety (ensuring the safety of the lives and the physical well-being of emergency personnel and the public)
- Incident stability (minimizing the incident's effect on the surrounding area while using resources efficiently)
- Property conservation (minimizing damage to property)

Persons on the scene who are familiar with the ICS will also be familiar with the following risk-benefit model:

Objective 9 ▶

"We will risk our lives a lot within a calculated plan for lives that are savable."

"We will risk our lives a little within a calculated plan for property that is savable."

"We will not risk our lives at all for lives or property that is already lost."

At the beginning of an incident, the Incident Commander will be the senior Emergency Medical Responder who arrives at the scene. As more resources arrive, command will be transferred to another person based on who has the primary authority for overall control of the incident. When command is transferred, the outgoing Incident Commander must give the incoming Incident Commander a full report and notify all staff of the change in command.

Depending on the size of the incident, the Incident Commander may assign to others the authority to perform certain activities. Scene operations may be broken down into groups. For example, a treatment group is assigned patient treatment, while an extrication group is responsible for extrication.

If you arrive on the scene of an MCI where the ICS has been established, report to the command post. Find out who the Incident Commander is. Identify yourself and your level of training. Follow the directions given by the Incident Commander about your assignment.

On The Scene

Wrap-Up

The fire captain on the first engine that arrives positions his truck to block the road behind the ambulance and assumes command of the scene. He tells the rescue squad to extricate the trapped patients. He establishes a staging area for incoming ambulances. He also asks the police to direct traffic and place flares to alert oncoming cars. As each ambulance crew arrives, you assign them a patient. Within 30 minutes, the last teen is en route to the local hospital. In the debriefing later, you discuss how the weather prevented the use of helicopter transport. Overall, everyone felt that all crews performed well and hoped that they are never again faced with such a scene. ■

Sum It Up

- As an Emergency Medical Responder, you should have the appropriate equipment and supplies with which to assess a patient, provide emergency care, and assist other healthcare professionals:
  - Personal protective equipment (PPE)
  - Basic wound care supplies
  - Instruments to measure blood pressure
  - Additional items as needed
- The six phases of a typical EMS response are the following:
  1. Detection of the emergency
  2. Reporting the emergency (the call made for assistance) and dispatch
  3. Response (medical resources sent to the scene)
  4. On-scene care
  5. Care during transport
  6. Transfer to definitive care

- Air medical transport may be necessary when the condition of one or more patients is critical. As an Emergency Medical Responder, you must observe the following safety considerations:
  - If your unit is designated to land the helicopter, you will need to locate a secure landing zone. You must locate an area that is easily controlled for traffic and pedestrians.
  - You should allow *at least* 100 feet by 100 feet to land any helicopter.
  - The area should be free of overhead obstacles, such as wires, trees, and light poles. It should also be free of debris and should be relatively level. The ground should be clear of rocks and grooves and must be firm enough to support the aircraft.
  - Mark the corners of the landing area with light sticks or cones. Alternately, you can use emergency vehicles with headlights directed toward the landing area (but not at the approaching aircraft).
  - If the landing area is dirt, lightly moisten the area with water, if possible.
  - Under no circumstances should anyone be allowed to enter the landing zone after it has been secured.
  - If you are the ground contact, you may be responsible for relaying important information to the responding flight crew about the patient's condition.
- *Extrication* is a means of freeing a trapped, or otherwise inaccessible patient, and getting him or her to a treatment area.
- As an Emergency Medical Responder, you will be responsible for giving necessary care to the patient before extrication. You will also make sure that the patient is removed in a way that minimizes further injury. Some Emergency Medical Responders are also responsible for extrication procedures.
  - All persons involved in an extrication operation must wear proper protective clothing. At least one member of the team should be in full protective clothing, including fire gear.
  - The two types of gaining access to a patient are simple and complex:
    - *Simple access* does not require equipment. Opening a door, rolling down a window, and having the patient unlock a door are examples of simple access.
    - *Complex access* requires the use of tools, special equipment, and special training.
  - After the patient is extricated, move him or her away from the incident area to an appropriate treatment area.
- *Disentanglement* is the moving or removal of material that is trapping a victim.
- As defined by the National Fire Protection Association (NFPA), a *hazardous material* is a substance (solid, liquid, or gas) that, when released, is capable of creating harm to people, the environment and property. Hazardous materials may be biological agents, other disease-causing agents, a waste, or a combination of wastes. These materials may be found in vehicle crashes, on railroads, in pipelines, in storage containers and buildings, in chemical plants, and in acts of terrorism. Hazardous materials can also be found in the home.
- A hazardous substance can be identified using a number of resources:
  - U.S. Department of Transportation (DOT) *Emergency Response Guidebook*
  - United Nations (UN) classification numbers
  - NFPA 704 placard system
  - UN/DOT placards
  - Shipping papers
  - Material safety data sheets

- The first phase of dealing with a hazardous materials incident is recognizing that one exists. As always, your personal safety is your priority in any emergency scene. Take the following steps in dealing with a hazmat emergency:
  1. Report the incident to an EMD so that the appropriate agencies can be notified.
  2. To maximize safety, approach and park uphill and upwind of a hazardous materials scene.
  3. Stage a minimum of 2,000 feet from a suspected hazardous materials incident. If possible, attempt to identify the material using placards or ID numbers through binoculars while remaining at a safe distance from the area.
  4. Avoid contact with the material. If there is no risk to you, remove patients to a safe zone.
  5. Note the following safety zones:
     - The *safe zone* (also called the *cold zone*) is an area safe from exposure or the threat of exposure.
     - The *warm zone* is a controlled area for entry into the hot zone. It also serves as the decontamination area after exiting the hot zone. All personnel in the warm zone must wear appropriate protective equipment.
     - The *hot zone* is the danger zone. The size of the hot zone depends on the characteristics of the chemical, the amount released (or spilled or escaped), local weather conditions, the local terrain, and other chemicals in the area.
- A *mass casualty incident (MCI)* may also be called a multiple-casualty incident or multiple-casualty situation (MCS). An MCI is any event that places a great demand on resources—equipment, personnel, or both.
- The *START triage system* is used by many systems in dealing with MCIs. It stands for ***S***imple ***T***riage ***A***nd ***R***apid ***T***reatment.
  - Four areas are evaluated during your initial assessment:
    1. The ability to walk (ambulation)
    2. Respirations
    3. Perfusion
    4. Mental status
  - Based on your assessment findings, you categorize each patient according to one of four categories. Color-coded triage tags that correspond with these categories are placed on the patient and used to identify the level of injury sustained:
    - Red—immediate
    - Yellow—delayed
    - Green—minor (ambulatory patients; "walking wounded")
    - Black—dead or dying
- The *JumpSTART triage system* was developed for use with children. It specifies how the four color-coded tags are applied to pediatric patients.
- The *National Incident Management System (NIMS)* was created to provide a consistent nationwide template that allows all government, private-sector, and nongovernment agencies to work together during domestic incidents.
  - The *Incident Command System (ICS)* is an important part of NIMS. The ICS is a standardized system developed to assist with the control, direction, and coordination of emergency response resources. The ICS can be used at an incident of any type and size.

- An *Incident Commander (IC)* is responsible for managing all operations at an incident site. The Incident Commander has three priorities:
  - Life safety
  - Incident stability
  - Property conservation

▶ At the beginning of an incident, the Incident Commander will be the senior Emergency Medical Responder who arrives at the scene. As more resources arrive, command is transferred to another person based on who has the primary authority for overall control of the incident.

- Depending on the size of the incident, the Incident Commander may assign to others the authority to perform certain activities. Scene operations may be broken down into groups, such as treatment and extrication.
- If you arrive on the scene of an MCI where the ICS has been established, report to the command post. Find out who the Incident Commander is. Identify yourself and your level of training. Follow the directions given by the Incident Commander about your assignment.

▶ Tracking Your Progress

After reading this chapter, can you	**Page Reference**	**Objective Met?**
• Discuss the medical and non-medical equipment needed to respond to a call?	512–513	☐
• List the phases of a prehospital call?	514–516	☐
• Discuss the role of the Emergency Medical Responder in extrication.	519	☐
• List various methods of gaining access to the patient?	520	☐
• Distinguish between simple and complex access?	520	☐
• Describe what the Emergency Medical Responder should do if there is reason to believe that there is a hazard at the scene?	521–522	☐
• State the role the Emergency Medical Responder should perform until appropriately trained personnel arrive at the scene of a hazardous materials situation?	522–523	☐
• Describe the criteria for a multiple-casualty situation?	523	☐
• Discuss the role of the Emergency Medical Responder in a multiple-casualty situation?	525	☐
• Summarize the components of basic triage?	523–524	
• Explain the rationale for having the unit prepared to respond?	516	☐

Chapter Quiz

Multiple Choice

In the space provided, identify the letter of the choice that best completes each statement or answers each question.

_____ **1.** The minimum size of a landing zone for a medical helicopter should be

a. 20 feet by 40 feet.
b. 100 feet by 100 feet.
c. 200 feet by 200 feet.
d. 500 feet by 500 feet.

_____ **2.** Which of the following definitions bests describes extrication?

a. stabilizing vehicles to prevent movement
b. protecting bystanders from injury at motor vehicle crash scenes
c. freeing patients from entrapment
d. sorting patients according to the severity of their injuries

_____ **3.** In using the START system, the initial treatment is limited to correcting which of the following conditions?

a. repositioning the airway and controlling bleeding
b. ventilating the patient by mouth-to-mask breathing and controlling bleeding
c. performing chest compressions and splinting fractures
d. repositioning the airway and ventilating the patient by mouth-to-mask breathing

_____ **4.** When triaging patients, how should the "walking wounded" be tagged?

a. immediate
b. delayed
c. minor
d. dead or dying

_____ **5.** At a hazardous materials scene, where should emergency vehicles be parked?

a. 100 feet from the scene
b. uphill and upwind from the scene
c. downhill and downwind from the scene
d. as close to the scene as possible

Short Answer

Answer each question in the space provided.

6. List the four categories used in the START triage system.

1. ______________________________
2. ______________________________
3. ______________________________
4. ______________________________

7. List the four areas evaluated during an initial assessment using the START triage system.

1. ______________________________
2. ______________________________
3. ______________________________
4. ______________________________

8. You are called to the scene of a mass casualty incident. The Incident Command System has been established. What should you do first when you arrive at the scene?

____

____

____

APPENDIX 1 Weapons of Mass Destruction: Awareness and Response

Note: This appendix is not intended to replace the need for a Hazardous Materials, Emergency Responder Course.

On The Scene

You are responding to a routine call for "difficulty breathing" at the high school. Dispatch notifies you that there are now several calls coming in—it appears there are multiple patients. As you arrive at the school, you see students streaming out of the building. They rush over to your vehicle, coughing, with tears in their eyes. You and your partner exchange a nervous glance as you pick up the radio and call for additional help. The students tell you they had a burning sensation in their eyes followed by coughing and a choking sensation. You direct them to go to the adjacent soccer field to wait for additional help. Your partner radios for the hazardous materials team to respond. He asks for all incoming units to stage at a parking lot a block away. Police support is requested to control access to the school—parents and reporters are already beginning to pour into the parking lot. ■

THINK ABOUT IT

As you read this appendix, think about the following questions:

- What type of terrorist agent may cause these signs and symptoms?
- Should you go into the building to check for additional patients?
- What are your priorities for patient care?

Introduction

Emergency Response in a Changing World

Our world has changed dramatically in just a few short years. Events that would have been unthinkable outside a movie theater now must be considered the early stages of a weapons of mass destruction (WMD) or hazardous materials event. **Weapons of mass destruction** are materials used by terrorists that have the potential to cause great harm over a large area.

Military experts agree that "incapacitating" a victim creates the need for a minimum of two healthcare professionals to begin any type of care.

B-NICCE is a simple way to remember the categories of WMD.

We must prepare for the "unthinkable" at all levels of training.

Terrorists use fear to bring about political change. They want to cause panic and disrupt normal activities. Their goal is to injure (incapacitate)—and not necessarily kill—large numbers of people. By injuring as many victims as possible, terrorists cause mass confusion and panic. This chaos could affect an already overloaded EMS system, bringing it to a standstill. Additionally, healthcare professionals and emergency responders are prime targets. Incapacitating them ensures that other victims do not recover.

There are six main categories of WMD:

- Biological
- Nuclear/radiological
- Incendiary
- Chemical
- Cyber/technological
- Explosive

Any material that has a harmful effect on the body can be used as a weapon of mass destruction or mass confusion. The sad reality is that there is an amazing amount of "terrorist" information available on the Internet. Fortunately, it is hard to "weaponize" most chemicals. For instance, in order to have a harmful effect, some biological agents must be dispersed into the air for them to then come into contact with a victim's lung tissue. Other types of materials, such as nerve agents, must come into contact with skin to have a harmful effect.

Types of Weapons of Mass Destruction

Biological Weapons

Biological weapons involve the use of bacteria, viruses, rickettsia, or toxins to cause disease or death (Figure A1-1). Diseases can be spread by the following means:

- Inhalation through the use of spray devices (aerosols)
- Ingestion of contaminated food or water supplies, after they are swallowed
- Absorption through direct skin contact with the substance
- Injection into the skin

Creating a biological weapon is not complicated. It can be done using materials purchased at a local hardware store and techniques learned in a high school chemistry course. Large quantities of biological weapons can often be produced in a few days to a few weeks.

Bacteria

Bacteria are germs that can cause disease in humans, plants, and animals. Bacteria can live outside the human body. They do not depend on other organisms to live and grow. Examples of diseases caused by bacteria that may be used as biological weapons include anthrax and tularemia (rabbit fever).

Rickettsias are very small bacteria that require a living host to survive. Rickettsias are transmitted by bloodsucking parasites, such as fleas, lice, and ticks. An example of a disease caused by rickettsias is Q fever.

FIGURE A1-1 ► Biological weapons involve the use of bacteria, viruses, rickettsia, or toxins to cause disease or death.

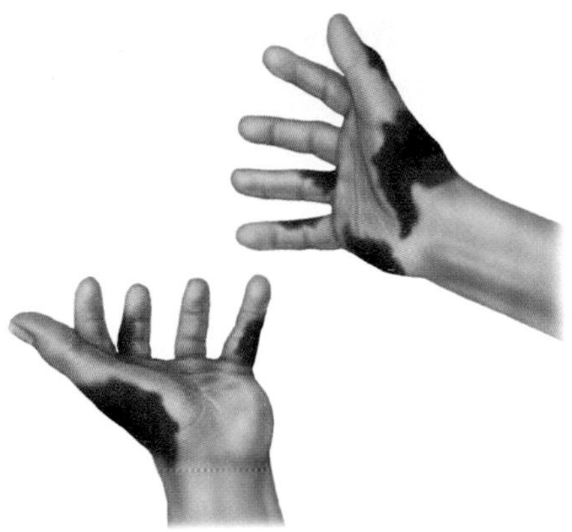

Bacteria: anthrax, tularemia (rabbit fever)

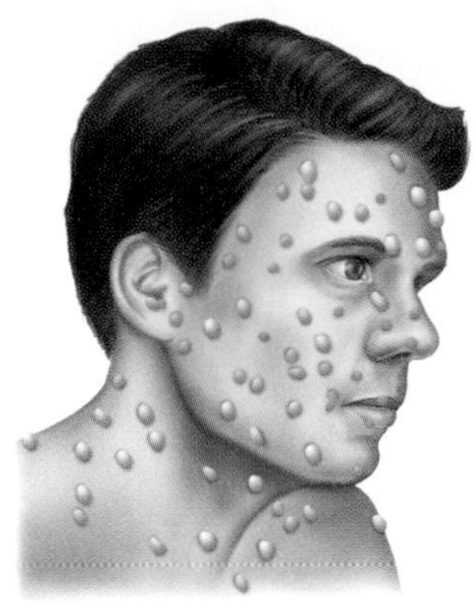

Virus: smallpox, Ebola virus

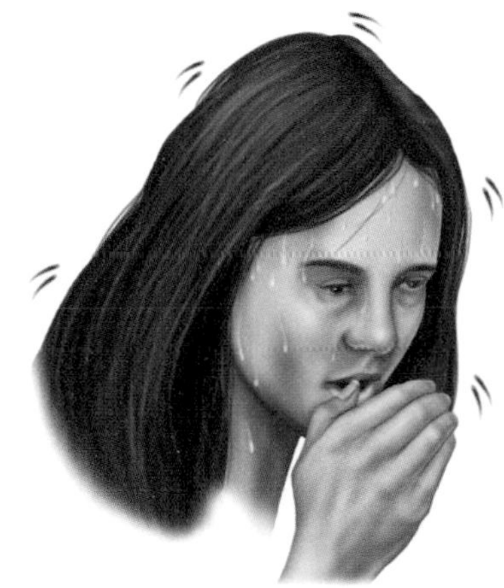

Rickettsia: Q fever

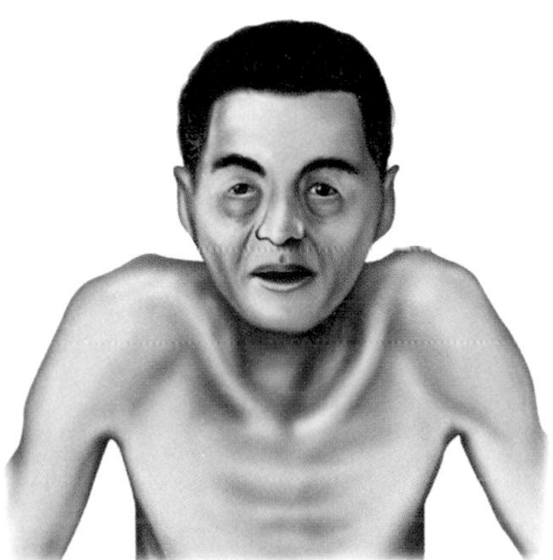

Toxin: ricin, botulism, enterotoxin B

Viruses

A **virus** is a type of infectious agent that depends on other organisms to live and grow. Viruses that could serve as biological weapons include smallpox and those that cause hemorrhagic fevers, such as the Ebola virus. Infection with a hemorrhagic virus causes bleeding from many body tissues. The person may die from shock or lack of oxygen in the lungs due to severe bleeding.

Toxins

Toxins are substances produced by an animal, a plant, or a microorganism. Toxins are not the same as chemical agents. Toxins are natural substances and are generally more deadly than chemical agents, which are humanmade. Toxins that could serve as biological weapons include ricin (made from the waste from processing castor beans), botulism (found in improperly canned food and contaminated water supplies, such as rivers and lakes), and enterotoxin B.

You Should Know

Indicators of Possible Biological Weapon Use

- Dead or dying animals, fish, or birds
- Unusual casualties
- Unusual illness not typical for the region

You Should Know

The Centers for Disease Control and Prevention (CDC) categorizes biological weapons according to their risk to national security. Category A diseases and agents are most likely to be used in an attack and include germs that are rarely seen in the United States. Category A diseases and agents include organisms that pose a risk to national security due to the following factors:

- They can be spread easily from person to person.
- They result in high death rates and have the potential for a major public health impact.
- They may cause public panic.
- They require special action for public health preparedness.

Category A diseases and agents include anthrax, botulism, plague, smallpox, tularemia, and viral hemorrhagic fevers.

Category B diseases and agents are the second-highest priority to the CDC, because they cause moderate amounts of disease and low death rates. They are fairly easy to spread. These weapons require specific public health action, such as improved diagnostic and detection systems. Category B agents include Q fever, brucellosis, glanders, ricin, enterotoxin B, viral encephalitis, threats to food and water safety, and typhus fever.

Category C diseases and agents include germs that could be engineered for future mass distribution, because they are fairly easy to obtain, produce, and spread. They can produce high rates of disease and death. Category C diseases and agents include Nipah virus and hantavirus.

Nuclear Weapons

Nuclear weapons may be used in the form of ballistic missiles or bombs. Nuclear power plants, nuclear medicine machines in hospitals, research facilities, industrial construction sites, and vehicles used to transport nuclear waste may be targets for terrorist groups.

Stop and Think!

You cannot see, smell, feel, or taste radiation. The longer you are exposed to it, the worse is its effect.

Nuclear Radiation

It is the charge that makes radiation an immediate problem. The charge disrupts cell function and structure.

Nuclear radiation gives off three main types of radiation: alpha, beta, and gamma (Figure A1-2).

Alpha Radiation

Alpha particles are large, heavy, and charged. They cannot penetrate very far into matter. Because clothing or a sheet of paper is thick enough to stop them, external exposure to alpha particles usually has no effect on people. The outermost, dead layer of your skin (epidermis) stops the particles from entering your body. However, if you eat, drink, or breathe in material that is contaminated with alpha-emitting particles, the alpha radiation can cause major damage to the live tissues inside your body.

FIGURE A1-2 ▶ Nuclear radiation gives off three main types of radiation: alpha, beta, and gamma.

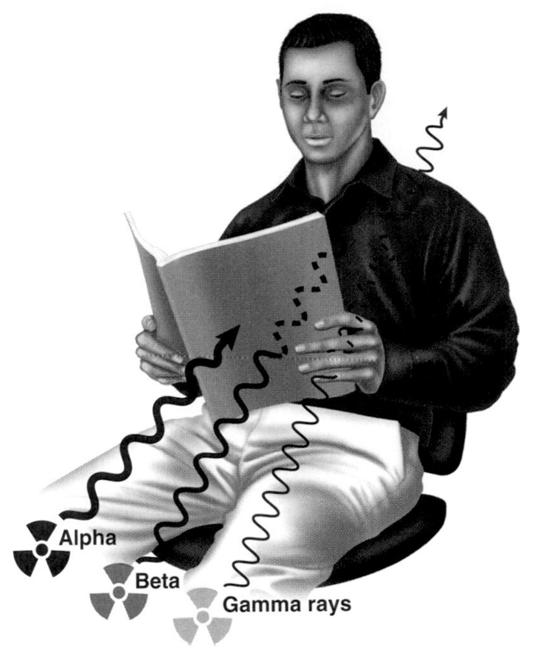

Beta Radiation

Beta particles are much smaller, travel more quickly, and have less charge than alpha particles. They can also penetrate more deeply than alpha particles. Beta particles can be stopped by layers of clothing. They can also be stopped by thin metal or plastic, such as several sheets of aluminum foil or Plexiglas. Generally, skin burns (called "beta burns") can occur if the skin is exposed to large amounts of beta radiation. Internal damage can occur if you eat, drink, or breathe in material that is contaminated with beta-emitting particles.

Gamma Radiation

Gamma rays are waves of very high energy, similar to light. These waves of energy penetrate very deeply and can easily go through a person. To reduce exposure from gamma rays, thick material, such as lead, must be used. Because gamma rays can penetrate tissues and organs, nausea, vomiting, high fever, hair loss, and skin burns may result if you are exposed to a large amount of gamma radiation in a short period of time.

Dirty Bombs

A dirty bomb is also known as a radiological weapon.

Any terrorist explosion or WMD incident can be caused by a "dirty bomb." According to the CDC, a dirty bomb is a mix of explosives, such as dynamite, with radioactive powder or pellets. When the dynamite or other explosives are set off, the blast carries radioactive material into the surrounding area. The impact of a dirty bomb depends on factors such as the size of the explosive, the amount and type of radioactive material used, and weather conditions.

Incendiary Weapons

Incendiary materials are substances that burn with a hot flame for a specific period. An incendiary system consists of the materials needed to start a fire:

- Initiator (the source that provides the first fire, such as a match)
- Delay mechanism (if needed)
- Igniter or fuse
- Incendiary (flammable) material or filler

Most terrorist attacks involve the use of explosives, improvised explosive devices, and incendiary materials. Incendiaries are used mainly to set fire to wooden structures and other burnable targets. Firebombs are examples of incendiaries. They range from a Molotov cocktail (bottle, gasoline, rag, and a match) to much larger and sophisticated bombs. Firebombs may contain napalm or other flammable fluid. They are usually ignited with a fuse. Some incendiaries are used to melt, cut, or weld metal.

Chemical Weapons

Remember that a hazardous materials incident is accidental. A terrorist attack is deliberate.

Chemical agents are poisonous substances that injure or kill people when inhaled, ingested, or absorbed through the skin or eyes. There are five broad categories of chemical weapons: nerve agents, blister agents, blood agents, choking (pulmonary) agents, and irritants (Table A1-1). The general symptoms of exposure vary by individual and depend on many factors, including the following:

- The substance involved
- The concentration of the substance

TABLE A1-1 Chemical Agents

Chemical Agents	Effects	Examples
Nerve agents	Interrupt nerve signals, causing a loss of consciousness within seconds and death within minutes of exposure	Tabun, Sarin, Soman, VX
Blister agents	Produce effects like those of a corrosive chemical, such as lye or a strong acid; result in severe burns to the eyes, skin, and tissues of the respiratory tract	Distilled mustard, forms of nitrogen mustard
Blood agents	Cause rapid respiratory arrest and death by blocking the absorption of oxygen to the cells and organs through the bloodstream	Cyanide, arsine, hydrogen chloride
Choking (pulmonary) agents	Inhaled chlorine mixes with the moisture in the lungs and becomes hydrochloric acid. The acid causes fluid to build up in the lungs (pulmonary edema); interferes with the body's ability to exchange oxygen and results in asphyxiation that resembles drowning.	Chlorine
Irritants	Results in immediate tearing of the eyes, coughing, difficulty breathing, nausea, and vomiting	Mace, pepper spray, tear gas

- The duration of exposure
- The number of exposures
- The route of entry (inhalation, ingestion, injection, or absorption)

Other factors that influence how an individual is affected include the person's age, gender, general health, allergies, smoking habits, alcohol consumption, and medications.

You Should Know

Indicators of Possible Chemical Weapon Use

- Dead or dying animals, fish, or birds
- Lack of insects
- Unexplained casualties
- Multiple victims
- Serious illnesses
- Unusual liquid, spray, vapor, or droplets
- Unexplained odors
- Low clouds or fog unrelated to the weather
- Suspicious devices or packages, including metal debris, abandoned spray devices, and unexplained weapons

Stop and Think!

Some chemical agents have a distinctive smell. Remember: If you can smell the chemical agent, you are too close.

Irritants are often used for personal protection and by police in riot control. Examples include Mace, pepper spray, and tear gas. These substances cause burning and intense pain to exposed skin areas. Exposure results in immediate tearing of the eyes, coughing, difficulty breathing, nausea, and vomiting.

Medical attention is needed for any of the following:

- Unconsciousness
- Confusion
- Lightheadedness
- Anxiety
- Dizziness
- Changes in skin color
- Shortness of breath
- Burning of the upper airway
- Coughing or painful breathing
- Drooling
- Chest tightness
- Loss of coordination
- Seizures
- Nausea, vomiting
- Abdominal cramping
- Diarrhea
- Loss of bowel or bladder control
- Dim, blurred, or double vision
- Tingling or numbness of the extremities

Treating a large number of patients with the same signs and symptoms at the same scene should trigger the thought of a WMD event.

All of these signs and symptoms can be indicative of some type of chemical exposure. They should be considered as the first warning signs that the call may be a WMD event. The reality of these types of situations is that responders may have already treated a large number of patients before recognizing that it is a WMD situation. Can you imagine the difficulty in recognizing the problem after patients have been transported to multiple hospitals over a period of several days? You must be conscientious in recognizing and reporting these types of scenes.

Cyber and Technological Weapons

Cyber and technological terrorism involves the use of computers to steal, alter, or destroy information. Cyber weapons include computer viruses and unauthorized access into computer systems. These weapons can cause computer systems to fail or malfunction. Computer hackers can alter who can access a computer system. They can also destroy or change important information stored in a computer or computer network.

Explosives

Explosives are associated with a very rapid release of gas and heat. Most terrorist attacks involve the use of explosives.

Terrorists often use various types of explosives, including the following:

- Grenades
- Rockets
- Missiles
- Mines
- Pipe bombs
- Vehicle bombs
- Package or letter bombs
- Bombs carried in devices, such as a knapsack or backpack

WMD Incident Response

A scene involving WMD is a crime scene. At a possible WMD incident, your primary responsibilities will be to do the following:

- Make sure that you, as well as additional responders, are safe
- Isolate the scene
- Preserve evidence and deny entry
- Ask for additional help and coordinate efforts with other responding fire, EMS, and law enforcement personnel
- Recognize the signs of a potential WMD incident and alert the proper authorities
- Recognize the potential of a secondary explosion and an attack on Emergency Medical Responders

Remember This!

Depending on the type of WMD incident, additional resources may be needed, including

- Law enforcement personnel
- Fire, hazardous materials, and other special rescue teams
- Gas, electric, and water companies
- Hospitals
- Environmental Protection Agency (EPA)
- Centers for Disease Control and Prevention (CDC)
- State health department
- Military
- Public transportation
- Disaster services (Red Cross, Salvation Army)

To work effectively, you must use standard operating procedures (SOP) and protocols according to your local emergency response plan (LERP). Try to assess the potential for an exposure using the following guidelines.

Remember This!

Because a terrorist event is a crime scene, it is important that you disturb the scene as little as possible.

Pre-Arrival Response

Pre-arrival information may be your only opportunity to recognize a WMD incident before you become part of the situation.

From the dispatch information you are given, listen for specific clues that indicate a possible terrorist incident, including

- Type of incident
- Incident location
- Number of reported casualties

Your knowledge of the terrain, local events, and local weather may be very important in recognizing a possible WMD event. For instance, knowing that a large, open-air event is going on in your response area should trigger the thought of the potential for a mass casualty incident in the event of an exposure.

Arrival Response

Scene Safety

Remember, *isolate and deny entry.*

As you approach the scene, consider the safest approach, such as uphill, upwind, or even upstream. Be aware of the terrain and try to avoid "bottlenecks" or traps. Do not become a victim yourself by rushing in haphazardly.

Incident Factors

Be prepared for a possible rush of contaminated patients.

Be alert for indicators of possible terrorist activity or WMD. Use the dispatch information provided, your senses, and any other information available. As you approach, you may smell odors that indicate a gas leak, chemical spill, or fire. Look for the following:

- An unusually large number of people with burns or "blast" injuries
- Large numbers of people running from the scene or on the ground
- Danger of fire, explosion, electrical hazards, or structural collapse

- Weapons, explosive devices
- Signs of corrosion
- Evidence of the use of chemical agents

Listen for the following:

- Screaming
- Explosion
- Breaking glass
- A hissing sound that indicates pressure releases
- Information from victims or bystanders

Stop and Think!

Remember that responders to the scene may be the target. This means *you.* Terrorists may use a secondary explosive device (equipped with a timer or trigger mechanism) designed to detonate after responders have arrived at a location. The intention is clear: to injure or kill responders.

Approach any large or special event with caution.

Incident Location The location of an incident may also be a clue to the type of problem. For example, targeted locations may include an abortion clinic, a religious function, or a political event. Other examples of high-risk targets include

- Landmarks—the White House, Hoover Dam, the Statue of Liberty
- Transportation sites—highways, railways, airports, bridges, tunnels
- Energy sources—nuclear power plants, oil or gas pipelines
- Financial institutions—the Federal Reserve, the Stock Exchange
- Government or public safety buildings—the military, EMS, police, fire
- High-attendance sites—amusement parks, concerts, sporting events, graduations
- Communications centers

Incident Date The anniversary of an event can be significant. For instance, the 1995 bombing of the Alfred P. Murrah Federal Building in Oklahoma City, Oklahoma, took place on the second anniversary of a 1993 standoff between Branch Davidians and the FBI near Waco, Texas. Unfortunately, the significance of a date may not be realized until after the incident has occurred.

Other Incident Factors Other factors to consider at a possible WMD incident include

- Time of day
- Temperature
- Wind intensity and direction
- Humidity
- Cloud cover
- Precipitation

These factors can be very important. For example, the time of day can be an indicator of the increased possibility of the use of a biological agent. In most cases, wind speed is slower at night and biological agents will not disperse or thin out as rapidly.

Think, Plan, Act, and Evaluate

Always err on the side of caution.

On arriving at the scene, use the "Think, Plan, Act, Evaluate" model to obtain scene control and establish a perimeter. Give dispatch the exact location of the incident or perimeter. Notify all responders of the location of the area of suspected contamination, safe routes for entry to the site, and where to stage (wait for instructions). Alert responders to potential hazards or danger.

Protective Equipment

A weapon of mass destruction is a hazardous material. If hazardous substances or conditions are suspected, the scene must be secured by qualified personnel wearing appropriate equipment. If you are not qualified and do not have the appropriate equipment, you may need to wait for additional help to arrive before you can attempt entry into the scene.

Safety Zones

If you have been trained to do so (and are properly equipped), identify and establish safety zones. The hot zone is the area of the incident that contains the hazardous material (contaminant). Areas around the contaminant that may be exposed to gases, vapors, mist, dust, or runoff are also part of the hot zone. The hot zone is a dangerous area. Only personnel with high-level personal protective equipment may enter this area. The warm zone serves as the entry and decontamination point. All personnel entering this area must wear appropriate protective gear. The cold zone is the safe zone and serves as the staging area for personnel and equipment. The Incident Command post is located in the cold zone.

Remember This!

The presence of hazardous materials is not always easy to detect. In a WMD incident, the presence of identifying placards may not be accurate because the placards may have been deliberately altered by terrorists.

National Incident Management System (NIMS)

Remember: Scene size-up is a continuous process. It allows the Incident Commander to review strategy and tactics periodically in order to effectively position more resources as necessary.

Initiate the National Incident Management System (NIMS) plan. Designate the Incident Commander and announce the location of the command post. The command post location may be determined by SOP or another resource. Generally, the command post should not be less than 300 feet away from the scene. When positioning emergency vehicles and other equipment, always be aware of the possibility of secondary devices and collapsing buildings. In most cases, apparatus should point away from the scene.

Try to identify quickly the type of incident (biological, nuclear, chemical, etc.). Relay the information to dispatch as soon as possible. Knowing the type of incident is important, so that you can take appropriate precautions when providing emergency care.

Approaching the Patient

Patient Access

Much of the information you will need to treat the patient properly may be gathered initially from a distance with the use of binoculars or spotting scopes.

Access to any patient must not occur without the proper personal protective equipment. Standard body substance isolation equipment may not be sufficient or appropriate for this type of response. In most respects, a contaminated patient is like any other patient, except that responders must protect themselves and others from dangers due to secondary contamination. The goals for emergency responders at a scene involving WMD include

- Terminating the patient's exposure to the contaminant
- Removing the patient from danger
- Providing emergency patient care
- Maintaining rescuer safety

In many instances, there will be no clear signals that the incident is a potential WMD event. Approach the scene with caution.

Emergency care in the hot zone is limited due to the risk of patient or rescuer exposure to hazardous substances or conditions.

Patient care must be performed only by trained personnel wearing the appropriate level of PPE, or the patient must have already been decontaminated.

Always assign the highest treatment priorities to the patient's airway, breathing, circulation, and decontamination. Remember to stay uphill and upwind as you approach any patient.

Determine if the scene has been secured to allow for your safe approach to the patient. Do not approach unless you are trained and equipped with appropriate PPE for the situation. *If you have not been trained and do not have the appropriate protective gear, you must stay out of the hot and warm zones.*

Patients who are unable to walk must be removed from the hot zone by trained personnel. This removal is usually done by fire department and/or hazardous materials personnel. Even if you have been trained and are properly equipped, emergency care in the hot zone must be limited to spinal stabilization, gross airway management (such as opening the airway and suctioning), and hemorrhage control. Remember that the patient will be further exposed to any airborne contaminants when you open the airway.

Patient Care and Assessment

You must first address life-threatening problems and gross decontamination before giving emergency care. Gross decontamination means removing all suspected contaminated clothing. Brush off any obvious contaminants. Remove the patient's jewelry and watch, if present. Cover wounds with a waterproof dressing after decontamination. If spinal stabilization appears necessary, begin it as soon as it is practical to do so.

Form a general impression and begin your initial assessment at the same time as decontamination. What is the patient's general appearance? Look for clues that suggest the presence of some type of exposure. Is he having a seizure? Seizure may alert you to the presence of some type of nerve agent. Is he twitching? What is his skin condition? Does he have visible secretions from his nose or mouth? Has he lost control of his bowels or bladder?

Assess the patient's level of responsiveness by shouting a question to him from a distance. If the patient responds to your voice or is moving, you can safely make some assumptions about the amount of blood flow to his brain. Look at the patient closely. Is he breathing? Can you see the rise and fall of his chest? Is his breathing regular, or is he gasping for air? Many nerve agents interfere with the breathing control centers in the brain. If you have not noted any unusual signs and symptoms or other suspicious activity, proceed cautiously and perform the rest of your initial assessment.

As you get closer to the patient, look at his body and the position of his limbs. Do you see any obvious signs of trauma, such as limbs in an abnormal position? This sign may indicate that some force has been applied to the patient's body. Is his clothing intact or has it been torn or shredded? Is there evidence of any foreign material on his clothing or skin? This sign may indicate that some type of explosive device was used. Request Advanced Life Support personnel if you suspect WMD contamination.

Complete a more detailed assessment as conditions allow. When treating patients, consider the chemical-specific information received from your poison control center and other information resources. In multiple-patient situations, begin proper triage procedures according to your local emergency response plan.

Stop and Think!

Rushing in to a possible WMD event only increases confusion and the potential for harm to yourself and other responders. Stay alert and remain suspicious of unusual events or circumstances.

Key Safety Points

Always consider the possibility of multiple hazards. Only emergency personnel wearing appropriate protective gear and actively involved in performing emergency operations should work inside a contaminated area.

Identify the materials involved in the incident *only* from a safe distance. Do not approach anyone coming from a contaminated area. She may be the perpetrator or may be contaminated.

Decontamination

The decon process should be directed at confining the contaminant in order to maintain the safety and health of response personnel, the public, and the environment.

At every incident involving hazardous materials, there is a possibility that personnel, their equipment, and members of the public will become contaminated. The contaminant poses a threat to the contaminated persons. It also poses a threat to other personnel who may subsequently be exposed to contaminated personnel and equipment. Decontamination (decon) is done to reduce and prevent the spread of contamination from persons and equipment at a hazardous materials incident by physical and/or chemical processes. Decon should be performed only by trained personnel wearing the appropriate level of PPE. Decontamination is usually performed in the warm zone. Decon procedures should be continued until they are determined or judged to no longer be necessary.

On The Scene

Wrap-Up

Because it is warm, arriving engines quickly set up decontamination tents outside. Most of the patients are feeling better now that they are out of the building. Several are still wheezing and need oxygen and drugs to improve their condition. You send 25 patients to the hospital for treatment. The hazmat team enters the building and finds that someone had dispersed chlorine gas in the ventilation system. Luckily, it was not a strong concentration, so all of your patients were treated and released from the hospital. Police are carefully evaluating the crime scene several hours later as you pack up your gear and prepare to leave the scene. ■

Appendix Quiz

Multiple Choice

In the space provided, identify the letter of the choice that best completes each statement or answers each question.

_____ **1.** A blister agent is an example of what type of weapon?

a. biological
b. chemical
c. nuclear
d. explosive

_____ **2.** Cyanide is an example of what type of agent?

a. nerve
b. blister
c. blood
d. choking

_____ **3.** When possible, what is the best positioning at an incident involving hazardous materials?

a. downhill and downwind
b. uphill and downwind
c. downhill and upwind
d. uphill and upwind

True or False

Decide whether each statement is true or false. In the space provided, write T for true or F for false.

_____ **4.** Nerve agents cause a loss of consciousness within seconds and death within minutes of exposure.

_____ **5.** Alpha radiation is more penetrating than gamma radiation.

_____ **6.** If you suspect a possible act of terrorism, you should notify the appropriate authorities as soon as possible.

Short Answer

Answer each question in the space provided.

7. List four common types of biological agents.

1. ______________________________
2. ______________________________
3. ______________________________
4. ______________________________

8. List six categories of weapons of mass destruction a terrorist might use.

1. ______________________________
2. ______________________________
3. ______________________________
4. ______________________________
5. ______________________________
6. ______________________________

APPENDIX

2 Rural and Frontier EMS

On The Scene

You are almost finished with your chores when your pager vibration signals an emergency call. The location of the emergency is vague; there are no street addresses in this part of the county. You immediately recognize that it is your second cousin's farm. It will take you 20 minutes to get there, but you realize you may be the closest Emergency Medical Responder. When you arrive, the sun is sinking behind the evening mist and it takes a minute before you see a person waving beside the tractor along the tree line. Carrying your rescue bags over your shoulder, you are winded by the time you reach the patient, your 57-year-old cousin. He is pale and his skin is wet and cool. He was pulling a stump with his tractor when the chain broke, striking him in the chest. He says that it is hard to catch his breath and his chest is painful. You quickly apply oxygen and start to get his vital signs.

If only there were cellular phone service here; you could call for a helicopter. His neighbor explains that he saw your cousin's tractor when he was coming in from the fields and went over to say hello when he found him. He had to leave him, ride home, and dial the seven-digit emergency number to report the situation. As you wait for other rescuers and an ambulance to arrive, you realize that your cousin's injuries will be complicated by the fact that he has high blood pressure and diabetes, which he just never has the time to take care of properly. Another half hour passes before you hear the whine of a siren echo off the rolling hills. Looking down on your now very quiet cousin, you realize that it may be too late. ■

THINK ABOUT IT

As you read this appendix, think about the following questions:

- What factors created a delay in the response to this emergency?
- Why might there be fewer resources in this rural area?
- How must the emergency team prioritize its care to improve the chance for this patient's survival?
- Why may there not be an Advanced Life Support response to this life-threatening emergency?

Introduction

Emergency Response in Rural and Frontier Areas

EMS is an important part of rural and frontier healthcare. Rural and frontier areas have been defined as the wilderness of woods, hills, mountains, plains, islands, and desert outside of urban and suburban centers. In most areas of the United States, when people place a 9-1-1 call for a medical emergency, they expect an immediate dispatch of an ambulance and/or fire equipment. In many areas of the United States, including many rural areas, EMS consistently meets this expectation. However, this expectation is not being met in some rural and frontier areas for a variety of reasons.

You Should Know

In 2004, the National Rural Health Association (NRHA), the National Organization of State Offices of Rural Health (NOSORH), and the National Association of State EMS Directors (NASEMSD) released the final draft of *Rural/Frontier EMS Agenda for the Future.* This document offers recommendations to support and improve emergency services in rural and frontier communities by focusing on restructuring, reimbursement, and recruitment issues. (Kevin K. McGinnis, MPS, WEMT-P, *Rural and Frontier Emergency Medical Services: Agenda for the Future.* Copyright © 2004 National Rural Health Association. www.NRHArural.org.)

The Challenges of Rural and Frontier EMS

Healthcare Resources

The number of hospital and medical practice closures in rural and frontier areas has increased. This increase has resulted in shrinking healthcare resources in these communities. Because of the heavy demands of rural healthcare (such as long hours and no backup), it is hard for many rural areas to recruit and retain doctors, nurses, and other healthcare personnel. Doctors and nurses who choose to work in rural and frontier areas often have limited contact with EMS personnel. They are often unfamiliar with the different levels of EMS professionals and their capabilities.

As the residents of rural and frontier areas age, their need for medical care increases. Residents must often travel great distances to see specialists. As their local healthcare resources disappear, residents of these areas call on EMS professionals for assistance. Requests for help may include an unofficial assessment, advice, or emergency care.

Some rural and frontier communities are using EMS professionals in doctors' offices, healthcare clinics, hospice, and home health settings. In some settings, EMS professionals are used between EMS calls to supplement the hospital staff. In others, they are used for regular shift coverage. Using EMS professionals in this way helps fill the gap in the community's healthcare resources.

Response Times

In urban areas, fire departments and ambulance services try hard to arrive at the patient's side within four to eight minutes of the patient's call for help. This goal is unrealistic in rural and frontier areas. Rural and frontier EMS professionals cover large, sparsely populated areas using minimal resources to respond to the scene. Response times in rural and frontier settings may be long due to the following:

- A delay in volunteers' response from home or work
- A failure to respond

- The physical distance that must be covered
- The type of transportation that must be used (land, air, water)
- The type and condition of the roadway, airway, or waterway
- Bad weather

Limited access to communications may delay the detection and reporting of a need for emergency care. When EMS professionals travel on land, remote locations and unpredictable road conditions (including unmarked roads) can delay their arrival on the scene.

EMS Workforce

Many rural and frontier EMS professionals often work a full-time job outside of their EMS roles. Many frequently volunteer their time to provide emergency medical care and transportation to members of their community. When a volunteer receives a request to respond to an EMS call, he or she leaves a full-time job to respond in his or her private vehicle. In areas where an emergency response vehicle is available, the volunteer must travel to the station, pick up the emergency vehicle, and then respond to the emergency. When an EMS call is over, the volunteer returns home, returns to his or her regular job, or goes back to the station to return the emergency vehicle. Rural and frontier EMS professionals

- Often know their patients
- Often know about patients' conditions
- Understand the environment in which patients live and work
- Know what patients need

Making a Difference

EMS professionals in rural and frontier areas have a different attitude about their job. It may be because while most of us talk about the possibility of providing EMS care for friends and family, these folks literally do. EMS for them is less a job and more a way of "giving back" to their community. Rural and frontier EMS professionals are often more open to education and technology than some of their urban counterparts. It may be because they are looking at a way to care not just for people but for people they know—their children's schoolmates, families they see at social gatherings, their colleagues, and so on.

In rural and frontier settings, the level of Emergency Medical Responder and Emergency Medical Technician (EMT) prehospital care is more likely to be available than is advanced-level care. This situation is partly due to the costs, time, and travel needed to obtain advanced-level training. Individuals who do become Advanced Emergency Medical Technicians and Paramedics often do not remain in the rural or frontier area after their training is finished. Low call volumes in some areas make it difficult for some advanced care professionals to keep up their skills. Continuing education opportunities may be limited and training resources (including qualified instructors) are often scarce.

You Should Know

Rural and frontier EMS systems rely heavily on volunteers. However, the increasing expectations of rural and frontier residents about the level and type of prehospital care may demand services that cannot be provided easily by volunteers.

States have been pressured to use EMT as the national minimum level of care for personnel who provide patient care on ambulances. Many of the volunteers in rural and frontier areas are Emergency Medical Responders. Some EMS leaders are concerned that increased training, testing, and certification requirements will jeopardize the interest and availability of their volunteers.

At the same time, the number of interested EMS volunteers may be decreasing due to the following factors:

- The increase in two-wage-earner households
- Limited or a lack of EMS pay
- An increasing exposure to the risks in providing EMS care
- The belief that there is increased personal liability when providing EMS care
- A lack of EMS leadership in the community
- Limited or a lack of funding for training, equipment, and supplies
- An increased number of nursing home and routine transfer calls instead of emergency calls

Illness and Injury

Many rural and frontier residents are employed in some of the most hazardous occupations in our country—logging, mining, farming, fishing, and hunting. Work-related deaths occur more frequently among these groups of workers than among workers as a whole.

A number of factors may contribute to the severity of injuries and the greater number of injury-related deaths seen in rural and frontier areas:

- There may be long delays between the time of the injury and its discovery by a passerby.
- It may take a considerable amount of time to get a patient from the scene of an accident to a hospital because of distances between the scene, the ambulance service, and the hospital.
- Prehospital care in many rural areas may be performed by volunteers who are unable to provide advanced airway management or fluid resuscitation.
- Emergency departments in small rural hospitals may be staffed by physicians who do not have the knowledge or skills needed to manage critical trauma patients.
- There may be relatively few trauma cases at a rural hospital, making it difficult for physicians and nurses to maintain their skills.
- Rural hospitals may not have 24-hour physician coverage. In addition, laboratory and X-ray services may not be available 24 hours a day.
- In situations involving multiple victims, delays may occur in the initial stabilization of patients because there are too few responders, physicians, or nurses available.
- Injuries from all-terrain vehicles, snowmobile collisions, and other recreational activities are common in rural settings.
- Injuries may occur due to farming activities. Adults and children may be injured while operating heavy machinery, operating dangerous tools, caring for large livestock, or handling dangerous pesticides or other chemicals. Responses to situations that involve large livestock can be unsafe for rescuers (Figure A2-1). Farm rescues may include hazards such as poisonous gases or low-oxygen atmospheres found in silos, confined-space situations, and unique extrication situations involving farm machinery.
- Industries located in rural and frontier areas may pose potential hazards (Figure A2-2).

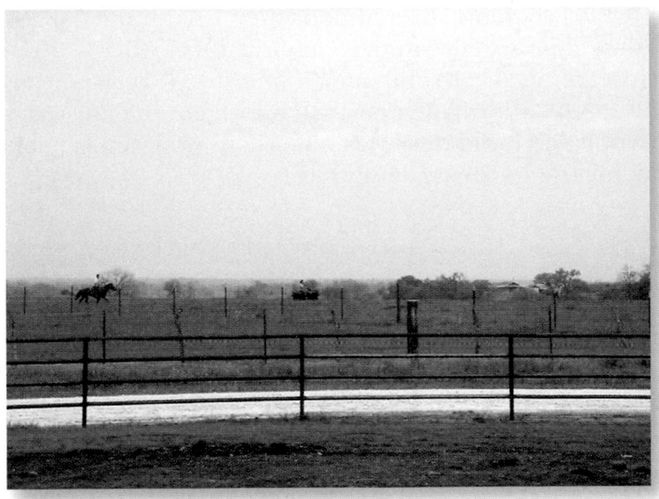

FIGURE A2-1 ▲ Adults and children may be injured due to farm activities. In this picture, a horse and an all-terrain vehicle are being used to herd cattle.

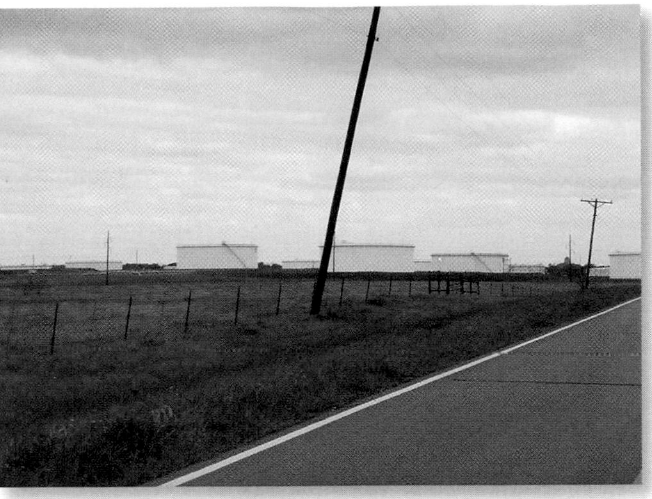

FIGURE A2-2 ▲ Industries located in rural and frontier areas may pose potential hazards.

- Rural emergencies may also include wilderness-related medical situations. These situations include envenomation from poisonous snakes; heat-, cold-, and water-related emergencies; and poisoning from plants.

Factors that may contribute to higher rates of motor vehicle–related injury and death in rural and frontier areas include

- Poor road conditions
- The absence of safety features (guard rails, appropriately placed shoulder reflectors)
- A greater likelihood of high-speed travel (65 mph or more)
- A greater use of utility vehicles and pickup trucks
- A lack of effective safety measures (seat belts)
- Greater distances between emergency facilities

A motor vehicle crash occurring along an infrequently traveled rural road may not be detected for hours. When the crash is detected, access to the EMS system may be further delayed because phones or other forms of communication may not be readily available. The patient may sustain injuries that require the use of specialized services, such as a trauma center. Trauma centers are usually not immediately available in rural and frontier areas. It is often necessary to contact an air medical service for patient transport. The air transport team may be located a distance from the accident site, which delays transporting the patient from the crash site to the hospital.

Making a Difference

In a rural or frontier EMS system, long distances, minimal resources, and road conditions that are less than optimal usually allow for a significant length of time for interaction between you and the patient. This prolonged patient contact time will give you an opportunity to talk with your patient, reassess his or her condition, perform additional skills, and provide frequent reassurance.

If a cardiac arrest occurs, CPR must be started as quickly as possible. Some rural and frontier communities have improved emergency cardiac care in their areas by providing citizen CPR programs. In addition, they have trained Basic Life Support personnel to use automated external defibrillators (AEDs). AEDs are particularly well suited to the needs of rural and frontier areas because they are easy to use. They are also more affordable now than ever before. Many states have grants and financial assistance programs available. These programs enable agencies to purchase AEDs for use in their community.

Making a Difference

If you will be working in a rural or frontier area, find out from your instructor how you can become a CPR instructor. Teaching CPR regularly and placing AEDs in public areas could save the life of a cardiac arrest patient in your community.

You Should Know

The Unique Training Needs of Rural and Frontier EMS Professionals

In some areas, organizations are working to develop and deliver training programs that meet the unique needs of rural and frontier EMS professionals. The following are examples of innovative programs:

- The Southern Coastal Agromedicine Center (SCAC), in collaboration with the North Carolina Forestry Association, has developed a Timber Medic program to improve logging injury outcomes.
- Cornell University offers a First on the Scene program that teaches farm family members, farm employees, and the general community how to make important decisions at the scene of a farm emergency. The program is intended for all farm groups, such as farm managers, employees, spouses, 4-H and Future Farmers of America groups, and others. Some of the available topics are tractor overturns, machinery entanglements, grain bin emergencies, and silo emergencies.
- The Farmedic Training Program, now housed at Cornell University, provides rural fire and rescue responders with a systematic approach to farm rescue procedures that addresses the safety of both patients and responders (Figure A2-3). This program has trained more than 22,000 students since it began in 1981. For more information, visit the following web site: http://www.farmedic.com/training/.

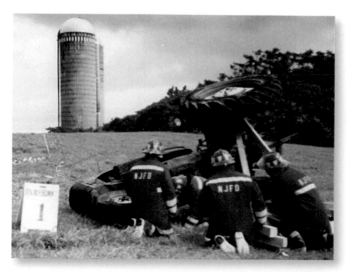

FIGURE A2-3 ▶ Farmedic Provider course in North Java, New York. The student team is stabilizing an overturned tractor to rescue the patient who is pinned under a tractor cowling. © www.farmedic.com. Cornell Farmedic Training Program. Cornell Agricultural Health and Safety Program. Cornell University, Ithaca, NY 14850. 1-800-437-6010.

On The Scene

Wrap-Up

By the time the EMTs on the ambulance bring their supplies across the field, your cousin is not breathing. You have placed an oral airway and are bagging him, trying hard to hold back the choking sobs that are causing your chest to heave. You and he grew up together, and you know that you'll be the one to have to break the news to his mother. She will be worried now, waiting alone in the farmhouse for him. By the time the EMTs place him on a spine board and carry him the long distance to the ambulance, the rapid, weak pulse you first felt is gone and you begin chest compressions. Although you quickly apply the AED, there is no shock advised. You stand and watch until the lights of the ambulance disappear in the swirling dust before you turn your truck toward your aunt's home. ■

Appendix Quiz

True or False

Decide whether each statement is true or false. In the space provided, write T for true or F for false.

_____ **1.** Prehospital care is provided in most rural and frontier areas of the United States by paid, full-time Paramedics.

_____ **2.** Logging, hunting, and fishing are among the least hazardous occupations in the United States.

Short Answer

Answer each question in the space provided.

3. List four reasons why the number of EMS volunteers in rural and frontier areas may be decreasing.

1. ______________________________

2. ______________________________

3. ______________________________

4. ______________________________

4. List two settings in which EMS professionals are being used in some rural and frontier communities.

1. ______________________________

2. ______________________________

5. List three reasons why the response time to a 9-1-1 call may be longer in a rural or frontier area than in an urban area.

1. ______________________________

2. ______________________________

3. ______________________________

APPENDIX

3 Special Populations

On The Scene

It's a beautiful spring day and the local park is full of students who are out for their last field trips of the year. As you watch a doe with her fawn, your peaceful thoughts are interrupted by the crackle of your radio. A deputy ranger tells you she has a report that a school bus has gone off the road and rolled onto its side. You radio for the local fire and ambulance companies before driving your first response truck to the collision.

As you round a hairpin turn, you see a small bus on its side. There appears to be minimal damage, so you sigh in relief. When you approach the bus, one adult has climbed out the window and rushes toward you. He tells you that this is a group of disabled students and they are very frightened. As you climb into the bus, you see two adults and six teenaged students; two are in mechanized wheelchairs, which are now lying on their sides. You quickly check and see that no one is unconscious. They all appear to have minor injuries, but your assessment of these patients will be challenging. The adult teachers who are with them tell you that one student has Down syndrome; two have cerebral palsy with severe spasticity and mental retardation; the three remaining students have developmental delays. ■

THINK ABOUT IT

As you read this appendix, think about the following questions:

- What strategies can you use to help communicate with the patients on this call?
- How can you minimize these patients' fear and anxiety?
- How will your ability to assess these patients be impaired?
- What must you consider if spinal stabilization is needed for the patients who have cerebral palsy?

Introduction

Caring for Special Needs Patients

As an Emergency Medical Responder, occasionally you will be faced with the need to provide care to a special needs patient. Special needs patients range from a person who has healthcare needs brought on by the normal aging process to a person who is severely emotionally or mentally disturbed.

You Should Know

Examples of Special Needs Patients

- Elderly patients
- Hearing-impaired patients
- Speech-impaired patients
- Vision-impaired patients
- Obese patients
- Quadriplegic patients
- Patients with mental illness
- Patients with Down syndrome
- Arthritic patients
- Patients with cancer
- Patients with cerebral palsy
- Patients with cystic fibrosis
- Patients with multiple sclerosis
- Patients with muscular dystrophy
- Patients with a previous head injury
- Patients with spina bifida
- Patients with myasthenia gravis
- Culturally diverse patients

Much of what we assume about a patient with special needs comes from some common misconceptions. The information presented in this appendix should correct these misconceptions and assist you in using a commonsense approach to assessing and treating special needs patients.

Making a Difference

Communicating with a special needs patient can be difficult. Communication difficulties can complicate assessing and treating these patients. Try to remember that these patients can be very independent and may resent any unwanted care. Having an arrogant attitude or "talking down" to a patient will usually cause him to become uncooperative. On the other hand, an honest and caring approach will go a long way toward lessening any problems that may arise.

Physical Disabilities

Geriatric Patients

The term *elderly* refers to persons 65 years of age and older.

In 2003, the number of persons in the United States age 65 years and older was estimated at 35.9 million. That number is projected to grow to almost 71.5 million by 2030. Elderly patients are rapidly becoming the largest group of patients encountered in the prehospital setting (Figure A3-1).

Making a Difference

Your patients are individuals of varying ages with a wide range of life experiences, knowledge, reasoning abilities, skills, and medical needs.

Technology-dependent patients have special healthcare needs. These patients depend on medical devices for their survival.

With advances in medical technology and treatment has come the problem of dealing with patients who have increased medical needs. Many older adults have at least one chronic medical condition. Some have multiple medical conditions, such as high blood pressure, heart disease, and arthritis. Many of these patients are on multiple medications. Some are technology-dependent. Although

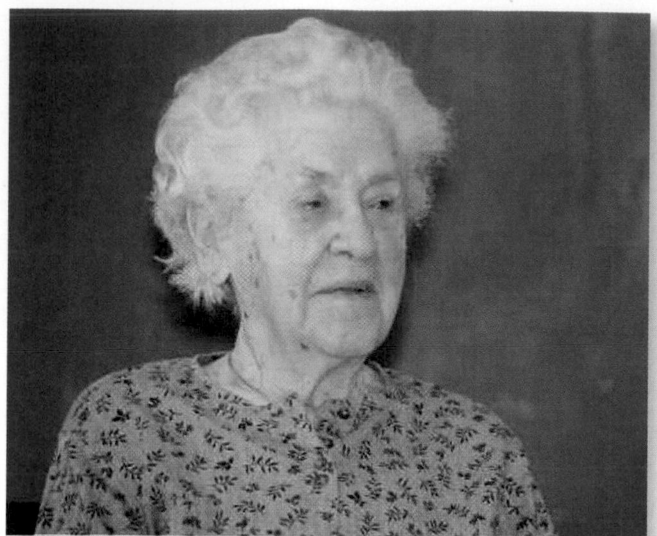

FIGURE A3-1 ▲ Elderly patients are rapidly becoming the largest group of patients that emergency personnel encounter in the prehospital setting. © Administration on Aging

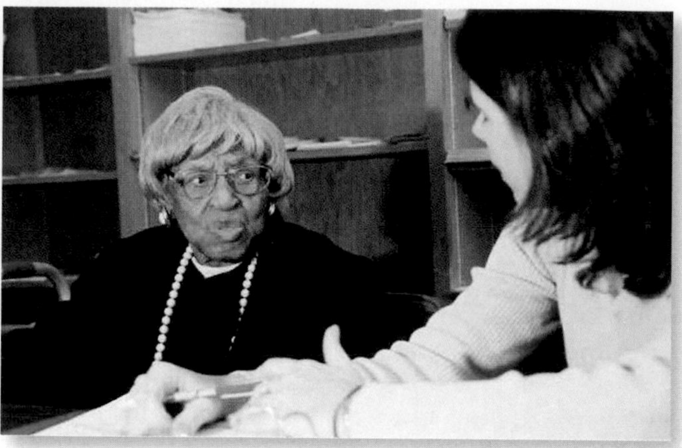

FIGURE A3-2 ▲ Be patient when speaking with an elderly person. Allow your patient time to process your questions. © Administration on Aging

some elderly patients have multiple medical conditions, do not assume that every elderly patient has age-related health problems. Many elderly patients are healthy and active into their later years.

You Should Know

Patients over the age of 65 are the largest population transported to the hospital by ambulance.

Many physical changes take place as we age, including changes associated with hearing, vision, taste, smell, and touch. In addition, reaction times are slowed due to changes in the central nervous system. Most muscle and organ systems also undergo changes. Because of these changes, your patient may be unable to communicate with you at the speed you would like. *Be patient.* Allow your patient time to process your questions (Figure A3-2). Do not be too hasty in assuming that she has a hearing impairment or does not understand. Speaking loudly to an elderly patient only distorts sounds. Stand directly in front of the patient and speak in a normal tone. Adjust the volume of your voice as necessary.

Making a Difference

When communicating with your patients, be respectful and willing to listen. You can build trust by letting the patient know that you are interested in what he or she has to say. Do not use terms such as *hon* or *dear* when speaking to an older adult. Terms such as these are disrespectful and unprofessional. Address your patient as Mr. __ or Mrs. __ unless the patient instructs you to do otherwise.

Ask the family, "What is different today? Is the patient confused? Behaving inappropriately? Having hallucinations?"

You may be called to assess an elderly patient with an altered mental status. One of your first goals must be to determine the patient's normal level of consciousness. It may be difficult for you to find out whether the patient's symptoms are due to a medical emergency, an ongoing (chronic) medical problem, or normal aging. To find out what the patient's normal mental status is, ask someone who knows the patient to give you this information. For example, ask a family member or neighbor how the patient appears to him today. Then ask the person providing information to compare how the patient appears today with how she was two or three days ago.

The elderly currently make up about 13% of the population and take almost 30% of all prescribed medications.

Some elderly patients are on several medications because they have multiple medical problems. If your elderly patient's chief complaint is unclear or does not seem to fall within the "normal" signs and symptoms of a particular disease, it may due to the fact that he has not been taking his medication as prescribed. The patient may not take his pills at all, may take them every now and then, or may accidentally overdose from taking too much medication.

A patient who is not taking his medication as prescribed may be doing so because he simply cannot afford it. Some prescribed medications are expensive. Many elderly patients are on fixed incomes and may have to choose between taking their medicine and paying for food and utilities. Some elderly patients see several doctors. If they fail to tell each doctor about the drugs another physician has prescribed, they may be prescribed drugs that can cause serious health problems when taken with the other medicines. Be respectful but firm when questioning patients about their medical history, including any prescribed medicines and their proper dosages.

Some of the medicines that geriatric patients take can hide the signs and symptoms of other illness. For example, some patients take heart or blood pressure medicines that keep the heart rate low. If they have a blood loss, the drug prevents the heart rate from increasing to compensate for the shock. When you assess them, you may think that they are stable because the heart rate remains normal despite shock.

Asking an elderly patient to rate his or her discomfort on a scale from 0 to 10 may not give a true picture of the pain he or she is experiencing.

If your elderly patient is complaining of pain or discomfort, ask carefully worded questions about the discomfort she is having. Because pain sensation can be lessened or absent in older adults, the patient can easily misjudge how serious her condition is. Elderly patients may live with chronic pain and underreport the discomfort associated with their current medical problem. The elderly patient may not tell you about important symptoms because she is afraid of being hospitalized. She may be afraid that, once she is at the hospital, she will never come home or she may not be able to make decisions about her care. Try to reassure the patient that she will receive the best of care at the hospital.

Remember This!

Look for visual cues that your elderly patient is in pain. For example, grimacing, wincing, or stiff muscles may be indicators that the patient is experiencing pain.

Remember to be sensitive to the patient's modesty.

Physical examination of the elderly patient can be a real challenge. Conduct your physical examination in the same general order as with patients in other age groups. Make sure to explain any procedure or exam that you are going to perform before actually performing it or touching the patient. This explanation is especially important when examining an older adult with a vision problem.

An older adult who has fallen and has lain on the floor for many hours may have a low body temperature.

Older adults often wear multiple layers of clothing, which can get in the way of your exam. Keep in mind that an elderly patient's temperature-regulating system becomes depressed. An elderly patient's temperature may generally be lower than normal due to a slower metabolic rate and decreased activity. In addition, the skin loses subcutaneous fat and becomes less effective at responding to changes in heat or cold. Some medications change the body's ability to control temperature. As a result of these factors, the elderly are more likely to be affected by environmental temperature extremes. They may also tire easily and have difficulty tolerating the exam.

An elderly patient's cough reflex is diminished, decreasing his or her ability to clear secretions.

It can be hard to tell the difference between the signs of a medical emergency and those of an ongoing medical condition. For example, the patient's breathing may be very quiet, because older adults often do not breathe as fast, breathe as deeply, and move as much air as younger persons. Patients may have an underlying respiratory problem that causes them to have noisy respirations.

On the other hand, these findings can also be signs of a respiratory emergency. Swelling of the legs may be due to poor circulation and inactivity, or it may be due to a heart problem.

Making a Difference

As many as 20% of older adults who seek emergency care are malnourished. The physical signs of malnutrition are not always easy to spot. While you are in a patient's home, take a moment to look around you. Does the patient have adequate food in the house? Is the patient able to prepare food? Also look for hazards in the home that can contribute to falls, such as extension cords, loose rugs, slick or wet floors, inadequate lighting, a lack of stair or bath rails, and uneven flooring. Be sure to let responding EMS personnel know your findings.

Use care when taking an elderly patient's blood pressure. An elderly patient's skin is often dry, thin, transparent, and wrinkled. Capillaries are fragile and the skin bruises easily. Your patient may also be on medications, such as steroids, that can cause the skin to become thin and tear easily.

The physical changes associated with aging must be considered when immobilizing an elderly patient or moving the patient from his home to an ambulance. As we age, bones become brittle. In addition, muscle fibers decrease in number and become weaker. The curves of the cervical and thoracic spine become more pronounced. Cartilage in the joints breaks down, resulting in stiffness and a loss of flexibility. Rough handling may cause tissue damage or even fractures. Padding a backboard may be necessary to allow for changes in the shape of the patient's spine. Use gentle care when moving your patient.

Hearing Problems

Not all hearing-impaired people hear the same sounds in the same way.

Because a patient has a hearing impairment does not mean that she lacks mental intelligence. Many deaf patients do not consider a lack of hearing a disability. In fact, they often resent being treated as if they have a disability. A common mistaken belief of some emergency care professionals is that you must speak more slowly and loudly for the patient to understand you. Not only does this not work, but it may actually confuse the patient. When you speak more slowly than normal, you tend to overemphasize the way you move your mouth when you speak. This can lead to a greater misunderstanding if the patient is trying to read your lips. Try not to drastically change the way you speak. Use your normal tone of voice and speak at your normal speed—as if you were carrying on a conversation with any other patient.

If the patient has a sound amplification device or hearing aid, you may need to help him put it in place (Figure A3-3). Family members are a good resource because they have experience communicating with the patient regularly. You may have to get your patient's attention with a gentle touch on the shoulder. Face your patient directly, so that he can see your face and mouth. Make sure that there is adequate lighting, so that the patient can see your face and mouth clearly. When speaking, do not move your head around. Doing so makes it difficult for the patient to follow what you are saying. If the patient has some limited ability to hear, try to reduce any unnecessary background noise. For example, shut off televisions, radios, dishwashers, or other noisy appliances while talking with the patient. You may even resort to using paper and pen to communicate.

Keep in mind that family members tend to reword your questions and the patient's answers.

When questioning your patient about his condition, think about the questions you want to ask. Then ask him short, direct questions that require a very specific

FIGURE A3-3 ▶ Examples of hearing aids.

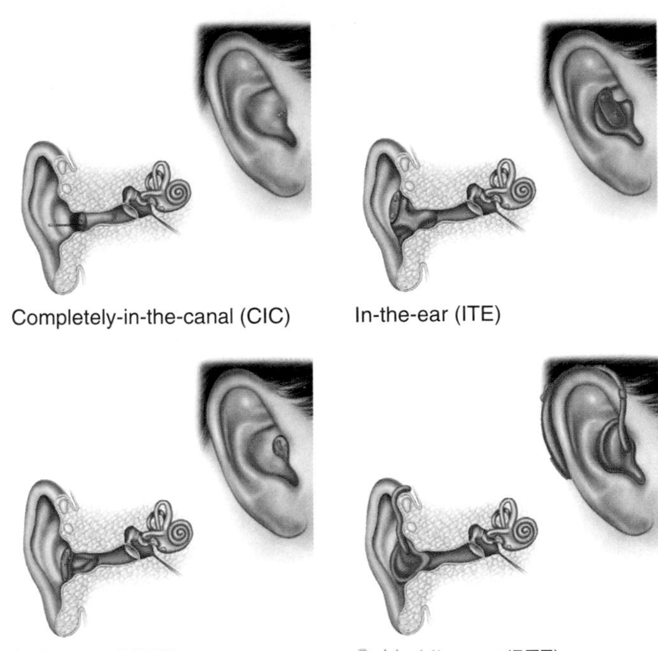

answer. Make sure to actually speak or say every word in your question. Ask one question at a time and follow up on the answer before starting another line of questioning. Doing so will allow you and the patient to focus on one problem at a time. It can even lead to a better interview. It is unlikely that the patient or a family member will understand confusing medical terms. Use common terms when asking questions and explaining the care you will provide. Avoid the use of sign language unless you are very skilled or an interpreter is present.

Your treatment of a hearing-impaired patient should be based on her medical condition. The care you provide will generally not require extraordinary changes in your usual treatment plan. Remember to explain any procedure before providing care. Inform arriving EMS personnel of the patient's hearing impairment. They will then contact the receiving facility to be sure an interpreter is available when they arrive.

Speech Impairments

Patients can experience speech difficulties due to a brain injury or a lack of oxygen to the brain. For example, a stroke patient may be unable to speak but may be able to understand your questions. You may be able to establish another means of communication, such as a hand squeeze or even eye blinks. If your patient appears to understand your questions but is unable to answer, stop asking the questions but continue to talk to the patient. Let him know that you understand he is unable to talk. It may be comforting to the patient to know that you are aware of his situation.

Making a Difference

Never assume that a person who cannot speak clearly lacks mental intelligence. A severe speech deficit can be completely unrelated to intelligence.

Children and adults may have language problems that stem from a hearing impairment, a congenital learning disorder, a speech delay, or cerebral palsy.

Sometimes a person's inability to say certain sounds or words is only temporary. For example, a person who has ingested too much alcohol or taken too many narcotics may slur his or her words, use words incorrectly, or be unable to recall some words.

Other speech problems may occur when a patient has difficulty with her speech pattern, such as stuttering. A patient who has cancer of the larynx may have a hoarseness or harshness in her voice. These patients may have only a limited ability to respond to your questions. Try to keep your questions short and to the point. In some situations, it may be helpful to ask questions that can be answered with a yes or no. Allow the patient time to respond and in her own way. Rushing the patient to answer may only increase her anxiety and frustration. Pay attention and listen carefully to what the patient has to say. She may even use hand gestures or a notepad to communicate her needs.

Your treatment of a patient with speech impairment should be based on her medical condition. The care you provide will generally not require unusual changes in your treatment plan. Remember to inform arriving EMS personnel of the patient's communication difficulty.

Vision Impairments

About 1 out of every 20 Americans has low vision. Five million Americans age 65 and older are blind or severely visually impaired.

A rapid loss of vision is *always* an emergency.

Every seven minutes, someone in America becomes blind or otherwise visually impaired.

Do not push, pull, or grab a blind patient.

The term *visual impairment* applies to a variety of vision disturbances. Visual impairments range from blindness and lack of usable sight to low vision. **Low vision** is a visual impairment that interferes with a person's ability to perform everyday activities. It cannot be corrected to normal vision with standard eyeglasses, contact lenses, medicine, or surgery. Low vision can result from a variety of diseases, disorders, and injuries that affect the eye.

A patient may have a visual impairment due to a medical emergency, a traumatic injury, or a preexisting condition. As a general rule, a patient who has a sudden change in vision needs immediate transport to the closest appropriate medical facility. Vision changes may be due to a lack of oxygen to the brain. They may also result from physical damage to the eyes, the optic nerve, or even the brain. If the vision disturbance is due to a preexisting condition, continue with your assessment and treatment.

When communicating with a blind patient, begin by identifying yourself in a normal voice. Most blind persons are not hearing impaired, so there is no need to raise your voice or shout when talking to them. If family members or others are present, address the patient by name so that it is clear to whom you are talking. Clearly explain any care you are going to provide before doing so. In this way, you do not surprise or startle the patient. Be sure to talk directly to the patient, not through a family member.

If the patient requires evaluation at the hospital, guide your patient carefully to the stretcher if he is able to walk. Offer the patient your arm and let him hold on just above your elbow. Guide the patient by leading him. It can be very helpful to verbalize the location of your equipment. When giving directions, indicate left and right according to the way the patient is facing.

A very strong bond can form between a visually impaired patient and his guide dog. Make every attempt to keep them together if at all possible. Do not pet or otherwise distract a guide dog. A blind person's safety depends on the animal's full attention. If the animal has been injured, contact your dispatcher for the appropriate care as soon as possible.

Obesity

It is estimated that as much as 50% of the population in the United States meets the medical criteria for obesity.

Obesity is an excess amount of body fat. Women who have more than 30% body fat are obese. Men with more than 25% body fat are obese. **Body mass index (BMI)** is a mathematical formula that expresses the relationship of weight to height. Individuals with a BMI of 25 to 29.9 are considered overweight. Individuals with a BMI of 30 or more are considered obese.

You Should Know

Medical Problems Linked to Obesity

Heart disease
Stroke
Diabetes
Gallbladder disease
Arthritis
Gout
Breathing problems
High cholesterol
High blood pressure

An obese patient can create a challenge for even the most experienced emergency care professional. The patient requires special attention in order for you to give her the appropriate care she deserves.

Obtain a thorough history and perform a physical examination. Much of the equipment used to take vital signs and treat the patient may be too small to obtain accurate measurements. For example, the largest size of blood pressure cuff may not reach around the patient's arm to allow you to get an accurate reading. In many cases, the obese patient will not be able to lay flat on her back. Laying the patient flat may cause her to have breathing difficulty. If you must move this patient while she is in a sitting position on a stretcher, keep in mind that the patient's center of gravity is much higher. This position can cause the patient to tip over much more readily. When lifting the patient, it is important to coordinate the move so that it is done safely and comfortably. Transporting an obese patient may require the use of additional personnel or even special equipment.

Spinal Cord Impairment

Quadriplegia is a loss of movement and sensation in both arms, both legs, and the parts of the body below an area of injury to the spinal cord. **Paraplegia** is the loss of movement and sensation in the body from the waist down.

Quadriplegia usually results when the spinal cord is injured in the area of the fifth to seventh cervical vertebrae. This injury can interfere with normal breathing, because stimulation of the muscles and organs necessary for breathing is drastically impaired. The quadriplegic patient may use a ventilator to help him breathe. This equipment may be complex and exceed the scope of practice of an Emergency Medical Responder. If the machine malfunctions, you may need to breathe for the patient using a bag-valve-mask device. Ask family members or other caregivers for help when treating a patient with quadriplegia. They are the experts about what is needed for the patient.

The quadriplegic patient cannot sense pain in any extremities. This patient will be unable to feel burns or even traumatic injuries if they occur. In some instances, these injuries may be severe or even life-threatening because the patient is not able to recognize the extent of the damage due to the loss of sensation.

Some patients with a lesser degree of paralysis may move with the help of supportive devices or splints. If these devices interfere with emergency care, they need to be removed. You may need to remove a patient from a wheelchair so that you can provide care.

Some patients depend on additional appliances, such as bladder or bowel collection devices. The patient's family or primary caregiver should be familiar with these devices and their proper care. When moving the patient, be careful not to pull or tug on the collection devices.

Making a Difference

Responding to Disabled Patients

Disabled persons pose many challenges to the Emergency Medical Responder. Begin by establishing trust between you and the patient. Ask the patient to help with his or her care and treatment by directing his or her moves and stating in what positions the patient is most comfortable. In the event that the patient is unable to communicate with you, ask family members or other patient caregivers to provide you with information.

Emergency Medical Responders must become familiar with safety issues regarding patients in wheelchairs. You must become familiar with how to lock brakes and move footrests so that you can assess, treat, and move the patient. Protect yourself from injury by using the lifting and moving techniques described in Chapter 5. You may also be able to "learn as you move" by taking direction from the patient or the patient's family members or caregivers.

Treat disabled patients as you would all other patients—with professionalism and respect. Don't be embarrassed to seek direction from the patient as it allows the patient to assist you with his or her care. Remember that most blind persons are not hearing impaired, so do not speak loudly to them. Persons who are unable to speak often write to communicate, so do not hesitate to ask a patient if he or she is hearing-impaired and can communicate in writing, If so, offer the patient a pen or pencil and paper.

Stay alert for sudden changes, be attentive, and never hesitate to provide compassionate care—the benefits to the patient and to you will be many.

Mental Illness

Remember that you must consider scene safety from the time you arrive at the scene of an emergency until you leave the scene.

Mental illness is a disorder that interferes with a person's thinking, feeling, moods, and ability to relate to others. There are many types of mental illness. When you are called to care for a patient with a mental illness, make sure of your own safety before taking any other action. Determine if the patient is a risk to herself or others, such as showing violent behavior or making statements about suicide. Look for signs of violence, substance abuse, or evidence of a suicide attempt. Be aware of potential weapons at the scene. If the patient is upset or agitated, wait for law enforcement personnel to arrive before approaching the patient.

Making a Difference

Responding to Suicidal Patients

As an Emergency Medical Responder, when you respond to an attempted suicide or threat of suicide, it is imperative that your safety comes first. Never enter a suicide scene alone—wait for backup from law enforcement personnel, just as you would on a domestic disturbance call.

If a suicide or an attempted suicide has occurred, take note of what the area looks like. All suicide scenes should be treated as crime scenes until investigators determine that no crime has occurred. When you treat the patient, make sure not to move anything that does not hamper your delivery of care.

If the patient has not attempted suicide but is threatening it, approach him or her cautiously. Stay calm. Never argue or shout at the patient. Be a truly active listener—look directly at the patient and make eye contact. Offer help and hope and avoid dominating the conversation. The patient is in crisis and needs to talk. Because "talk buys time," the more you allow the patient to talk, the less urgent the desire to commit suicide becomes. Often, a patient will move from having thoughts of wanting to die to wondering if he or she needs to die. Reinforce to the patient that you care. It is important to deal compassionately with the patient, so that he or she gains trust in you.

In treating suicidal patients, follow local protocol during assessment and treatment. Make sure to seek stress debriefing afterward if the suicide affects you emotionally.

Some patients may refuse to talk to you or may be very talkative. Others may be insulting. If the patient appears distracted, say her name, so that you can get her attention. Then speak to her in a calm voice. Be sure to allow time for the patient to answer you. When finding out about the patient's history, do not be afraid to ask about a history of mental illness or prescription medicines. If the patient has been prescribed medications for her condition, ask if she is taking them as prescribed. You should also ask the patient if she has ingested alcohol or drugs.

Treat a patient with a mental illness the same as any other patient who needs medical help. Remember that patients who have a mental illness also experience heart attacks, diabetes, and all of the illnesses and injuries that other patients experience.

Making a Difference

Responding to Mentally Ill Patients

Mentally ill patients can pose a great danger to Emergency Medical Responders, especially when a mentally ill patient is unstable and in crisis. Size up the scene just as you would a call for a suicide or domestic disturbance. Enter the scene only when law enforcement backup is available.

To remain safe, you must remain calm and observant. Look for signs of aggression from the patient. Pay attention to the patient's tone of voice and inflexion as well as the patient's body language. Clenched fists, distended neck veins, and flushed skin are indications that the patient is agitated. Keep a safe distance and maintain a calm tone of voice. Be prepared for quick changes in emotion from the patient, including increased aggression. If the patient is a danger to him- or herself, before providing treatment or care, make sure law enforcement personnel are available to restrain the patient.

Follow-up care at the hospital will benefit from complete and accurate documentation from the scene. Thorough documentation allows the medical team to make an accurate diagnosis. You should not document that the patient has a particular mental condition. Instead, you should only describe the patient's behavior, such as his or her demeanor, actions, words, and response to care. Ask family members or others who are familiar with the patient about the patient's history, including the treating physician and medication information.

Developmental Disabilities

Research suggests that the developmentally disabled are at an increased risk for physical or emotional abuse.

Persons with developmental disabilities have impaired or insufficient development of the brain, which causes an inability to learn at the usual rate. You may find it hard to recognize that your patient has a developmental disability.

Your attitude and the way you treat this patient may make the difference between a very confusing call and the delivery of optimal care. Listen to what the patient has to say. You may have to rely on the family or the patient's caregiver to help you find out what the patient's chief complaint is. You may also need their help in finding out about the patient's past medical history, medications, and current symptoms. In some cases, your very presence inside the patient's home may be upsetting. Be as calm and comforting as possible. The need to transport this patient for further care may increase his fear or anxiety. He may not understand why you need to take him away from his home and why you must provide emergency care. When EMS transport personnel arrive, they may want a family member or the patient's caregiver to accompany the patient to the hospital to help keep him calm. In many instances, an honest, caring approach to this patient will alleviate many potential problems.

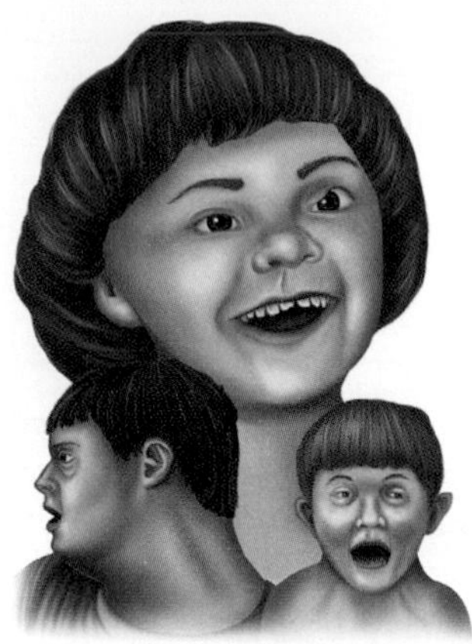

FIGURE A3-4 ▲ A patient with Down syndrome has characteristic physical features.

Approximately 25% of Down syndrome patients have a heart defect at birth.

Down Syndrome

Down syndrome is a genetic condition that causes mild to severe mental retardation and delays in physical development. A patient with Down syndrome has characteristic physical features (Figure A3-4):

- Eyes that slope up at the outer corners
- Folds of skin on each side of the nose that cover the inner corners of the eyes
- A small face and features
- A large, protruding tongue
- Flattening on the back of the head
- Hands that are short and broad

Most patients with Down syndrome are very trusting and loving. They may be frightened by you and the care you need to provide. To ease the patient's fears, try showing what you need to do on yourself or the patient's caregiver before performing it on the patient. In most cases, the patient's caregiver should go with the patient to the hospital.

Diseases and Special Injuries

Arthritis

The word *arthritis* is often used to refer to a group of more than 100 diseases that can cause pain, stiffness, and swelling in the joints and other parts of the body, including muscles, bones, tendons, and ligaments.

Technically, the word ***arthritis*** means inflammation of a joint. However, arthritis may affect not only the joints but also other parts of the body, including muscles, bones, tendons, and ligaments.

A patient with arthritis often has joint pain, stiffness, swelling, and redness of the surrounding area. These symptoms usually limit the patient's daily activities and may limit your ability to perform a physical examination. For example, the patient may be unable to straighten her arms, interfering with your evaluating her blood pressure.

A patient with arthritis may have difficulty moving about. If the patient requires immobilization or transport to the hospital, pad all voids with blankets, pillows, or trauma dressings.

Make your equipment fit the patient. Don't make the patient fit your equipment.

Cancer (Malignant Tumor)

Patients being treated for cancer can develop sudden, life-threatening complications, such as an infection.

The most basic definition of cancer is the uncontrolled growth of cells that invade surrounding tissue. These cells may even move to distant body sites and begin to grow there as well. The type of problems that the patient experiences will depend on the body part affected. You will need to obtain a thorough history from the patient, including as much information about the cancer as possible. The patient may be on pain medication or may be undergoing chemotherapy or radiation treatments. Extreme nausea is a common side-effect of these treatments and may mask the underlying problem for which you were called.

When performing a physical examination, make sure to locate and note any pain medication patches. These medications are absorbed through the skin and can affect you if it comes into contact with your skin. Calm, comfort, and offer emotional support to the patient.

Cerebral Palsy

Mental retardation occurs in about 75% of all people with cerebral palsy.

Cerebral palsy is a disorder that affects the body's ability to control voluntary muscles. It occurs because of a brain defect or an injury present at birth or soon after. This disorder can lead to stiffness and the contraction of groups of muscles, which may be seen as involuntary, squirming movements. The patient may also have a loss of coordination and balance.

A patient with cerebral palsy may need suctioning due to increased oral secretions. When preparing the patient for transport, pad the patient's limbs if they are in a twisted position. Do not force the limbs to move. Use extra pillows, trauma pads, or blankets to pad any limbs that are not in proper alignment.

Cystic Fibrosis

Patients with CF have an abnormality in the glands that produce or secrete sweat and mucus.

Cystic fibrosis (CF) is an inherited disease. A defective gene causes the body to produce abnormally thick, sticky mucus that affects multiple organs, including the lungs and digestive system. Breathing problems are common in these patients. They may need supplemental oxygen but may not tolerate an oxygen mask. Blow-by oxygen may be the only way to give them extra oxygen. If the patient shows signs of a severe breathing difficulty, you may need to breathe for the patient using a BVM. One-hundred percent oxygen should be used if it is available and you have been trained to use it.

Nearly 40% of the people with CF are age 18 and older.

While advances in medical technology have greatly increased the life expectancy of these patients, most of the patients you will treat will be children or young adults. In general, these patients have had many contacts with medical professionals. They may be afraid of one more trip to the hospital and one more procedure that must be performed. You may need to explain the importance of going to the hospital. Do not hesitate to call for an Advanced Life Support unit when needed.

Multiple Sclerosis

Do *not* have a patient with multiple sclerosis walk to the stretcher.

Multiple sclerosis is a disease of the central nervous system. In this disease, the message-transmitting fibers in the brain and spinal cord are progressively destroyed.

If the patient's speech has been affected by the disease, communication may be hard. Try to talk with the patient first. If this is not helpful, try to get the information you need from the family or the patient's caregiver. You may need help moving the patient to a stretcher for transport.

It may be hard to figure out if the patient's signs and symptoms are a new problem, such as a stroke, or are related to the multiple sclerosis.

You Should Know

Common Signs and Symptoms of Multiple Sclerosis

- Tiredness
- Dizziness
- Clumsiness
- Muscle weakness
- Slurred speech
- An inability to speak
- Blurred or double vision
- Numbness, weakness, or pain in the face
- Tingling or a feeling of constriction in any part of the body
- Limbs that feel heavy and become weak

Muscular Dystrophy

Muscular dystrophy is a group of inherited muscle disorders of unknown cause. In this disorder, there is a slow but progressive degeneration of muscle fibers. Some types of muscular dystrophy eventually affect the respiratory and cardiovascular systems, leading to the patient's death. The patient may need respiratory support and advanced cardiac care. Do not hesitate to call for Advanced Life Support personnel if you think the patient needs advanced care.

Patients with Previous Head Injuries

It may be difficult to recognize a patient who has had a previous head injury. There may be few, if any, outward signs of the previous injury. You must obtain a good medical history to find out if the reason you were called today is because of a new event or if it is related to the patient's previous injury. The patient who has had a prior head injury may have speech problems, short-term memory loss, and problems moving. You may find that some patients show signs similar to those of a stroke patient. Perform a thorough physical exam to find out if the patient has any obvious signs of new or recent trauma. Treat the patient based on medical need without being distracted by the previous injury.

Spina Bifida

Spina bifida is a congenital defect in which part of one or more vertebrae fails to develop, leaving a portion of the spinal cord exposed to the external environment. This condition can lead to paralysis of the lower limbs and a lack of bladder and bowel control. A large number of patients with spina bifida may have latex allergies due to repeated exposure. Try to remember to use nonlatex gloves and equipment when caring for these patients. A patient with spina bifida should not be expected to walk, although most can.

Myasthenia Gravis

Myasthenia gravis is a disorder in which muscles become weak and tire easily. The cause of this disorder is not known. The eyes, face, throat, and extremity muscles are most commonly affected. As the disease progresses, the patient may develop drooping eyelids, double vision, and difficulty speaking, chewing, and swallowing. In addition, movement of the limbs may be difficult and breathing muscles may become weak. You may need to provide supportive respiratory care, such as suctioning and supplemental oxygen, if it is available and you have been trained to use it. Consider the need for Advanced Life Support personnel to transport the patient to an appropriate facility.

Culturally Diverse Patients

Ethnicity, religion, gender, and homelessness are issues you may encounter when trying to provide care to your patients. Cultural differences can include patients' use of home remedies and treatments that you may be unfamiliar with. Try to familiarize yourself with the alternative treatments of the cultures in your area. Families from other cultures may respond differently than you do to the death of a loved one. As long as their behaviors are not harmful to themselves or others, be respectful and support their grieving.

Patients who speak a language other than English have unique challenges. They may be unfamiliar with the customs, care, and general expectations of the society that they are now a part of. It is your job to provide competent medical care to your patients without regard to race, creed, or cultural differences. Treat every patient with respect. When possible, obtain permission to provide treatment. Use an interpreter, such as a family member, when necessary. The receiving facility should be notified as soon as possible if an interpreter will be needed.

One of the most difficult problems that you may face is a patient who does not want your care. He or she may refuse your care based on cultural or religious beliefs. Carefully document the patient's refusal of your care.

Terminally Ill Patients

You must remember that the process of dying is an extremely emotional time for the patient and the family.

In many cases, a terminally ill patient will be cared for by hospice and should not need your assistance. However, families enrolled in hospice or who have DNR orders often still call 9-1-1 as their loved one nears death due to the following reasons:

- They are fearful.
- They do not want to be alone during the death.
- They do not know what to do.
- They fear that their family member is suffering.

In some instances, the patient's family will call for help in a desperate attempt to extend the patient's life. Listen carefully to determine the needs of the patient and family. Treat them with the care and compassion that they may desperately need. Even if the patient has Do Not Resuscitate orders, these orders do not mean "no care." Provide care to the best of your abilities and offer emotional support to the family members. If you have been called to the home of a hospice patient who has died, you must remember that the family members are now your patients. Call for appropriate resources to help them begin the grieving process.

Patients with Financial Challenges

A large portion of the U.S. population does not have health insurance. In addition, the homeless problem has increased at an alarming rate. Many patients in our communities rely on the 9-1-1 system and emergency departments for all of their medical care. This situation has caused a significant increase in the call volume for prehospital professionals in most areas of the country. This circumstance may impact the number of calls you run in any one shift. However, it should not change the care you provide these patients. They need your compassion, your understanding, and your care. Try not to make value judgments about the patients you meet. Provide care based on their medical need, not their ability to pay for services.

On The Scene

Wrap-Up

You know that your first challenge will be to calm the students. In a normal tone of voice, you tell them your name and that everyone is okay. You reassure them that the fire department is going to come and help them out of the bus. You face each student, address each by name, and ask if he or she is hurt. The patient with Down syndrome is very frightened when you attempt to assess her pulse, so you first show her a pulse check by checking her caregiver's pulse. That eases her fear and your assessment proceeds as well as you could expect.

The students appear to have minor cuts and bruises. However, because of their inability to communicate effectively, they must be immobilized and taken to the hospital. Since their teachers deny any injuries, you send one in each ambulance to calm their students. Immobilizing the patients who have cerebral palsy is very challenging. With time and much creative padding, each student is secured on a backboard. When the last ambulance departs the scene, you heave a sigh of relief, thankful that the bus stopped short of the steep cliff leading to the river below. ■

Appendix Quiz

Multiple Choice

In the space provided, identify the letter of the choice that best completes each statement or answers each question.

_____ **1.** You are called to the scene of a possible suicide attempt. You are greeted at the end of the driveway by a hysterical woman who identifies herself as the patient's mother. The mother states that her 30-year-old son has been depressed lately over the recent loss of his job and a breakup with his girlfriend. Her son told her he "can't deal with this anymore" and locked himself in the bathroom with a gun. The patient was last seen 30 minutes ago. Although she has not heard a gunshot, her son stopped answering her 10 minutes ago. You should now

a. contact your dispatcher for advice about what you should do.
b. enter the patient's home and try to talk with him through the bathroom door.
c. enter the patient's home, break down the door, and attempt to talk with him.
d. wait for the arrival of law enforcement personnel before entering the patient's home.

_____ **2.** Patients with an abnormality in the glands that produce or secrete sweat and mucus suffer from which one of the following diseases?

a. arthritis
b. cystic fibrosis
c. cerebral palsy
d. muscular dystrophy

True or False

Decide whether each statement is true or false. In the space provided, write T for true or F for false.

_____ **3.** When communicating with a hearing-impaired patient, speak more slowly and loudly so that the patient can understand you.

_____ **4.** When you are trying to speak with a patient who has a limited ability to hear, he or she will usually benefit from having background noise reduced, such as turning off a television or loud appliances.

_____ **5.** If a stroke patient is unable to speak, he or she will be unable to understand your questions.

_____ **6.** A rapid loss of vision is *always* an emergency.

Matching

Match the key terms in the left column with the definitions in the right column by placing the letter of each correct answer in the space provided.

_____ **7.** Down syndrome
_____ **8.** Low vision
_____ **9.** Cystic fibrosis
_____ **10.** Paraplegia

a. Loss of movement and sensation in both arms, both legs, and the parts of the body below an area of injury to the spinal cord
b. Excess body fat
c. Inherited muscle disorder of unknown cause in which there is slow but progressive degeneration of muscle fibers

_____ 11. Muscular dystrophy

_____ 12. Obesity

_____ 13. Quadriplegia

_____ 14. Multiple sclerosis

d. Progressive disease of the central nervous system in which the message-transmitting fibers in the brain and spinal cord are progressively destroyed

e. Loss of movement and sensation in the lower half of the body from the waist down

f. Disease in which a defective gene causes the body to produce abnormally thick, sticky mucus that affects multiple organs

g. Genetic condition that causes mental retardation

h. Visual impairment that cannot be corrected to normal vision with standard eyeglasses or contact lenses

Short Answer

Answer each question in the space provided.

15. A 75-year-old man is complaining of a sudden onset of chest pain. The patient is blind. Describe how you will approach this patient and begin communicating with him.

____

____

____

16. What is meant by the term *body mass index?*

____

____

____

17. List four medical problems that are linked to obesity.

1. _____________________

2. _____________________

3. _____________________

4. _____________________

Sentence Completion

In the blanks provided, write the words that best complete each sentence.

18. _____________ is an inflammation of a joint.

19. _____________ _____________ is a neuromuscular disorder that affects the ability to control voluntary muscles.

20. _____________ _____________ is a congenital defect in which part of one or more vertebrae fails to develop, leaving a portion of the spinal cord exposed to the external environment.

Glossary

A

Abandonment: terminating patient care without ensuring that care will continue at the same level or higher

Abdomen: the part of the body trunk below the ribs and above the pelvis

Abdominal cavity: the body cavity located below the diaphragm and above the pelvis; contains the stomach, intestines, liver, gallbladder, pancreas, and spleen

Abnormal behavior: a manner of acting or conducting oneself that is not consistent with society's norms and expectations, interferes with the individual's well-being and ability to function, or is harmful to the individual or others

Abortion: the delivery of the products of conception early in pregnancy

Abrasion: a superficial wound caused by rubbing or scraping, resulting in partial loss of the skin surface

Abruptio placenta: the condition that occurs when a normally implanted placenta separates prematurely from the wall of the uterus during the last trimester of pregnancy

Accessory muscles: the muscles between the ribs, above the collarbones, or in the abdomen used during inhalation or exhalation to assist breathing

Acrocyanosis: blueness of the hands and feet

Active rewarming: adding heat directly to the surface of the patient's body

Advance directives: legal documents that specify healthcare wishes when people become unable to make decisions for themselves

Airborne diseases: infections spread by droplets produced by coughing or sneezing

Air embolism: bubbles of air in the bloodstream

Airway adjuncts: devices used to help keep a patient's airway open

Altered mental status: a change in a patient's level of awareness

Alveoli: grapelike sacs at the end of bronchioles where oxygen and carbon dioxide are exchanged between the air and blood

Amniotic sac: the sac of fluid that surrounds the fetus inside the uterus

Amputation: the separation of a body part from the rest of the body

Anaphylactic shock: shock due to a severe allergic reaction

Anatomical position: a person standing, arms to the sides with the palms turned forward, feet close together, the head pointed forward, and with the eyes open

Anatomy: the study of the structure of an organism (such as the human body)

Angulation: the abnormal position of an extremity

Anterior: the front portion of the body or body part

Anxiety: a state of worry and agitation that is usually triggered by a vague or an imagined situation

Anxiety disorder: a more intense state of worry and agitation than normal anxiety

Aorta: the largest artery in the body

Appendicular skeleton: the upper and lower extremities (arms and legs), the shoulder girdle, and the pelvic girdle

Arteries: blood vessels that carry blood away from the heart to the rest of the body

Arterioles: the smallest branches of arteries leading to the capillaries

Arthritis: inflammation of a joint

Aspiration: the breathing of a foreign substance into the lungs

Assault: threatening, attempting, or causing fear of offensive physical contact with a patient or another individual

Atria: the two upper chambers of the heart (singular = *atrium*)

Auscultate: the process of listening to body sounds with the aid of a stethoscope

Automated external defibrillator (AED): a machine that analyzes the heart's rhythm for any abnormalities and, if necessary, directs the rescuer to deliver an electrical shock

AVPU scale: a memory aid used to identify a patient's mental status. Each letter of the scale refers to a level of awareness. *A* = alert, *V* = responds to verbal stimuli, *P* = responds to painful stimuli, *U* = unresponsive. A patient who is oriented to person, place, time, and event is said to be "alert and oriented × ('times') 4" or "A and O × 4."

Avulsion: the tearing off or tearing away of a patch of skin or other tissue from the body

Axial skeleton: the part of the skeleton that includes the skull, spinal column, sternum, and ribs

B

Bacteria: germs that can live outside the human body and do not depend on other organisms to live and grow

Bandage: material that holds a dressing in place over a wound

Baseline vital signs: an initial set of vital sign measurements against which later measurements can be compared

Battery: the unlawful touching of another person without consent

Battle's sign: a bluish discoloration behind the ear that is a sign of a possible skull fracture

Behavior: the manner in which a person acts or performs

Behavioral emergency: a situation in which the patient displays abnormal behavior that is unacceptable or intolerable to the patient, family members, or the community

Bilateral: pertaining to both sides

Bipolar disorder: a brain disorder that causes unusual shifts in a person's mood, energy, and ability to function

Birth canal: the vagina and lower part of the uterus

Bloodborne diseases: infections spread by contact with the blood or body fluids of an infected person

Blood pressure: the force exerted by the blood on the walls of the arteries

Blood volume: the total amount of blood circulating within the body

Bloody show: mucus and blood that may come out of the vagina as labor begins

Blunt trauma: any mechanism of injury that occurs without actual penetration of the body

Body: the main part of a skeletal muscle

Body cavity: a hollow space in the body that contains internal organs

Body mass index (BMI): a mathematical formula that expresses the relationship of weight to height

Body mechanics: the way we move our bodies when lifting and moving

Body substance isolation (BSI) precautions: self-protection against all body fluids and substances (blood, urine, semen, feces, vaginal secretions, tears, saliva, cerebrospinal fluid, etc.); also referred to as standard precautions, universal precautions

Body temperature: the balance between the heat produced by the body and the heat lost from the body

Brainstem: the portion of the brain that consists of the midbrain, pons, and medulla oblongata

Breathing: the mechanical process of moving air into and out of the lungs

Breech delivery: a delivery in which the presenting part of the infant is the buttocks or feet instead of the head

Bronchioles: small, thin-walled branches of a bronchus

Bronchus: large passageway for air to and from the alveoli

Bruise: a collection of blood under the skin due to bleeding capillaries

C

Capillaries: the very thin blood vessels that connect arteries and veins

Cardiac arrest: the temporary or permanent cessation of the heartbeat

Cardiac muscle: involuntary muscle found only in the heart

Cardiogenic shock: shock that occurs when the heart muscle fails to generate enough force to pump oxygenated blood effectively to all parts of the body

Cardiopulmonary failure: respiratory failure that occurs with shock

Cardiopulmonary resuscitation (CPR): a combination of rescue breathing and external chest compressions to oxygenate and circulate blood when the patient is in cardiac arrest

Carpals: wrist bones

Cells: the basic building blocks of the body

Centers for Disease Control and Prevention (CDC): the agency of the U.S. government that promotes health and quality of life by preventing and controlling disease, injury, and disability

Central nervous system: the brain and spinal cord

Central pulse: a pulse found close to the trunk of the body

Cephalic (head) delivery: a delivery in which an infant emerges head first from the birth canal

Cerebellum: the second largest part of the human brain; responsible for the precise control of muscle movements and the maintenance of posture and equilibrium

Cerebral palsy: a neuromuscular disorder that affects the body's ability to control voluntary muscles

Cerebrospinal fluid (CSF): a clear liquid that acts as a shock absorber for the brain and spinal cord and provides a means for the exchange of nutrients and wastes among the blood, brain, and spinal cord

Cerebrum: the largest part of the brain, made up of two hemispheres

Certification: a designation as having met predetermined requirements to perform a particular activity

Cervix: the narrow opening at the lower end of the uterus; connects the uterus to the vagina

Chief complaint: the reason EMS has been called, usually in the patient's own words

Childbirth: the emergence of an infant from its mother's uterus

Child maltreatment: an act or a failure to act by a parent, a caregiver, or another person as defined by state law that results in physical abuse, neglect, medical neglect, sexual abuse, and/or emotional abuse; an act or a failure to act that presents an impending risk of serious harm to a child

Circulatory system: the cardiovascular and lymphatic systems

Clavicle: collarbone

Cleaning: the process of washing a contaminated object with soap and water

Closed wound: an injury in which damage occurs to the soft tissues under the skin, but the surface of the skin is not broken; also called a closed soft-tissue injury

Communicable disease: a disease that can be spread from one person or animal to another, either directly or indirectly

Competence: the patient's ability to understand the questions you ask and understand the implications of the decisions he or she makes concerning his or her care

Concussion: a temporary loss of function in part or all of the brain

Conduction: the transfer of heat between objects that are in direct contact

Consent: permission

Contusion: a wound in which the epidermis remains intact, but the cells and blood vessels in the dermis are injured; a bruise

Convection: the transfer of heat by the movement of air or water current

Cranial cavity: the body cavity located in the head that contains the brain

Cranium: the skull

Crepitation (crepitus): a crackling sensation heard and felt beneath the skin; caused by bone ends grating against each other or air trapped between layers of tissue

Critical incident: events that interfere, or have the potential to interfere, with an individual's psychological ability to cope

Critical Incident Stress Debriefing (CISD): a group meeting led by a mental health professional and peer support personnel to allow rescuers to share thoughts, emotions, and other reactions to a critical incident

Critical Incident Stress Management (CISM): a comprehensive program developed to assist emergency workers in coping with stressful situations and to accelerate the normal recovery process after experiencing a critical incident

Crowning: the stage of birth when the presenting part of the infant remains visible at the vaginal opening

Cumulative stress: repeated exposure to smaller stressors that accumulate over time; burnout, occupational stress

Cyanosis: blue skin

Cystic fibrosis: a disease in which a defective gene causes the body to produce abnormally thick, sticky mucus that affects multiple organs

D

Defibrillation: the delivery of an electrical shock to the heart

Defusing: a shorter, less formal version of a debriefing for rescuers, held immediately or within a few hours after a critical event

Delivery: the birth of the baby at the end of the second stage of labor

Delusions: false beliefs that a person believes are true, despite facts to the contrary

Denial: a stage of the grief process in which the patient or a family member does not believe what is happening related to the patient's illness or injury

Dependent lividity: a sign of the settling of blood in dependent areas (those areas on which the body has been resting)

Depression: a state of mind characterized by feelings of sadness, worthlessness, and discouragement

Diaphragm: the dome-shaped muscle below the lungs; the primary muscle of respiration

Diastolic blood pressure: the pressure in the arteries when the heart is at rest

Diencephalon: the part of the brain between the cerebrum and the brainstem; contains the thalamus and hypothalamus

Dilate: widen

Direct ground lift: a non-urgent move used to lift and carry a patient with no suspected spine injury from the ground to a bed or stretcher

Direct pressure: firm pressure applied to a bleeding site with gloved hands or bandages to control bleeding

Disentanglement: the moving or removal of material that is trapping a victim

Disinfecting: cleaning with chemical solutions such as alcohol or chlorine

Dislocation: the displacement of the ends of bones from their normal positions in a joint

Distal: farthest away from the midline, or center area, of the body

Do Not Resuscitate order: a written physician order that instructs medical professionals not to provide medical care to a patient who has experienced a cardiopulmonary arrest

Down syndrome: a genetic condition that causes mild to severe mental retardation and delays in physical development

Draw sheet: a narrow sheet placed crosswise on a bed under a patient; used to assist in moving a patient or in changing soiled bed sheets

Dressing: absorbent material placed directly over a wound

Duty to act: a formal contractual or an implied legal obligation to provide care to a patient requesting services

E

Eclampsia: a condition of pregnancy characterized by high blood pressure, swelling, protein in the urine, and seizures

Emergency Medical Responder: a person who has the basic knowledge and skills necessary to provide lifesaving emergency care while awaiting the arrival of additional EMS help

Emergency Medical Services (EMS) system: a coordinated network of resources that provides emergency care and transportation to victims of sudden illness and injury

Emergency move: a move used because there is an immediate danger to the patient or rescuer

Emergency transportation: the process of moving a patient from the scene of an emergency to an appropriate receiving facility

Empathy: understanding, being aware of, and being sensitive to the feelings, thoughts, and experience of another

Enhanced 9-1-1: a 9-1-1 telephone system that indicates the telephone number and location of 9-1-1 calls

Epiglottis: a flap of cartilage that covers the trachea when swallowing, so that food and liquids do not enter the lungs

Erect: standing upright

Esophagus: the muscular tube about 9 inches long (in adults) that is a passageway for food

Ethics: principles of right and wrong, good and bad, and the consequences of human actions; what a person *ought* to do

Evaporation: a loss of heat by vaporization of moisture on the body surface

Evisceration: the protrusion of an organ through an open wound

Exhalation (expiration): the process of breathing out and moving air out of the lungs

Exposure: contact with infected blood, body fluids, tissues, or airborne droplets, either directly or indirectly

Expressed consent: a type of consent in which a patient gives express authorization for the provision of care and transport

External bleeding: bleeding that you can see

Extrication: a means of freeing a trapped or otherwise inaccessible patient and getting him or her to a treatment area

F

Fallopian tubes: a pair of tubes that receive and transport the egg from the ovary to the uterus after ovulation

False ribs: rib pairs 8 through 10; these ribs attach to the cartilage of the seventh ribs

Femur: the thigh bone; extends from the hip to the knee

Fibula: the bone that lies next to the tibia along the outer side of the lower leg

First responder: an individual with medical training who is the first to arrive at the scene of an emergency, such as a motor vehicle crash, life-threatening medical situation, or disaster

Flail chest: a condition in which three or more adjacent ribs are fractured in two or more places or when the sternum is detached. The section of the chest wall between the fractured ribs becomes free-floating because it is no longer in continuity with the thorax. This free-floating section of the chest wall is called the flail segment.

Floating ribs: ribs that have no attachment to the sternum (rib pairs 11 and 12)

Foodborne diseases: infections spread by the improper handling of food or by poor personal hygiene

Foramen magnum: the large opening in the base of the skull through which the spinal cord passes

Fowler's position: lying on the back with the upper body elevated at a 45- to 60-degree angle

Fracture: a break in a bone

G

Glottis: the space between the vocal cords

Grief: intense sadness caused by the loss of someone or something that had great meaning to the individual

Grieving: a response that helps people cope with the loss of someone or something that had great meaning to them

Growth plate: an area of growing tissue near each end of a long bone in children and adolescents

Gurgling: bubbling noise

H

Hallucinations: false sensory perceptions

Hazardous material: "a substance (solid, liquid, or gas) that, when released, is capable of creating harm to people, the environment, and property"

Healthcare system: a network of people, facilities, and equipment designed to provide for the general medical needs of the population; also referred to as healthcare delivery system

Health Insurance Portability and Accountability Act (HIPAA): a law passed by Congress in 1996 to ensure the confidentiality of a person's health information

Hematoma: a localized collection of blood beneath the skin due to a tear in a blood vessel

Hemoglobin: the iron-containing protein in red blood cells that carries oxygen from the lungs to the tissues

Hemophilia: a disorder in which the blood does not clot normally

Hemorrhage (major bleeding): an excessive loss of blood from a blood vessel; may be internal or external

Hemorrhagic shock: shock caused by severe bleeding

High-Fowler's position: patient sitting upright at a 90-degree angle

Homeostasis: the property of an organism to regulate its internal processes to maintain a constant internal environment; steady state

Host: a plant, a person, or an animal capable of harboring and providing nourishment for another organism

Humerus: the upper arm bone

Hypothermia: a core body temperature of less than 95°F (35°C)

Hypovolemic shock: shock caused by a loss of plasma, blood, or another body fluid

I

Impaled object: an object embedded in an open wound

Implied consent: consent assumed from a patient requiring emergency intervention who is mentally, physically, or emotionally unable to provide expressed consent

Incendiary materials: substances that burn with a hot flame for a specific period

Incident Command System (ICS): a standardized system developed to assist with the control, direction, and coordination of emergency response resources

Incompetent: a patient's inability to understand the questions asked of him or her or to understand the implications of the decisions he or she makes regarding his or her care

Infection: the invasion and growth of germs in a host, with or without detectable signs of illness

Infectious disease: a communicable disease caused by microorganisms, such as bacteria

Inferior: in a position lower than another

Informed consent: consent in which the patient understands the risks and benefits of care

Inhalation (inspiration): the process of breathing in and moving air into the lungs

In-line stabilization: a technique used to minimize movement of the head and neck

Insertion: the movable attachment to a bone

Internal bleeding: bleeding that occurs inside body tissues and cavities

J

Joint: a place where two bones come together

K

Kinematics: the science of analyzing the mechanism of injury and predicting injury patterns

Kinetic energy: the energy of motion; the amount of kinetic energy an object has depends on the mass of the object and the speed (velocity) of the object

L

Labor: the time and process beginning with the first uterine muscle contraction until delivery of the placenta

Laceration: a cut or tear in the skin of any length, shape, and depth

Larynx: the voice box

Lateral: toward the side of the body

Lateral recumbent position: lying on the side; left side = left lateral recumbent position, right side = right lateral recumbent position

Licensure: the granting of a written authorization by an official or legal authority to perform medical acts and procedures not permitted by persons without such authorization

Ligament: the connective tissue that joins the end of one bone with another

Limb presentation: a delivery in which the presenting part of the infant is an arm or a leg instead of the head

Log roll: a technique used to move a patient from a face down to a face up position while maintaining the head and neck in line with the rest of the body

Low vision: visual impairment, not correctable by standard glasses, contact lenses, medicine, or surgery, that interferes with a person's ability to perform everyday activities

Lungs: spongy, air-filled organs that bring air into contact with the blood so that oxygen and carbon dioxide can be exchanged in the alveoli

M

Major bleeding: life-threatening bleeding

Manubrium: the uppermost portion of the breastbone; connects with the clavicle and first rib

Mechanism of injury: the manner in which an injury occurs and the forces involved in producing the injury

Medial: toward the midline of the body

Mediastinum: the part of the thoracic cavity between the lungs that contains the heart, major vessels, esophagus, trachea, and nerves

Medical director: a physician who provides medical oversight and is responsible for ensuring that actions taken on behalf of ill or injured people are medically appropriate

Medical neglect: a type of maltreatment caused by a caregiver's failure to provide for the appropriate healthcare of a child although financially able to do so

Medical oversight: the process by which a physician directs the emergency care provided by EMS personnel to an ill or injured patient; also referred to as medical control or medical direction

Medical patient: a patient whose condition is caused by an illness

Medical practice acts: state laws that grant authority to provide medical care to patients and determine the scope of practice for healthcare professionals

Menstruation: the periodic discharge of blood and tissue from the uterus

Mental illness: a disorder that interferes with a person's thinking, feeling, moods, and ability to relate to others

Metacarpals: the bones that form the support for the palm of the hand

Metatarsals: the bones that form the part of the foot to which the toes attach

Microorganism: an organism too small to be seen with the unaided eye; bacteria, some fungi, and protozoa are microorganisms

Midline: an imaginary line drawn through the middle of the body from the nose to the umbilicus (navel) that divides the body into right and left halves

Mottling: an irregular or a patchy discoloration of the skin that is usually a mixture of blue and white; usually seen in patients in shock or cardiac arrest

Multiple sclerosis: a disease of the central nervous system in which the message-transmitting fibers in the brain and spinal cord are progressively destroyed

Muscle tone: the constant tension produced by muscles of the body over long periods

Muscular dystrophy: a group of inherited muscle disorders of unknown cause in which there is slow but progressive degeneration of muscle fibers

Myasthenia gravis: a disorder in which muscles become weak and tire easily

N

Nasal flaring: excessive widening of the nostrils with respiration

Nasal septum: a wall of tissue that separates the right and left nostrils

Nasopharyngeal airway: a soft, rubbery device that is inserted into the nose of an unresponsive or semi-responsive patient to help keep the airway open

Nature of the illness (NOI): the medical condition that resulted in the patient's call to 9-1-1

Neglect: the failure to provide for a child's basic needs

Negligence: deviation from the accepted standard of care, resulting in further injury to the patient

Non-urgent move: a patient move used when no immediate threat to life exists and the patient's safety, and that of the prehospital crew, are the primary concerns

O

Obesity: an excess amount of body fat

Obstetric emergency: an emergency related to pregnancy or childbirth

Occlusive: airtight

Occupational Safety and Health Administration (OSHA): the branch of the federal government responsible for safety in the workplace

Off-line medical direction: medical supervision of EMS personnel through the use of policies, protocols, standing orders, education, and quality management review; also called indirect, retrospective, or prospective medical direction

On-line medical direction: direct communication with a physician (or his or her designee) by radio or telephone, or face to face communication at the scene, before performing a skill or administering care

Open (compound) fracture: a broken bone that penetrates the skin

Open soft-tissue injury: an injury in which the skin surface is broken

Open wound: an injury in which the skin surface is broken

Organ: at least two different types of tissue that work together to perform a particular function; examples include the brain, stomach, and liver

Organ system: tissues and organs that work together to provide a common function; examples of organ systems include the respiratory system and nervous system

Origin: the stationary attachment of a muscle to a bone

Oropharyngeal airway (OPA): a curved device made of rigid plastic that is inserted in the mouth of an unresponsive patient without a gag reflex to help keep the airway open

Osteoporosis: a skeletal disorder that develops when the rate of old bone removal occurs too quickly or if old bone replacement occurs too slowly

Ovaries: paired, almond-shaped organs in a woman's body that produce eggs; located on each side of the uterus in the pelvic cavity

Ovulation: the release of an egg from an ovary

P

Palpate: to feel

Panic attack: an intense fear that occurs for no apparent reason

Paranoia: a mental disorder characterized by excessive suspiciousness or delusions

Paraplegia: the loss of movement and sensation in the body from the waist down

Passive rewarming: warming a patient without the use of additional heat sources beyond the patient's own heat production; methods include placing the patient in a warm environment

Patella: the flat, triangular, movable bone that forms the anterior part of the knee; kneecap

Patent: open

Pathogens: germs capable of producing disease

Pathophysiology: the study of changes in the body caused by disease

Patient assessment: the process of evaluating a person for signs of illness or injury

Patient history: the part of the patient assessment during which facts are obtained about the patient's medical history

Pelvic cavity: the body cavity below the abdominal cavity; contains the urinary bladder, part of the large intestine, and reproductive organs

Pelvic girdle: the bones that enclose and protect the organs of the pelvic cavity; provides a point of attachment for the lower extremities and major muscles of the trunk and supports the weight of the upper body

Pelvis: the bony ring formed by three separate bones that fuse to become one in an adult

Penetrating trauma: any mechanism of injury that causes a cut or piercing of the skin

Perfusion: the flow of blood through an organ or a part of the body

Pericardial cavity: the body cavity containing the heart

Perineum: the area between the vaginal opening and the anus

Personal protective equipment (PPE): specialized clothing or equipment worn by an individual for protection against a hazard; general work clothes (e.g., uniforms, pants, shirts, or blouses) not intended to function as protection against a hazard are not considered personal protective equipment

Personal space: the invisible area immediately around each of us that we declare as our own

Phalanges: the bones of the fingers and toes

Pharynx: the throat

Phobia: an irrational and constant fear of a specific activity, object, or situation

Physical abuse: physical acts that have caused or could have caused physical injury to a child

Physiology: the study of the normal functions of an organism (such as the human body)

Placenta: a specialized organ through which the fetus exchanges nourishment and waste products during pregnancy

Placenta previa: the condition that occurs when part or all of the placenta implants in the lower part of the uterus, covering the opening of the cervix

Plasma: the liquid portion of the blood

Pleurae: serous (oily), double-walled membranes that enclose each lung

Pleural cavities: body cavities that contain the lungs; the right lung is located in the right pleural cavity; the left lung is located in the left pleural cavity

Pleural space: a space between the visceral and parietal pleura, filled with a small amount of oily fluid, which allows the lungs to glide easily against each other

Position of function: the natural position of the hand or foot at rest

Posterior: the back side of the body or body part

Postictal phase: the recovery period after a seizure

Power grip (underhand grip, supinated grip): a method of placing your hands on an object that is designed to take full advantage of the strength of your hands and forearms

Power lift: a technique used to lift a heavy object

Preeclampsia: a condition of high blood pressure and swelling that occurs in some women, usually during the third trimester of pregnancy

Presenting part: the part of an infant that emerges from the birth canal first during delivery

Pressure bandage: material, such as roller gauze, that is applied snugly to create pressure on a wound and hold a dressing in place over it

Prone: face down

Prospective medical direction: activities performed by a physician before an emergency call, such as the development of treatment protocols and standing orders

Protected Health Information (PHI): information that relates to a person's physical or mental health, treatment, or payment that identifies the person or gives a reason to believe that the individual can be identified or is transmitted or maintained in any form

Protocols: written instructions to provide emergency care for specific health-related conditions

Proximal: closer to the midline or center area of the body

Psychological maltreatment: a pattern of caregiver behavior that conveys to children that they are worthless, flawed, unloved, unwanted, endangered, or only valued in meeting another's needs

Pulse: the rhythmic contraction and expansion of the arteries with each beat of the heart

Putrefaction: the decomposition of organic matter, such as body tissues

Q

Quadriplegia: a loss of movement and sensation in both arms, both legs, and the parts of the body below an area of injury to the spinal cord

Quality management: a system of internal and external reviews and audits of all aspects of an EMS system to identify those aspects needing improvement to ensure that the public receives the highest quality of prehospital care

R

Raccoon eyes: the bluish discoloration around the eyes that suggests a possible skull fracture

Radiation: the transfer of heat, as infrared heat rays, from the surface of one object to the surface of another without contact between the two objects

Radius: the bone on the thumb (lateral) side of the forearm

Rapid trauma assessment: a quick, head-to-toe examination performed on a trauma patient with significant mechanism of injury to determine life-threatening injuries

Recovery position: the position an unresponsive patient who is breathing and in no need of CPR (and in whom trauma is not suspected) is placed—on his or her side to help keep his or her airway open

Regression: a return to an earlier developmental state

Respiration: the act of breathing air into the lungs (inhalation) and out of the lungs (exhalation); the exchange of gases between a living organism and its environment

Respiratory arrest: absent breathing

Respiratory distress: an increased work of breathing (respiratory effort)

Respiratory failure: a condition in which there is an inadequate amount of oxygen in the blood and/or ventilation to meet the demands of body tissues

Retrospective medical direction: activities performed by a physician after an emergency call, such as reviewing the documentation pertaining to an emergency call

Rigor mortis: the rigidity of body muscles that occurs after death

S

Scapula: one of a pair of large, essentially flat, triangular bones on the back of the chest; shoulder blade

Scene safety: an assessment of the scene and surroundings to ensure the well-being of the first responder, other rescuers, the patient(s), and bystanders

Scene size-up: the first phase of patient assessment that includes taking body substance isolation precautions, evaluating scene safety, determining the mechanism of injury or nature of the patient's illness, determining the total number of patients, and determining the need for additional resources

Schizophrenia: a group of mental disorders

Scope of care (scope of practice): the specific medical procedures and functions that can be performed by a licensed or certified healthcare professional

Seizure: a temporary change in behavior or consciousness caused by abnormal electrical activity of one or more groups of brain cells

Self-splint (anatomic splint): using a part of the body as a rigid support

Semi-Fowler's position: patient sitting up with his head at a 45-degree angle and legs out straight

Septic shock: shock due to a severe infection

Septum: a wall of tissue

Sequence of survival: the ideal sequence of events that should take place immediately following the recognition of an injury or the onset of sudden illness

Sexual abuse: inappropriate adolescent or adult sexual behavior with a child

Sexually transmitted diseases: infections spread by either blood or sexual contact

Shock: the inadequate flow of blood through an organ or a part of the body

Shock position: lying on the back, with the feet elevated approximately 8 to 12 inches

Shoulder girdle: the bony arch formed by the collarbones (clavicles) and shoulder blades (scapulae)

Sign: any medical or trauma condition displayed by the patient that can be seen, heard, smelled, measured, or felt

Skeletal muscles: voluntary muscles; most skeletal muscles are attached to bones

Smooth muscle: involuntary muscle found in many internal organs (except the heart)

Snoring: noisy breathing through the mouth and nose during sleep

Soft tissues: the layers of the skin and the fat and muscle beneath them

Sphygmomanometer: a blood pressure cuff

Spina bifida: a congenital defect in which part of one or more vertebrae fail to develop

Spinal cavity: the body cavity that extends from the bottom of the skull to the lower back and contains the spinal cord

Spinal precautions: precautions made to stabilize the head, neck, and back in a neutral position to prevent movement that could cause injury to the spinal cord

Splint: a device used to limit the movement of an injured arm or leg to reduce pain and further injury

Spontaneous abortion: the loss of a fetus due to natural causes, usually before the 20th week of pregnancy

Sprain: the stretching or tearing of a ligament, the connective tissue that joins the end of one bone with another

Stage: to wait a safe distance away from the patient until the scene has been made safe for you to enter

Standard of care: the minimum level of care expected of similarly trained healthcare professionals; based on education, experience, laws, and protocols

Standing orders: written instructions that authorize EMS personnel to perform certain medical interventions before establishing direct communication with a physician

Status epilepticus: a seizure that lasts longer than 30 minutes or a series of seizures occurring over a 30-minute period in which the patient remains unresponsive between seizures

Statutes: laws established by Congress, the legislative branch of the federal government, and state legislatures

Sterilizing: a process that uses boiling water, radiation, gas, chemicals, or superheated steam to destroy all of the germs on an object

Sternum: the breastbone; the flat bone that joins the clavicles (collarbones) and the first seven pairs of ribs

Stethoscope: an instrument used to hear sounds within the body, such as respirations; also used to measure blood pressure

Stoma: a surgical opening in the neck

Strain: a twist, pull, or tear of a muscle or tendon

Stridor: a high-pitched sound that is usually heard on inhalation; a sign of upper airway obstruction

Stress: a chemical, physical, or emotional factor that causes bodily or mental tension

Stressor: any event or condition that has the potential to cause bodily or mental tension

Subluxation: a dislocation that fully or partially returns to its normal alignment without intervention

Suctioning: a procedure used to remove vomitus, saliva, blood, food particles, and other material from a patient's airway

Sudden cardiac death: the unexpected loss of life occurring either immediately or within one hour of the onset of cardiac symptoms

Sudden Infant Death Syndrome (SIDS): the sudden and unexpected death of an infant that remains unexplained after a thorough case investigation, including performance of a complete autopsy, examination of the death scene, and review of the clinical history

Suicide: any willful act designed to end one's own life

Superior: above or in a higher position than another portion of the body

Supine: lying face up

Surfactant: a thin substance that coats each alveolus and prevents the alveoli from collapsing

Swathe: a piece of soft material used to secure an injured extremity to the body

Symptom: any condition described by the patient, such as shortness of breath, nausea, and dizziness

Systolic blood pressure: the pressure in the arteries when the heart is pumping blood

T

Tarsals: the bones of the heel and back part of the foot

Tendons: strong cords of connective tissue that stretch across joints; when muscles contract, they create a pull between bones

Terminal illness: an illness or injury for which there is no reasonable expectation of recovery

Thoracic (chest) cavity: the body cavity located below the neck and above the diaphragm; contains the heart, major blood vessels, and lungs

Tibia: shinbone; the larger of the two bones of the lower leg

Tissues: a group of similar cells that cluster together to perform a specialized function

Torso: the back and trunk; the trunk includes the chest and abdomen

Tourniquet: a tight bandage that surrounds an arm or a leg that is used to stop the flow of blood in the extremity

Trachea: the windpipe; the tube through which air passes to and from the lungs; extends down the front of the neck from the larynx and divides in two to form the mainstem bronchi

Traction: maintaining a continuous, steady pull on a bone or extremity to relieve spasm, pain, or pressure or align parts

Traction splint: a device used to immobilize a closed fracture of the femur (thighbone)

Trauma patient: a patient who has experienced an injury from an external force

Treatment protocol: a list of steps to be followed when providing emergency care to an ill or injured patient

Trendelenburg position: lying on the back, with the head of the bed lowered and the feet raised in a straight incline

Triage: sorting patients by the severity of their illness or injury

True ribs: rib pairs 1–7 attached anteriorly to the sternum by cartilage

U

Ulna: the bone on the medial side of the forearm

Umbilical cord: an extension of the placenta, through which the fetus receives nourishment while in the uterus

Uterus (womb): a hollow, muscular organ of the female reproductive system where a fertilized egg implants and develops into a fetus

Uvula: the small piece of tissue that looks like a punching bag and that hangs down in the back of the throat

V

Vagina (birth canal): a muscular tube that serves as a passageway between the uterus and the outside of the body

Vasoconstriction: the narrowing of a blood vessel

Vasodilation: the widening of a blood vessel

Veins: blood vessels that return blood to the heart

Ventricles: the two lower chambers of the heart

Ventricular fibrillation (VF): an abnormal heart rhythm that prevents effective heart contractions

Venules: the smallest branches of veins leading to the capillaries

Virus: a type of infectious agent that depends on other organisms to live and grow

Vital organs: the organs essential for life, such as the brain, heart, and lungs

Vital signs: assessments of breathing, pulse, skin, pupils, and blood pressure

W

Weapons of mass destruction: materials used by terrorists that have the potential to cause great harm over a large area

Wheezing: a high-pitched whistling sound heard during breathing caused by air moving through narrowed airway passages

Womb: the hollow, muscular organ of the female reproductive system, in which a fertilized egg implants and develops into a fetus; also called the uterus

Wound: an injury to the soft tissues

X

Xiphoid process: a piece of cartilage that makes up the inferior portion of the breastbone

Chapter Quiz Answers

Chapter 1—Introduction to the EMS System

Multiple Choice

1. b
2. d
3. b
4. c
5. b
6. c
7. c
8. a
9. d
10. b
11. c
12. b
13. a
14. d

True or False

15. F

Matching

16. i
17. l
18. g
19. h
20. k
21. j
22. d
23. e
24. a
25. b
26. c
27. f

Short Answer

28. The 10 essential components of an Emergency Medical Services (EMS) system are
    1. Regulation and policy
    2. Resource management
    3. Human resources and training
    4. Transportation
    5. Facilities
    6. Communications
    7. Public information and education
    8. Medical oversight
    9. Trauma systems
    10. Evaluation
29. The five responsibilities of an Emergency Medical Responder are
    1. Personal health and safety
    2. Composure and a caring attitude
    3. Neat, clean, professional appearance
    4. Up-to-date knowledge and skills
    5. Current knowledge of local, state, and national issues affecting EMS
30. An Emergency Medical Responder is the first person with medical training who arrives at the scene of an emergency. An Emergency Medical Responder provides initial emergency care, including assessing for life-threatening conditions. A Paramedic is the most advanced level of EMS professional. A Paramedic has received additional education in patient assessment, IV fluid and medication administration, advanced airway procedures, ECG monitoring, diseases, physical examination techniques, and invasive procedures. A Paramedic can perform all the skills of an Emergency Medical Responder, an Emergency Medical Technician, and an Advanced Emergency Medical Technician.
31. The six phases of a typical EMS response are
    1. Detection of the emergency
    2. Reporting the emergency (the call made for assistance, dispatch)
    3. Response (medical resources sent to the scene)
    4. On-scene care
    5. Care during transport
    6. Transfer to definitive care
32. Presenting a neat, clean, professional appearance invites trust, instills confidence, enhances cooperation, and brings a sense of order to an emergency situation.

Chapter 2—The Well-Being of the Emergency Medical Responder

Multiple Choice

1. c
2. a
3. a
4. a
5. b
6. c

True or False

7. T

Matching

8. j	16. q	24. n
9. k	17. m	25. i
10. w	18. f	26. r
11. o	19. h	27. a
12. v	20. b	28. s
13. x	21. e	29. p
14. c	22. u	30. l
15. d	23. g	31. t

Short Answer

32. People react differently to situations involving illness and injury. The child's mother may express anger, rage, despair, crying, or feelings of guilt, or she may show little reaction.
33. Despite your best efforts to resuscitate a patient, you may experience emotions such as anger, anxiety, frustration, fear, grief, and helplessness when a patient dies. These emotions are common and expected, and you should not feel embarrassed or ashamed when a situation like this affects you.
34. Examples of stressful situations include the following (any six):
    - Mass casualty incidents
    - Infant and child trauma
    - Death, terminal illness
    - Amputations
    - Violence
    - Death of a child
    - Infant, child, elder, or spousal abuse
    - Death or injury of a coworker or other public safety personnel
    - Emergency response to the illness or injury of a friend or family member
35. The five Stages of Grief are
    1. Denial
    2. Anger
    3. Bargaining
    4. Depression
    5. Acceptance
36. Personal protective clothing that should be worn in this situation includes the following (any four):
    - Puncture-proof gloves
    - Turnout gear
    - Helmet
    - Eye protection (such as heavy goggles)
    - Boots with steel toes
37. Develop good dietary habits, exercise, and practice relaxation techniques.

Chapter 3—Legal and Ethical Issues

Multiple Choice

1. b	2. c	3. d

True or False

4. T	6. F	8. T
5. T	7. F	

Matching

9. e	12. b	15. c
10. h	13. a	16. d
11. f	14. g	

Short Answer

17. Patient care may be transferred to another healthcare professional if that person accepts the patient and the other healthcare professional's medical qualifications are equal to or greater than yours.
18. The four elements that must be proved in a negligence case are the following:
    1. You had a duty to act.
    2. You breached that duty.
    3. Injury/damages were inflicted.
    4. Your actions or lack of actions caused the injury/damage.
19. You must inform the patient of the following:
    - The nature of his injury
    - The treatment that needs to be performed
    - The benefits of that treatment
    - The risks of not providing that treatment
    - Any alternatives to treatment
    - The dangers of refusing treatment (including transport)
20. To obtain expressed consent, you must
    - Identify yourself and your level of medical training
    - Explain all treatments and procedures to the patient
    - Identify the benefits of each treatment or procedure
    - Identify the risks of each treatment or procedure

Sentence Completion

21. Scope of care (also called scope of practice) consists of the emergency care and skills an Emergency Medical Responder is legally allowed and expected to perform when necessary.
22. A written document specifying a person's healthcare wishes when he or she becomes unable to make decisions for him- or herself is known as a(n) advance directive.

Chapter 4—The Human Body

Multiple Choice

1. b
2. d
3. b
4. a
5. a
6. b
7. c

True or False

8. T
9. T

Matching

10. h
11. f
12. b
13. g
14. b
15. d
16. c
17. a
18. g
19. c
20. h
21. i
22. a
23. k
24. e
25. f
26. b
27. l
28. j
29. d
30. i
31. h
32. g
33. f
34. a
35. d
36. e
37. b
38. c

Short Answer

39. The three formed elements of the blood are
    1. Red blood cells
    2. White blood cells
    3. Platelets
40. The two parts of the central nervous system are
    1. Brain
    2. Spinal cord

Chapter 5—Lifting and Moving Patients

Multiple Choice

1. c
2. d
3. b
4. b

True or False

5. T

Matching

6. f
7. e
8. h
9. g
10. b
11. c
12. d
13. i
14. j
15. a

Short Answer

16. The greatest danger to this patient is aggravating a spinal injury.
17. The stretcher should be placed at a 90-degree angle to the bed, with the head end of the stretcher at the foot of the bed.

Sentence Completion

18. When dragging a patient, avoid reaching more than 15–20 inches in front of your body.

Chapter 6—Airway and Breathing

Multiple Choice

1. d
2. a
3. a
4. b
5. d
6. a

True or False

7. F
8. F

Matching

9. e
10. c
11. f
12. h
13. d
14. b
15. a
16. g

Short Answer

17. OPAs are available in a variety of sizes. To select the correct size, hold the OPA against the side of the patient's face. Select an OPA that extends from the corner of the patient's mouth to either the tip of the earlobe or the angle of the jaw.
18. The signs of inadequate breathing include (any five)
    1. An anxious appearance and concentration on breathing
    2. Confusion and restlessness
    3. A breathing rate that is too fast or slow for the patient's age
    4. An irregular breathing pattern

5. A depth of breathing that is unusually deep or shallow
6. Noisy breathing (snoring, gurgling, wheezing)
7. A patient who is sitting upright and leaning forward to breathe
8. An inability to speak in complete sentences
9. Pain with breathing
10. Skin that looks flushed, pale, gray, or blue or that feels cold or sweaty

19. Chest thrusts may be used to relieve an upper airway obstruction in the following patients:
1. An obese adult
2. A woman in the later stages of pregnancy
3. An infant

20. The three categories of airway obstruction are
1. Partial airway obstruction with good air exchange
2. Partial airway obstruction with poor air exchange
3. Complete airway obstruction

21. The two methods that may be used to open an airway are
1. Head tilt–chin lift
2. Jaw thrust without head tilt

22. The following methods are used to deliver positive-pressure ventilation (any three):
1. Mouth-to-mask ventilation
2. Mouth-to-barrier device ventilation
3. Mouth-to-mouth ventilation
4. Bag-valve-mask ventilation

23. The tongue is the most common cause of upper airway obstruction in an unresponsive patient.

24. The gases that are exchanged during the process of breathing are oxygen and carbon dioxide.

Sentence Completion

25. The largest cartilage of the larynx is the thyroid cartilage, also called the <u>Adam's apple</u>.

26. OPA stands for <u>oropharyngeal</u> <u>airway</u>.

27. When providing rescue breathing for an infant or a child, give 1 breath every <u>3</u> to <u>5</u> seconds, which is <u>12</u> to <u>20</u> breaths/minute.

28. When providing rescue breathing for an adult, give 1 breath every <u>5</u> to <u>6</u> seconds, which is <u>10</u> to <u>12</u> breaths/minute.

Chapter 7—Circulation

Multiple Choice

1. d **2.** b **3.** c **4.** c **5.** b **6.** b **7.** d **8.** b

True or False

9. T **10.** F

Matching

11. g **12.** i **13.** l **14.** j **15.** m **16.** p **17.** c **18.** r **19.** e **20.** b **21.** a **22.** o **23.** f **24.** d **25.** h **26.** q **27.** n **28.** k

Chapter 8—Patient Assessment

Multiple Choice

1. a **2.** c **3.** b **4.** a **5.** c **6.** b **7.** d **8.** c

True or False

9. F **10.** T

Matching

11. f **12.** d **13.** k **14.** h **15.** i **16.** g **17.** e **18.** j **19.** b **20.** l **21.** c **22.** a

Short Answer

23. Common hazards found at the scene of a trauma patient include the following (any three):
1. Traffic
2. Unstable vehicle, aircraft, or machinery
3. Leaking fluids
4. Downed power lines
5. Fire, smoke, or potential fire hazards
6. Entrapped victims

24. It is important to find out the number of patients on the scene in order to request additional resources if necessary.

25. Assessing circulation in a patient younger than six includes
    1. Checking the patient's pulse
    2. Looking for severe bleeding
    3. Assessing skin temperature, color, and condition
    4. Assessing capillary refill
26. The signs of adequate breathing include the following (any four):
    1. Breathing effort (work of breathing) is quiet, relaxed, and effortless.
    2. Breathing rate is within normal limits for age.
    3. Breathing pattern is regular.
    4. Both sides of the chest rise and fall equally.
    5. Depth of breathing is adequate.
    6. Skin color is normal; skin is warm and dry.
27. *D*eformities, *O*pen injuries, *T*enderness, *S*welling
28. The term *spinal precautions* refers to stabilizing the head, neck, and back in a neutral position. This stabilization is done to minimize movement that could cause injury to the spinal cord.

Sentence Completion

29. Blunt trauma is any mechanism of injury that occurs without actual penetration of the body.
30. A trauma patient is a person who has experienced an injury from an external force.

Chapter 9—Medical Emergencies

Multiple Choice

1. b
2. b
3. c
4. c
5. b

True or False

6. T
7. T

Short Answer

8. The causes of an altered mental status include the following (any five):
    1. *A*lcohol, abuse
    2. *E*pilepsy (seizures)
    3. *I*nsulin (diabetic emergency)
    4. *O*verdose
    5. *U*remia (kidney failure)
    6. *T*rauma (head injury), temperature (fever, heat- or cold-related emergency)
    7. *I*nfection
    8. *P*sychiatric conditions
    9. *P*oisoning (including drugs and alcohol)
    10. *S*hock, stroke
9. A local cold injury may be early (superficial) or late (deep).
10. Young children are at an increased risk for hypothermia because they have less subcutaneous fat for body insulation. Their large surface area relative to their overall size also results in a more rapid heat loss. Children's ability to shiver may be inadequate because of their small muscle mass. Newborns are unable to shiver. Infants and very young children are unable to protect themselves from the cold. They cannot put on additional clothes and cannot move to warm surroundings without help.
11. Assess the patient's general temperature by placing the back of your hand between the patient's clothing and the patient's abdomen.
12. Local cold injury (also called frostbite) involves tissue damage to a specific area of the body. It occurs when a body part (such as the nose, ears, cheeks, chin, hands, or feet) is exposed to prolonged or intense cold.
13. The three main types of heat emergencies are heat cramps, heat exhaustion, and heat stroke.
14. In documenting the reason for the restraints, you should include the following information:
    - The number of personnel used to restrain the patient
    - The type of restraint used
    - The time the restraints were placed on the patient
    - The status of the patient's ABCs and distal pulses before and after the restraints were applied
    - The reassessment of the patient's ABCs and distal pulses

Chapter 10—Bleeding and Soft-Tissue Injuries

Multiple Choice

1. c
2. b
3. b
4. c

True or False

5. T
6. F
7. T
8. T

Matching

9. e
10. c
11. a
12. b
13. i
14. g
15. j
16. d
17. h
18. f

Short Answer

19. The following six methods may be used to control bleeding:
    1. Apply direct pressure to the wound.
    2. Elevate the affected extremity.
    3. Apply pressure to an arterial pressure point.
    4. Apply a splint to immobilize the extremity.
    5. Apply a pressure (air) splint.
    6. Apply a tourniquet.
20. The signs or symptoms of early shock include the following (any four):
    1. Anxiety, restlessness
    2. Thirst
    3. Nausea/vomiting
    4. Increased respiratory rate
    5. Slight increase in heart rate
    6. Pale, cool, moist skin
    7. Delayed capillary refill in an infant or a young child
    8. Blood pressure in the normal range
21. You should perform ongoing assessments for a patient in shock at least every five minutes.
22. The most common causes of internal bleeding are
    1. Injured or damaged internal organs
    2. Fractures, especially fractures of the femur and pelvis
23. The types of open wounds are the following (any four):
    1. Abrasion
    2. Laceration
    3. Penetration/puncture wound
    4. Avulsion
    5. Amputation
    6. Open crush injury
24. a. Evisceration

    b. Do not touch or try to replace the exposed organ. Carefully remove clothing from around the wound. Cover the exposed organs and wound by applying a thick, moist dressing lightly over the organs and wound. Secure the dressing in place with a large bandage to retain moisture and prevent heat loss. Place the patient in a position of comfort if no spinal injury is suspected. Keep the patient warm. Assess for signs of shock and treat if present.
25. A chemical burn is the most urgent eye injury. The damage to the eye depends on the type and concentration of the chemical, the length of exposure, and the elapsed time until treatment.
26. The signs and symptoms that suggest a possible airway problem include the following (any four):
    - Facial burns
    - Soot in the nose or mouth
    - Singed facial hair or nasal hair
    - Swelling of the lips or the inside of the mouth
    - Coughing
    - Inability to swallow secretions
    - A hoarse voice
27. Have him sit up and lean his head forward. This will help keep blood from draining into the back of his throat. Pinch the fleshy part of his nostrils together with your thumb and two fingers for 15 minutes.

Sentence Completion

28. A contusion (bruise) is the most common type of closed wound.
29. A superficial (first-degree) burn affects only the epidermis and results in only minor tissue damage.
30. An occlusive dressing prevents air from entering a wound.

Chapter 11—Injuries to Muscles and Bones

Multiple Choice

1. d
2. a
3. b
4. d
5. b
6. c

True or False

7. T
8. F
9. T
10. F

Matching

11. f
12. d
13. g
14. a
15. b
16. e
17. h
18. c

Short Answer

19. The musculoskeletal system gives the body its shape, provides a rigid framework that supports and protects internal organs, provides for body movement, maintains posture, helps stabilize joints, and produces body heat.

20. A dislocation occurs when the ends of bones are forced from their normal positions in a joint.

21. Ice reduces blood flow into the affected area, which reduces swelling.

22. RICE stands for *R*est, *I*ce, *C*ompression, and *E*levation.

23. The three most common signs and symptoms of a musculoskeletal injury are pain, deformity, and swelling.

24. The reasons for splinting include the following (any four):

1. Limit the motion of bone fragments, bone ends, or dislocated joints
2. Lessen the damage to muscles, nerves, or blood vessels caused by broken bones
3. Help prevent a closed injury from becoming an open injury
4. Lessen the restriction of blood flow caused by bone ends or dislocations compressing blood vessels
5. Reduce bleeding due to tissue damage caused by bone ends
6. Reduce pain associated with the movement of the bone and the joint
7. Reduce the risk of paralysis due to a damaged spine

25. The hazards of improper splinting include the following (any three):

1. Compressing nerves, tissues, and blood vessels from the splint
2. Delaying transport of a patient with a life-threatening injury
3. Reducing distal circulation due to the splint's being applied too tightly to the extremity
4. Aggravating the musculoskeletal injury
5. Causing or aggravating tissue, nerve, vessel, or muscle damage from excessive bone or joint movement

26. A traction splint is a device used to immobilize a closed fracture of the femur (thighbone).

27. Before and after applying a splint, you should assess distal pulses, movement, and sensation (PMS) in the injured extremity.

28. The types of splints include the following (any three):

1. Anatomic/self-splint
2. Rigid/semi-rigid splints
3. Soft splints
4. Pneumatic splints
5. Traction splints

29. The three most commonly injured areas of the spine are the following:

1. Cervical (neck) spine—most commonly injured
2. Thoracic (chest) spine
3. Lumbar (low back) spine

Sentence Completion

30. Cardiac muscle is an <u>involuntary</u> muscle.

31. The three major parts of a skeletal muscle are the <u>insertion</u>, the body, and the <u>origin</u>.

32. The two main divisions of the skeleton are the <u>axial</u> and the <u>appendicular</u> skeleton.

33. A shoulder injury typically involves three bones: the <u>collarbone (clavicle)</u>, the <u>shoulder-blade (scapula)</u>, and the <u>upper-arm bone (humerus)</u>.

34. Splinting an elbow injury requires immobilization of the <u>humerus</u> (the bone above the injury) and the <u>radius</u> and <u>ulna</u> (the bones below the injury).

Chapter 12—Childbirth

Multiple Choice

1. d	**6.** c	**11.** d
2. d	**7.** d	**12.** c
3. b	**8.** d	**13.** b
4. a	**9.** b	
5. c	**10.** a	

True or False

14. T **15.** F

Matching

16. g	**19.** b	**22.** a
17. f	**20.** e	**23.** c
18. h	**21.** d	

Short Answer

24. The placenta is responsible for the following functions (any three):
    1. The exchange of oxygen and carbon dioxide between the blood of the mother and the fetus (the placenta serves the function of the lungs for the developing fetus)
    2. The removal of waste products
    3. The transport of nutrients from the mother to the fetus
    4. The production of a special hormone of pregnancy that maintains the pregnancy and stimulates changes in the mother's breasts, cervix, and vagina in preparation for delivery
    5. Maintaining a barrier against harmful substances
25. Avoid positioning the mother completely flat on her back because compression of the inferior vena cava and aorta can lower her blood pressure and decrease perfusion of the uterus.
26. If the bag of waters does not break or has not broken, use your gloved fingers to tear it. Push the sac away from the infant's head and mouth as they appear.
27. Newborns lose heat very quickly because they are wet and suddenly exposed to an environment that is cooler than that inside the uterus. Quickly dry the baby's body and head to remove blood and amniotic fluid. Immediately remove the wet towel or blanket from the infant and then quickly wrap the baby in a clean, warm blanket. Because most body heat is lost through the head, remember to cover the baby's head as soon as possible.
28. The signs that indicate separation of the placenta include a gush of blood, a lengthening of the umbilical cord, a contraction of the uterus, and an urge to push. Encourage the mother to push to help deliver the placenta.

Sentence Completion

29. A full-term baby's respiratory rate is normally between <u>30</u> and <u>60</u> breaths per minute.
30. A full-term baby's heart rate is normally between <u>100</u> and <u>180</u> beats per minute.
31. A breech birth occurs when the baby's <u>buttocks</u> or <u>feet</u> come out of the uterus first.

Chapter 13—Infants and Children

Multiple Choice

1. b
2. d
3. a
4. c
5. b
6. c
7. a

Short Answer

8. An increased heart rate in an infant or a child can be caused by bleeding, vomiting, diarrhea, shock, fever, anxiety, or pain.
9. The signs of physical abuse include the following (any four):
    1. Multiple bruises in various stages of healing
    2. Human bite marks
    3. Inflicted burns—stockinglike burns with no associated splash marks, usually present on the buttocks, genitalia, or extremities
    4. Circular burns from a cigarette or cigar
    5. Rope burns on the wrists
    6. Burns in the shape of a household utensil or appliance, such as a spoon or an iron
    7. Fractures
    8. Head, face, and oral injuries
    9. Abdominal injuries
    10. An injury inconsistent with the history or developmental level of the child
10. Possible causes of an altered mental status include the following (any five):
    1. Low blood oxygen level (hypoxia)
    2. Head trauma
    3. Seizures
    4. Infection
    5. Shock
    6. Low blood sugar
    7. Drug or alcohol ingestion
    8. Abuse
    9. Fever
    10. Respiratory failure

Chapter 14—EMS Operations

Multiple Choice

1. b
2. c
3. a
4. c
5. b

Short Answer

6. The four categories used in the START triage system are the following:
   1. Red—immediate
   2. Yellow—delayed
   3. Green—minor (ambulatory patients; "walking wounded")
   4. Black—dead or dying
7. When using the START system, four areas are evaluated during the initial assessment: (1) the ability to walk (ambulation), (2) respirations, (3) perfusion, and (4) mental status.
8. If you arrive on the scene of a mass casualty incident where the ICS has been established, report to the command post. Find out who the Incident Commander is and identify yourself and your level of training. Follow the directions given by the Incident Commander about your assignment.

Appendix 1—Weapons of Mass Destruction: Awareness and Response

Multiple Choice

1. b 2. c 3. d

True or False

4. T 5. F 6. T

Short Answer

7. The four common types of biological agents are the following:
   1. Bacteria
   2. Viruses
   3. Rickettsias
   4. Toxins
8. The six categories of WMD a terrorist might use are
   1. Biological
   2. Nuclear
   3. Incendiary
   4. Chemical
   5. Cyber or technological
   6. Explosive

Appendix 2—Rural and Frontier EMS

True or False

1. F 2. F

Short Answer

3. The number of interested EMS volunteers may be decreasing due to the following factors (any four):
   1. The increase in two-wage-earner households
   2. Limited or a lack of EMS pay
   3. An increasing exposure to the risks in providing EMS care
   4. The belief that there is increased personal liability when providing EMS care
   5. A lack of EMS leadership in the community
   6. Limited or a lack of funding for training, equipment, and supplies
   7. An increased number of nursing home and routine transfer calls instead of emergency calls
4. Some rural and frontier communities are using EMS professionals in doctors' offices, healthcare clinics, hospices, and home health settings.
5. Response times in a rural or frontier setting may be long due to the following (any three):
   1. A delay in volunteers' response from home or work
   2. A failure to respond
   3. The physical distance that must be covered
   4. The type of transportation that must be used (land, air, water)
   5. The type and condition of the roadway, airway, or water
   6. Bad weather

   Limited access to communications may delay the detection and reporting of a need for emergency care. When EMS professionals travel on land, unpredictable road conditions (including unmarked roads) can delay their arrival on the scene.

Appendix 3—Special Populations

Multiple Choice

1. d 2. b

True or False

3. F
4. T
5. F
6. T

Matching

7. g
8. h
9. f
10. e
11. c
12. b
13. a
14. d

Short Answer

15. Begin by identifying yourself in a normal voice. Most blind persons are not hearing impaired, so there is no need to raise your voice or shout when talking to them. If family members or others are present, address the patient by name so that it is clear to whom you are talking. Clearly explain any care you are going to provide before doing so. In this way, you do not surprise or startle the patient. Be sure to talk directly to the patient, not through a family member.
16. Body mass index (BMI) is a mathematical formula that expresses the relationship of weight to height. Individuals with a BMI of 25 to 29.9 are considered overweight, while individuals with a BMI of 30 or more are considered obese.
17. Medical problems linked to obesity include the following (any four):
    1. Heart disease
    2. Stroke
    3. Diabetes
    4. Gallbladder disease
    5. Arthritis
    6. Gout
    7. Breathing problems
    8. High blood cholesterol
    9. High blood pressure

Sentence Completion

18. Arthritis is an inflammation of a joint.
19. Cerebral palsy is a neuromuscular disorder that affects the ability to control voluntary muscles.
20. Spina bifida is a congenital defect in which part of one or more vertebrae fails to develop, leaving a portion of the spinal cord exposed to the external environment.

Index

C

D

E

F

G

H

I

J

K

L

M

N

O

P

Q

R

S

T

U

V

W

X

Z